DISORDERS OF

HAIR GROWTH

Diagnosis and Treatment

To Jenny and Kent, my loving children, whose patience and support of my efforts transcend their ages

CONTENTS

CONTRIBUTORS

Edward Abell, M.D., Department of Medicine, St. Francis Hospital, Pittsburgh, Pennsylvania

Wilma F. Bergfeld, M.D., Head, Clinical Research, Department of Dermatology, Head, Dermatopathology, Department of Pathology, Cleveland Clinic Foundation, Cleveland, Ohio

Arthur P. Bertolino, M.D., Ph.D., Associate Clinical Professor of Dermatology; Director, Hair Consultation Unit, The Ronald O. Perelman Department of Dermatology, New York University Medical Center, New York, New York

Richard L. DeVillez, M.D., Professor of Medicine/Dermatology, University of Texas Health Science Center at San Antonio, San Antonio, Texas

Maj. Dirk M. Elston, M.C., U.S.A., Dermatology Service, Brooke Army Medical Center, Fort Sam Houston, Texas; Clinical Assistant Professor of Medicine (Dermatology), University of Texas Health Science Center at San Antonio, San Antonio, Texas

Virginia C. Fiedler, M.D., Professor and Associate Head, Dermatology; Chief of Clinical Research, University of Illinois Medical Center, Chicago, Illinois

Karyn L. Grossman, M.D., Resident in Dermatology, Harvard Affiliated Hospital Program, Harvard Medical School, Boston, Massachusetts

Abdul Hafeez, M.D., Resident in Dermatology, University of Illinois Medical Center, Chicago, Illinois

Maria K. Hordinsky, M.D., Associate Professor, Department of Dermatology, University of Minnesota, Minneapolis, Minnesota

Claude L. Hughes, Jr., Ph.D., M.D., Associate Professor; Director, Reproductive Hormone Lab, Division of Reproductive Endocrinology and Infertility, Department of Obstetrics and Gynecology, Duke University Medical Center, Durham, North Carolina

Joseph C. Kvedar, M.D., Assistant Professor of Dermatology, Harvard Medical School, Boston, Massachusetts

Andrew G. Messenger, M.D., FRCP, Consultant Dermatologist, Royal Hallamshire Hospital, Sheffield, England

Marianne Nelson O'Donoghue, M.D., Associate Professor of Dermatology, Rush Presbyterian–St. Luke's Medical Center, Chicago, Illinois

W. Michael O'Guin, Ph.D., Assistant Professor of Dermatology, The Ronald O. Perelman Department of Dermatology, New York University Medical Center, New York, New York

Elise A. Olsen, M.D., Associate Professor of Medicine; Director, Dermatopharmacology Study Center, Division of Dermatology, Department of Medicine, Duke University Medical Center, Durham, North Carolina

Walter P. Unger, M.D., FRCP(C), FACP, Associate Professor of Medicine [Dermatology], University of Toronto, Toronto, Ontario, Canada

David A. Whiting, M.D., FACP, FRCP(ED), Clinical Professor of Dermatology and Pediatrics, The University of Texas Southwestern Medical Center at Dallas; Medical Director, Baylor Hair Research and Treatment Center, Dallas, Texas

Wesley S. Wilborn, M.D., Associate Clinical Professor of Dermatology, Emory University School of Medicine, Atlanta, Georgia

PREFACE

I first became interested in writing and editing a book on disorders of hair growth after giving a particularly well-received lecture on the subject to our dermatology residents several years ago. The residents expressed surprise at never having seen the information I presented capsulized in print and asked me for appropriate references to expand their knowledge. Having pieced my own lectures together from bits of knowledge gathered from a variety of sources, I realized that there was no one source that would serve to explore the basic mechanisms, clinical presentation and therapy of hair disorders. As my approach to the treatment of patients with hair loss or hair overgrowth, like my approach to the practice of medicine in general, has always been to ground myself in the pathophysiology and clinical expression of a disorder, which then makes the treatment options seem obvious, I thought a textbook that would approach each problem of hair growth from this perspective could be of great service to practicing physicians.

Alopecia is a particularly vexing problem for physicians and patients alike. Physicians, who have been traditionally schooled to treat illnesses, often trivialize the complaints of hair loss in an otherwise healthy-appearing patient. This may be because the hair loss is imperceptible to the observer or is perceived as a natural component of aging, the patient's psychological overlay appears out of proportion to the problem, the perception is that there is no effective therapy for alopecia, or the physicians believe that hair is a cosmetic concern of beauticians and laymen and not one warranting the attention of physicians. For all of the above reasons as well as the perceived lack of medical understanding of the cause of these disorders, patients with hair loss are similarly frustrated upon seeing most physicians. As opposed to patients with a systemic illness or a chronic skin condition who commonly ask, "why me?," patients with alopecia typically look on the problem as unwarranted and are exasperated by the physician's inability to immediately "cure" the problem.

All of the concerns noted above by both physicians and patients have some validity and make the treatment of patients with alopecia challenging. However, they also overlook three major points. First, most cases of alopecia *can* be diagnosed by the combination of history, physical examination, microscopic examination of affected hairs, and appropriate directed laboratory tests. Second, hair loss or hair overgrowth may be a manifestation of systemic disease or the necessary clue to an otherwise elusive multisystemic disorder or syndrome. Physicians have a tremendous opportunity here to make an important diagnosis through noninvasive testing. Third, physicians *can* effectively treat most patients with alopecia, although treatment may not necessarily include the ability to restore a full head of hair. Halting further progression of the hair loss, reassurance about the lack of systemic complications, and surgical correction or education about effective use of hair protheses may be just as important and worthwhile as griseofulvin is for tinea capitis.

This book offers the dermatologist, the internist or family physician, the endocrinologist, the pediatrician, the obstetrician-gynecologist and, indeed, any physician who sees hair loss or overgrowth in regular practice the opportunity to understand the basic pathophysiology, clinical presentation, and effective treatment options for patients with hair growth disorders. Tools for establishing a working differential diagnosis are discussed after the normal embryology, anatomy, specifics of hair production, and control of normal hair growth are presented. The chapters that follow are organized according to hair growth disorders that share like presentations or overlapping features. Rather than exhaustively listing syndromes within the text that have the physical sign of hair loss or overgrowth, liberal use of tables is employed to facilitate recognition of these uncommon or rare syndromes; this is particularly true in the chapters on hair shaft defects, hair loss in childhood, and hypertrichosis. This book is meant to be all-encompassing in terms of clinical practice and to obviate the need to refer to other information sources for specifics of therapy. Although not a histology textbook, most clinical descriptions of alopecia are accompanied by color photomicrographs of pertinent histology; this is particularly important in the realm of scarring or permanent alopecia. Clearly, this latter subdivision of alopecia highlights the need for further work on the basic etiology of these and other common hair growth disorders. Current knowledge and future avenues of research are also discussed in this book.

It is hoped that the general mission of this textbook, i.e., to make the diagnosis and treatment of hair disorders concise, clear and eminently practical, has been accomplished.

ACKNOWLEDGMENTS

I would like to thank Norma Longo for her tireless commitment to excellence on behalf of this project: she was intimately involved in the organization, typing and editing of this textbook and deserves the title of "editorial assistant *par excellence.*" I would also like to thank the other members of my Duke Dermatopharmacology Study Center team who have helped on this project: Shirley Blalock, Mary Ellen Sherron, Cynthia Tuttle, and Mark Sampson. My gratitude is also expressed to all the individual authors of this textbook, many of whom reviewed chapters other than their own and made helpful suggestions, and to William Lamsback at McGraw-Hill and John Fitzpatrick at Editorial Services of New England, Inc., who aided and supervised the production of this textbook.

Elise A. Olsen

DISORDERS OF

HAIR GROWTH

Diagnosis and Treatment

Chapter

1

EMBRYOLOGY AND ANATOMY OF THE HAIR FOLLICLE

Edward Abell

INTRODUCTION

Before undertaking a comprehensive description of the development and anatomy of the hair follicle, it is appropriate to give some consideration to the purposes for which these structures were evolved. In this way, the descriptive process can be related, as far as is possible, to the functional requirement of the structure. Central to this consideration is the requirement for a structure that will elaborate a hair shaft and then allow it to escape from the site of production in a continuous flow to emerge through the skin surface and extend substantially beyond. Though this may seem a facile statement, it is, nonetheless, the major function of the hair follicle. There are other functions in which the hair follicle is involved, but there can be no doubt that this anatomical structure was evolved to produce and extrude a hair shaft.

Production of hair is peculiar to mammals. In most mammals with substantial quantities of body hair, the major purpose is that of conservation of body heat. The mat of hair fiber trapping warm air close to the body surface provides protection from extremes of cold. That many animals adapt their insulation layer to the seasonal climatic change by various patterns of molting illustrates that this function provides for considerable adjustment. Thick mammalian pelts probably also serve to protect the animal from outside injury from claw and thorn and many other minor but common hazards of a wild existence. Such functions are clearly of little relevance to modern humans in whom, from an evolutionary point of view, the growth of body hair has diminished greatly in importance.

There is no evidence in man that the complete loss of body hair, whether this occurs as a congenital or acquired abnormality, produces any significant biologic impairment to the individual or reduction in life expectancy. The development of specialized hairs in humans, as in other mammals, still serves tactile and protective functions (eyelashes and nasal hairs), and though we may be at considerable pains to eliminate the odor created on axillary and pubic hair, these structures still act as a vector for apocrine secretion.

For the most part, therefore, it seems that in humans it is the secondary roles that hair has come to serve that have become important, at least in a social sense. These roles might be considered as analogues of the devices used for social organization seen in many animal species. Though humans no longer make use of hair for protection, heat retention, or camouflage, it still remains a very important means by which individuals display and are recognized. Appropriate appearance and grooming are still very important in social organization and sexual signaling, as may be attested to by the vast commercial efforts developed to sustain, promote, and augment the residual human pelt.

A knowledge of follicular anatomy and development is of considerable importance to physicians who wish to be involved in the care of patients with hair problems, for without these basic tools, it is impossible to gain insight into this complex field of medicine.

EMBRYOLOGY

Development

The earliest stage of human embryonic life at which organization of the primitive epidermis leads to the development of hair structures is between 9 and 12 weeks.[1–3] These changes begin in the areas of the developing chin, eyebrow, and upper lip. At this stage, the primitive ectoderm consists of only three or four cell layers—the basal layer, one or two layers of intermediate cells, and the periderm. More or less simultaneously, a gathering or crowding of cell nuclei in the primitive basal zone occurs, together with a corresponding gathering of cells in the primitive mesoderm immediately below, the so-called *pregerm* (Fig. 1-1*A,B*). It is not known with certainty which of these two changes occurs first. The cells in the basal zone become elongated and begin to grow downward into the primitive mesoderm to form the *hair germ* (Fig. 1-1*C*). This downgrowth continues, with the gathered mesoderm cells remaining in front of the ectoderm (the *hair* peg) (Fig. 1-1*D,E*). The mesodermal cells will ultimately form the fibrous sheath of the follicle as well as the hair papilla.

The hair peg continues its downward path into the mesoderm as an oblique extension, and subsequently the deepest portion of the ectoderm enlarges into a bulbous mass which encloses the primitive hair papilla: the *bulbous hair peg* (Fig. 1-1*F*). This hair peg development is in no way an invagination of the primitive ectoderm but occurs through cellular growth and division to form a solid core of epithelial cells. During the development of these hair structures, the ectodermal and mesodermal elements remain in intimate contact and reflect the association which will continue throughout the life of the follicular apparatus.

Hair follicle development progresses in a cephalocaudal direction to cover the entire body surface of the embryo. In many, if not most, areas, hairs usually develop in clusters of three, although clusters of two to five (or occasionally more) are also found. Hair germ development is delayed considerably on the trunk and limbs, which may not show germ organization until as late as the sixteenth week. However, all embryonic follicular development is complete by about the twenty-second week. It is, therefore, apparent that overall follicular development may be seen in very many stages of evolution at any given time. Indeed, follicles may be producing hair on the scalp while hair germs are just beginning to develop on the legs. The development of the hair germs follows a symmetrical pattern over the body surface. The downgrowth into the dermis also grows at more or less the same oblique angle in the same body areas, and this angulation creates an identifiable anterior and posterior aspect to each follicle.

The next stage in follicular growth is the development of epithelial buds on the posterior aspect (the side which forms an obtuse angle) of the bulbous hair germ. The more superficial of these will evolve into one or more sebaceous glands. The more inferior, larger one (termed "Wulst," or *bulge,* by Stöhr) will act as the epithelial attachment or contact area for the arrector pili muscle (Fig. 1-1*F*). It is apparent that the arrector pili muscle evolves in the primitive mesoderm without contact with the developing follicle to which it will be associated. This muscle also develops at an oblique angle in the posterior aspect of the hair in such a position as to elevate the hair on the skin surface when thrown

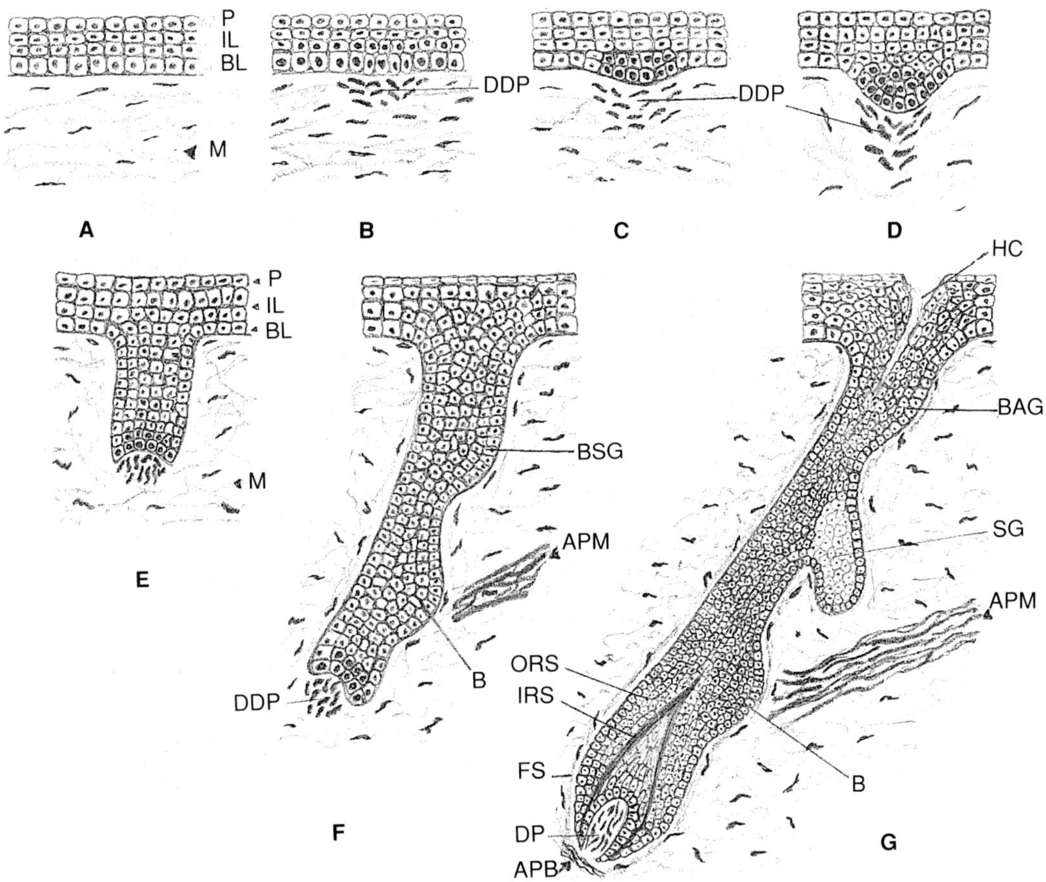

Figure 1-1 Diagrammatic representation of embryologic development of the hair follicle: (*A*) Primitive ectoderm before pre-germ development. (*B*) Pregerm development. (*C*) Hair germ. (*D*) and (*E*) Downgrowth of hair germ into mesoderm (hair peg). (*F*) Bulbous hair germ. (*G*) Fully developed hair follicle. APB = Arao-Perkins body, APM = arrector pili muscle, B = bulge (insertion APM), BAG = bulge (apocrine gland potential), BL = basal layer, BSG = bulge (sebaceous gland), DP = dermal (hair) papilla, DDP = developing dermal papilla, FS = follicular sheath, HC = hair canal, IL = intermediate layer, IRS = inner root sheath, M = mesoderm, ORS = outer root sheath, P = periderm, SG = sebaceous galnd.

into contraction (Fig. 1-2). Evidence has been found in recent years that the bulge area of the inferior bud may carry the stem-cell capacity for follicular generation.[4,5] In this respect, it is interesting that it is to this site that follicular regression occurs during catagen, thus bringing the effete hair bulb into close or perhaps intimate contact with the epithelial cells of the bulge site of arrector pili insertion.

In many follicles, a third bud appears on the posterior aspect of the hair germ in a more superficial location to that of the sebaceous gland bud. This third bud will develop into a rudimentary apocrine gland in some areas. However, these buds involute completely in most body areas. Development of mature apocrine glands occurs on the scalp, some areas of the face, axilla, groin, genital skin, and around the anus, in the external ear canals, eyelids, the areola of the breasts, and in some random areas of the trunk and limbs.

Mesenchymal cells condense around the cylindrical germ and elaborate the follicular fibrous sheath. Beneath the bulbous portion of the hair germ, these cells form a distinct pad of tissue which is in direct contact with the hair papilla through a small gap in the epithelial cells of the developing hair bulb (Fig. 1-1*G*). This pad will develop a rich elastic tissue network to be-

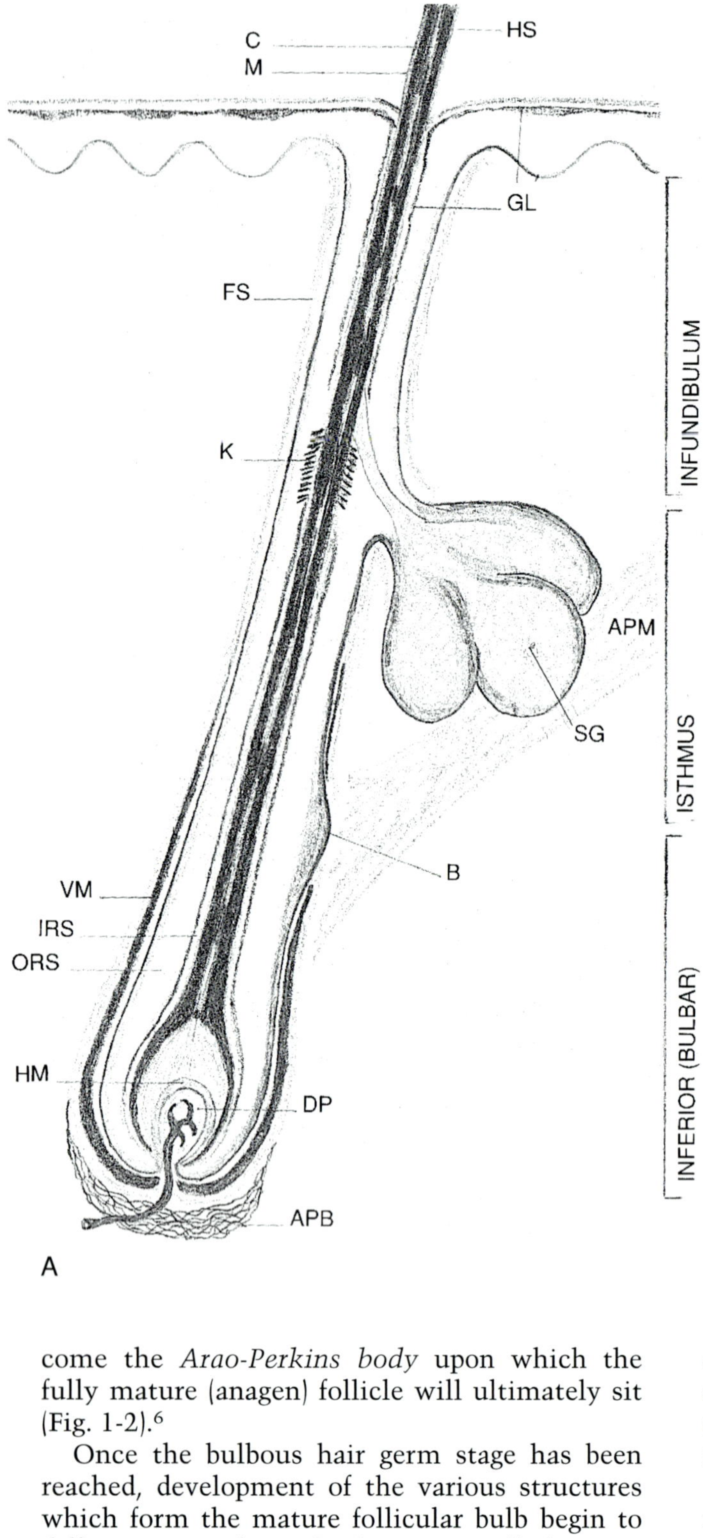

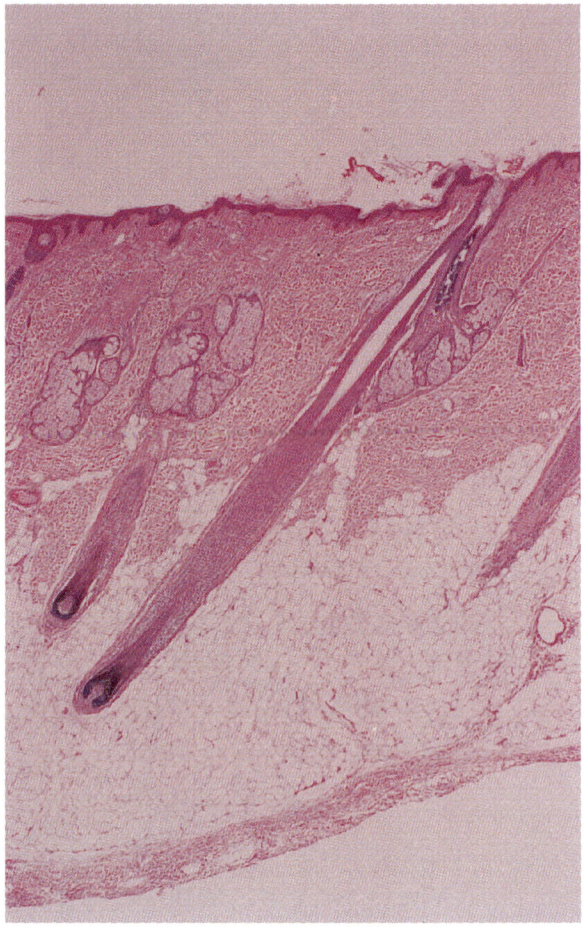

Figure 1-2 (*A*) Diagrammatic representation of an intermittently medullated terminal hair and follicular structures. APB = Arao-Perkins body, APM = arrector pili muscle, B = bulge, C =hair cortex, DP = dermal papilla, FS = follicular sheath, GL = glandular layer, HM = hair matrix, HS = hair shaft, IRS = inner root sheath, KZ = keratinizing zone, M = hair medulla, ORS = outer root sheath, SG = sebaceous gland, VM = vitreous membrane. (*B*) Photomicrograph of anagen terminal hair follicle (H&E × 10.) (*Photo courtesy of Dr. Hideko Kamino.*)

come the *Arao-Perkins body* upon which the fully mature (anagen) follicle will ultimately sit (Fig. 1-2).[6]

Once the bulbous hair germ stage has been reached, development of the various structures which form the mature follicular bulb begin to differentiate to form the *hair cone.* All elements of the inner and outer root sheaths together with the hair shaft are identifiable in the embryo. Even though these changes occur, the direction of epithelial growth remains downward into the developing dermis as the follicle has still not achieved its full size. Only after this has been achieved is the direction of cellular growth significantly upward.

It seems probable that the hair papilla plays an important role in orchestration of follicular growth and function and perhaps on differentiation also.[7–9] That apparently identical epithelial cells in the mature hair matrix are able to elaborate cells of such disparate appearance and function as those found in the outer and inner root sheaths and hair shaft speaks for very high levels of control. In recent years, information concerning control factors for follicular development and growth have been reported. These studies are reviewed in Chapter 3.

Melanocytic cells of the developing epidermis, derived by migration from the neural crest, become distributed relatively randomly in the early hair germ, but functionally active melanocytes become concentrated only in the area of the epithelial portion of the bulbous germ that will ultimately become the hair bulb matrix.[10]

Lumen formation in the cylinder of cells forming the mature hair germ occurs in two distinct patterns. In the lower portion below the sebaceous gland bud, a lumen forms by the necrosis of germ cells without their undergoing keratinization. By complete contrast, the upper portion, which will form the infundibulum, undergoes both necrosis and keratinization. This is the first site in which keratinization can be identified in the developing epidermis, occurring before that of the surface epithelium.[11] This developmental process indicates particularly clearly that the infundibular epithelium is a territory distinct from the surface epidermis.

Intrauterine Follicular Function

Embryonic hair follicles may be producing hair by the sixteenth to twentieth weeks. The initial product is lanugo hair, fine nonpigmented hairs which cover the whole body. Growth of this type of hair is usually complete by birth and, under normal circumstances, does not persist significantly into postuterine life. Lanugo hair is shed into the amniotic fluid between the thirty-second and thirty-sixth weeks, and subsequent hair growth on the scalp, eyebrows, and lashes is of a more substantial type. Lanugo hair growth continues on the rest of the body and is shed between the third and fourth month post partum, after which time subsequent hair growth is unsynchronized and of more substantial type.

FOLLICULAR ANATOMY

Overview

Each hair structure is made up of either two or three elements, depending upon whether the hair is of sufficient size to develop a central medulla[12,13] (Fig. 1-3). The major structure, forming the bulk and strength of the shaft, is the cortex. This is covered by a single layer of overlapping keratinized cells which form an imbricated coating called the *cuticle.* This structure appears to play a vital protective role, for, if the cuticle is severely damaged or lost, the integrity of the cortical cells is rapidly breached. In many large hairs, there is a central zone of more loosely organized keratinized material, the *medulla.*[14] The medulla, more easily appreciated under polarized microscopy, is only partially keratinized and may be continuous or interrupted along the hair shaft.

Gross Anatomy

It is clear from direct observation that there is a very large number of variations of hair type in respect to color, length, coarseness, and distribution pattern, not only in different body locations but also between individuals and different racial groups, and at different ages of life.

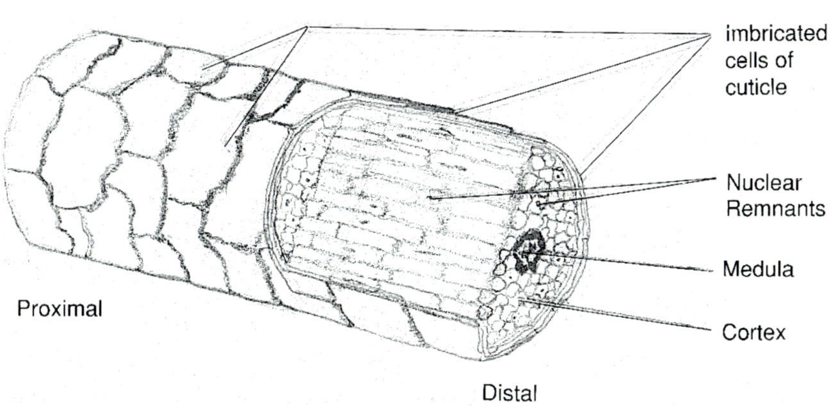

Figure 1-3 Diagrammatic representation of the ultrastructure of the hair shaft.

After uterine life, hairs are divided, by size, into two major types. Terminal hair is described as being substantial or large in size, pigmented, and frequently medullated; it can grow to considerable length (from 1 to 100 cm, approximately). Terminal hair shaft diameter is about 60 μm, and terminal hair bulbs in anagen on the scalp are situated in the subcutaneous fat. Terminal hair is the typical hair of the scalp throughout life in normal individuals. Vellus hairs are smaller, more lightly pigmented, and nonmedullated, and do not normally grow more than 2 cm in length. They generally have a diameter of less than 30 μm, and vellus anagen hair bulbs are situated in the reticular dermis. Variation in pigment and length may be appreciated but does not determine the hair type: some terminal hairs (e.g., eyelashes, eyebrows, and nasal and ear canal hairs) are quite short. As hair growth rates are relatively similar in these areas, it is clear that these differences in length are brought about by alterations in the duration of anagen. Shortening of anagen is compensated by lengthening of the resting phase (telogen). Vellus hairs of the male beard, axillary, and pubic hair areas transform to terminal hair at puberty in response to increased androgen production.

The curvature of hair shows enormous variation. Hair shafts may be absolutely straight or, at the other extreme, very tightly curled, and a complete range exists between these two extremes. The more curved or curled the hair shaft, the more likely it is that the dermal and/or subcutaneous hair follicle will show a curved path. How the curvature of the follicle imparts the curl to the shaft is not clear, but it has been suggested that the developing hair shaft "sets" in the mold. The cross section of Caucasian hair is round, oval, or elliptic, but that of Negroid shafts is more elliptical or flattened.

The appearance of hair density is more complex. It seems clear that there is some difference in follicular density between individuals, and direct histological measurements show a range of values.[15] Whether there are significant differences between racial groups is not clear, but it appears that Oriental races have a reduced number of total body follicles. However, most of the apparent variation in density is more substantially attributed to variation in hair shaft size.

Hair follicles and their attendant sebaceous glands develop in clusters which form the follicular unit. It is now well-documented that the follicular units do not appear randomly in the scalp. The use of histological sections cut in the transverse plane parallel to the epidermal surface, clearly demonstrates a regular mosaic pattern of follicular units separated by trabeculae of connective tissue (Fig. 1-4).[16] In the sebaceous follicles of the neck and upper chest, the formation of regular bilaterally symmetrical patterns of follicular units is obvious to direct inspection. These sebaceous follicles generally have tiny vellus hairs but large superficial sebaceous glands. Clinically, these create small beaded papules which allow easy detection of the follicular units through the epidermis.

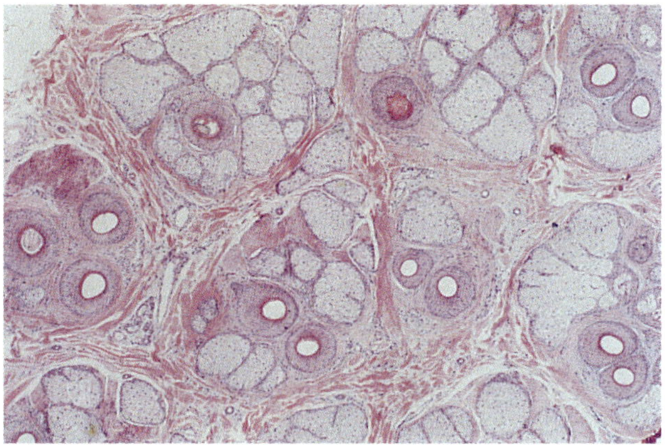

Figure 1-4 Low power photomicrograph of scalp biopsy sectioned in the horizontal plane, showing grouped follicles and sebaceous glands separated by connective tissue trabeculae (H&E × 25).

Tables 1-1 and 1-2 present the various aspects of follicular measurement and function in various anatomic sites.

Microscopic Anatomy

A fully mature anagen hair follicle can be divided into three segments. These divisions are useful as they recognize not only the major anatomic parts but also the functional divisions of the follicle, which are of major significance in the structural alterations that occur repeatedly as the follicle goes through the different cycles of growth. These segments divide the follicle into three approximately equal parts which, from superficial to deep, are the infundibulum, the isthmus, and the inferior or bulbar segment (Fig. 1-2). A fourth segment of the pilosebaceous follicular unit would comprise the sebaceous gland.

Table 1-1
FOLLICULAR DATA[12,15,39]

Total body hair follicles	5 million (estimated)
Total scalp hair follicles	100,000–150,000
Anagen follicles (adult)	90%
Telogen follicles (adult)	10%
Anagen follicles (child)	95%
Telogen follicles (child)	5%
Growth rate hair	
Scalp (1cm/month)	0.37–0.44 mm/day
Body and beard	0.27 mm/day
Follicular density	
At birth	1135/cm^2
1 year	795/cm^2
15 years	615/cm^2
30 years +	485/cm^2
80 years	435/cm^2
Mean terminal hair shaft diameter of adult male scalp	70 μm (range 60–84 μm)

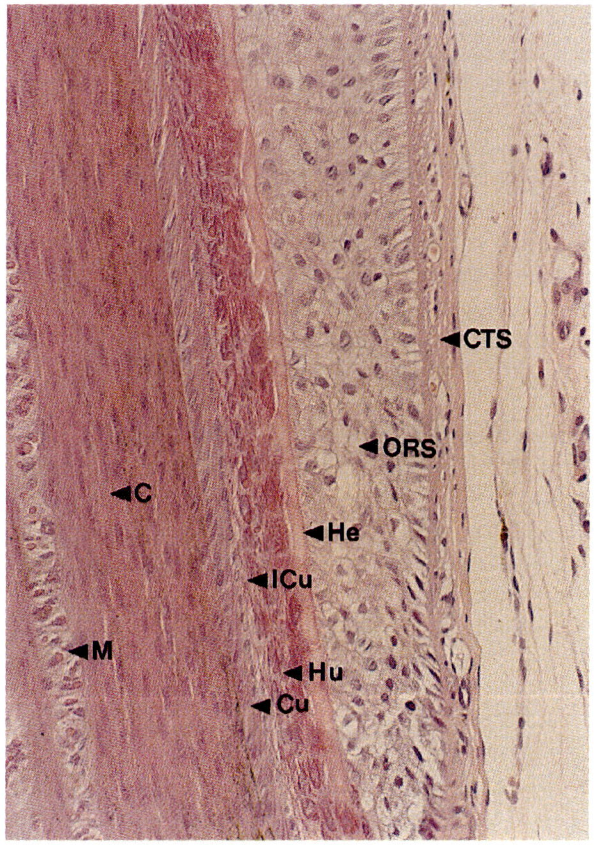

Figure 1-5 Vertical cross section of anagen hair at level of keratinization (i.e., junction of superior bulbar region and isthmus). (H&E × 260). M = medulla; C = cortex; CU = cuticle; ICU = inner root sheath (IRS) cuticle; HU = Huxley's layer of IRS; HE = Henle's layer of IRS; ORS = outer root sheath; CTS = connective tissue sheath.

A transverse or vertical section of the hair follicle at the infundibulum, sebaceous gland, isthmus, or bulbar segment will show structural variations in the hair shaft and the surrounding organizational units. These are fairly typical for a particular anatomical level and for a given stage in the hair follicle growth cycle. The basic units of the follicle are (from central to peripheral) the hair shaft, the hair shaft cuticle, the inner root sheath (including the inner root sheath cuticle, Huxley's layer, and Henle's layer), the outer root sheath, and the connective tissue sheath (Fig. 1-5). Each structural unit will be discussed in this chapter in the context of its role in hair shaft formation and release.

Only the upper third of the follicle, or infundibulum, does not take part in the follicular adaptation to the growth cycle but remains stable throughout life. The infundibulum acts as a conduit for the hair shaft, the product of the sebaceous glands and shed keratin material. The bulbar segment is elaborated during anagen for the production of not only the hair shaft but all elements of the inner and outer root sheaths. It is then almost completely broken down preparatory to a period of sustained inactivity (telogen). This breakdown process is called *catagen,* and when this occurs, there is a simultaneous adaptive change in the middle third, or isthmus, segment of the follicle which allows for retention of the hair shaft during telogen. The hair shaft is anchored to the remnant of the outer root sheath by a specialized keratinization process. Once the follicle has been regenerated in anagen, the isth-

Table 1-2
Hair Growth Cycle[12,39]

Adult scalp	
Anagen period	2–8 y
Telogen	2–4 mo
Catagen	2–4 wk
Length of anagen other sites (young male)	
Legs	5–7 mo
Arms	1.5–3 mo
Fingers	1–3 mo
Eyelashes	1–6 mo
Normal scalp hair loss (adult)	50–100 hairs/day

mus segment remains relatively inert throughout the rest of anagen and appears to function largely as a structural support for the developing hair shaft.

It should be clear from this brief introduction that the anatomy of the follicle is not static or rigid but is dependent upon the phase of the growth cycle in which it is examined. Anatomy and growth cycle are so intimately related that their description can only be considered together. The following description is that of a typical adult anagen scalp hair.

THE INFUNDIBULUM

Though developed as a distinct and separate structure from the surface epidermis, when fully formed, these structures are in direct continuity (Fig. 1-6). Indeed, they both share the same pattern of stratification and keratinization. However, the infundibulum lacks the organization of the dermal interface into a rete ridge pattern and, therefore, the neurovascular supply lacks the papillary pattern of the surface. Instead, the infundibulum is a straight tube of epithelium bounded on its outer wall by simple cuboidal basal cells. Maturation follows the pattern of the surface epithelium by formation of polygonal squamous cells prior to the appearance of keratohyalin granules in a well-developed granular layer. Fully keratinized squamous cells several layers thick line the surface of the lumen, and this stratum corneum is formed without loss of continuity with that of the surface epithelium. The lumen of the follicle will normally contain the hair shaft as well as some keratin material shed from the wall, variable amounts of sebaceous excretion, and the organisms that normally colonize this nidus (bacteria, lipophilic yeasts, and, particularly on the head, neck, and upper trunk, *Demodex* mites). The infundibulum extends from the follicular orifice to the site of insertion of the sebaceous duct.

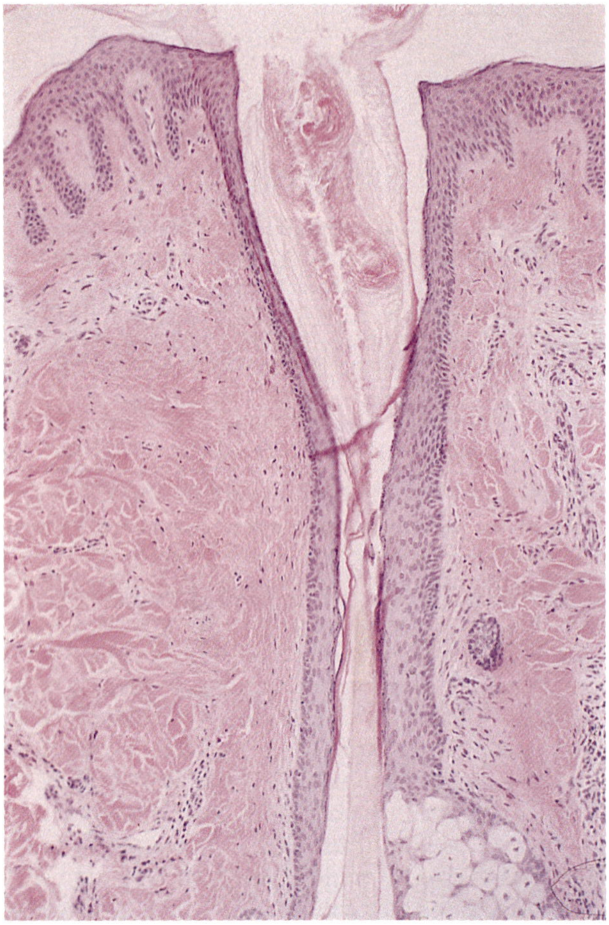

Figure 1-6 Photomicrograph of follicular infundibulum extending from skin surface to insertion of the sebaceous duct: note continuity of granular zone throughout the entire structure (H&E × 65).

THE SEBACEOUS GLAND

At first, the sebaceous gland is a solid hemispheric knob at the posterior wall of the follicle, but gradually the central cells take on a foamy appearance typical of lipid-filled cells. The anterior wall is lined by keratinizing cells of infundibular character. When the gland shows lobulation, a carina-like septum finally defines a sebaceous duct separate from the tube for the hair shaft.[1]

THE ISTHMUS

The middle third of the follicle begins below the sebaceous duct and extends to the bulge or area of attachment for the arrector pili muscle (Fig. 1-2). This latter site is often anatomically inconspicuous in adult follicles. Its separation from the bulbar segment of the follicle is, therefore, imprecise and as the formation of this structure is so closely related to the activity of the hair bulb, it is appropriate to consider it as a direct extension of the lower third of the follicle. The isthmus consists of a tube of epithelial cells which, in hematoxylin and eosin–stained tissue, have clear cytoplasm: this is due to a substantial deposition of glycogen. Peripherally, the isthmus is limited by the fibrous sheath of the follicle

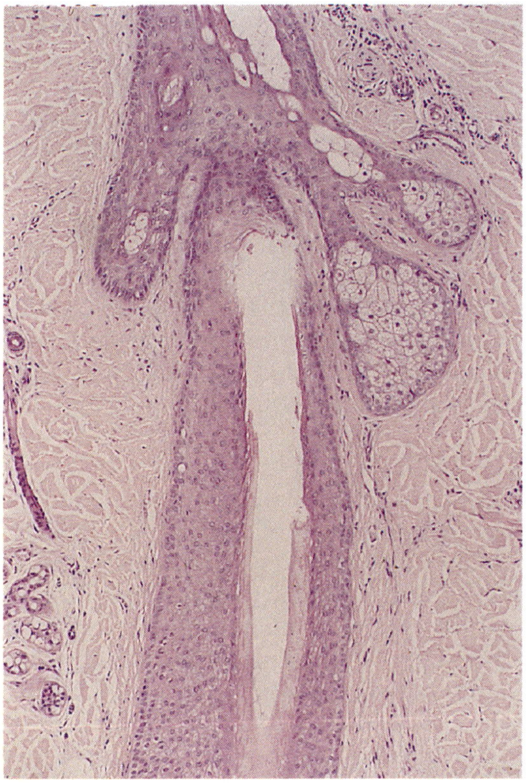

A

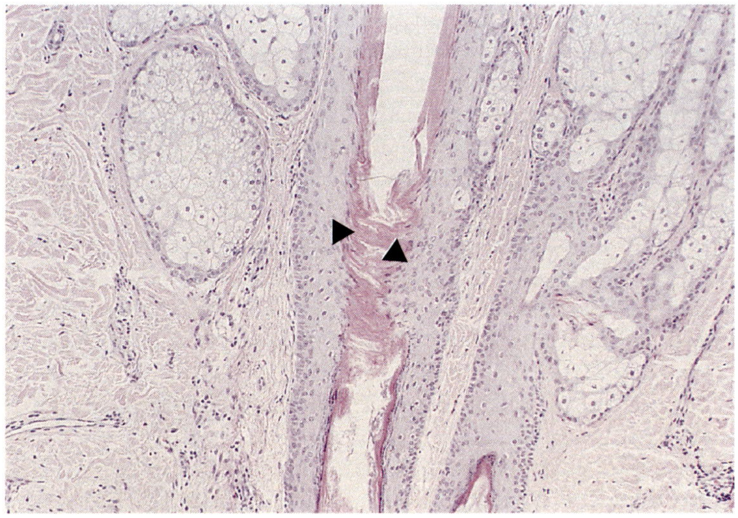

B

Figure 1-7 Photomicrographs of follicular isthmus: (*A*) the outer root sheath with fully keratinized inner root sheath on luminal surface. When the inner root sheath disintegrates, the outer root sheath cells are able to keratinize terminally (H&E × 65). (*B*) Close-up of this site of trichilemmal keratinization (*arrow*) (H&E × 65).

and, at the internal margin and toward the distal end, by the fully keratinized and disintegrating inner root sheath. At this level, Huxley's and Henle's layers of the inner root sheath lose their staining characteristics, fuse, and wane.[17]

The isthmus also differs from the infundibulum in its apparent lack of keratinization of the cells of the outer root sheath. Terminal differentiation of the outer root sheath cells is found in the most superficial portion of the isthmus immediately below the sebaceous duct insertion (Fig. 1-7). This very restricted area is the site of tricholemmal or pilar keratinization,[18] which appears to occur at this site only following destruction of the inner root sheath. This destruction of the inner root sheath seems to be an active process rather than a passive one, as the zone shows an alteration of staining properties associated with detectable protease activity.

Within the adventitial tissue immediately surrounding the isthmus, the fibrous sheath shows a particularly dense mat of small nerve fibers. This structure is probably the site which mediates the sensory perception of tactile appreciation.

THE BULBAR OR INFERIOR REGION

The lower third of the follicle is the site of the majority of activity in the hair follicle. It consists of the hair bulb, containing the hair matrix which surrounds the hair papilla, and the deepest part of the straight portion of the follicle. The bulbs of terminal scalp hairs in anagen may lie deep in the subcutaneous tissue, but the bulbs of smaller terminal follicles in anagen at other sites, or any follicles in telogen, lie in the dermis. Some small vellus follicles may have their bulbs in the uppermost reticular dermis.

The hair matrix, situated in the very center of the bulb, consists of those epithelial cells which lay directly upon the superficial and lateral aspects of the hair papilla (Fig. 1-8). A line arbitrarily drawn across the hair bulb at the widest part of the dermal papilla marks the *critical level of Auber.* The cells of the matrix under the line of Auber remain undifferentiated and have a high mitotic rate, while those cells above the line have low mitotic activity but differentiate into the cells of the hair matrix and inner root sheath.[19] Matrix cells appear to be uniform despite the highly varied products which are ultimately derived from their proliferation. Numerous large, dendritic melanocytic cells also occupy the basal layer, their dendrites arborizing into the intercellular areas of the bulb.[20] Melanin incorporation into matrix cells is very sharply controlled, as pigment is found only in the hair shaft and cuticle.

The division and maturation of matrix cells produces columns of cells which stream superficially into the central part of the bulb and then enter the straight linear portion of the follicle. Appropriate tissue stains identify the various products of cell differentiation, and how, in precise symmetry, the elements of the hair shaft, inner root sheath, and the peripheral outer root sheath are elaborated (Fig. 1-8). Those cells in the central part of the matrix will form the hair shaft, consisting of the medulla (where present), the cortex, and the hair shaft cuticle.

The constituents of the inner root sheath are elaborated immediately peripheral to the hair cuticle. Immediately adjacent is the single cell layer which forms the cuticle of the inner root sheath. Continuing peripherally are three or four cell layers which make up Huxley's layer, and beyond this is the single cell layer of Henle. Beyond the inner root sheath are cells which differentiate from a single layer on the margin of the bulb into the multicellular tube of clear cells which form the outer root sheath.

Figure 1-8 Photomicrograph of bulbar portion of follicle with hair papilla, matrix, and the various elements elaborated from the matrix. The fibrous pad of the Arao-Perkins body (*arrow*) lies beneath the papilla (H&E × 130).

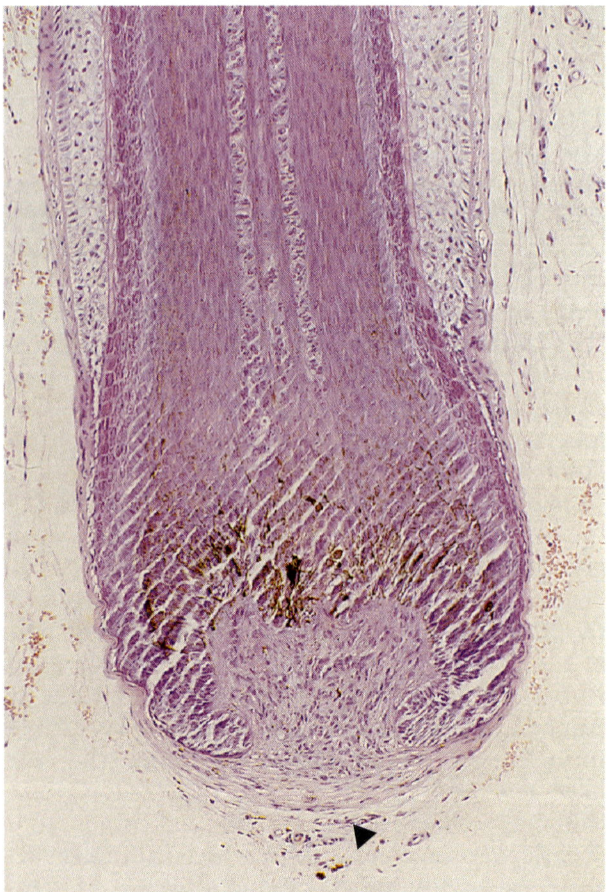

THE HAIR PAPILLA

The hair papilla, almost totally encapsulated by the matrix epithelium, consists of an oval or rounded mass of spindle cells (fibroblasts) set in a mucopolysaccharide-rich connective tissue within which sparse collagen fibers may be present (Fig. 1-8).[21] A basement lamina of 5-µm thickness lies between the papilla and the matrix epidermal cells, and this is in direct continuity with the vitreous membrane structures of the follicular sheath. The fibroblasts show abundant cytoplasm and appear to be metabolically active during anagen, but these cells undergo considerable cytoplasmic reduction in catagen, suggesting a more quiescent state. Nerve fibers and small blood vessels pass into the papilla through the small gap in the base of the hair matrix epithelium. Directly beneath the papilla and in continuity with it is the fibroelastic pad (the Arao-Perkins body).

The size of the hair papilla correlates directly with the size of the follicle and the hair produced. The larger the papilla, the larger the follicle and the thicker the hair produced.[22] It is considered probable that the papilla induces and coordinates follicular function. Transplant experiments suggest that the papilla is capable of inducing follicular development and the formation of the hair shaft when placed in proximity to follicular epithelium.[8,23]

THE FOLLICULAR SHEATH

This structure surrounds the entire length of the follicle and is made up of two significant elements. A basement membrane invests the epithelial cells of all segments of the follicle. This is substantially thickened around the outer root sheath of the bulbar portion of the follicle, shows more periodic acid–Schiff (PAS)-positive staining, and is known as the *hyaline* or *vitreous (glassy) membrane*. In the early stages of catagen, this eosinophilic staining structure crumbles as the outer root sheath collapses and serves as a striking marker of this stage of the growth cycle.

Outside the basement membrane is a connective tissue sheath which develops late in fetal life and is apparent around the entire follicle. In the lower portion of the follicle, the connective tissue sheath is clearly a two-layer structure, with collagen fibers in the innermost layer arranged circularly and the collagen fibers arranged longitudinally in the outer layer. In the upper follicle, collagen fibers are arranged only longitudinally.[24] There are prominent elastic filaments arranged longitudinally above the bulge area of the follicle but few in number below this region.[24]

THE NEUROVASCULAR SUPPLY

Dermal arteriolar vessels feed into a dense network of interconnecting small vessels which ensheath the bulbar portion of the follicle. In the isthmus zone, a thinner network of small vessels runs mainly longitudinally in the direction of the follicle, but a more complex network is reestablished in the area of the sebaceous gland duct. The vessels of the infundibular area are in communication with the superficial plexus vessels of the papillary dermis of which they are an integral part. These vessels are most readily demonstrated by alkaline phosphatase enzyme histochemical staining.[25,26]

Follicular vascularization is directly related to follicular size, with the larger structures showing larger and more abundant vessels. The larger hair papillae will usually show a small arteriolar vessel entering through the gap in the base of the matrix. The arteriole branches into smaller vessels which are dispersed through the papilla. Smaller papillae show only a capillary vascular supply.[27] This relatively complex vascular network is substantially preserved during early to mid catagen. Only in late catagen does there seem to be some reduction of the vasculature.[28] The blood vessels are an integral part of the fibrous sheath remnant down which the next anagen follicle will develop.

The entire length of the follicle is covered by a fine network of sensory nerves.[29] Large nerve fibers from the deep dermis or subcutaneous tissue approach from all quadrants and converge on the hair follicle at the level of the sebaceous duct.[29] Although larger follicles have a greater number of associated fibers, nerves around hair follicles assume many different patterns which have no particular relation to the size of the follicle.[29] Vellus hairs possess vertically oriented nerve fibers, the terminal branches forming a palisade underneath horizontally oriented nerves (Fig. 1-9). Branching of this vertical layer of nerve fibers forms a collar at the level of the infundibulum. Around large follicles, one finds many horizontally and vertically oriented nerves but no clear corona of palisade endings in the inner vertical layer.[30] This perifollicular network of nerves and end organs greatly extends the range of cutaneous sensory perception.

THE PROCESS OF HAIR SHAFT FORMATION AND RELEASE

During the anagen growth phase, the matrix cells maintain a constant high mitotic rate which provides a rapid stream of cells into the central portion of the bulb and then outward to the surface.[31,32] To a variable degree, these cells become elongated, especially those which form the hair cortex and the two cuticles. The cortex cells become densely packed and lamellated and usually are heavily melanized. Those hairs which develop a medulla show some central disorganization of this linear stream of cells, which leads to the formation of a loosely organized hair shaft core containing small cavities.

The cells of the hair cuticle lie somewhat obliquely against those of the cortex and intimately interdigitate with the cuticle cells of the inner root sheath so that their narrow ends abut one another and these two layers grow out together.[33] This organization requires the hair cuticle cells to partially overlap one another (and, of course, so do those of the inner root sheath cuticle), and it is this arrangement which produces the characteristic imbrication of the hair shafts.

Peripheral to the hair shaft and inner root sheath cuticle lie the three or four cell layers of Huxley, which show a very prominent pattern of keratinization (Fig. 1-10). These cuboidal cells elongate into a columnar shape before developing large, angular cytoplasmic masses which stain brightly eosinophilic. These eosinophilic masses are the trichohyaline granules, a specific marker of root sheath keratinization. All components of the inner root sheath show this form of

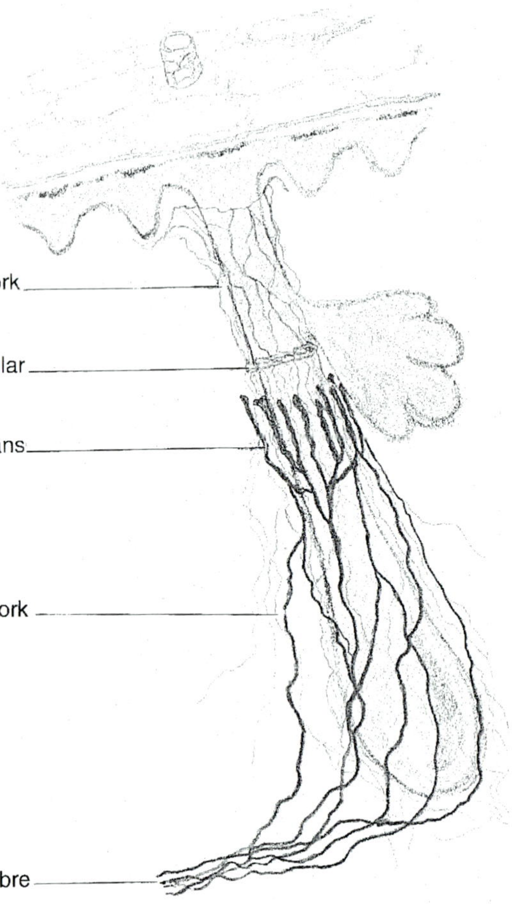

Figure 1-9 Diagrammatic representation of innervation of the hair follicle.

keratinization, but it is characteristically most prominent in Huxley's layer.[34] Huxley's layer is the last structure in the inner root sheath to terminally differentiate.

In the outermost component of the inner root sheath is the single layer of Henle. These cells undergo complete keratinization very rapidly and are the first product of the matrix to be terminally differentiated.[34,35] None of the products of the inner root sheath become incorporated into the hair shaft.

The elaborate and complex keratinization occurring in the inner root sheath has doubtless evolved for a specific purpose. The emergence of the hair shaft from the bulb is associated with the keratinization and terminal differentiation of the cells in Huxley's layer. It is at this precise level that the two columns of tightly interlocked cuticle cells are seen to separate (like the teeth in two cog wheels) (Fig. 1-10). It would appear, therefore, that this complex mechanism of keratinization and differentiation has been elaborated as a means of allowing the developing and rapidly outgrowing hair shaft to disassociate itself from the more permanent structures of the follicle and to continue freely through the follicular lumen to the exterior. Without the detachment of the two cuticles, the hair outgrowth would tear away the root sheath structures. The complex keratinization of the inner root sheath seems to function as a means of achieving this disassociation.

THE GROWTH CYCLE

Human hair grows in a continuous cyclic pattern[12,31,35] (Fig. 1-11). Periods of growth (anagen) are followed by relatively brief periods in which the bulbar portion of the follicle is almost totally degraded (catagen) preceding the resting phase (telogen). The duration of anagen varies

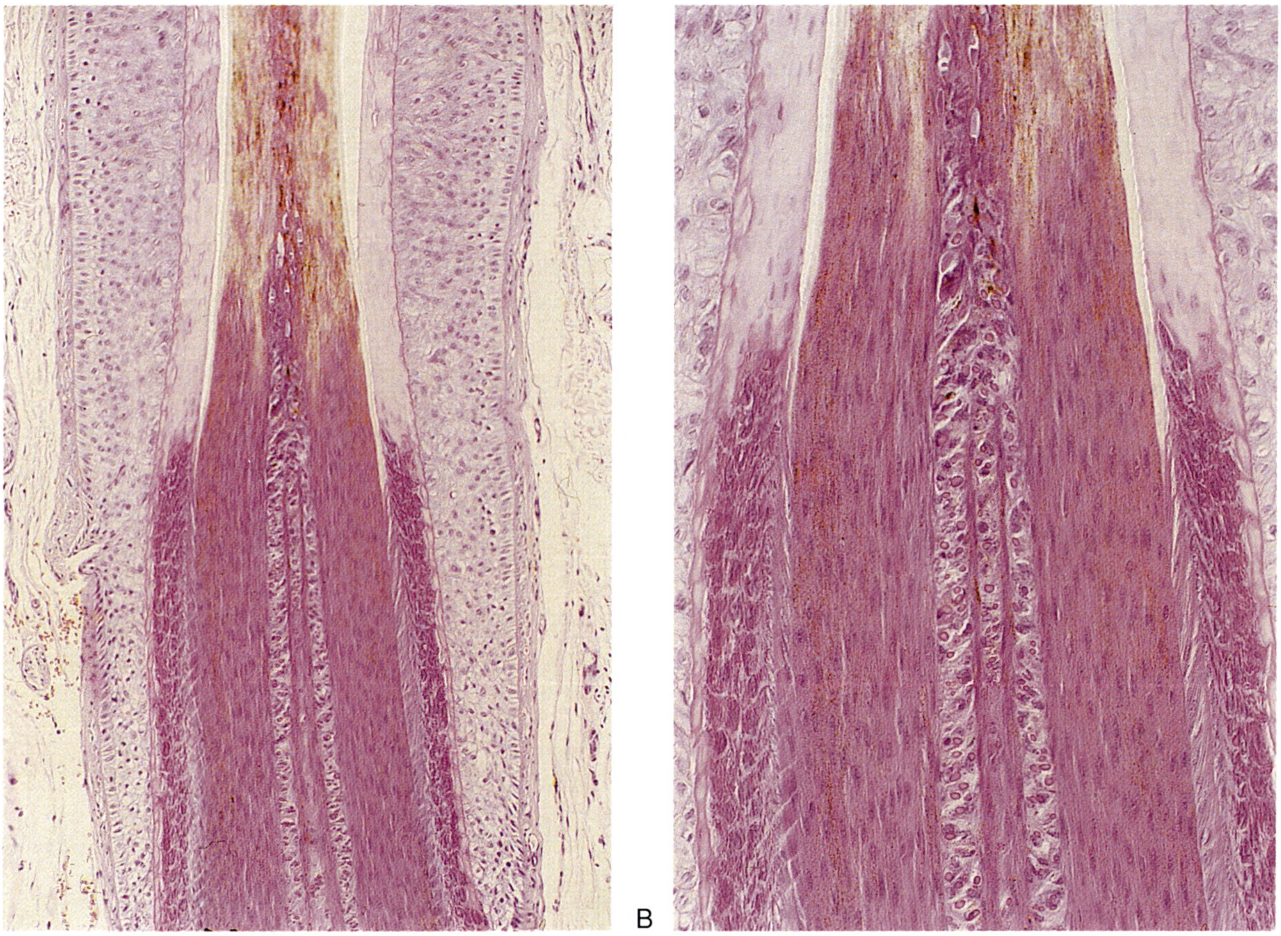

A B

Figure 1-10 Photomicrographs of the junction of the bulbar and isthmus zones of a medullated hair shaft and its inner root sheath where these structures are going through the process of terminal differentiation. (*A*) Terminal keratinization of cuticle cells and those of Huxley's layer allow separation of the hair shaft which now lies free in the follicular canal (H&E × 130). (*B*) A high-power view demonstrates the order of the keratinization of the various follicular elements; note the organization of the two layers of cuticle cells as this process proceeds (H&E × 260).

substantially by anatomic site (Table 1-2) and to a lesser extent for catagen and telogen. Under normal conditions, hair growth is randomized or nonsynchronized. Only in certain physiological states, such as the postpartum period or after episodes of significant systemic disease, will synchronization of the hair cycle be precipitated. With the synchronization of catagen, the ultimate result is a delayed hair shedding (molt) at a period equivalent to the combined time of catagen and telogen. Curiously, where this type of synchronization occurs, the affected follicles rapidly revert to a random pattern of cycling.

The hair shaft is normally retained in the follicle during catagen and telogen unless extracted by vigorous grooming. Shedding of the hair occurs only after the next anagen cycle has been established to a degree that a new hair shaft is beginning to enter the follicular canal. Not more than 10 percent of follicles are in telogen at any time (Table 1-2). This figure represents the maximal figure for telogen: in most normal scalps, the telogen count is probably substantially lower, being in the range of 6 to 8 percent.

It is both conventional and appropriate to describe the physiological changes of catagen first and then follow the follicle through to the next fully established anagen period (Fig. 1-12). What

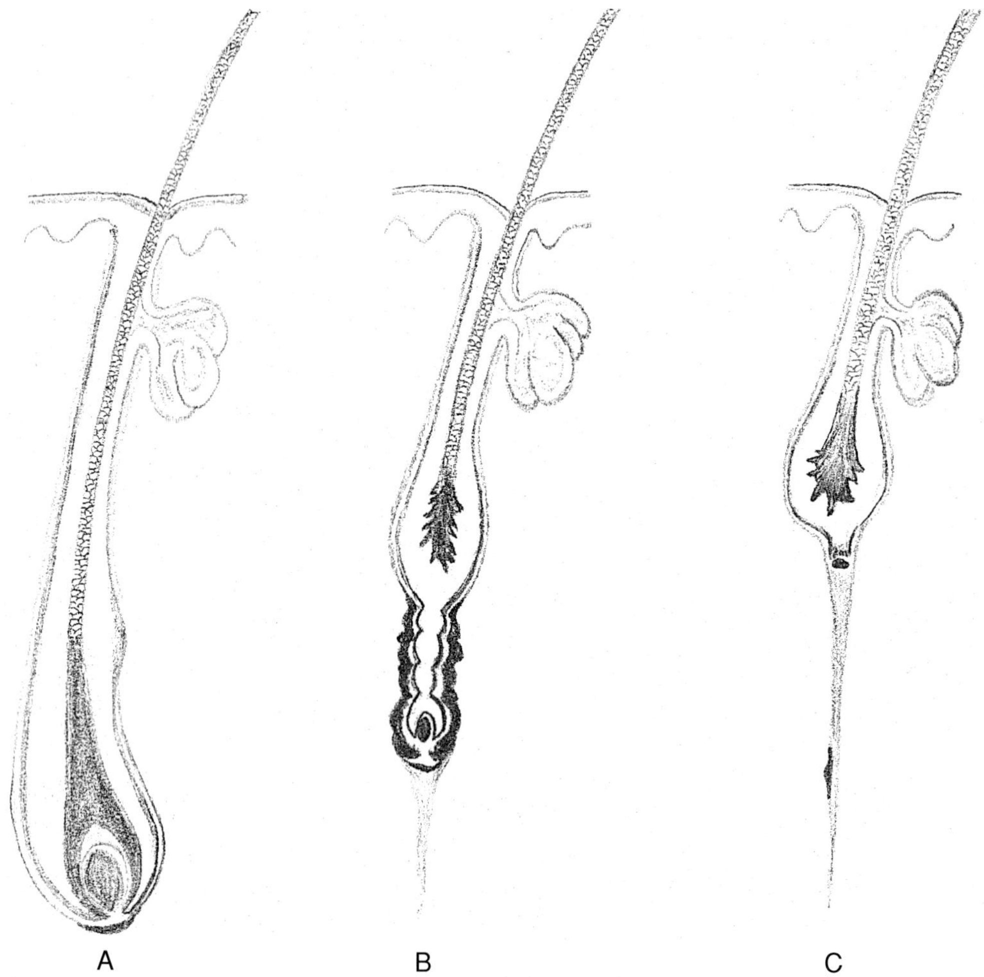

Figure 1-11 Diagrammatic representation of phases of the hair growth cycle. (*A*) Anagen. (*B*) Catagen (mid-catagen stage). Note developing "club" structure as the outer root sheath collapses and withdraws up the follicular sheath, the dermal papilla keeping in close contact. The Arao-Perkins body is also drawn some way up the sheath. (*C*) Telogen. Note fully developed "club" with dermal papilla lying just below the involuted remnant of the bulbar portion of the follicle, which has retracted up the sheath to lie at the level of the bulge. The empty follicular sheath trails below in the dermis. Note position (*arrow*) of the Arao-Perkins body.

signals the onset of catagen and cessation of matrix cell division is not fully understood, but a complex system must be involved. The melanocytes in the matrix are the first cells to show changes indicating the onset of catagen. Pigment production ceases before the final portion of the hair shaft is constructed, producing a proximal "end" which is without pigment. This last element of the shaft also appears less well compacted when compared with the rest of the hair, and as a result, the end becomes slightly enlarged. These are some of the changes responsible for the club shape characteristic of a fully developed telogen hair.[36] Because the "club" hair is retained in the resting or telogen period of the cycle and shed at the time of anagen recovery, the shed club hair becomes a marker for the follicle's recent passage through the telogen phase. Identification of an increased number of club hairs in a plucked hair sample, therefore, indicates a relative shift of the growth cycle into telogen during the recent past.

Catagen is established by cessation of mitosis of the bulb matrix cells. This coincides, more or less, with the appearance of scattered but numerous prematurely keratinized cells throughout the

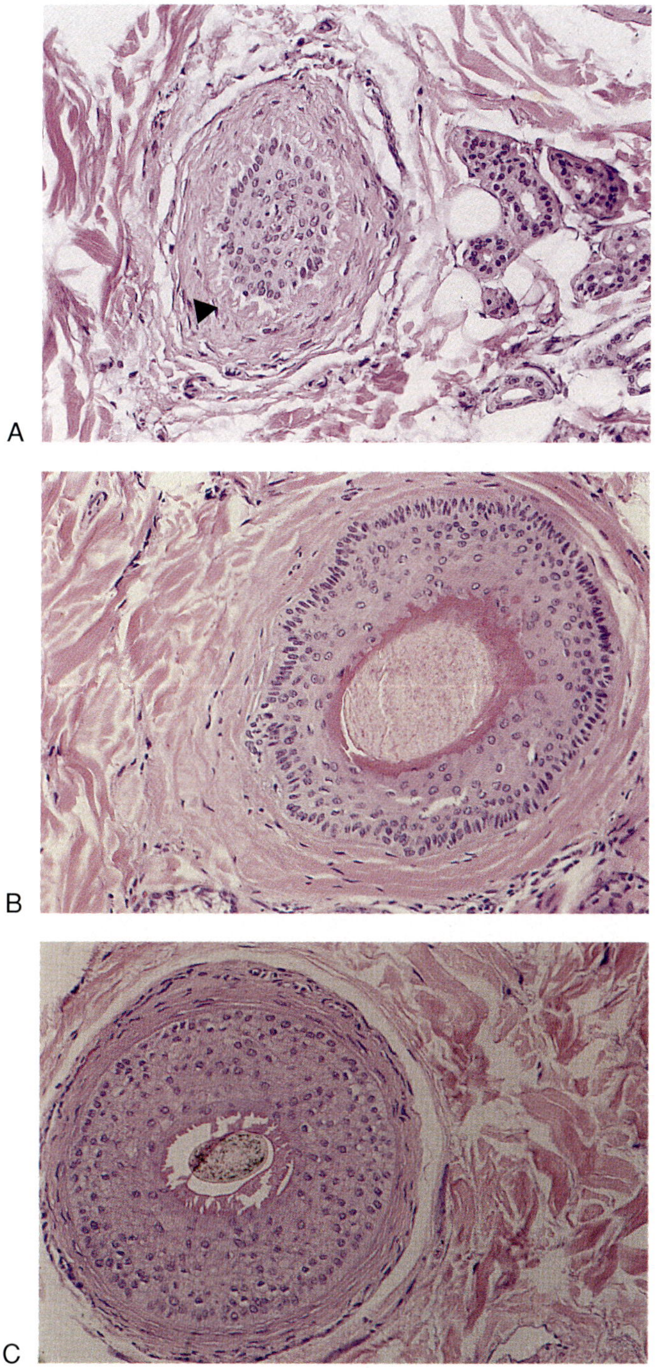

Figure 1-12 Composite photomicrographs of hair follicles as presented in horizontal section (*A*) A mid catagen follicle sectioned at the level of the eccrine glands in the deeper dermis: note involuting outer root sheath remnant and crumpled vitreous membrane (*arrow*). (*B*) A telogen hair at the level of the upper reticular dermis (note developed club structures). (*C*) Anagen follicle sectioned at the isthmus. Note fully keratinized inner root sheath around the hair shaft and the follicular sheath around the outer root sheath. The follicular sheath is much better appreciated in this type of section (H&E × 260).

outer root sheath epithelium. Cells in catagen undergo marked condensation and fragmentation and are then engulfed by adjacent viable epithelial cells, a process called *apoptosis.* These cytoplasmic apoptotic bodies may contain nuclear remnants, facilitating recognition and differentiation from autophagic vacuoles (Fig. 1-13).[37] The cessation of cell production in the matrix and the loss of outer root sheath cells through apoptotic degeneration leads to a dramatic collapse of the bulbar portion of the follicle. The rapid reduction of hair bulb volume creates shrinkage of the bulb epithelium superficially upward within the fibrous sheath, and the sheath collapses around the receding follicle. The vitreous or glassy membrane becomes crumpled and very prominent, because of the follicular collapse and/or the accumulation of increasing quantities of PAS-positive mucopolysaccharide material (Fig. 1-14). The remarkable shrinkage of the epithelial component of the bulb leads to the hair papilla becoming exposed once again. However, it follows the effete matrix tissue in its upward journey in the follicular sheath, maintaining close contact at all times through catagen and telogen. The Arao-Perkins fibrous pad appears to partially follow this path of retreat. In subsequent anagen cycles, the elastic component of these pads can be found in the side wall of follicular sheaths (Fig. 1-15), new ones being formed below the reactivated papilla.

Figure 1-13 Photomicrograph of three hair follicles in horizontal section. The central follicle is a terminal anagen follicle (the hair shaft is lost in sectioning), and the other two follicles are in late catagen. Note the developing club structures as well as the numerous apoptotic cells in the outer root sheath epithelium (H&E × 260).

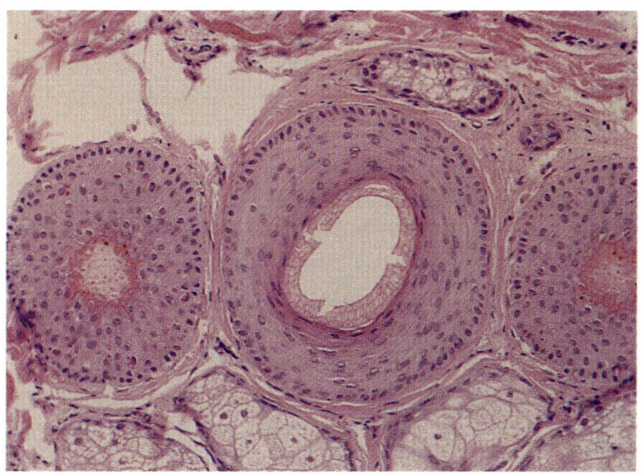

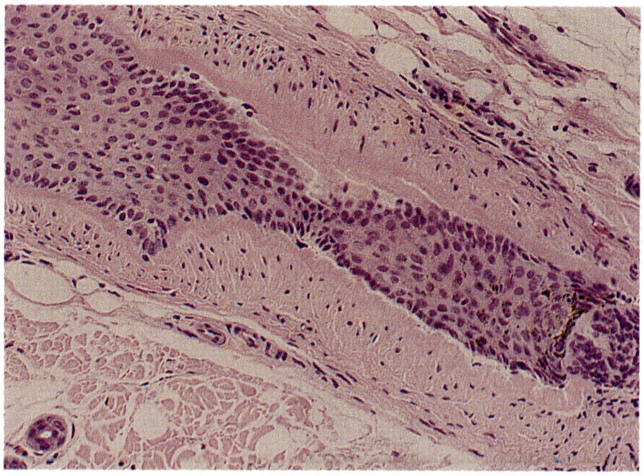

Figure 1-14 Photomicrograph of an early catagen hair follicle in vertical section. Note the collapsing outer root sheath epithelium, the thick vitreous membrane of the follicular sheath, and the way in which the hair papilla maintains its position with the shrinking epithelial elements (H&E × 130).

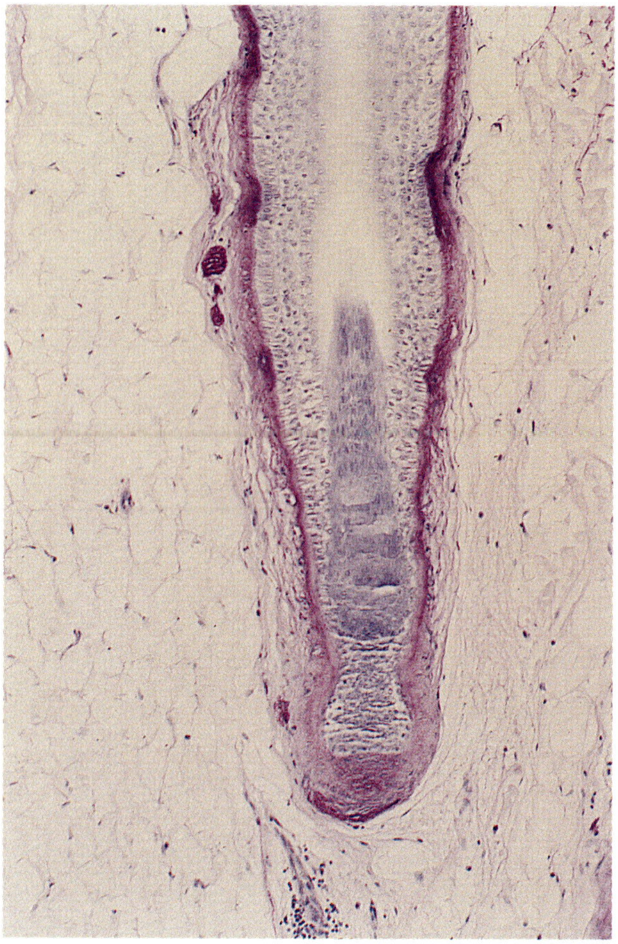

Figure 1-15 Photomicrograph of the bulbar part of an anagen follicle: note the elastic pad (Arao-Perkins body) below the hair papilla and the remnants of old Arao-Perkins bodies lying in the side wall of the follicular sheath at a higher level in the dermis. (Luna elastic stain × 65).

Ultimately, the epithelial collapse and involution leads to a reduction of all of the bulbar portion of the follicle. Only the hair papilla and the residue of the matrix remain, situated more or less at the site of the bulge for arrector pili muscle attachment (proposed site of follicular stem cells). Between one-third and one-half of the follicular length is lost in the catagen process.

While these dramatic changes are taking place, there is active change occurring in the isthmus portion of the outer root sheath. This area becomes rounded and distended around the somewhat expanded terminal portion of the hair shaft. Tricholemmal keratinization of the most distal part of the outer root sheath remnant creates an irregular corona around the hair shaft which interdigitates with the proximal part of the outer root sheath cells (Fig. 1-16), producing an anchorlike structure by which the hair is tethered in the follicle until displaced by the regeneration of anagen. This fully developed structure is the club hair (in situ) which, when complete, identifies the beginning of the telogen part of the cycle.[36] However, it seems quite clear that, though the criteria may suggest that there is a precise moment of transfer from catagen to telogen, this is not biologically accurate: one sees follicles with fully developed club structures in which it is quite clear that the catagen process is still ongoing. It seems more appropriate to consider that catagen and telogen blend into one another.

After catagen involution is complete and the club hair fully formed, telogen is a period of apparent complete inactivity. The follicle seems to be completely stable: no obvious structural changes are known to occur until anagen returns. Telogen usually lasts at least a few months.

Melanocytes can be identified in the quiescent hair matrix though they remain inactive. Control of the melanocyte activity in the hair cycle seems to be very precise (see Chapter 3 for information on control of follicular melanogenesis).

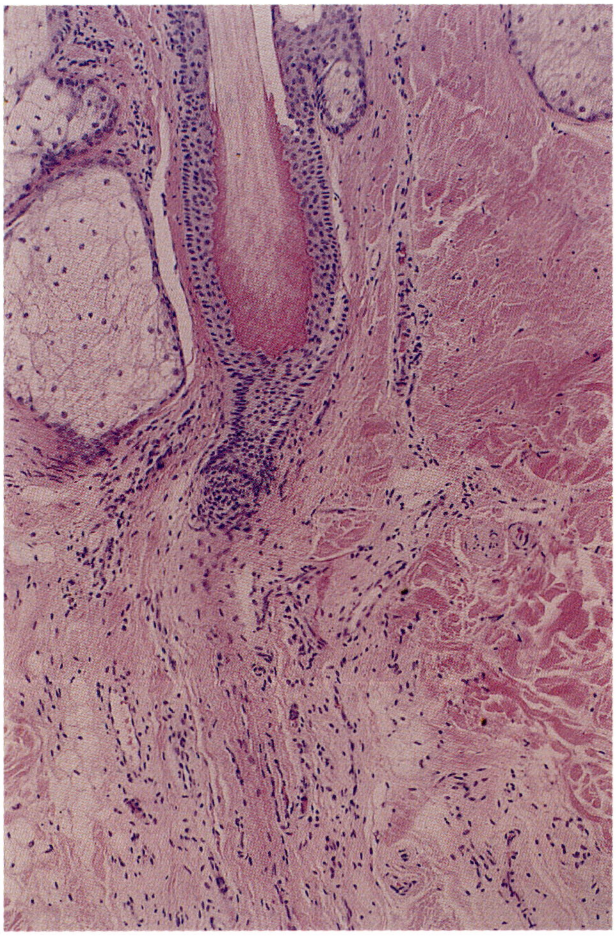

Figure 1-16 Photomicrograph of a telogen follicle with elaborated club structures. Note the fully formed trichilemmal keratin material (anchor for the terminal portion of the hair shaft) and also the position of the dormant hair papilla (H&E × 130).

Despite the intense periods of frantic melanocytic activity followed by complete quiescence in repeated cycles, the hair matrix appears to be a site of considerable privilege for these cells. No descriptions of melanocytic neoplasia, either benign or malignant, are known to be associated with the follicular matrix.

It should be noted that in albino patients, nonfunctioning melanocytes are present in the hair matrix. However, in contrast, the process of graying and ultimately whitening of the hair which occurs with aging is associated with partial and then complete loss of melanocytes.[38] In the event of further confirmation of a follicular stem-cell focus at the site of the arrector pili muscle insertion, it may be determined that this stem-cell zone is responsible for the production of a new hair matrix. Should this be so, melanocytes may then need to migrate into this new germinal site in order to reestablish contact with the new matrix epithelial germ.

The return of the anagen stimulus rapidly leads to development of an active hair cone in much the same way as was described in the embryonic stage of development. Indeed, elaboration of all the constituents of the hair bulb occurs again, while the cellular proliferation at the same time pushes the reforming bulb back down the collapsed follicular sheath. The detailed stages of regeneration of mature anagen are presented in Table 1-3 and shown in Figure 1-17.

CONCLUDING REMARKS

From a combined ectodermal and mesenchymal origin, hair follicles evolve into organs capable of repetitively undergoing regression and re-formation of anatomical parts. The ebb and flow of these anatomic parts serve as markers for stages of activity in follicular growth and suggest areas for control. Knowledge of the normal embryology and anatomy of the hair follicle, moreover, facilitates recognition of pathological follicular growth and development.

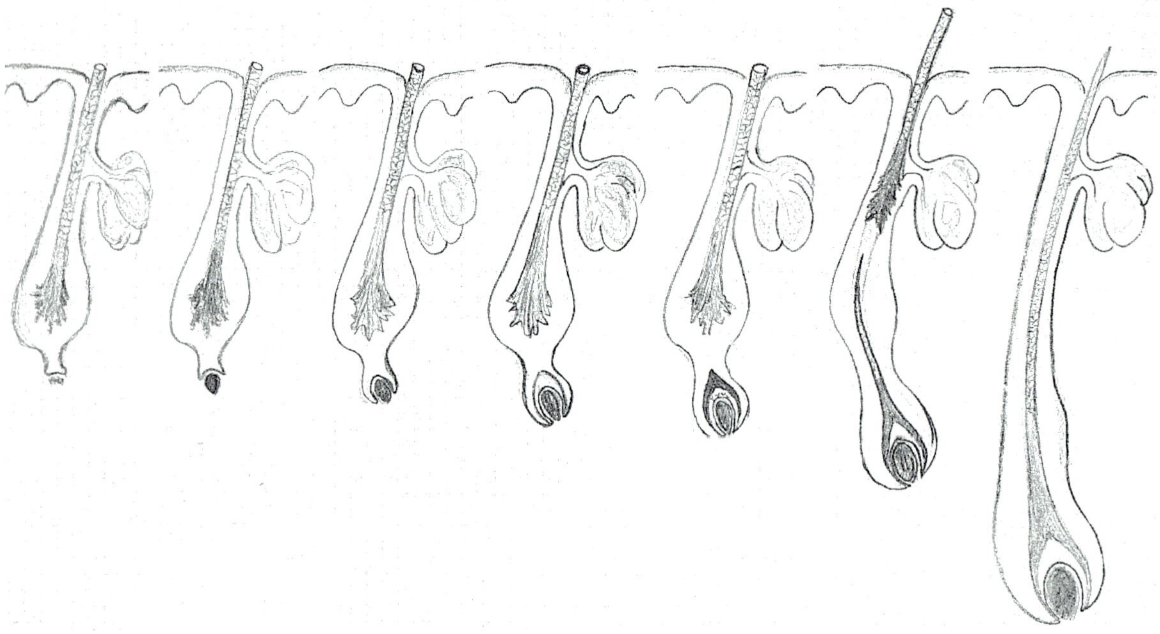

Figure 1-17 Diagrammatic representation of the stages of follicular anagen development. *Stage I:* Growth of hair papilla which is associated with an increase of metabolic activity. Increased mitotic activity occurs in the hair bulb matrix. *Stage II:* Hair bulb begins descent into dermis within the empty follicular sheath. The bulb matrix cells begin to envelop the papilla and also start the differentiation of the various follicular components. *Stage III:* Bulb matrix cells achieve differentiation of all follicular components. *Stage IV:* Matrix melanocytes reactivate and melanin distribution restarts. Hair shaft remains within hair cone. *Stage V:* Hair shaft emerges from hair cone and grows alongside old club hair which then begins to dislodge from the outer root sheath remnant. The old hair is usually shed before stage VI. *Stage VI:* New hair shaft emerges from the skin surface. *Stage VII:* Continued stable growth phase until onset of catagen.

REFERENCES

1. Pinkus H: Embryology of hair. In Montagna W, Ellis RA (eds): *The Biology of Hair Growth.* New York, Academic Press, 1958, pp 1–32.
2. Breathnach AS, Smith J: Fine structure of the early hair germ and dermal papilla in the human foetus. J Anat 102:511–526, 1968.
3. Hashimoto K: The ultrastructure of the skin of human embryos: IX. Formation of the hair cone and intraepidermal hair canal. Arch Klin Exp Dermatol 238:333–345, 1970.
4. Cotsarelis G, Sun T-T, Lavker RM: Label retaining cells reside in the bulge area of pilosebaceous unit: Implication for follicular stem cells, hair cycle, and skin carcinogenesis. Cell 61:1329–1337, 1990.
5. Murphy GF, Lavker RM, Whitaker D, Korngold R: Cytotoxic folliculitis in GvHD, evidence for follicular stem cell injury and recovery. J Cutan Pathol 18:309–314, 1991.
6. Arao T, Perkins EM: The interrelation of elastic tissue and human hair follicles. In Montagna W, Dobson RL (eds): *Advances in Biology of Skin,* vol. 9: *Hair Growth.* Oxford, Pergamon Press, 1969, pp 433–440.
7. Sengel R: Role of extracellular matrix in the development of skin and cutaneous appendages. In Lash JQ, Saxen L (eds): *Development Mechanisms: Normal and Abnormal.* New York, Alan R. Liss, 1985, p 123.
8. Oliver RF: The experimental induction of whisker growth in the hooded rat by implantation of dermal papillae. J Embryol Exp Morphol 18:43–51, 1967.
9. Kollar EJ: The induction of hair follicles by embryonic dermal papillae. J Invest Dermatol 55:374–378, 1970.
10. Mishima Y, Widlan S: Embryonic development of melanocytes in human hair and epidermis. J Invest Dermatol 46:263–277, 1966.
11. Holbrook KA, Odland GF: Structure of the human fetal hair canal and initial hair eruption. J Invest Dermatol 71:385–390, 1978.
12. Montagna W, Parakkal PF: *The Structure and Function of the Skin,* 3d ed. New York, Academic Press, 1974, pp 172–258.

13. Pinkus H: Anatomy and histology of skin. In Graham JH, Johnson WC, Helwig EB (eds): *Dermal Pathology.* Hagerstown, MD, Harper & Row, 1972, pp 1–24.
14. Garn SM: The examination of hair under the polarizing microscope. Ann NY Acad Sci 53:649–652, 1951.
15. Headington JT, Novak E: Clinical and histologic studies of male pattern baldness treated with topical minoxidil. Curr Ther Res 36:1098–1106, 1984.
16. Headington JT: Transverse microscopic anatomy of the human scalp. Arch Dermatol 120:449–456, 1984.
17. Pinkus H, Mehregan AH: Normal structure of skin. In *A Guide to Dermatohistopathology,* 2d ed. Appleton, Century, Crofts, 1976, pp 7–51.
18. Pinkus H: "Sebaceous cysts" are trichilemmal cysts. Arch Dermatol 99:544–555, 1969.
19. Auber L: The anatomy of follicles producing wool-fibres, with special reference to keratinization. Trans R Soc Edinb 62:191–254, 1952.
20. Starrico RG: The melanocytes and the hair follicle. J Invest Dermatol 35:185–194, 1960.
21. Johnson WC, Helwig EB: Histochemistry of the acid mucopolysaccharides of skin in normal and in certain pathologic conditions. Am J Clin Pathol 40:123–131, 1963.
22. Arao T: Connective tissue hair sheath especially on the structure and the development of elastic tissues. In Kobori T, Montagna W (eds): *Biology and Disease of the Hair.* Baltimore, University Park Press, 1976, pp 15–22.
23. Schinckel PG: Mitotic activity in wool follicle bulbs. Aust J Biol Sci 14:659–676, 1961.
24. Oliver RF: The induction of follicle formation in the adult hooded rat by vibrissa dermal papillae. J Embryol Exp Morphol 23:219–236, 1970.
25. Kopf AW, Orentreich N: Alkaline phosphatase in alopecia areata. Arch Dermatol 76:288–295, 1957.
26. Cormia F: Vasculature of the normal scalp. Arch Dermatol 88:692–701, 1963.
27. Durward A, Rudall KM: The vascularity and patterns of growth of hair follicles. In Montagna W, Ellis RA (eds): *The Biology of Hair Growth.* New York, Academic Press, 1958, pp 189–218.
28. Ellis RA, Moretti G: Vascular patterns associated with catagen hair follicles in the human scalp. Ann NY Acad Sci 83:448–457, 1959.
29. Winkelmann RK: The innervation of a hair follicle. Ann NY Acad Sci 83:400–407, 1959.
30. Montagna W, Giacometti L: Histology and cytochemistry of human skin: XXXII. The external ear. Arch Dermatol 99:757–767, 1969.
31. Kligman AM: The human hair cycle. J Invest Dermatol 33:307–316, 1959.
32. Epstein WL, Maibach HL: Cell proliferation and movement in human hair bulbs. In Montagna W, Dobson RL (eds): *Advances in Biology of Skin,* vol. 9: *Hair Growth.* Oxford, Pergamon Press, 1969, pp 83–98.
33. Bandmann HJ, Bosse K: Histologie und Anatomie des Haarfollikels im Verlauf des Haarcyclus. Arch Klin Exp Dermatol 227:390–409, 1966.
34. Parakkal PF, Motoltsy AG, Geodeon A: A study of the differentiation products of the hair follicle cells with the electron microscope. J Invest Dermatol 43:23–34, 1964.
35. Pinkus H: Embryology and anatomy of skin. In Helwig EB, Mostofi FK (eds): *The Skin.* International Academy of Pathology Monograph. Baltimore, Williams & Wilkins, 1971, pp 1–27.
36. Pinkus H: Factors in the formation of club hair. In Brown AC, Crounse RG (eds): *Hair, Trace Elements and Human Illness.* New York, Praeger, 1980, pp 147–154.
37. Weedon D, Strutton G: Apoptosis as the mechanism of the involution of hair follicles in catagen formation. Acta Derm Venereol (Stockh) 61:335–369, 1981.
38. Herzberg J, Gusek W: Das Ergrauen des Kopfhaares. Arch Klin Exp Dermatol 236:368–384, 1970.
39. Ebling FJG: The biology of hair. Dermatol Clin 5:407–481, 1987. Dermatol Clin.

Chapter

2

DIFFERENTIATION OF THE HAIR SHAFT

Arthur P. Bertolino
and
W. Michael O'Guin

INTRODUCTION

Differentiation is the biologic process by which an organism or a tissue, organ, and so forth, within an organism is modified in structure and/or function during the course of development. Thus, differentiation of the hair shaft may appropriately refer to the original process by which it is formed as well as its cyclic regeneration. The hair follicle is the biologic "factory" within which production of the hair shaft is accomplished.

Our current understanding of the hair follicle, in general, is still rudimentary, with our level of knowledge extending little beyond the stage of cataloging its components and recognizing select biologic interrelationships. Nevertheless, sufficient information has been acquired to formulate a meaningful overview of hair shaft differentiation. While only certain aspects of the involved processes have been elucidated, they provide a foundation for further investigations.

The hair shaft and its differentiation may be viewed from a number of levels. First, there is the macroscopic view, which focuses upon the gross features of the hair fiber. Second, there is the cellular view, which unveils a complex organization of varied cell types biologically orchestrated into specialized compartments within the follicle. Finally, there is the molecular vantage from which structures are appreciated and constituent biomolecules and genes assume central importance. In this chapter, we focus on the cellular and molecular aspects of differentiation and the current knowledge of genetic regulation of this differentiation.

HAIR SHAFT CELLULAR AND MOLECULAR DIFFERENTIATION

The hair shaft is composed of a number of distinct cellular compartments, and its differentiation is influenced by the complex array of cells

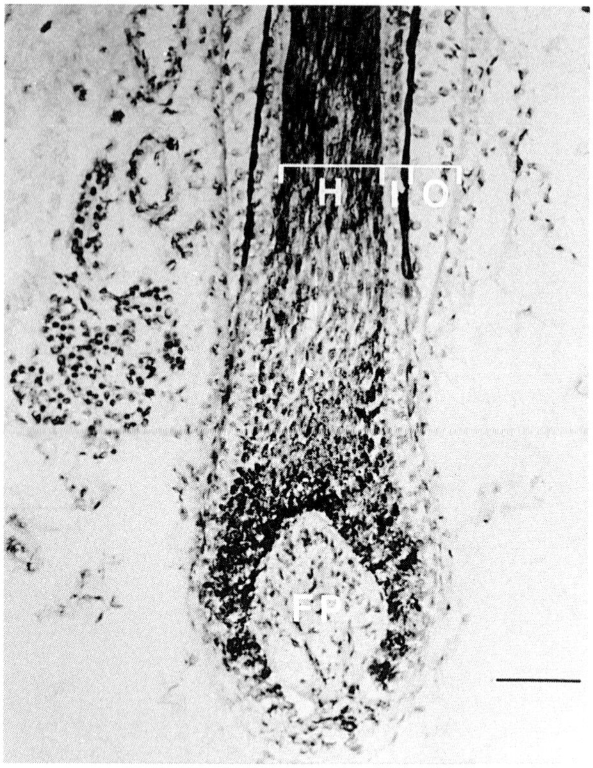

Figure 2-1 Histologic section of human scalp. The lower two-thirds of a hair follicle is shown in longitudinal section in the center of the field. H = hair shaft; I = inner root sheath; O = outer root sheath; FP = follicular papilla. (Scale bar = 100 mm)

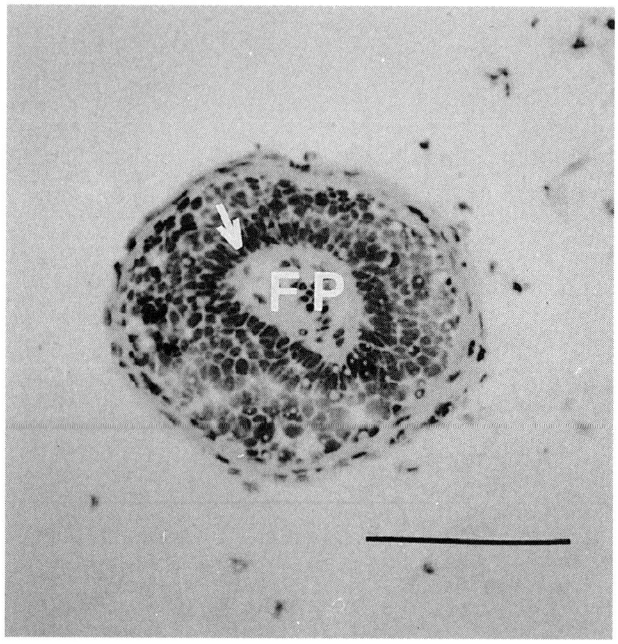

Figure 2-2 Human scalp hair bulb (histologic cross-section). The hair bulb portion of the follicle is the annular structure in the central portion of the field. Arrowhead = matrix cells which appear as a distinct ring of cells immediately surrounding the follicular papilla (FP). (Scale bar = 100 μm)

that form the hair follicle. Perhaps the most logical cell type with which to begin a discussion of differentiation would be the follicular stem cell. However, as only a presumptive population of stem cells has been identified in the area of the follicular bulge, little has yet been confirmed regarding their role in hair shaft differentiation.[1] Therefore, a more appropriate current approach to this subject relies upon the classic method of describing the cellular composition of the *hair shaft* proper, the surrounding *inner root sheath,* which forms an integral role in hair shaft formation, and the peripheral *outer root sheath,* which, although somewhat removed from the population of cells differentiating into the hair shaft, forms the surrounding mass of follicular tissue (Fig. 2-1).

The process of follicular differentiation begins deep within the hair follicle with a group of apparently uniform epithelial cells (the matrix cells) found in the hair bulb immediately adjacent to the follicular papilla (Fig. 2-2). In the rapidly growing, or anagen, follicle these matrix cells constitute a multipotent, germinative population which is highly active and gives rise not only to the hair cortex but also, through a poorly understood, complex pattern of differentiation, to the medulla, cuticle, and inner root sheath. The outer root sheath does not appear to arise from the matrix. Each portion of this multipartite, follicular structure is morphologically distinguishable and undergoes a distinct process of terminal differentiation.

The Hair Shaft

Cortex and Medulla

The progenitor cells of the hair cortex are a group of highly mitotically-active matrix cells found adjacent to the distal portion of the follicular papilla. These cells are present in anagen, undergo apoptosis (programmed cell death) during catagen, and are absent in telogen. If a medulla is present, the matrix cells at the apex of the papilla will give rise to this lineage. The morphology of the matrix cells is unremarkable, with no apparent distinction among cells des-

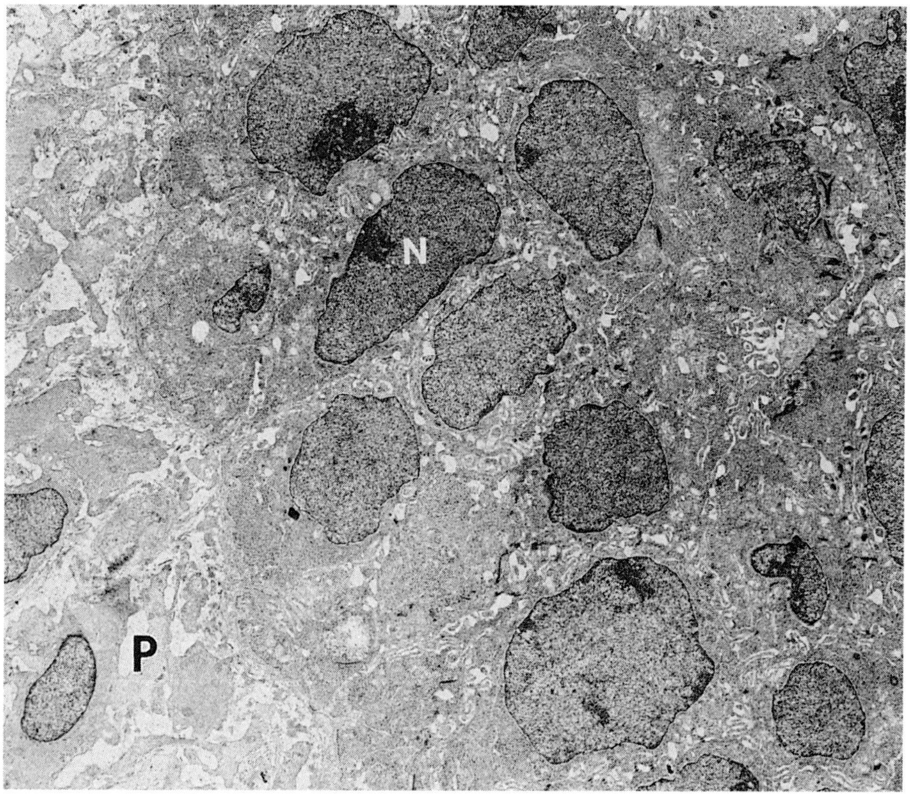

Figure 2-3 Matrix cells. Matrix cells display a simple profile typical of primitive epithelial cells. N = nucleus of one of the many matrix cells filling most of the field; P = follicular papilla which occupies the lower left corner of the field. Note relatively few intermediate filaments, numerous mitochondria, well-developed golgi, and a relatively large nuclear-to-cytoplasmic volume ratio. (Electron micrograph ×7500) (*Courtesy of Dr. Ken Hashimoto.*)

tined to give rise to any of several distinct layers of matrix-derived follicular compartments. At the electron-microscopic level, the matrix cells have a fairly simple profile typical of primitive epithelial cells (Fig. 2-3).[2,3] There are relatively few intermediate filaments, numerous mitochondria, well-developed golgi, and a relatively large nuclear-to-cytoplasmic volume ratio.

Intermediate filaments, 8 to 10nm protein structures that form a major part of the cytoskeleton of most cells, are differentiation products of the cortex and are represented by a family of keratins in this tissue. The process of hair keratin filament formation (Fig. 2-4) probably begins as soon as the presumptive cortical matrix cells leave the basement membrane. Keratins are peptides of 40,000 to 68,000 molecular weight that are each a product of a unique gene.[4] There are two keratin subfamilies,[5] one of larger peptides with a more basic isoelectric point (type II) and the other of smaller peptides with a more acidic isoelectric point (type I). The hair-specific keratins (hard, or "low-sulfur," keratins) have been divided into the type Ia (acidic) and type IIa (basic) proteins that are defined by highly conserved amino acid homologies unique to each class. Epithelial keratins (soft keratins) are similarly divided into type Ib (acidic) and IIb (basic) proteins. All keratins possess a central alpha-helical domain, which actually consists of four distinct alpha-helical segments separated by nonhelical segments.[6,7] Keratin filaments are obligate copolymers[8] and are expressed as pairs containing one member from each subfamily. With aggregation, keratins assume a coiled-coil helical structure with the alpha-helical domain in the core and the nonhelical terminal domains toward the periphery.[9] According to x-ray diffraction measurements, the diameter of the alpha helix approximates 9.8 Å and its pitch (repeat distance for coiling) is 5.1 Å, which corresponds to a polypeptide chain link of 3.6 amino acids (Fig. 2-5).[10]

As the precortical matrix cells divide and move distally away from the immature matrix cells into the hair shaft elongation zone, they begin to express increasing amounts of keratin filaments oriented along the longitudinal axis of the developing hair[2,11] (Fig. 2-6). Following the model for the soft keratins (Fig. 2-7), the type Ia and IIa polypeptides join to form a heterodimer. The heterodimers almost immediately join to

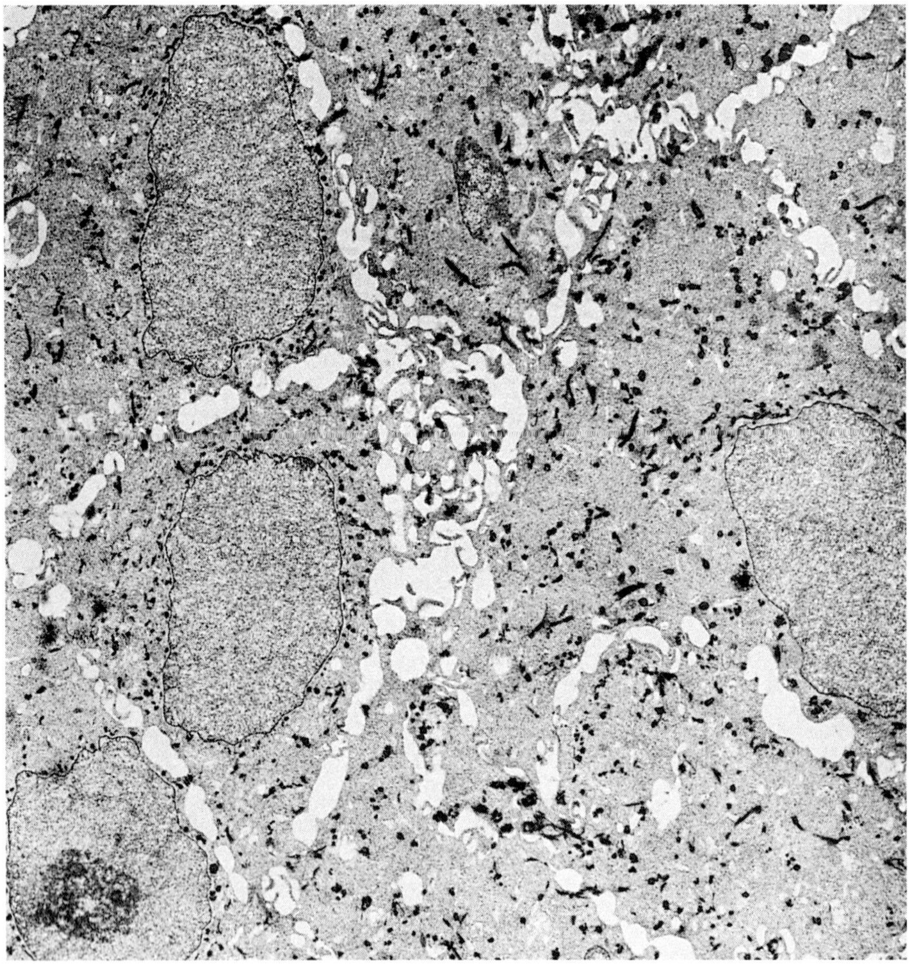

Figure 2-4 Early keratinization in cortical cells. Early filament formation is evident in numerous cytoplasmic foci. (Electron micrograph ×10,000) (*Courtesy of Dr. Ken Hashimoto.*)

form heterotetramers containing two type Ia subunits and two type IIa subunits. The heterotetramers, and possibly other small oligomers, are the functional building blocks of a keratin protofilament, which will join noncovalently as antiparallel coiled-coil pairs in the 8nm intermediate filament. As differentiation proceeds toward the keratogenous zone, cellular organelles degenerate, and the keratin filaments become more numerous and begin to organize into higher-ordered filament bundles which form the microfibrils, fibrils, and macrofibrils observed by electron microscopy (Fig. 2-8). These large aggregates eventually fill the entire cytoplasm (Fig. 2-9). Above the keratogenous zone, the cells shrink and are composed almost entirely of tightly packed keratin fibrils embedded in an amorphous matrix (Fig. 2-10).

In the keratin filaments, stability depends on covalent cystine cross-links, coulombic interactions between side-group chains, hydrogen bonds between neighboring groups, and hydrophobic interactions.[10] The covalent cystine linkages average one per four turns of the coil and, although they contribute most of the strength to the alpha-helical structure, they are most susceptible to chemical modification by oxidants and reducing agents. Coulombic interactions, or salt links, occur every two turns of the coil and are electrovalent unions of acidic and basic side-chain residues. The strength of these cross-links is highly dependent on the isoelectric point of the keratin fiber and is decreased in an acidic or alkaline dielectric (e.g., H_2O) medium. Hydrogen bonds occur between the oxygen and hydrogen atoms of the carboxy and amino terminal groups in the polypeptide chain and can be disrupted by insertion of water molecules between the pep-

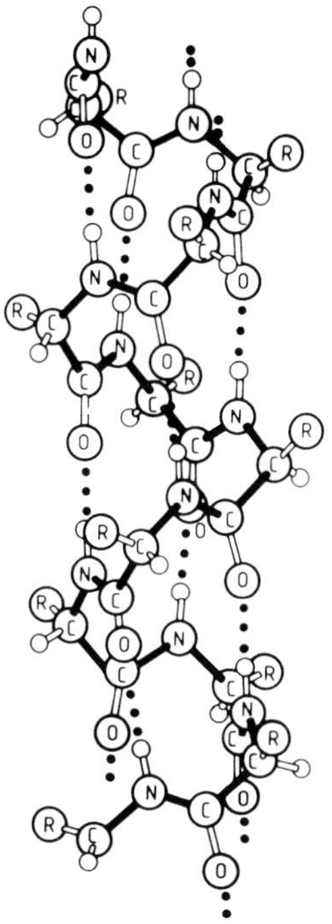

Figure 2-5 Keratin polypeptide structure. Note the alpha-helical conformation. (*Reproduced from Zviak and Dawber.*[10])

tide chains. Hydrophobic interactions are weak bonds that result from the tendency of nonpolar hydrocarbon side chains to come together in the presence of the polar compound, water.

The increased organization and packing of these keratin subunits are coordinated with the expression of a number of matrix proteins which are chemically distinct from the keratin subunits. Data derived from hair keratin DNA and protein sequence analyses suggest that specific sequences flanking the filament-forming domain of keratin are likely to protrude beyond the surface of the keratin structure, making them likely domains for specific interaction with various matrix proteins.[12] The matrix proteins form the intermediate filament-associated protein (IFAP) group: the cysteine-rich "high-sulfur proteins," the cysteine-rich "ultrahigh-sulfur proteins," and the "high-glycine–tyrosine proteins." A major type of covalent keratin matrix interaction is through the formation of disulfide bonds involving the cysteine residues on the matrix molecules and cysteine residues on the keratin filaments.

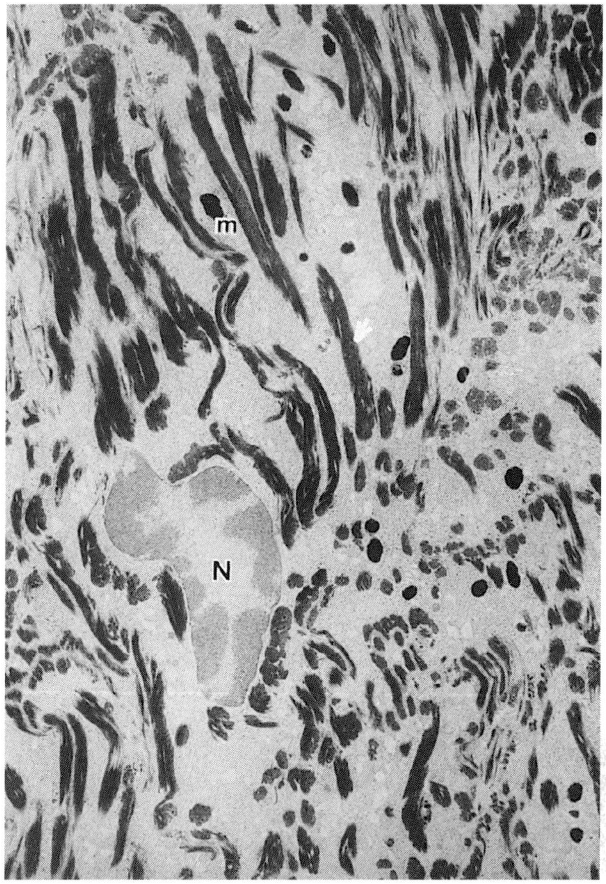

Figure 2-6 Keratin filaments in developing hair cortex. Filaments appear as bundles along the longitudinal axis (vertical) of cells. N = nucleus; m = melanosome. (Electron micrograph ×10,000) (*Courtesy of Dr. Ken Hashimoto.*)

The presence of a medulla is a variable feature in human hairs and can range from complete absence to a well-developed, continuous structure in very coarse hairs (Fig. 2-11). Although the medulla is more often present in larger-diameter hairs, it is not clear what determines whether or not a medulla will develop. The differentiating medulla is characterized by the presence of large numbers of amorphous, eosinophilic granules known as *trichohyalin granules* (Fig. 2-12). Trichohyalin granules are composed primarily of a 220-kd protein called *trichohyalin,* which, when released from the granules, specifically interacts with the intermediate filaments. However, unlike the trichohyalin-containing cells of the inner root sheath, the medulla contains few, if any, intermediate filaments. The terminally differentiated medulla contains a hardened trabecular

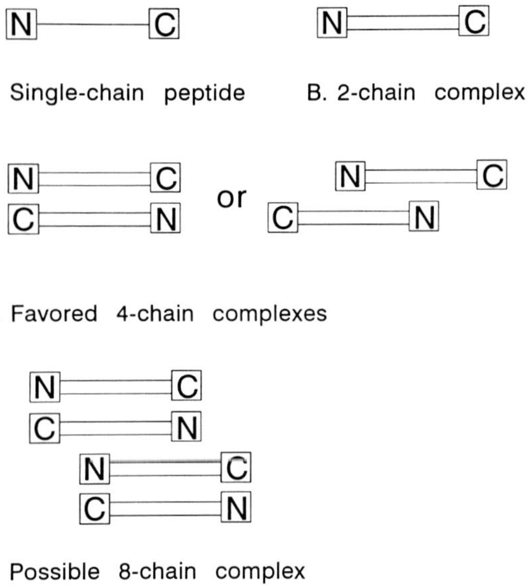

Figure 2-7 Model of keratin filament formation. N,C = amino-terminal and carboxy-terminal ends of peptides, respectively. See text for details. (*Adapted from Steinert and Roop.*[4])

network which forms when the trichohyalin granules aggregate into large masses which become highly vacuolated.[2] Trichohyalin will be addressed further in the discussion of the inner root sheath.

Cuticle of the Hair Shaft

The developing cortical matrix cells are surrounded by a single, somewhat cuboidal, cell layer which is destined to become the cuticle of the hair shaft (Fig. 2-13). As the presumptive cuticle cells differentiate, they become increasingly elongated and flattened. The end result of these morphological changes is the development of the overlapping layers of cuticle cells, which resemble multiple layers of scales or roof tiles (Fig. 2-14).[11] Each mature cuticle cell becomes very compact and contains a distinctly ordered cellular structure (Fig. 2-15). The outer cell membrane becomes very thick (5 to 25 nm). Beneath this thickened membrane are three distinguishable layers—the electron-dense, cystine-rich A layer, the less electron dense exocuticle layer, and the relatively electron-lucent endocuticle. In areas where several cuticle cells are overlapping, this cellular organization produces a multilayered, lamellar structure surrounding the entire hair.[11] The outermost layer of cuticle cells interacts with the cuticle of the inner root sheath (see later text) in such a manner as to physically anchor the developing hair in the base of the follicle.

Combined biochemical and immunohisto-

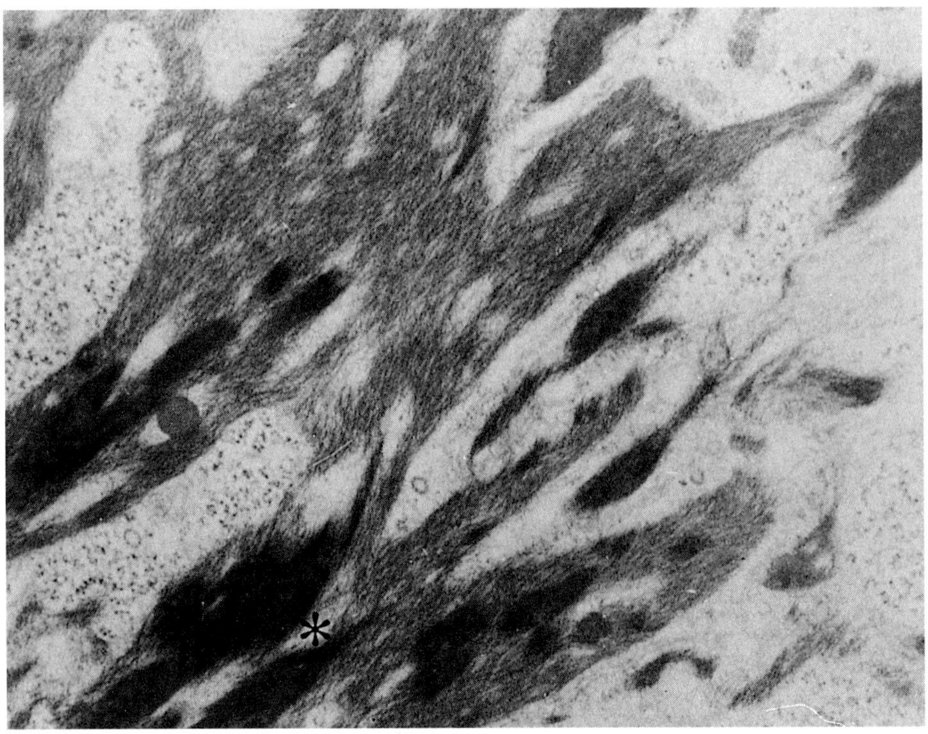

Figure 2-8 Aggregates of keratin filaments in hair cortex. Progressively larger aggregates are formed by lateral association of filaments. The asterisk (*) marks a focus of condensed keratin filaments. (Electron micrograph ×30,000) (*Courtesy of Dr. Ken Hashimoto.*)

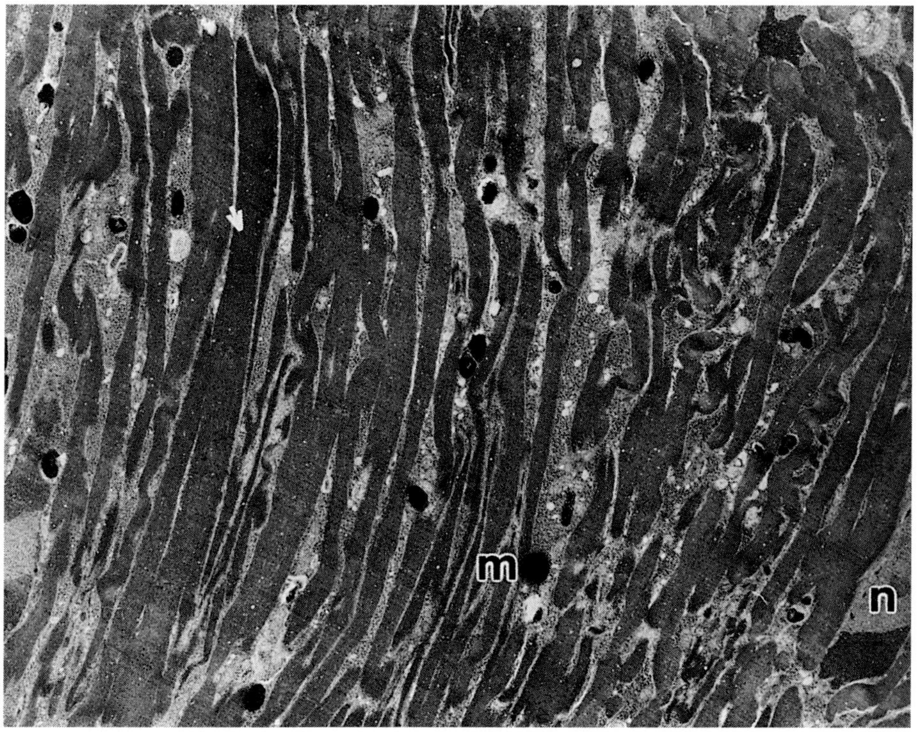

Figure 2-9 Keratin filaments fill the cortical cytoplasm. As cortical cells mature, an orderly array of large keratin aggregates is produced and interfibrillary matrix is deposited. m = melanosome; n = degenerating nucleus. (Electron micrograph ×12,500) (*Courtesy of Dr. Ken Hashimoto.*)

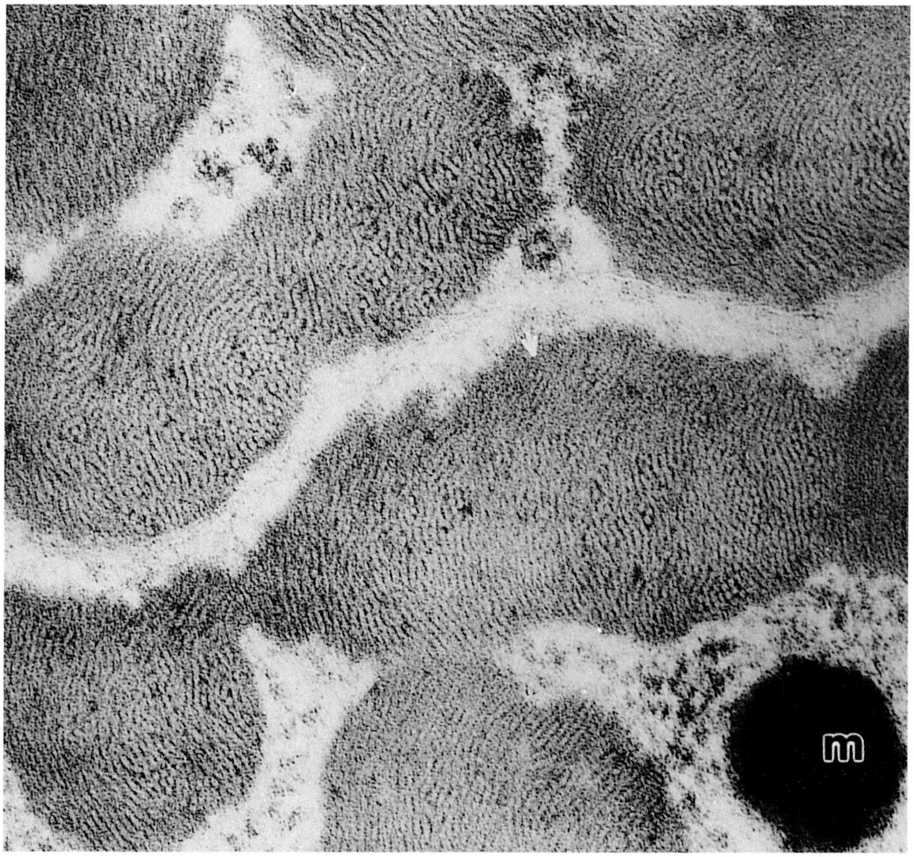

Figure 2-10 Mature cortical cell cytoplasm. Cross-sectional view demonstrating fingerprintlike pattern of keratin fibrils (arrowhead). m = melanosome. (Electron micrograph ×200,000) (*Courtesy of Dr. Ken Hashimoto.*)

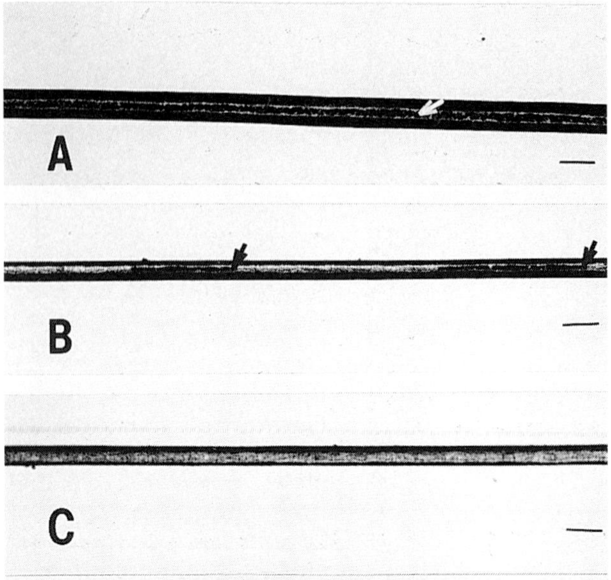

Figure 2-11 Hair shaft medulla. A = continuous medulla (arrowhead) in a pigmented hair; B = intermittent medulla (arrowheads) in a gray hair; C = absent medulla in a gray hair. (Scale bars = 100 μm)

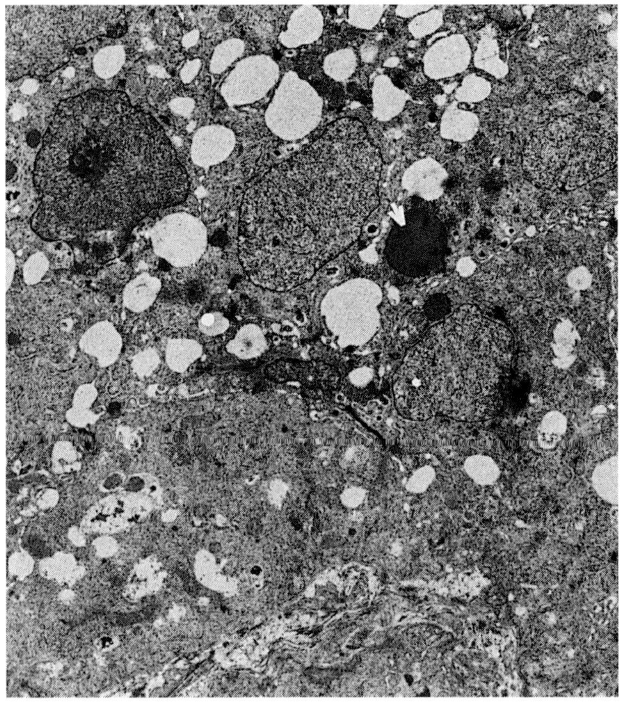

Figure 2-12 Differentiating medulla. Trichohyalin granules (arrowhead) begin to appear in large numbers. (Electron micrograph ×7500) (*Courtesy of Dr. Ken Hashimoto.*)

chemical studies have demonstrated that the type Ia and type IIa keratin proteins are restricted to the cortex and the cuticle layers of the human hair follicle.[13–15] The cuticle cells of the hair shaft express hair keratin beginning at the midbulb region. These keratins are not unique to the hair follicle but are specifically associated with the "hard-type" keratinization associated with the hair shaft and are also found in other, related tissues such as the nail plate and certain highly specialized cells of the dorsal tongue.[13,16,17]

Inner Root Sheath

As one moves circumferentially away from the cuticle of the hair shaft, the next three layers constitute the inner root sheath: the cuticle of the inner root sheath, Huxley's layer, and Henle's layer, respectively (Fig. 2-13). The matrix cells destined to give rise to the inner root sheath layers are located deeper in the hair bulb on the lateral aspects of the follicular papilla but are morphologically indistinguishable from the more central hair shaft matrix cells. The process of terminal differentiation in the inner root sheath is frequently referred to as *cornification* or *hardening* but is a unique process which is very different from the events that occur in the epidermis.

The major hallmark of inner root sheath differentiation is the presence of large numbers of eosinophilic cytoplasmic inclusions known as trichohyalin granules.[18–20] Small trichohyalin granules are first seen in the primitive cells of Henle's layer and represent one of the earliest markers of hair follicle differentiation (Fig. 2-13). As the three layers become morphologically distinguishable, it can be seen that trichohyalin granules are present in all of the cells, with those of Henle's layer exhibiting the most advanced differentiation. As the cells further differentiate and move away from the matrix, the trichohyalin granules continue to accumulate and increase in size. The development of trichohyalin granules is accompanied by the accumulation of increasing numbers of intermediate filaments in the cytoplasm, which are arranged parallel to the longitudinal axis of the follicle. In the suprabulbar inner root sheath, the process of hardening occurs first in Henle's layer and subsequently in Huxley's layer and the cuticle. When this stage of inner root sheath differentiation occurs, the cellular organelles degenerate, the trichohyalin granule material is completely dispersed, and the cytoplasm is filled with tightly

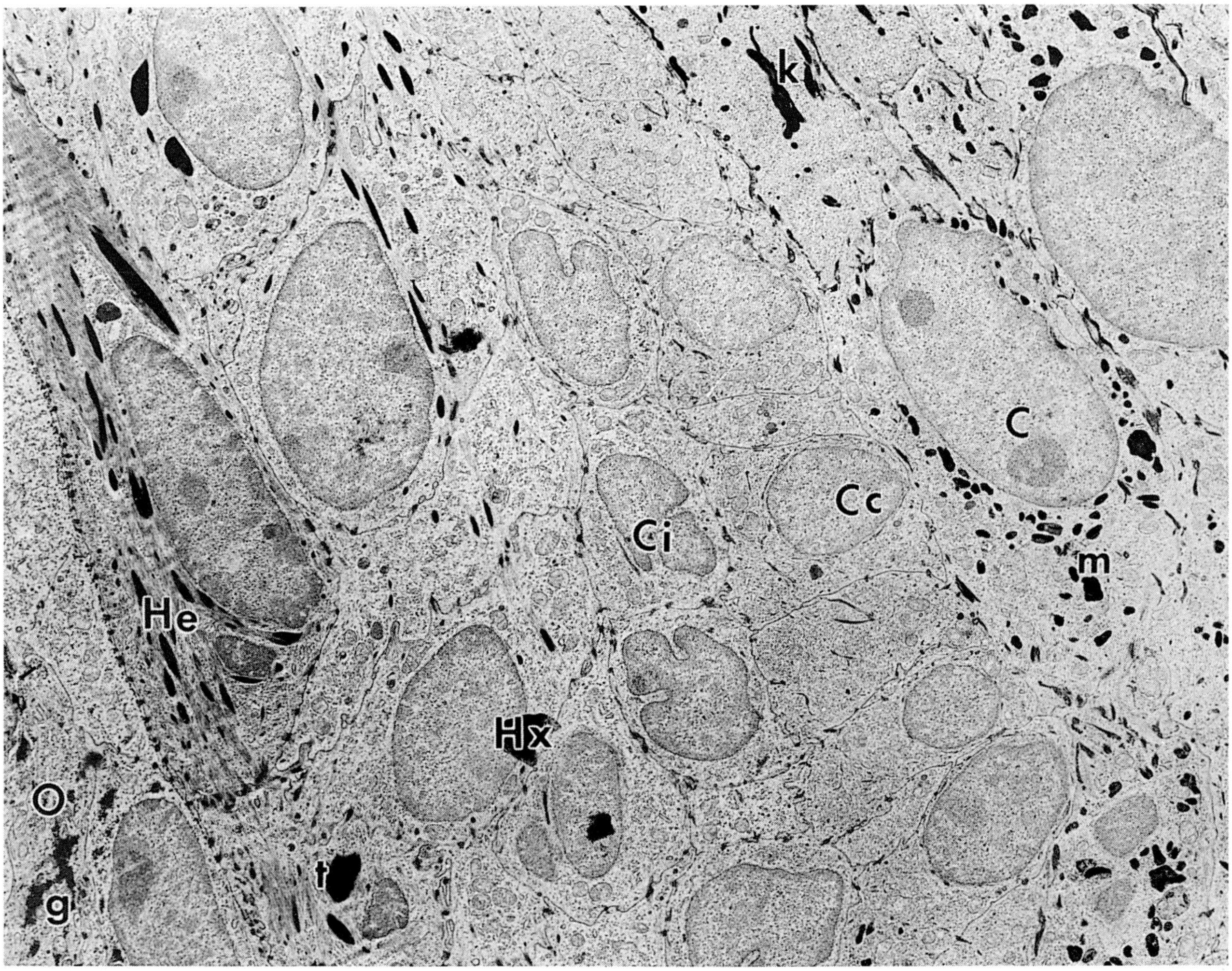

Figure 2-13 Select follicular histologic compartments. C = cortex; Cc = cortical cuticle (hair shaft); Ci = cuticle of the inner root sheath; Hx = Huxley's layer of the inner root sheath; He = Henle's layer of the inner root sheath; O = outer root sheath; g = glycogen granule; t = trichohyalin granule; k = keratin filaments. (Electron micrograph ×10,000) (*Courtesy of Dr. Ken Hashimoto.*)

packed, parallel arrays of intermediate filaments apparently embedded in an amorphous matrix derived from the trichohyalin granules. This process has been described as involving the periodic bridging of parallel bundles of intermediate filaments in a manner which aligns the filaments with the longitudinal axis of the follicle. It is at this level that two significant enzyme activities become involved in the final hardening process. Trichohyalin is extensively cross-linked by transglutaminase, to itself as well as to the intermediate filaments (Fig. 2-16). This provides the stable, hardened characteristic of the inner root sheath. Subsequent to this covalent cross-linking, peptidyl-arginine deiminase converts many of the arginines found in trichohyalin to citrulline, thus accounting for the abundance of this otherwise rare amino acid in the hair.[21,22]

As the cells of the inner root sheath cuticle harden, they become thinner and overlap in a manner opposite to the direction of follicle growth. This permits the inner root sheath cuticle to form a template for the opposing cuticle of the cortex in a way that allows the two cuticles to become interlocked much like a zipper. The hardened layers of the inner root sheath do not contribute to the hair proper but serve to anchor and direct the growth of the developing hair. At the level of the hair follicle roughly correspond-

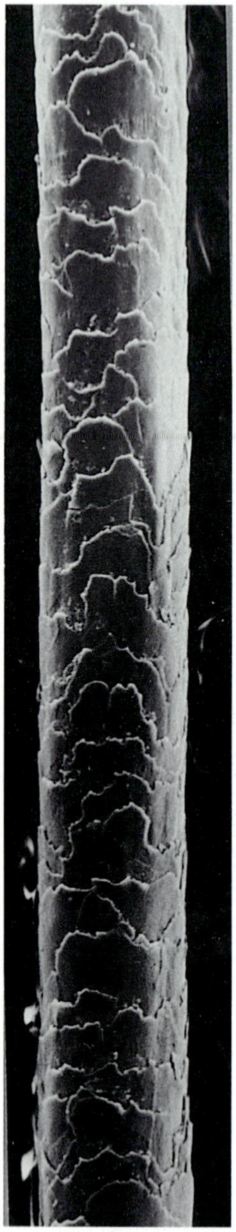

Figure 2-14 Hair shaft surface. Note the scalelike array of overlapping cuticular cells. (Scanning electron micrograph ×600) (*Courtesy of Dr. Ken Hashimoto.*)

ing to the sebaceous gland duct, the inner root sheath layers degenerate and are sloughed, thus freeing the developed hair shaft from further interaction with the follicle.

Outer Root Sheath

The progenitor outer root sheath cells have not been precisely located but appear not to be among the matrix cells proper. They may be located among the basal cells along the lateral basement membrane (glassy membrane), but this has not been firmly established. In the bulbar region of the follicle, the outer root sheath cells divide and move distally, up the follicle. At the suprabulbar area, a second proliferative population of outer root sheath cells is seen in the area where the outer root sheath layer abruptly increases in thickness. At this level, the cells migrate both distally and centripetally. The innermost layer of the outer root sheath is the most highly differentiated, as determined by its lack of proliferative activity and increase in cytoplasmic filaments. In the follicular infundibulum, above the sebaceous duct, the outer root sheath cells become increasingly stratified and exhibit a parakeratotic cornification (tricholemmal keratinization). Above the infundibulum, the outer root sheath is continuous with, and indistinguishable from, the interfollicular epidermis.

HAIR PROTEIN GENES AND THEIR REGULATION

Overview of Genes

Over the last 40 years, the basic concept of an individual's genetic program has evolved from an unapproachably complex array of chromosomes and genes to defined DNA sequences. Today, we have the modern tools of molecular biology, which have enabled us not only to approach these formerly formidable realms of biologic science but also to unravel many of the molecular aspects of their normal operation and pathologic malfunctions. In simplistic terms, the library of an individual's genetic information is stored in the DNA sequences of his or her genes. Carefully regulated transcription of these genes results in messenger RNAs, which carry this information from the nucleus to the cytoplasm of cells, where translation of the messengers produces specific proteins. These proteins, in turn, perform the majority of key cellular functions.

While much is still to be learned about the molecular aspects of biologic mechanisms, many general aspects of gene structure and function have been elucidated and many of the details regarding specific genes are emerging. Genes are located on chromosomes in areas called *loci*. In some circumstances, groups of related genes are

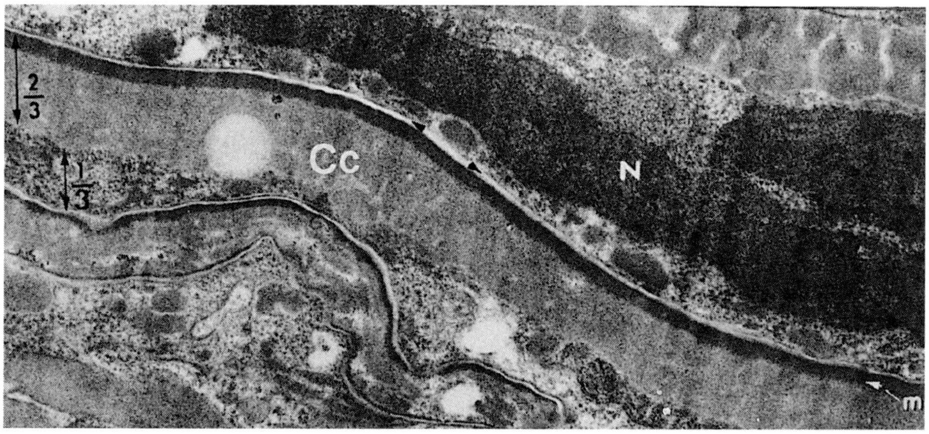

Figure 2-15 Hair shaft cuticle. Distinctive cellular architecture in the mature cortical cuticle (Cc) cell is composed of a thickened cell membrane (arrowheads); a marginal band (m), or A layer; the exocuticle, which is electron-light and represents approximately two-thirds of the lateral portion of the cytoplasm; and the endocuticle, which is more electron-dense and represents the inner one-third of the cytoplasm. N = nucleus in adjacent less mature cell. (Electron micrograph ×52,500) (*Courtesy of Dr. Ken Hashimoto.*)

clustered in one locus while others may be distributed in the genome. Genes are composed of structural information segments (exons) which carry the code for the gene end product (protein) and also of segments which support management of the structural segments. These noncoding segments often include introns of variable sizes between the exons. Introns, also known as *intervening sequences,* are transcribed into RNA but removed enzymatically before translation so that the exons are in a continuous coding sequence. The noncoding segments also routinely include upstream (5′) and downstream (3′) segments flanking the exon-intron aggregate domain. While regulatory elements may be located in any of the noncoding segments, promoters (the basic gene turn-on regulatory elements) are typically located just upstream from the first exon initiation codon (ATG). Other up- and down-regulatory elements are often located upstream from the promoters. Regulation of gene function is commonly modulated by interaction of proteins called *transcription factors* with these regulatory elements.

Figure 2-16 Isopeptide cross-links. Transglutaminase catalyzes cross-linking of peptides between glutamine and lysine residues.

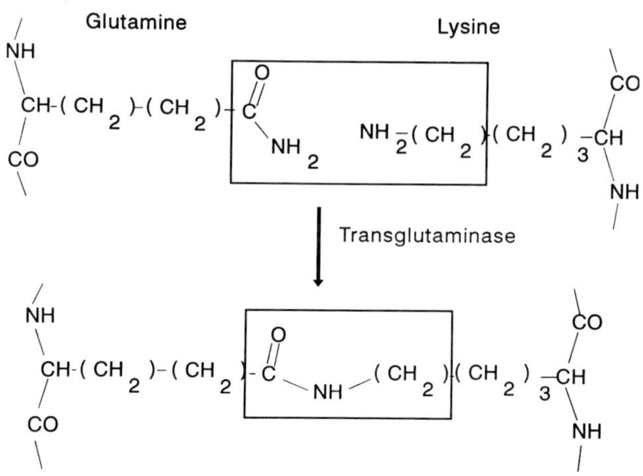

The available molecular biologic techniques have allowed investigators not only to isolate and characterize genes but to decode sequences of encoded proteins from DNA sequences and to prepare molecular probes. Such molecular probes have been useful in elucidating pathways and controls of related genes and other macromolecules. In the sections that follow, we discuss accumulated data regarding the major hair protein genes and their regulation.

The Hair Protein Genes

Representative genes from most of the major classes of hair proteins have been isolated. In some instances, multiple genes have been characterized from an individual species and similar genes from different species have been examined. As only a few human genes have been isolated, much of what is known about the hair genes

Table 2-1
CHARACTERIZED CONSTITUENT HAIR PROTEIN GENES

Group	Family	No. of Genes (Est. Total)	Average Gene Size (kb)	Species
IF	*Hair keratins*			
	Type Ia	5	4–5	S,M,H*
	Type IIa	5	7–9	S
IFAP	*High-sulfur*			
	B2	7	0.9	S
	BIIIA	11	0.9	S
	BIIIB	4	0.8	S
IFAP	*Ultrahigh-sulfur*			
	Cortex	10	1	S,M
	Cuticle	6	1	S,H
IFAP	*High-gly–tyr*			
	Type I F	1	0.6	S
	Type I C2	1	0.6	S
	Type II	10	0.6	S
	Trichohyalin	1?	> 6	R

*S = sheep; M = mouse; H = human; R = rabbit.
Source: Modified from Powell et al.[46] and expanded.

originates from studies of nonhuman hair-bearing animals.

The relevant genes may be grouped according to the following protein types: the "low-sulfur proteins" [the hair-type keratin intermediate filament (IF) proteins], the "high-sulfur proteins" [intermediate filament-associated protein (IFAP group)], the "ultrahigh–sulfur proteins" (IFAP group), and the "high-glycine/tyrosine proteins" (IFAP group). Each of these four major classes may be further subdivided into several subclasses.[23,24] The currently characterized genes are summarized in Table 2-1. The IF group includes the hair keratin (HK) genes; the IFAP group classically includes the high-sulfur (HS) protein genes, the ultrahigh–sulfur (UHS) protein genes, and the high-glycine/tyrosine (HGT) protein genes. The trichohyalin (TH) gene remains in a separate group, as its product has not been definitively associated with any of the currently defined intermediate filaments,[24] although it is a filament-associated protein.[19,20,24]

HAIR KERATIN GENES

A number of hair keratin genes have been isolated and characterized. They include type Ia genes from sheep,[25] mice,[26] and humans[27] and a type IIa gene from sheep.[28] Murine gene-localization studies[29] have shown that most, if not all, type Ia and IIa genes are clustered in the Krt-1 locus (chromosome 11) and Krt-2 locus (chromosome 15), respectively. By analogy, the human genes would be expected to cluster at the corresponding loci on chromosomes 17 and 12, respectively. This clustered arrangement is corroborated by the finding of multiple hair keratin genes on DNA segments from genomic clones.[30] However, the detailed organization of the various genes in the clusters, as well as the sequences of most of the individual genes, remains to be determined.

At least five type Ia and five type IIa distinct genes are predicted.[15,31] The structural portions of the characterized type Ia genes span 4 to 5 kb, whereas the span is approximately 7 to 9 kb for type IIa genes. The type Ia genes have seven exons and six introns, whereas the type IIa genes have nine exons and eight introns. Intron-exon boundaries appear conserved within those genes of the same hair keratin type. In addition, corresponding genes from various species have been highly conserved.

HIGH-SULFUR PROTEIN GENES

There are numerous genes corresponding to the high-sulfur proteins, and most of what is known about these genes has emerged from sheep studies.[32,33] As is presented in Table 2-1, these genes are all relatively small, approximately 0.8 to 0.9 kb. This reflects the fact that they typically lack introns. Due to significant sequence homologies also present among members of this gene family, cDNA probes corresponding to individual proteins have been useful for isolation of multiple genes.[32] As with the hair keratins, these genes also seem to be located in clusters; some genes have been found within a couple of kilobases of each other.

ULTRAHIGH-SULFUR PROTEIN GENES

The ultrahigh–sulfur protein genes also are numerous and have been studied in several species including sheep,[34] mice,[35] and humans.[34] They are quite unusual in that they encode proteins with an extremely high cysteine content (approximately one-third of the amino acids). While the genes are less highly expressed in sheep than in mice or humans, an interesting feature is that expression may be dramatically up-regulated by increased dietary cysteine. The subgrouping of members of this family relates to distribution of gene expression within cortex or cuticle of the hair shaft (Table 2-1). Members within subgroups share high sequence homology. As with the high-sulfur protein genes, the ultrahigh–sulfur protein genes also lack introns and span approximately 1 kb. At least several genes have been isolated on cloned DNA segments, suggesting clustering of members in this gene family. In situ hybridization studies with human DNA have suggested localization to chromosome 11.[36]

HIGH-GLYCINE/TYROSINE PROTEIN GENES

Also constituting a multigene family (Table 2-1), the high-glycine/tyrosine protein genes[37] are divided into two subgroups: type I and type II. Unlike studies of the other multigene families, studies of subgroup members have revealed negligible nucleotide sequence homologies. Nevertheless, as with other IFAP genes, these genes also lack introns and have an average size of approximately 0.6 kb. Somewhat less information has been gathered regarding these genes as compared with those from the other groups.

TRICHOHYALIN GENES

The only trichohyalin gene that has currently been characterized is of rabbit origin.[24] It is presumably composed of three exons and two introns, although the first exon represents an untranslated sequence and has not been located; the second exon contains 22 bp of the 5′-noncoding region and 138 bp of the coding region; the third exon contains the remaining 4083 bp of the coding region and the complete 3′-noncoding region (1051 bp). The gene product has 1407 amino acids and a predicted size of 183,870 daltons.

Differential Gene Expression

The wide array of hair protein genes expressed in the follicle makes orchestration of their expression potentially complex. We are still gaining insight regarding differential expression of these genes by examination of the distribution of gene products within the follicle. Immunohistologic approaches for examining gene product distributions within the hair follicle utilizing specific antibody probes have been only partially applicable, due to the high-sequence homologies present among members of some of the major hair protein families. Studies with various antibodies to trichohyalin[20,38] have demonstrated detailed features of its expression during differentiation in follicular cells. While group-specific antibodies have been prepared for a number of the other proteins,[39–43] relatively few monospecific antibodies have been developed.[44,45] Thus, only limited data have been produced in this fashion.

More comprehensive studies have recently utilized nucleic acid probes for in situ hybridizations to determine the follicular distributions of various hair protein messenger RNAs.[28,46] These studies have revealed differential expression of the groups of hair proteins as well as some individual members within certain groups. Striking sequential and spatial patterns of hair protein expression have been demonstrated within the fine wool follicles of merino sheep (Figs. 2-17 and 2-18). The first group of hair protein genes to be activated are the IF genes, which appear in all cortical cell types. Next, the HGT genes are expressed in cells of one-half of the cortex. A little later, the HS and UHS genes are expressed in the complementary half of the cortex. As differentiation proceeds, most cortical cells produce the HGT and HS proteins, but UHS gene expression remains restricted to half of the cortex. The last hair proteins expressed are those from the UHS subgroup that localize to the cuticle of the hair shaft. Specific nucleic acid probes for individual IF messenger RNAs have also been used; these studies have demonstrated sequential transcriptional activation of certain of the subgroup genes during differentiation.[28] It remains to be determined if the sequential and spatial patterns of

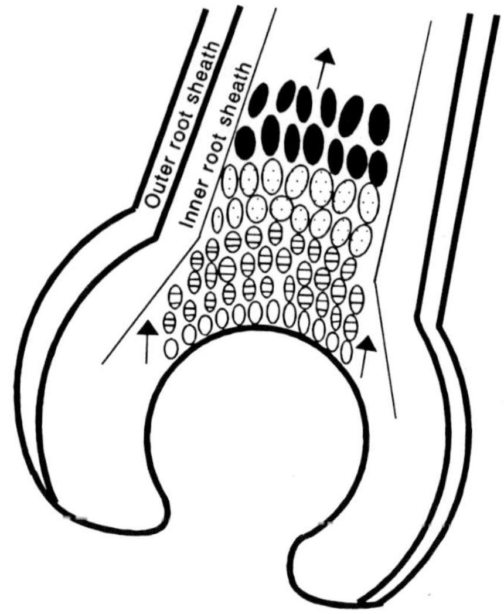

Figure 2-17 Sequential hair keratin expression. In situ hybridization studies using cDNA probes for specific type IIa hair keratin mRNAs have demonstrated sequential expression of these proteins in sheep. In particular, one gene is first to be activated (cells with horizontal bars). This is followed by activation of two other genes (stippled cells) and, finally, a fourth member of the gene family (black cells). (*Adapted from Powell et al.*[28])

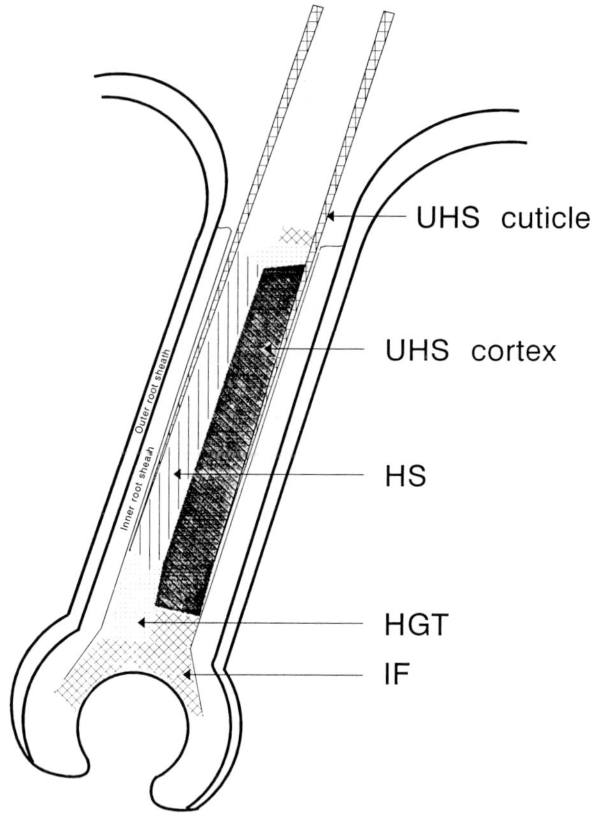

Figure 2-18 Patterns of hair protein expression. Gene expression in a sheep hair follicle shows overlapping and discrete patterns. See text for details. (*Adapted from Powell et al.*[46])

hair protein gene expression demonstrated in sheep follicles are as dramatic in other species, as the sheep hair cortex is rather uniquely compartmentalized into paracortex and orthocortex.

Gene Regulation

We are now at the stage at which an understanding of the molecular aspects of hair protein gene regulation may begin to be realized. This is possible due to the recent isolation and characterization of a number of relevant genes. In addition to sequence analyses and comparisons, some of the genes have been expressed in host cells[45] and others have been successfully used to generate transgenic animals which express native proteins or various reporter molecules.[47,48] Prior to these studies, the most dramatic observations of regulation involved dietary influences of certain amino acids upon UHS protein expression.[24,49–51]

The typical TATA box element, which is commonly found in eukaryotic genes and serves as the binding site for RNA polymerase II, has been identified in all of the hair genes examined. Likewise, the common CAAT box which serves as a transcriptional activator is present in all of these genes. In addition, the AP-1 and AP-2 sites have also been identified in some of these genes.[46] Thus, a number of ubiquitous regulatory motifs have been demonstrated in the hair genes.

Multiple potential regulatory elements in the promoter regions of the genes have also been recognized through sequence comparisons (Table 2-2). These range from 7 to 12 nucleotides in length. Although some appear to be slightly degenerate in their conserved sequences, the variations are small and not unusual in that other regulatory elements have also displayed similar degeneracy. Whether or not these putative regulatory motifs have biologic significance remains to be determined by careful expression studies designed to test these elements.

Recent studies of human[52] and mouse[26] type Ia hair keratin genes have also suggested that some regulatory elements may exist within introns. This possibility was first recognized by the observation of conserved sequences. Further sup-

Table 2-2
POTENTIAL HAIR PROTEIN GENE REGULATORY MOTIFS*

Gene	*HK-1* (*CTTTGAAGA*)	*HGT-1* (*TCAGTTT*)	*HGT-2* (*TAATCAGA*)	*HS-1* (*CCAAAGGCAAAG*)	*HS-2* (*ACAAAAGCAGGA*)	*HS-3* (*AAAAATGCT*)	*UHS-1* (*ACAAGGAAA*)	*CU-1* (*CAGGAGGAAGG*)
IF type Ia	✓ (8/9)							✓ (10/11)
IF type IIb	✓							
	2 ✓ (8/9)			✓ (10/12)				
HGT type I C2	✓	✓	✓					
HGT type I F	✓	✓	✓				✓ (7/9)	
HGT type II		✓	2 ✓				✓ (8/9)	
Rabbit								
HS B2A				✓	✓ (11/12)	2 ✓ (8/9)		
HS B2C				✓ (10/12)	✓ (11/12)	3 ✓ (2x8/9)		
HS B2D	✓ (8/9)			✓ (11/12)	✓ (11/12)	✓ (8/9)	✓ (8/9)	
HS BIIIA 9								
HS BIIIB 4					✓ (9/12)			
UHS cortex								
Rabbit							✓	
Mouse					✓ (9/12)		✓	2 ✓ (9/11)
								(10/11)
UHS cuticle								
Human							✓	✓
Sheep					✓ (9/12)			2 ✓ (10/11)

* Where a motif is identified (✓) the preceding number indicates two or more copies and the numbers in parentheses show the match to the consensus if there are differences. Thus, (8/11) indicates that 8 nucleotides match the 11-nucleotide consensus.
Source: Modified from Powell et al.[46]

portive evidence was obtained by intron-deletion studies utilizing a host cell transient expression system. As with other putative regulatory motifs, additional careful studies must be performed to establish whether these findings are biologically meaningful.

CONCLUDING REMARKS

In review, our current perspectives regarding differentiation of the hair shaft span the macroscopic, cellular, and molecular vantages. We have the benefit of understanding the basic features of hair shaft shape in normal and pathologic conditions. The cellular complexities of the hair shaft and follicle have also been fairly clearly defined. More recently, the molecular aspects of hair follicle function have entered the realm of practical investigation. Although considerable information has been gathered, we still have much to learn about the processes involved in differentiation of this unique tissue.

REFERENCES

1. Cotsarelis G, Sun TT, Lavker RM: Label-retaining cells reside in the bulge area of pilosebaceous unit: Implications for follicular stem cells, hair cycle, and skin carcinogenesis. Cell 61:1329–1337, 1990.
2. Rogers GE: Structural and biochemical features of the hair follicle. In Montagna W, Lobtiz W (eds): *The Epidermis.* New York, Academic Press, 1964, p. 179
3. Roth SI: Hair and nail. In Zelickson AS (ed): *Ultrastructure of Normal and Abnormal Skin.* Philadelphia, Febiger, 1967, p 105.
4. Steinert PM, Roop DR: The molecular and cellular biology of intermediate filaments. Annu Rev Biochem 57:593–625, 1988.
5. Sun TT et al.: Classification, expression, and possible mechanisms of evolution of mammalian epithelial keratins: A unifying model. In Levine A et al (eds): *Cancer Cells,* vol. 1: *The Transformed Phenotype.* Cold Spring Harbor, N.Y., Cold Spring Harbor Lab, 1984, p 169.
6. Hanukoglu I, Fuchs E: The cDNA sequence of a type II cytoskeletal keratin reveals constant and variable structural domains among keratins. Cell 33:915–924, 1983.
7. Steinert PM et al.: Complete amino acid sequence of a mouse epidermal keratin subunit and implications for the structure of intermediate filaments. Nature 302:794–800, 1983.
8. Steinert PM, Idler WW: Self-assembly of bovine epidermal keratin filaments *in vitro.* J Mol Biol 108:547–567, 1976.
9. Steven AC et al.: Epidermal keratin filaments assembled *in vitro* have masses-per-unit length that scale according to average subunit mass: Structural basis for homologous packing of subunits in intermediate filaments. J Cell Biol 97:1939–1944, 1983.
10. Zviak C, Dawber RPR: Hair structure, function, and physicochemical properties. In Zviak C (ed): *The Science of Hair Care.* New York, Marcel Dekker, 1986, pp 1–44.
11. Hashimoto K: The structure of human hair. Clin Dermatol 6(4):7–21, 1988.
12. Rogers GE: Synthesis and cross-linking in the structure and growth of hair keratins. Clin Dermatol 6(4):26–31, 1988.
13. Lynch MH et al.: Acidic and basic hair nail ("hard") keratins: Their colocalization in upper cortical and cuticle cells of the human hair follicle and their relationship to "soft" keratins. J Cell Biol 103:2593–2606, 1986.
14. Ito M et al.: Immunological characteristics and histological distribution of human hair fibrous proteins studied with anti-hair keratin monoclonal antibodies, HKN-2, HKN-4 and HKN-6. J Histochem Cytochem 34:269–275, 1986.
15. Heid HW, Moll I, Franke WW: Patterns of expression of trichocytic and epithelial cytokeratins in mammalian tissues. I. Human and bovine hair follicles. Differentiation 37:137–157, 1988.
16. Dhouailly D et al.: Expression of hair-related keratins in a soft epithelium: Subpopulations of human and mouse dorsal tongue keratinocytes express keratin markers for hair-, skin-, and esophageal-types of differentiation. Exp Cell Res 181:141–158, 1989.
17. O'Guin WM, Dhouailly D, Manabe M, Sun TT: Specific keratins and their associated proteins as markers for hair follicle differentiation. In Rogers GE, Reis PI, Marshall RC (eds): *Biology of the Wool and Hair.* New York, Chapman Hall, 1989, p 37.
18. Vorner H: Uber trichohyalin. Ein Beitrag zur Anatomic des Haares und Wurzelscheiden. Dermatol Z (Berlin) 10:357, 1903.
19. Rothnagel JA, Rogers GE: Trichohyalin, an intermediate filament-associated protein of the hair follicle. J Cell Biol 102:1419–1429, 1986.
20. O'Guin WM, Sun TT, Manabe M: Interaction of trichohyalin with intermediate filaments: Three immunologically defined stages of trichohyalin maturation. J Invest Dermatol 98:24–32, 1992.
21. Rogers GE, Harding HW, Llewellyn-Smith IJ: The origin of citrulline-containing proteins in the hair follicle and the chemical nature of trichohyalin, an intracellular precursor. Biochim Biophys Acta 495:159–175, 1977.
22. Rogers GE: The occurrence of citrulline structural proteins of the hair follicle. In Goldsmith LA (ed): *Biochemistry and Physiology of the Skin.* New York, Oxford University Press, 1983, p 475.
23. Powell BC, Rogers GE: Hair keratin, composition, structure and biogenesis. In Bereiter-Hahn J, Matoltsy AG, Richards KS (eds): *Biology of the Integument.* Berlin, Springer-Verlag, 1986, X, p 675.
24. Rogers GE, Fietz MJ, Fratini A: Trichohyalin and matrix proteins. Ann NY Acad Sci 642:64–81, 1991.
25. Wilson BW et al.: Complete sequence of a type-I microfibrillar wool keratin gene. Gene 73:21–31, 1988.
26. Kaytes PS et al.: Hair-specific keratins: Characterization and expression of a mouse type I keratin gene. J Invest Dermatol 97:835–842, 1991.

27. Yu J et al.: Isolation and characterization of a human type Ia hair keratin gene. J Invest Dermatol 96:542, 1991.
28. Powell B, Crocker L, Rogers G: Hair follicle differentiation: Expression, structure and evolutionary conservation of the hair type II keratin intermediate filament gene family. Development 114:417–433, 1992.
29. Compton JG et al.: Chromosomal localization of mouse hair keratin genes. Ann NY Acad Sci 642:32–43, 1991.
30. Powell BC, Cam GR, Fietz MJ, Rogers GE: Clustered arrangement of keratin intermediate filament genes. Proc Natl Acad Sci 83:5048–5052, 1986.
31. Heid HW, Werner E, Franke WW: The complement of native alpha-keratin polypeptides of hair-forming cells: A subset of eight polypeptides that differ from epithelial cytokeratins. Differentiation 32:101–119, 1986.
32. Powell BC, Sleigh MJ, Ward KA, Rogers GE: Mammalian keratin: Organisation of genes coding for the B2 high-sulphur proteins of sheep wool. Nucleic Acids Res 11:5327, 1983.
33. Frankel MJ et al.: The keratin BIIIB gene family: Isolation of cDNA clones and structure of a gene and a related pseudogene. Genomics 4:182–191, 1989.
34. MacKinnon PJ, Powell BC, Rogers GE: Structure and expression of genes for a class of cysteine-rich proteins of the cuticle layers of differentiating wool and hair follicles. J Cell Biol 111:2587–2600, 1990.
35. McNab AR et al.: An ultra high sulfur keratin gene is expressed specifically during hair growth. J Invest Dermatol 92:263–266, 1989.
36. MacKinnon PJ et al.: An ultrahigh sulfur keratin gene of the human hair cuticle is located at 11q13 and cross hybridizes with sequences at 11p15. Mamm Genome 1:53–56, 1991.
37. Kuczek ES, Rogers GE: Sheep wool (glycine + tyrosine)-rich keratin genes: A family of low sequence homology. Eur J Biochem 166:79–85, 1987.
38. Manabe M, O'Guin WM: Existence of trichohyalin-keratohyalin hybrid granules in non-follicular epithelia: The co-localization of two major intermediate filament-associated proteins. Differentiation. (In press, 1993.)
39. Hamilton EH, Payne RE, O'Keefe EJ: Trichohyalin: Presence in the granular layer and stratum corneum of normal human epidermis. J Invest Dermatol 96:666–672, 1991.
40. French PW, Hewish DR: Localization of low-sulfur keratin proteins in the wool follicle using monoclonal antibodies. J Cell Biol 102:1412–1418, 1986.
41. Ito M et al.: Cell differentiation in human anagen hair and hair follicles studied with anti-hair keratin monoclonal antibodies. J Invest Dermatol 86:563–569, 1986.
42. Hewish DR, Robinson CP, Sparrow LG: Monoclonal antibody studies of alpha-keratin low-sulfur proteins. Aust J Biol Sci 37:17, 1984.
43. Hewish DR, French PW: Monoclonal antibodies to a subfraction of merino wool high-tyrosine proteins. Aust J Biol Sci 39: 341, 1986.
44. Bertolino AP et al.: Differential expression of type I hair keratins. J Invest Dermatol 94:297–303, 1990.
45. Yu DW et al.: Transient expression of mouse hair keratins in transfected HeLa cells: Interactions between "hard" and "soft" keratins. J Invest Dermatol 97:354–363, 1991.
46. Powell BC, Nesci A, Rogers GE: Regulation of keratin gene expression in hair follicle differentiation. Ann NY Acad Sci 642:1–20, 1991.
47. Vogeli G et al.: High-sulfur protein gene expression in a transgenic mouse. Ann NY Acad Sci 642:21–31, 1991.
48. Powell BC, Rogers GE: Cyclic hair-loss and regrowth in transgenic mice overexpressing an intermediate filament gene. EMBO J 9:1485–1493, 1990.
49. Reiss PJ, Schinkel PG: Some effects of sulfur-containing amino acids on the growth and composition of wool. Aust J Biol Sci 16:218, 1963.
50. Gillespie JM, Reis PJ: The dietary-regulated biosynthesis of high sulfur wool proteins. Biochem J 98:669–677, 1966.
51. Reis PJ, Tunks DA, Downes AM: The influence of abomasal and intravenous supplements of sulphur-containing amino acids on wool growth rate. Aust J Biol Sci 26:249, 1973.
52. Yu DW, Yu J, Freedberg IM, Bertolino AP: *In vitro* expression of a human hair keratin gene. J Invest Dermatol 98:559, 1992.

Chapter

3

THE CONTROL OF HAIR GROWTH AND PIGMENTATION

Andrew G. Messenger

INTRODUCTION

Hair has several functions. In many mammals, hair is of vital importance for thermal insulation, a property which has probably played an important role in the animals' evolutionary success. Hair is also concerned with social and sexual communication, both visually and as a means for dispersing scents secreted by skin glands, and, in some mammals, with providing camouflage. Certain hairs, e.g., vibrissae, have specialized sensory functions. Man is relatively hairless compared with other primates, and human hair has no known significance for survival of the species. However, it remains an important cosmetic asset, and perceptions about cultural norms and departures therefrom give rise to great distress and multi-million-dollar industries.

The diversity in function means that the mechanisms controlling hair growth are unlikely to be identical in all follicles. For the most part, we know little of the finer points of hair growth control, although certain broad principles have been established. For example, we have a reasonable understanding of the tissue interactions which lead to hair follicle development at a cellular level but know much less about the molecular basis for these events. In addition to its role as a producer of hair, the hair follicle is an instructive structure from a general biological standpoint. Many physiological processes, including the control of cell growth, mesenchymal-epithelial interactions, epithelial differentiation, and hormone action, are encapsulated in this readily accessible structure, making the hair follicle a valuable model for scientific research and discovery in fields other than dermatology.

HAIR FOLLICLE DEVELOPMENT

Embryogenesis

The hair follicle is derived from both epidermal and dermal tissue. The dermal component is

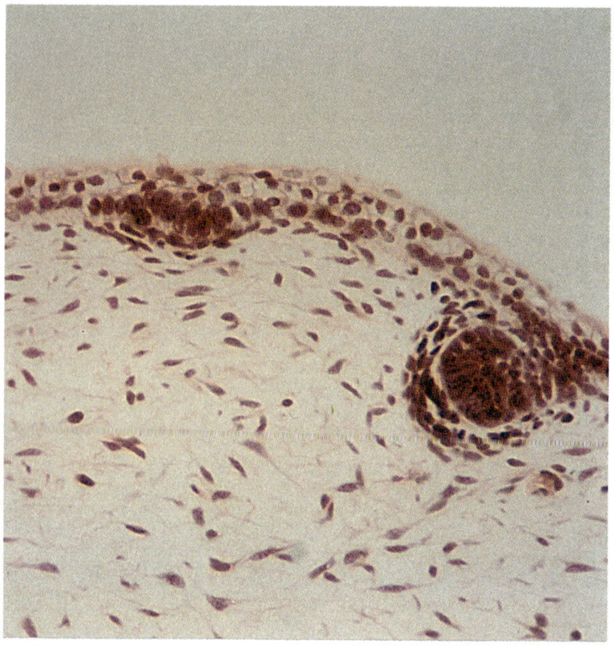

Figure 3-1 Early stages of hair follicle development in human fetal skin. The follicle on the left is at the placode stage; that on the right is at the hair peg stage and shows a well-developed mesenchymal component.

formed as an aggregate of mesenchymal cells directly beneath the developing epithelial placode (Fig. 3-1). The epidermal component grows downward to form the hair peg and then, by a process of continued cell division and differentiation, the hair bulb matrix, the hair fiber, and its surrounding root sheaths. Concomitantly, the mesenchymal aggregate organizes into the dermal papilla, invaginating the base of the follicle and the dermal sheath surrounding the lower part of the follicle. In rodent pelage and vibrissa follicles, cell division in the dermal papilla ceases at an early stage of development,[1] and the cellular population of the papilla is thought to remain stable thereafter, throughout successive adult hair cycles.

Tissue-recombination experiments have shown that hair follicle development depends on a series of messages between the dermis and the overlying epidermis.[2–4] The initial message is derived from the dermis and instructs the epidermis to form an appendage. This signal is common to all classes of vertebrates; thus, mouse dermis is able to instruct chick epidermis to initiate development of a feather follicle. This is followed by a less well-defined but class-specific signal from the epidermis which instructs the dermis to form a dermal papilla. Finally, a second dermal message stimulates the epidermal placode to form the class-specific appendage. As well as its inductive role in follicle development, the dermis also appears to be responsible for determining the position or pattern of follicles and the follicle type.

Much current research is aimed at identifying the molecular basis for these developmental events. Present evidence indicates that follicle development depends on a complex series of interactions involving extracellular matrix, growth factors and other soluble signals, cell adhesion molecules, and direct cell-cell contacts.[3] Epidermal growth factor (EGF) was the first growth factor to be implicated, as its administration to newborn mice delays hair follicle development.[5] Transforming growth factor alpha (TGFα), which binds to the same receptor as EGF, also inhibits murine hair growth.[6] EGF peptide has been identified in fetal sheep skin by immunohistochemistry, where it was localized to the periderm and the intermediate layers of the epidermis. There was no staining of the epithelial or mesenchymal cells of developing hair follicles until late in development, when staining was present in the sebaceous gland and the outer root sheath.[7] The distribution of EGF receptors (EGF-Rs) in embryonic skin has been investigated in several studies using ^{125}I-EGF or immunohistochemistry.[8–10] During early development in rat and human skin, EGF-Rs are absent in the placode and hair germ but present in the adjacent interfollicular epidermis. Later on, EGF-Rs are expressed in the outer root sheath and sebaceous epithelium and, in some species, in the hair bulb, although they are consistently absent in the dermal papilla. Together these observations suggest that EGF (or TGFα) is involved in hair follicle development; this is supported by one study in which administration of antibodies to EGF accelerated growth of the first coat in newborn mice.[11]

Transcripts for several members of the transforming growth factor beta (TGFβ) family, including TGFβ-1, TGFβ-2, TGFβ-3, bone morphogenetic protein-2 (BMP-2), and BMP-4, have also been identified in different distributions in developing hair follicles.[12,13] The expression of mRNA for BMP-4 is particularly interesting as it occurs transiently in the mesenchyme at sites thought to correspond to mesenchymal aggregates but before aggregation is morphologically apparent. This is the earliest molecular event yet described in follicle development and may relate to the first dermal message.

Intrinsic Control of the Hair Growth Cycle

In man, local regulatory mechanisms predominate in hair cycle control, and systemic factors are relatively unimportant. Several hypotheses have been advanced to explain the intrinsic rhythmic activity of the hair follicle, although none has yet been established with any certainty.

CHALONE HYPOTHESIS

It has been known for many years that plucking of resting hairs from telogen follicles advances the onset of anagen. This led to the idea that the hair cycle is controlled by a locally active inhibitor which accumulates during anagen, causing entry into catagen when present in sufficient concentration (the *chalone hypothesis*).[48,49] It was proposed that the inhibitor disperses during telogen and that this could be accelerated by plucking resting hairs. This idea has been disputed because the plucking of resting hairs from follicles which have already entered anagen does not prolong the anagen in progress, although it does advance the onset of the next anagen cycle.[35] In support of the chalone hypothesis, it has recently been reported that murine skin contains a factor which inhibits hair growth in vivo and in vitro. This inhibitory factor appeared to derive from the epidermis and was present in telogen skin but not in anagen skin.[50] It has not been characterized further, although, in a previous study, a lectinlike hair growth inhibitor was isolated from rat skin.[51]

GROWTH FACTORS

The ideas embodied in the chalone hypothesis live on in current concepts of paracrine and autocrine regulation of cell growth and differentiation by growth factors and cytokines. Using the polymerase chain reaction, Sutton and colleagues studied the expression of mRNAs for a number of growth factors in mouse skin during the hair growth cycle.[52] Transcripts for TGFβ-1, TGFβ-2, TGFβ-3, basic fibroblast growth factor (bFGF), TGFα, and EGF were detected in whole-skin samples. The levels of TGFβ-1, TGFβ-2, and TGFα remained the same during the cycle, whereas the signals for TGFβ-3 and bFGF were present in anagen but much weaker in catagen. EGF levels were more variable but also tended to be lower at the end of the cycle. The physiological significance of these observations is not known, although there is some evidence implicating EGF in control of the hair cycle. In addition to its effect on hair follicle development (see earlier text), the administration of large doses of mouse EGF to adult sheep causes follicles to enter catagen, with cessation of hair growth and loss of the fleece.[53,54] Subsequently, EGF has been found to induce a catagenlike change in cultured human hair follicles.[55] Both EGF[7] and bFGF[10] have been immunolocalized in the outer root sheath of mature sheep follicles. The distribution of bFGF was more peripheral than that of EGF and, in some follicles, extended around the hair bulb; neither growth factor was found in the dermal papilla. In contrast, immunoreactivity for TGFβ-1 in rat follicles has been reported to be confined to the dermal papilla during anagen.[56] The distribution suggested an association with the extracellular matrix, and the staining for TGFβ was lost as the follicles entered catagen.

Growth factors have diverse effects on cell proliferation and differentiation. Their biologic activity also depends on a number of factors, including posttranslational modification, interactions with the extracellular matrix and other signaling molecules, and receptor expression. Although a number of growth factors have been detected in the hair follicle, we are largely ignorant of the significance of these observations in terms of growth-factor function.

ROLE OF THE DERMAL PAPILLA IN HAIR CYCLE CONTROL

The anagen phase of the hair cycle can be considered as a developmental process in which the aim is in the production of a club hair. The dermal papilla provides the inductive stimulus for anagen-type differentiation of the follicular epithelium, and it seems likely that interactions involving the dermal papilla and neighboring epithelial cells are also involved in regulating the hair growth cycle. Once established during embryonic development, the cellular population of the dermal papilla is thought to remain little changed throughout successive hair growth cycles in the adult animal. The evidence for this belief is limited and is based largely on autoradiographic studies which have shown that, unlike the hair bulb matrix, radiolabeling with tritiated thymidine in the dermal papilla during the hair growth cycle is low and probably restricted to endothelial cells.[57] It seems probable that changes in papilla cell number do occur during vellus-terminal transition and vice versa, but this has yet to be documented. Nevertheless, major changes do take place in the dermal papilla during the hair growth cycle in terms of cell morphology, vascularization, and in the composition and volume of the extracellular matrix.[58,59] During anagen, dermal papilla cells contain prominent golgi apparatus and endoplasmic reticulum and show vigorous pinocytic activity indicative of protein synthesis. They lie in an extensive extracellular matrix which differs from that of the interfollicular dermis (see later text). The extracellular matrix diminishes in volume during catagen to become almost nonexistent in telogen, where the dermal papilla appears as a tightly packed ball of cells immediately below the lower pole of the follicular epithelium. There is also a change in the morphology of dermal papilla cells. As the follicle enters telogen, the dermal papilla cells become more compact and their cytoplasm contains few organelles. The capillary loops, present in larger dermal papillae during anagen, are also lost. Thus, during anagen the papilla appears to be an active vascularized synthetic structure, whereas in telogen it is nonvascularized and quiescent.

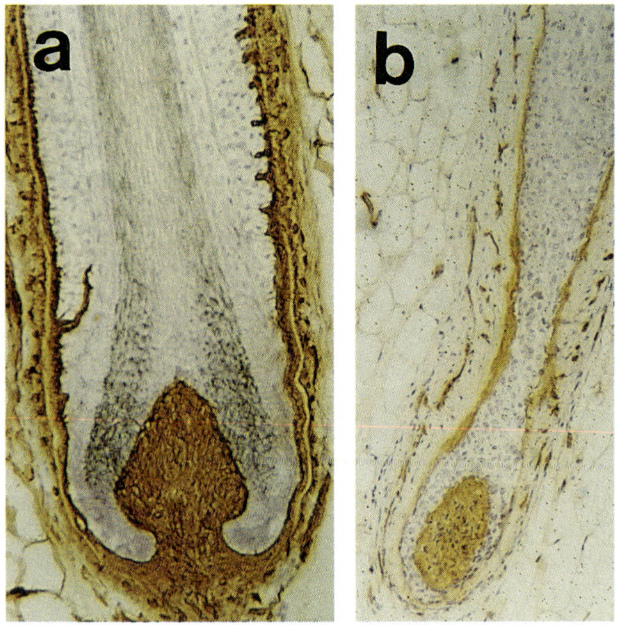

Figure 3-6 Immunoperoxidase staining for (*A*) type IV collagen in a human anagen follicle and (*B*) laminin in a catagen follicle. Staining for both basement membrane proteins is seen throughout the dermal papilla and is not restricted to structural basement membranes.

The dermal papilla extracellular matrix also has a distinctive composition and, in addition to the volumetric changes, the expression of some extracellular matrix molecules varies in concert with the hair growth cycle. A number of basement membrane molecules, including type IV collagen, laminin, and heparan sulfate proteoglycan, have been immunolocalized in the dermal papilla.[60–64] They are present throughout the hair growth cycle and are not restricted in their distribution to epithelial and vascular basement membranes (Fig. 3-6). The cellular source of basement membrane molecules in the dermal papilla extracellular matrix is uncertain, but it seems likely that dermal papilla cells are a major contributor as these cells synthesize type IV collagen in vitro,[62,64] and interrupted basement membranelike structures may be seen closely associated with dermal papilla cells at the ultrastructural level.[65] The dermal papilla extracellular matrix also stains for fibronectin during anagen, and staining diminishes during catagen.[61,65] Reexpression of fibronectin occurs at the papilla-epithelial interface in very early anagen and may relate to cell migration occurring at this stage of the hair growth cycle. In contrast, the expression of bullous pemphigoid antigen, a normal component of the epidermal basement membrane, is limited to the basement membrane of the follicular epithelium and is not seen in the dermal papilla.[60,64] It is also discontinuous, both during embryonic development, where staining for bullous pemphigoid antigen is lost at an early stage of embryonic development around the base of the follicle, and in the adult follicle. During anagen, the outer root sheath basement membrane stains for bullous pemphigoid antigen down to the lower tip of the hair bulb, but staining is absent from the hair bulb matrix basement membrane surrounding the dermal papilla. However, bullous pemphigoid antigen is expressed at the papilla-epithelial interface in late catagen and telogen. In the epidermis, bullous pemphigoid antigen is associated with hemidesmosomes, and its absence in the anagen hair bulb matrix basement membrane may reflect the paucity of hemidesmosomes in this site.

It has also been known for many years that the dermal papilla contains an abundance of proteoglycans (mucopolysaccharides) by virtue of its histochemical staining properties.[58] More recently, chondroitin and chondroitin sulfate (glycosaminoglycan side chains on proteoglycan molecules) have been demonstrated in the dermal papilla and dermal sheath of anagen follicles in both man and rat using specific monoclonal antibodies.[62,63,66] Neither is demonstrable in the dermis using these techniques, although chondroitin-6-sulfate proteoglycan is found in the epidermal basement membrane. Staining for chondroitins diminishes during catagen and is absent from telogen follicles (Fig. 3-7). Reexpression occurs when the follicle reenters anagen.

Little is known of the function of extracellular matrix in the dermal papilla, although many properties are ascribed to extracellular matrix in other tissues which may well be relevant to hair growth. These include structural organization, facilitation of cell migration, and modulation of differentiation. Various growth factors (e.g., TGFβ, bFGF) are known to bind to extracellular matrix, which may then serve to filter or localize their activity. Extracellular matrix molecules also interact directly with cells by binding to specific cell-surface receptors and can activate second messenger systems. There is some evidence to implicate proteoglycans in hair growth in addition to their changing pattern of expression during the hair cycle. Injection of glycosaminoglycans into the skin has been reported to stimulate hair growth in rabbits.[67] The accumulation of proteoglycans in the skin in certain pathologic states such as pretibial myxedema is also sometimes associated with hypertrichosis. Conversely, feather development in chick embryos is disrupted in the presence of β-xyloside (which inhibits assembly of glycosaminoglycans on the proteoglycan core protein).[68] Recently it has been proposed that extracellular matrix proteoglycans may have an immunoprotective role in the hair follicle. The expression of class I major histocompatibility antigens by epithelial cells in the lower part of the follicle is very low or undetectable,[69] making them a potential target for natural killer cells. Westgate and colleagues[70] suggested that proteoglycans in the dermal sheath and dermal papilla form a protective barrier, preventing this putative immune attack. The loss of proteoglycans during catagen is associated with an accumulation of activated macrophages around the regressing epithelial column and an increase in epithelial class I expression. However, it is not yet clear whether macrophage infiltration is a primary event in

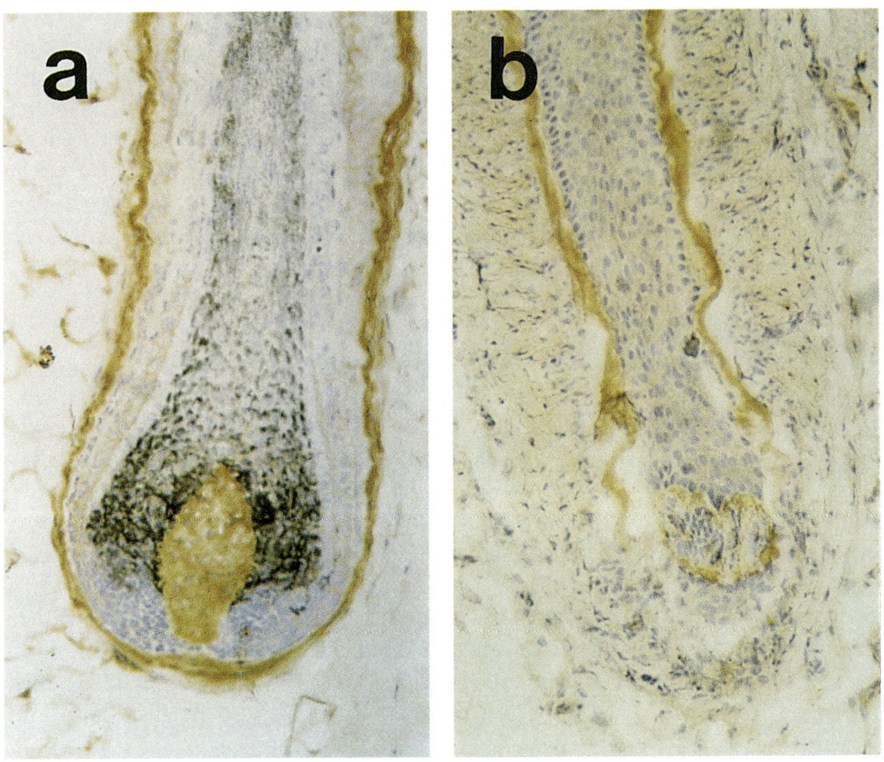

Figure 3-7 Immunoperoxidase staining for chondroitin 6-sulfate in human follicles. During anagen (*A*) chondroitin 6-sulfate is present in the dermal papilla and the dermal sheath. In catagen (*B*), staining diminishes in the dermal papilla and the lower part of the dermal sheath. (*Courtesy of Dr. A. J. G. McDonagh.*)

catagen or whether it is simply a "mopping-up" operation.

Although we do not fully understand the function of the hair follicle extracellular matrix, there is evidence that it is essential for maintaining growth. Link and colleagues[71] showed that treatment of cultured vibrissa follicles with dispase, an enzyme which degrades type IV collagen and fibronectin, caused condensation of the dermal papilla and impaired thymidine labeling in matrix epithelium.

HAIR FOLLICLE STEM CELLS

All self-renewing tissues are believed to contain a population of stem cells. These cells have a number of characteristic features—they are relatively undifferentiated, they have a great proliferative potential, and they are usually found in well-protected and highly vascularized areas. Stem cells are normally slow-cycling but, following certain growth stimuli, they can be induced to enter the proliferative pool, where they undergo cell division, giving rise to transient amplifying cells. These transient amplifying cells have a limited mitotic potential before they become terminally differentiated. The location of stem cells in the hair follicle is still the subject of some controversy, but a number of lines of evidence point to their being situated in the outer root sheath close to the insertion of the arrector muscle. This site, termed the *bulge* region or *Wulst,* is derived from the lower of two bulges to one side of the developing embryonic follicle (the upper bulge will form the sebaceous gland). The evidence for there being a stem-cell population in the bulge region is as follows:

1. Immunohistochemical studies show that basal cells in the Wulst express keratin 19.[72] Keratin 19 expression has been associated with regions containing stem cells and having a risk of malignant transformation.
2. Increased proliferative activity and morphological irregularities are seen in this site, together with expansion of keratin 19–positive cells during epidermal regeneration.
3. The lower follicle retracts to this site in telogen in most follicle types (though not all—the vibrissa follicle undergoes very little shortening in catagen).
4. In murine follicles, a population of slow-cycling cells has been demonstrated in the bulge region.[73] These cells were identified by autoradiography following repeated injections of ^{3}H-thymidine. Rapid uptake of label occurred in the hair bulb matrix, but only cells in the bulge region retained label for a prolonged period. Retention of thymidine labeling is thought to be a characteristic of stem cells, which typically are slow-cycling. Cotsarelis and colleagues[73] suggested that entry into anagen occurs when stem cells in the bulge region are activated by signals from the dermal papilla. The daughter transient-amplifying cells form the hair bulb matrix and ultimately its differentiated cell products. As a transient-amplifying population, cells in the hair bulb matrix would have a finite proliferative potential which, once exhausted, would result in cessation of growth and entry into catagen.

The concept that stem cells reside in the bulge region also explains certain aspects of hair follicle pathology. In alopecia areata, a disease in which follicles are not destroyed, the inflammatory infiltrate is concentrated in and around the hair bulb. In the scarring alopecias, on the other hand, the inflammatory infiltrate affects the upper part of the follicle, extending down to the arrector insertion, thus including the putative stem-cell region. The "bulge hypothesis" also implies that cell movement in the outer root sheath during early anagen occurs in a downward direction rather than upward from the matrix. While it is difficult to subject it to direct examination, the idea that cell movement in the outer root sheath is downward has been forcefully argued from the results of recombinant studies on the vibrissa follicle.[29]

ANDROGENS

Androgens are the most important systemic modulators of human hair growth. They are necessary for conversion of vellus hair on the body and the beard region to terminal hair, a process which starts at puberty and continues for several decades.[74] The response of hair follicles to androgens varies with body site; the growth of pubic and axillary hair occurs earliest, reaches a peak during the third decade, and then declines. Beard growth is maximal during the fourth decade and remains much the same thereafter. Growth of chest hair peaks even later, and that of terminal hairs in the nares and the external auditory meatus is a feature of late middle age. The growth of hair on the scalp is not androgen-dependent but, paradoxically, androgens are necessary for the development of balding. Man is not the only mammal to show androgen-induced changes in hair growth; the mane in lions and in male red deer is also stimulated by male hormones; several other primates, such as the macaque and the uacari, show balding on the scalp. The importance of androgens in beard growth and balding was first recognized by Hamilton.[74,75] He observed that men castrated before the age of puberty neither grew beards nor went bald unless they were treated with testosterone. Castration of older men prevented the progression of balding but did not reverse it. Beard growth appeared to be partially reversed by castration, the reversibility being greatest in those who had been castrated at an early age. The occurrence of hirsutism and balding in women with hyperandrogenic disorders provides further evidence for the importance of androgens in hair growth.

In order to respond to androgens, hair follicles must possess androgen receptors. Genetic males who lack androgen receptors (testicular feminization) have testes and normal or high levels of circulating testosterone. However, they have female external genitalia and, in the complete form of the syndrome, fail to develop pubic and axillary hair, do not grow beards, and do not go bald. Some pubic and axillary hair may be present in incomplete forms of testicular feminization. Pharmacologic blockade of androgen receptors with cyproterone acetate will partly reverse hirsuties[76] and induce some recovery of hair growth in women with androgenetic hair loss,[77] although, as would be predicted from Hamilton's observations, antiandrogen treatment does not completely reverse hair growth to a prepubertal state.

There is a pronounced genetic influence on androgen-dependent hair growth, particularly in respect to balding, which tends to run in families. However, genetic factors are also important in beard growth. This is most evident in racial differences—for example, beard growth in Caucasian men is greater than in Japanese men.[75] These genetic differences are presumably determined at the level of the hair follicle, as they do not reflect differences in circulating androgen levels.

Mechanism of Action of Androgens

The wide range of responses to androgens, depending on body site, suggests the specificity of the response is determined locally in the skin. This is well-illustrated by the success of hair transplantation, where follicles from relatively nonresponsive occipital skin retain the behavior of the donor site when transplanted into bald scalp. Moreover, the development of micrografting, where individual follicles are transplanted, indicates that androgen responsiveness is at the level of the follicle itself.

Androgens circulate in the blood either free or bound to proteins, especially sex hormone–binding globulins. It is believed that free steroid diffuses into the cell, where it binds to a specific nuclear receptor.[78] Interaction between the receptor hormone complex and nuclear DNA activates the relevant genes to regulate the appropriate RNA. Understanding how androgens affect hair growth is complicated by the fact that they may undergo extensive intracellular conversion in the target tissue[79] (Fig. 3-8). The weak androgen dehydroepiandrosterone can be converted to androstenedione, which itself can be reversibly converted to testosterone. The metabolism of testosterone to the more potent androgen 5α-dihydrotestosterone (DHT) by the enzyme 5α-reductase appears to be an important step in many androgen-responsive tissues (though not all). Men who are deficient in 5α-reductase (type II pseudohermaphroditism) have testes and normal or high levels of testosterone production but have ambiguous external genitalia. Following puberty they show a male pattern of skeletal muscle development and a female distribution of pubic and axillary hair growth. However, beard growth is sparse and the frontal hair line does not recede.[80] Thus, the response of pubic and axillary follicles to androgens does not require the formation of DHT (neither does skeletal muscle). However, 5α-reductase activity does appear to be necessary for the full expression of secondary sexual hair characteristics elsewhere on the body, in the beard, and on the scalp. This conclusion is supported by animal studies of 5α-reductase inhibitors. In the macaque, topical treatment with the 5α-reductase inhibitor 4MA

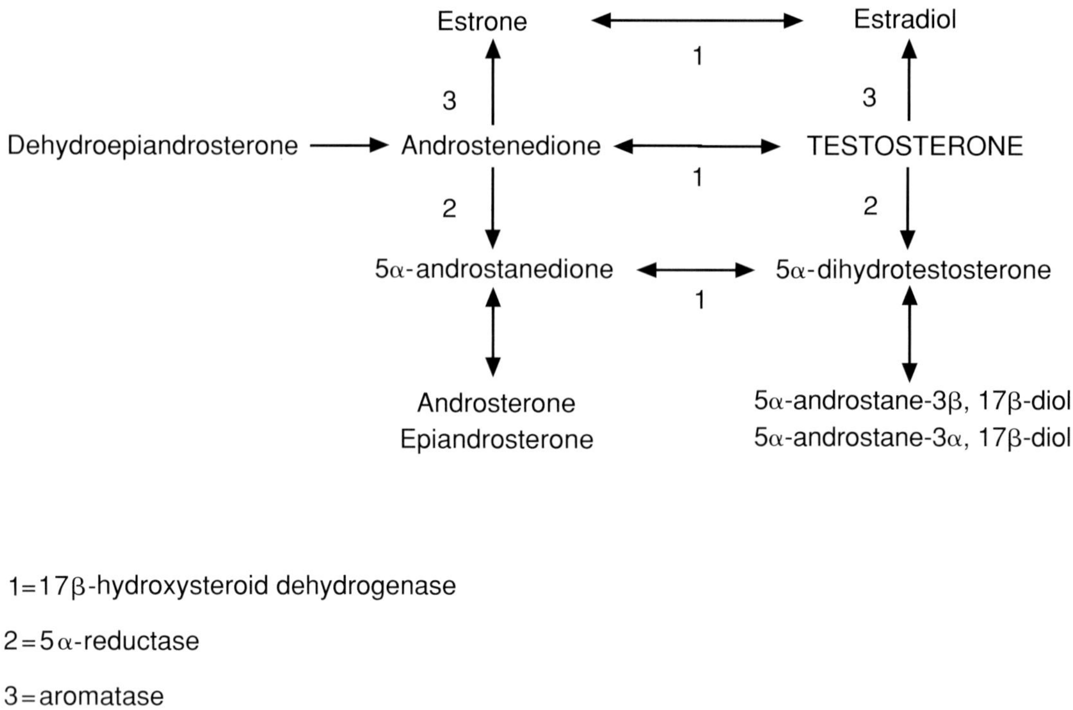

Figure 3-8 Possible pathways of androgen metabolism in the skin.

prevented the development of balding.[81] More recently, the oral administration of finasteride, another 5α-reductase inhibitor, has been shown to increase scalp hair growth in balding macaques.[82]

Several studies, most using plucked hairs as a source of tissue, have looked at the ability of human hair follicles to metabolize androgens.[83,84] These have shown that hair roots have both hydroxysteroid dehydrogenase and 5α-reductase activity. In studies where testosterone was the starting material, the major metabolite was androstenedione and, although testosterone was also metabolized to DHT, the level of 5α-reductase activity did not correlate well with the site-dependent secondary sex characteristics of the hair. Testosterone and androstenedione may also be aromatized to estrogens, and the P_{450} aromatase enzyme has recently been identified by immunostaining in the outer root sheath of hair follicles.[85] The conversion of androstenedione to estrogens has been demonstrated in plucked hair roots,[86] but the level of aromatase activity was very low and the relevance of this metabolic pathway is unknown.

Site of Androgen Action in the Hair Follicle

Androgens alter the size of the hair follicle and the diameter of the hair fiber. They also modify the duration of the hair growth cycle. Treatment of hirsute women with cyproterone acetate reduced the final length of thigh hairs. This was due to a shortening of the anagen phase of the hair cycle rather than a reduction in linear growth rate.[76] Based on morphometric data, Van Scott and Ekel suggested that hair follicle size was dependent on the volume of the dermal papilla,[87] an idea which has some experimental support. Using the rat vibrissa model, Ibrahim and Wright confirmed Oliver's observation that a new dermal papilla was reconstituted from the dermal sheath when the hair bulb was amputated. They also found that the volume of hair fiber growing from such a follicle, after regeneration of the hair matrix, correlated with the volume of the reconstituted dermal papilla.[88] If follicle size and, as has been discussed earlier, the hair cycle are regulated by the dermal papilla, could androgen-dependent changes be due to a

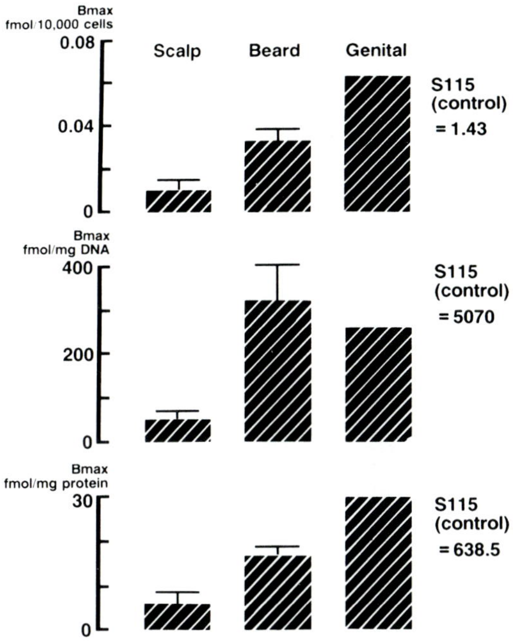

Figure 3-9 Androgen receptor concentrations (Bmax) in cultured human dermal papilla cells from different body sites. Androgen receptors are present in all cells, but the levels are higher in cells derived from beard and pubic follicles than in cells from the scalp. (*From Randall et al.*[94])

primary action on the dermal papilla rather than on the epithelium? This idea is not without precedent, as androgen action in some other tissues is via a primary effect on the mesenchyme.[89–91] If this is also true for the hair follicle, it must follow that dermal papilla cells express androgen receptors. That this is the case has now been shown using two different methods. First, androgen receptors have been demonstrated in the nuclei of dermal papilla cells by immunohistochemical staining of tissue sections.[92] Immunoreactive androgen receptors were also identified in interfollicular keratinocytes and dermal fibroblasts, in sweat glands and sebaceous glands, and in the hair follicle infundibulum. However, there was no staining in epithelial cells in the lower part of the hair follicle. Second, androgen receptors have been identified in cultured human dermal papilla cells by classic binding studies using the synthetic nonmetabolizable androgen mibolerone.[93] Dermal papilla cells from all the body sites so far studied contain saturable androgen receptors, and the receptor concentration is higher in cells from beard and pubic follicles than in those from occipital scalp follicles (Fig. 3-9).

Two studies have shown that cultured human dermal papilla cells are also able to metabolize testosterone in a physiologically relevant way. In dermal papilla cells cultured from occipital scalp follicles and from axillary follicles, the main metabolite of testosterone was androstenedione and there was little or no 5α-reductase activity, whereas in beard dermal papilla cells, the major metabolite was DHT.[95,96] DHT production by beard cells was about fourfold greater than that in cells from occipital scalp or axillary follicles and in reticular dermal fibroblasts from beard skin (Table 3-1). The pattern of testosterone metabolism in cultured dermal papilla cells, in contrast to plucked hair follicles, is therefore in keeping with that expected from the hair distribution in 5α-reductase–deficient individuals, although there is no information yet available on androgen metabolism in dermal papilla cells from balding scalp.

If the dermal papilla is the primary target of androgen action, how does it respond to androgens in order to communicate a growth-regulatory effect on the follicular epithelium? Androgens might act simply by changing the volume of the dermal papilla to alter the area over which matrix cells interact with the papilla. Such changes in papilla volume undoubtedly take place, although we do not know if this reflects a change in cell number, in the volume of the extracellular matrix, or both. Two studies have suggested that cultured beard dermal papilla cells,

Table 3-1
5α-REDUCTASE ACTIVITY IN CULTURED CELLS (PMOL/MG PROTEIN PER HOUR + /– SEM)

Cells	*Beard*	*Occipital Scalp*	*Axilla*
Dermal papilla cells	3.89 ± 0.33	1.08 ± 0.05	1.24 ± 0.27
Dermal fibroblasts	1.14 ± 0.05	0.99 ± 0.05	0.97 ± 0.07

Source: From Itami et al.[97]

but not scalp papilla cells, release mitogenic factors in response to testosterone. Medium conditioned by beard papilla cells cultured in the presence of testosterone stimulated the growth of other dermal papilla cells.[96] Also, the growth of cultured outer root sheath keratinocytes was enhanced when cocultured with beard dermal papilla cells in the presence of testosterone but not by testosterone in the absence of dermal papilla cells.[97] The nature of this androgen-induced mitogenic activity has not yet been determined.

In spite of the progress made in understanding how androgens influence hair growth, it remains a mystery why the same hormones produce opposite effects in different body sites. At this stage, we should not assume that these effects are necessarily due to the same mechanism operating at different levels.

PIGMENTATION

The color of mammalian hair is determined mainly by melanin pigmentation, although its appearance may be modified by other physical characteristics of the hair shaft. Hair melanin is formed by the pigment-producing cells known as *melanocytes,* which are derived embryologically from the neural crest. In the adult follicle, these cells are found within the hair bulb epithelium around the upper half of the dermal papilla (Fig. 3-10). Melanocytes are also present in the basal layer of the infundibulum and, in small numbers, in the outer root sheath of the lower part of the follicle. These latter cells are normally DOPA-negative and nonmelanized and appear to form a melanocyte reservoir in the skin. Under certain circumstances, for example during repigmentation of vitiligo, outer root sheath melanocytes proliferate and migrate to the epidermis.[98] Hair bulb melanocytes donate pigment almost exclusively to cells undergoing early differentiation to form the hair cortex. This is well-illustrated in Figure 3-7*A*. Melanocytes are rarely found in the lower part of the epithelial matrix, where cells are destined mainly to form the inner root sheath, and it is also unusual to find pigment in the hair cuticle. There is, therefore, a close spatial and functional relationship between hair bulb melanocytes and the cells which act as pigment receptors (cortical keratinocytes).

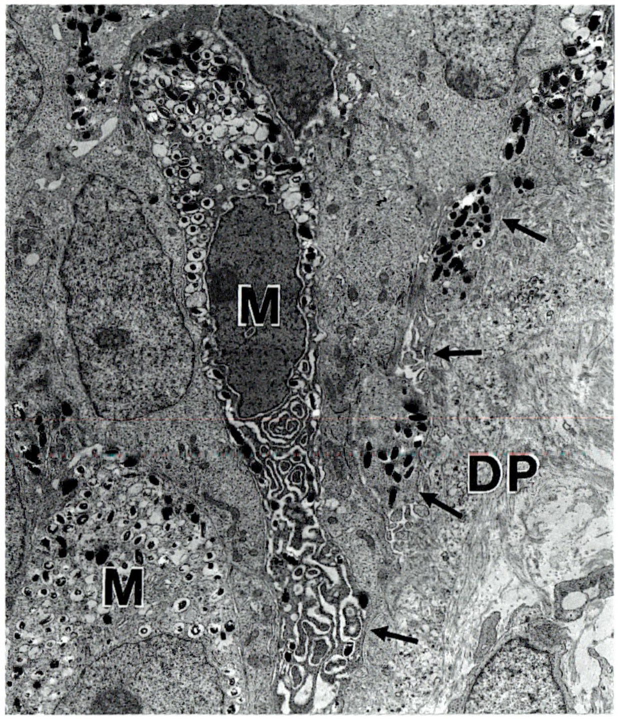

Figure 3-10 Electron micrograph showing two melanocytes (M) adjacent to the epithelial basement membrane (arrows) in the upper hair bulb. DP = dermal papilla. (×4500)

Ultrastructurally, hair bulb melanocytes appear more melanogenic than epidermal melanocytes and their population density is much greater than in the epidermis (approximately one melanocyte to four basal keratinocytes in the upper hair bulb compared to a ratio of 1:25 in the basal layer of the epidermis.[99] Is this due to the effect of different environments on the same cell type, or are hair bulb and epidermal melanocytes separate populations of cells? Perhaps the best evidence to support the former view comes from tissue-recombinant studies in rats. Amputation of the hair bulb of vibrissa follicles effectively removed all hair bulb melanocytes, yet when these follicles regenerated, they often grew pigmented hairs.[20] Even more striking was the demonstration that combinations of cultured pelage dermal papilla cells with glabrous footpad epidermis also resulted in follicles growing pigmented hair.[29] The most probable source for hair bulb melanocytes in these latter follicles is the epidermis. Although a dermal papilla origin cannot be entirely excluded, melanocytes have never been found in this site, and it is also very unlikely that they would survive the several subcultures experienced by the dermal papilla cells. On the other hand, epidermal or hair bulb melanocytes can be lost independently of each other. In vitiligo, hair pigmentation may be retained in the absence of melanocytes in the epidermis, and the reverse is true of senile graying.

Pigmentation and the Hair Growth Cycle

Melanogenic activity varies during the course of the hair growth cycle. "Inactive" melanocytes have been identified in the secondary germ region of murine telogen follicles, and it is assumed that these cells are the precursors of active melanocytes during the next anagen phase.[100] Melanogenesis occurs after epithelial proliferation has started and coincides with the onset of morphological evidence of cortical differentiation. Tyrosinase activity becomes apparent in anagen III, and pigment transfer to cortical epithelium begins in the anagen IV stage of development.[101,102] In pigmented hair follicles, intense melanogenesis continues throughout the remainder of anagen (anagen V and VI) and then ceases with the onset of catagen. Indeed, cessation of pigmentation has been stated to be the earliest sign of impending catagen, preceding the characteristic changes in follicular morphology.[103] It is not clear whether some melanocytes in the hair bulb survive catagen to form the source of cells for the next anagen or whether there is a melanocyte stem-cell population, perhaps in the outer root sheath, which serves this purpose.

Control of Melanogenesis

The genetic regulation of hair pigmentation has been studied extensively in the mouse, where a great number of variants have arisen spontaneously or through selective breeding.[104] These mutations have been mapped to over 50 loci in the mouse genome, a few of which have a large number of alleles. Genetic control is exerted at several points in the pigmentary pathway, including melanocyte migration and proliferation, melanocyte-dermal interactions in the hair bulb, melanocyte morphology, and enzyme activity.

Melanocytes originate in the neural crest, whence their precursors (melanoblasts) migrate to the skin and other body sites. This process is disturbed in several mouse mutant strains, the first of which to be studied was the W mutant. Heterozygous animals (*W*/+) have a white belly spot and mixed pigmented and nonpigmented hairs elsewhere. Homozygotes show other features, including severe anemia, and they lack germ cells in the gonads. A similar phenotype occurs in mutations at a second locus, Steel (*Sl*). In both *W* and *Sl* mutants, melanocytes are absent from hair follicles due to failure of migration during embryogenesis. It has subsequently been established that the *W* locus encodes a tyrosine kinase cell membrane receptor, known as c-kit, and *Sl* encodes the c-kit ligand, stem-cell factor (also known as mast-cell growth factor). C-kit is expressed by hemopoietic stem cells, mast cells, and melanocytes. In the bone marrow, stem-cell factor (SCF) is derived from stromal cells. Direct evidence that c-kit/SCF interaction is necessary for colonization of hair follicles by melanocytes during embryogenesis comes from the studies of Nishikawa and coworkers.[105] They showed that injection of c-kit antibody into pregnant mice caused dilution of hair pigment in the offspring. The timing of injection was critical, the maximal effect occurring with administration of c-kit antibody at 14.5 days post coitum, probably coinciding with melanocyte migration into the skin. In newborn mice, injection of c-kit antibody caused extensive dilution of hair pigment. In adult mice, there was no loss of hair pigment at the site of injection, but small areas of depigmentation appeared more than a month later elsewhere on the skin, possibly corresponding to sites where follicles were in early anagen at the time of injection. This latter experiment strongly implicates the c-kit/SCF pathway in regulating hair pigmentation during the adult hair cycle, as well as in melanocyte migration and skin colonization during embryogenesis.

Two types of melanin are present in mammalian hair, the black-brown pigment eumelanin and the yellow-red pheomelanin. Both are synthesized from tyrosine, which is converted to dopaquinone by the enzyme tyrosinase (Fig. 3-11). Dopaquinone then undergoes a series of oxidative reactions to form either eumelanin or pheomelanin. Subsequent steps in the eumelanin pathway may also be under tyrosinase control. Later events in pheomelanin synthesis appear to rely on the availability of -SH compounds and are independent of tyrosinase. Eumelanin and pheomelanin production have been studied most extensively in mice, where the relative propor-

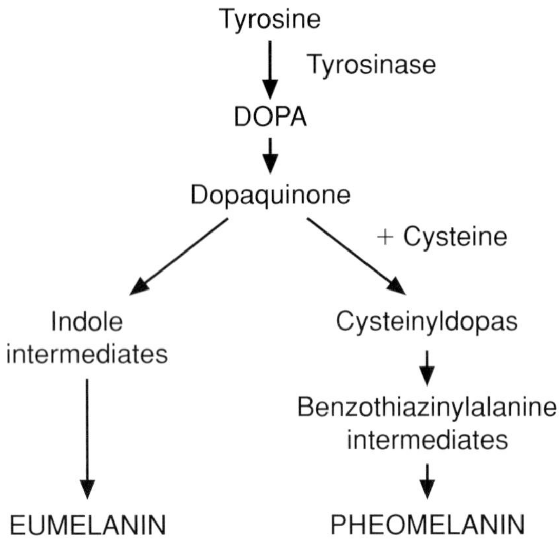

Figure 3-11 Pathways of melanin synthesis.

tions of the two pigments are controlled by alleles at two loci, nonagouti (*a*) and extension (*e*).[104] The *a*-locus phenotype appears to be mediated through the genotype of the hair bulb, not the melanocyte, whereas the effect of *e* is autonomous to the melanocyte, a relationship which is similar to that of *Sl* and *W*, suggesting a receptor-ligand mechanism. Both *a* and *e* loci are multiallelic, and their phenotypic expression varies from a pure yellow coat (pheomelanin) to black (eumelanin). Intermediate phenotypes may show either regional variation in coat color or banded yellow and black pigmentation on a single hair, implying a switch between eumelanogenesis and pheomelanogenesis during a single hair cycle, or they may produce black hairs during one cycle and yellow hairs during the next. In eumelanic follicles, melanocytes contain ellipsoidal melanosomes with a characteristic lamellar internal structure (eumelanosomes). Pheomelanogenesis is associated with melanocytes containing spherical melanosomes which have a less well defined internal structure containing granules or vesicles (pheomelanosomes). Human hair also contains both eumelanin and pheomelanin.[99,106] The highest levels of pheomelanin are found in fire-red hair, although the relationship between hair color and eumelanin-pheomelanin ratios is not clear-cut. Melanocytes in human follicles with highly pheomelanized hairs contain typical pheomelanosomes.[106] In other hair colors, melanocytes have eumelanosomes, even though pheomelanin is present in the hair.

Tyrosinase activity is undoubtedly an important factor in hair pigmentation, and much is known about its regulation in other systems, notably in melanoma cells. In agouti mice, tyrosinase activity is higher in follicles during eumelanogenesis than during pheomelanogenesis.[107] However, tyrosinase mRNA and synthesis levels are the same, suggesting that the lower level of tyrosinase activity during pheomelanogenesis is due to posttranslational regulation.[108] A number of studies have shown that α-melanocyte stimulating hormone (α-MSH) stimulates tyrosinase activity and pigmentation in murine hair follicles.[107,109] In agouti mice, α-MSH stimulates tyrosinase activity during eumelanogenesis but not during pheomelanogenesis. However, α-MSH does not increase tyrosinase activity in human hair follicles,[110] and it is not known whether melanotrophic peptides are normally involved in hair pigmentation.

In some mammalian species living at high latitudes (e.g., snow hares, stoats, some lemmings, and some hamsters), the color of the pelage changes to white in the winter. As in seasonal control of the hair growth cycle, this change in coat color is probably mediated by the pineal gland. In several species, melatonin implants inhibit pigmentation of new hair growth following the spring molt, although it is not clear whether this is a direct effect on follicular melanogenesis.[111] Melatonin is a potent inhibitor of melanogenesis in short-term cultures of hair follicles from the Siberian hamster, although it does not inhibit tyrosinase activity. This latter property of melatonin is in keeping with the observation that the growth of a pigmented coat following the spring molt in the Siberian hamster and growth of a white coat following the autumn molt are associated with a peak in tyrosinase activity of similar magnitude. Thus, in this species melatonin appears to inhibit melanogenesis at a post-tyrosinase stage in the pathway. However, not all animals respond to melatonin in this way, even those showing seasonal changes in coat color, and it is unknown whether melatonin has any physiological role in hair pigmentation in man.

Graying of Hair

Graying of hair is one of the most obvious manifestations of aging in man, yet it has received relatively little research attention compared with other cutaneous features of aging. Simple observation, particularly of younger people, suggests that usually what appears to be gray hair is, in fact, a mixture of white hair and pigmented hair. True gray hairs can be found but are not common until old age. It is also very uncommon to see hairs which show progressive loss of pigment along the length of the hair shaft. Therefore, it seems likely that in the early stages of graying, pigmentation is lost abruptly in individual follicles, and this takes place at some stage in the interval between successive anagen phases or in early anagen prior to the onset of melanogenesis.

In 1921, Bloch showed that the DOPA reaction is negative in white hair bulbs and reduced in true gray hairs.[112] Subsequently, it has been shown by autoradiography that tyrosinase activity is reduced in gray hairs and absent in white hairs.[102] In the most recent study, Nanninga and coworkers found that plucked pigmented hair roots contained specific α-MSH binding sites, whereas white hairs did not.[113] Several ultrastructural studies have failed to identify melanocytes in white hair bulbs.[114–116] However, the identification of melanocytes relies on biochemical or ultrastructural markers, the absence of which does not absolutely exclude melanocytes being present. Sato and coworkers found dendritic "indeterminate" cells in the upper part of white hair bulbs which they suggested may represent effete melanocytes.[116] There are a number of anecdotal reports of repigmentation of senile white hair, sometimes after many years.[117,118] This phenomenon has also been observed following electron beam therapy (E. Olsen, personal communication), and the author has seen this repigmentation in an elderly woman with porphyria cutanea tarda. It is possible, therefore, that graying is not necessarily irreversible, giving hope that one of the more obvious manifestations of aging may yet be conquered.

CONCLUDING REMARKS

Recent years have seen a number of advances in hair biology. In particular, considerable progress has been made in understanding the tissue interactions involved in hair follicle development in both embryonic and adult skin. The emphasis on epithelial or dermal influences fluctuates, but it is gradually becoming clearer that each compartment has an important part to play in regulating events during development and during the hair growth cycle. Such tissue interactions crop up repeatedly and now appear to include androgen-regulated responses and hair follicle pigmentation. We are also beginning to understand the molecular basis of hair growth control, although the picture is still far from clear. The use of models in which the function of specific molecules can be tested is likely to play an increasingly important part in this area. Techniques such as embryonic skin culture, in vitro recombinant cultures, organ cultures, and transgenic constructs are already being used for this purpose in hair biology. However, we are little nearer to understanding one of the most intriguing features of the hair follicle: What is the nature of the "clock" which controls the hair growth cycle and where in the follicle is it situated?

REFERENCES

1. Wessells NK, Roessner KD: Nonproliferation in dermal condensations of mouse vibrissae and pelage hairs. Dev Biol 12:419–433, 1965.
2. Sengel P: *The Morphogenesis of Skin.* Cambridge, Cambridge University Press, 1976.
3. Hardy MH: The secret life of the hair follicle. Trends Genet 8:55–61, 1992.
4. Kollar EJ: The induction of hair follicles by embryonic dermal papillae. J Invest Dermatol 55:374–378, 1970.
5. Moore GP, Panaretto BA, Robertson D: Epidermal growth factor delays the development of the epidermis and hair follicles of mice during growth of the first coat. Anat Rec 205:47–55, 1983.
6. Tam JP: Physiological effects of transforming growth factor in the newborn mouse. Science 229:673–675, 1985.
7. Du Cros DL, Isaacs K, Moore GPM: Localization of epidermal growth factor immunoreactivity in sheep skin during wool follicle development. J Invest Dermatol 98:109–115, 1992.
8. Green MR, Couchman JR: Distribution of epidermal growth factor receptors in rat tissues during embryonic skin development, hair formation, and the adult hair growth cycle. J Invest Dermatol 83:118–123, 1984.
9. Nanney LB et al.: Immunolocalization of epidermal growth factor receptors in normal developing human skin. J Invest Dermatol 94:742–748, 1990.
10. Moore GP et al.: Hair growth induction: Roles of growth factors. Ann NY Acad Sci 642:308–325, 1991.
11. Zshiesche W, Eckert K: Effects of anti-EGF serum on newborn mice. Experientia 44:249–251, 1988.
12. Lyons KM, Pelton RW, Hogan BLM: Organogenesis and pattern formation in the mouse: RNA distribution patterns suggest a role for bone morphogenetic protein-2A (BMP-2A). Development 109:833–844, 1990.
13. Jones CM, Lyons KM, Hogan BLM: Involvement of bone

morphogenetic protein-4 (BMP-4) and Vgr-1 in morphogenesis and neurogenesis in the mouse. Development 111:531–542, 1991.
14. Hardy MH, Van Exan RJ, Sonstergard KS, Sweeny PR: Basal lamina changes during tissue interactions in hair follicles—An *in vitro* study of normal dermal papillae and vitamin A-induced glandular morphogenesis. J Invest Dermatol 80:27–34 1983.
15. Chuong C-M, Ting SA, Widelitz RB, Lee Y-S: Mechanism of skin morphogenesis: II. Retinoic acid modulates axis orientation and phenotypes of skin appendages. Development 115:839–852, 1992.
16. Hirai Y, Nose A, Kobayashi S, Takeichi M: Expression and role of E- and P-cadherin adhesion molecules in embryonic histogenesis: II. Skin morphogenesis. Development 105:271–277, 1989.
17. Chuong C-M, Chen H-M, Jiang T-X, Chia J: Adhesion molecules in skin development: Morphogenesis of feather and hair. Ann NY Acad Sci 642:263–280, 1991.
18. Hirai Y et al.: Epimorphin: A mesenchymal protein essential for epithelial morphogenesis. Cell 69:471–481, 1992.
19. Cohen J: The transplantation of individual rat and guinea-pig whisker papillae. J Embryol Exp Morphol 9:117–127, 1961.
20. Oliver RF: Whisker growth after removal of the dermal papilla and lengths of follicle in the hooded rat. J Embryol Exp Morphol 16:231–244, 1966.
21. Oliver RF: The experimental induction of whisker growth in the hooded rat by implantation of dermal papillae. J Embryol Exp Morphol 18:43–51, 1967.
22. Oliver RF: The induction of follicle formation in the adult hooded rat by vibrissa dermal papillae. J Embryol Exp Morphol 23:219–236, 1970.
23. Oliver RF: Local interactions in mammalian hair growth. In Spearman RIC, Riley PA (eds): *The Skin of Vertebrates.* Linnean Society Symposium Series, no. 9. 1980, pp 199–210. London, Academic Press.
24. Jahoda C, Oliver RF: The growth of vibrissa dermal papilla cells *in vitro.* Br J Dermatol 105:623–627, 1981.
25. Messenger AG: The culture of dermal papilla cells from human hair follicles. Br J Dermatol 110:685–689, 1984.
26. Jahoda CA, Oliver RF: Vibrissa dermal papilla cell aggregative behaviour *in vivo* and *in vitro.* J Embryol Exp Morphol 79:211–224, 1984.
27. Messenger AG, Senior HJ, Bleehen SS: The *in vitro* properties of dermal papilla cell lines established from human hair follicles. Br J Dermatol 114:425–430, 1986.
28. Jahoda CA, Horne KA, Oliver RF: Induction of hair growth by implantation of cultured dermal papilla cells. Nature 311:560–562, 1984.
29. Reynolds AJ, Jahoda CAB: Inductive properties of hair follicle cells. Ann NY Acad Sci 642:226–241, 1991.
30. Reynolds AJ, Jahoda CAB: Hair follicle stem cells? A distinct germinative epidermal cell population is activated *in vitro* by the presence of hair dermal papilla cells. J Cell Sci 99:373–385, 1991.
31. Chase H, Montagna W, Malone J: Changes in the skin in relation to the hair growth cycle. Anat Rec 116:75–82, 1953.
32. Ebling FJ, Hale PA: The composition of female rat skin in relation to region, age, hair growth cycle and hormones. J Endocrinol 36:177–201, 1966.
33. Hansen LS, Coggle JE, Wells J, Charles MW: The influence of the hair cycle on the thickness of mouse skin. Anat Rec 210:569–573, 1984.
34. Durward A, Rudall KM: Studies on hair growth in the rat. J Anat 83:325–335, 1949.
35. Ebling FJG: The hormonal control of hair growth. In Orfanos CE, Happle R (eds): *Hair and Hair Diseases.* Berlin, Springer-Verlag, 1990, pp 267–299.
36. Pecoraro V, Astore I, Barman JM: Cycle of the scalp hair of the new-born child. J Invest Dermatol 43:145–147, 1964.
37. Johnson E: Environmental influences on the hair follicle. In Orfanos CE, Montagna W, Stuttgen G (eds): *Hair Research.* Berlin, Springer-Verlag, 1981, pp 183–194.
38. Allain D, Rougeot J: Induction of autumn moult in mink (Mustela vison Peale and Beauvois) with Melatonin. Reprod Nutr Dev 20:197–201, 1980.
39. Badura LL, Goldman BD: Prolactin-dependent seasonal changes in pelage: Role of the pineal gland and dopamine. J Exp Zool 261:27–33, 1992.
40. Martinet L, Allain D, Weiner C: Role of prolactin in the photoperiodic control of moulting in the mink (Mustela vison). J Endocrinol 103:9–15, 1984.
41. Maurel D, Coutant C, Boissin J: Effects of photoperiod, melatonin implants and castration on molting and on plasma thyroxine, testosterone and prolactin levels in the European badger (Meles meles). Comp Biochem Physiol [A] 93:791–797, 1989.
42. Rose J, Oldfield J, Stormshak F: Apparent role of melatonin and prolactin in initiating winter fur growth in mink. Gen Comp Endocrinol 65:212–215, 1987.
43. Smale L, Dark J, Zucker I: Pineal and photoperiodic influences on fat deposition, pelage, and testicular activity in male meadow voles. J Biolog Rhythms 3:349–355, 1988.
44. Maurel D, Coutant C, Boissin J: Thyroid and gonadal regulation of hair growth during the seasonal molt in the male European badger, Meles meles L. Gen Comp Endocrinol 65:317–327, 1987.
45. Randall VA, Ebling FJ: Seasonal changes in human hair growth. Br J Dermatol 124:146–151, 1991.
46. Lynfield YL: Effect of pregnancy on the human hair cycle. J Invest Dermatol 35:323–327, 1960.
47. Kligman AM: Pathologic dynamics of human hair loss. Arch Dermatol 83:175–198, 1961.
48. Chase HB, Eaton GJ: The growth of hair follicles in waves. Ann NY Acad Sci 83:365–368, 1959.
49. Bullough WS: Mitotic control in mammalian tissues. Biol Rev 50:99–127, 1975.
50. Paus R, Stenn KS, Link RE: Telogen skin contains an inhibitor of hair growth. Br J Dermatol 122:777–784, 1990.
51. Frater R: Inhibition of growth of hair follicles by a lectin-like substance from rat skin. Aust J Biol Sci 36:411–418, 1983.
52. Sutton R et al.: myc Protooncogenes of wool and hair growth. Ann NY Acad Sci 642:326–338, 1991.
53. Moore GPM, Panaretto BA, Carter NB: Epidermal hyperplasia and wool follicle regression in the skin of sheep infused with epidermal growth factor. J Invest Dermatol 84:172–175, 1985.
54. Hollis DE, Chapman RE: Apoptosis in wool follicles during mouse epidermal growth factor (mEGF)-induced catagen regression. J Invest Dermatol 88:455–458, 1987.

55. Philpott MP, Green MR, Kealey T: Human hair growth *in vitro.* J Cell Sci 97:463–471, 1990.
56. Green MR: Distribution of TGFb-1 during the hair growth cycle: Relationship with the connective tissue sheath and dermal papilla. J Invest Dermatol 92:434, 1989.
57. Pierard GE, de la Brassinne M: Modulation of dermal cell activity during hair growth in the rat. J Cutan Pathol 2:35–41, 1975.
58. Montagna W, Chase HB, Malone JD, Melaragno HP: Cyclic changes in polysaccharides of the papilla of the hair follicle. Q J Microscop Sci 93:241–245, 1952.
59. Young RD, Oliver RF: Morphological changes associated with the growth cycle of vibrissal follicles in the rat. J Embryol Exp Morphol 36:597–607, 1976.
60. Westgate GE, Shaw DA, Harrap GF, Couchman JR: Immunohistochemical localization of basement membrane components during hair follicle morphogenesis. J Invest Dermatol 82:259–264, 1984.
61. Couchman JR, Gibson WT: Expression of basement membrane components through morphological changes in the hair growth cycle. Dev Biol 108:290–298, 1985.
62. Couchman JR: Rat hair follicle dermal papillae have an extracellular matrix containing basement membrane components. J Invest Dermatol 87:762, 1986.
63. Couchman JR, King JL, McCarthy KJ: Distribution of two basement membrane proteoglycans through hair follicle development and the hair growth cycle in the rat. J Invest Dermatol 94:65–70, 1990.
64. Messenger AG, Elliott K, Temple A, Randall VA: Expression of basement membrane proteins and interstitial collagens in dermal papillae of human hair follicles. J Invest Dermatol 96:93–97, 1991.
65. Messenger AG, Elliot K, Westgate GE, Gibson WT: Distribution of extracellular matrix molecules in human hair follicles. Ann NY Acad Sci 642:253–262, 1991.
66. Westgate GE, Messenger AG, Watson LP, Gibson WT: Distribution of proteoglycans during the hair growth cycle in human skin. J Invest Dermatol 96:191–195, 1991.
67. Mayer K, Kaplan D, Steigleder GK: Effect of mucopolysaccharides on hair growth in the rabbit. Proc Soc Exp Biol Med 108:59–63, 1961.
68. Goetinck PF, Carlone DL: Altered proteoglycan synthesis disrupts feather pattern formation in chick embryonic skin. Dev Biol 127:179–186, 1988.
69. Harrist TJ, Rutter DJ, Mihm MC Jr, Bhan AK: Distribution of major histocompatibility antigens in normal skin. Br J Dermatol 109:623–633, 1983.
70. Westgate GE, Craggs RI, Gibson WT: Immune privilege in hair growth. J Invest Dermatol 97:417–420, 1991.
71. Link RE et al.: Epithelial growth by rat vibrissa follicles *in vitro* requires mesenchymal contact via native extracellular matrix. J Invest Dermatol 95:202–207, 1990.
72. Lane EB, Wilson CA, Hughes BR, Leigh IM: Stem cells in hair follicles: cytoskeletal studies. Ann NY Acad Sci 642:197–213, 1991.
73. Cotsarelis G, Sun TT, Lavker RM: Label-retaining cells reside in the bulge area of pilosebaceous unit: Implications for follicular stem cells, hair cycle and skin. Cell 61:1329–1337, 1990.
74. Hamilton JB: Male hormone is a prerequisite and an incitant in common baldness. Am J Anat 71:451–480, 1942.
75. Hamilton JB: Age, sex and genetic factors in the regulation of hair growth in man: A comparison of Caucasian and Japanese populations. In Montagna W, Ellis RA (eds): *The Biology of Hair Growth.* New York, Academic Press, 1958, pp 399–433.
76. Ebling FJ et al.: Effect of cyproterone acetate on hair growth, sebaceous secretion and endocrine parameters in a hirsute subject. Br J Dermatol 97:371–381, 1977.
77. Mortimer CH, Rushton DH, James KC: Effective medical treatment for common baldness in women. Clin Exp Dermatol 9:342–350, 1984.
78. King RJB: The structure and function of steroid receptors. J Endocrinol 114:341–349, 1987.
79. Strauss JS, Pochi PE: The hormonal control of the pilosebaceous unit. In Toda K, Ishibashi Y, Yori Y, Morikawa F (eds): *Biology and Disease of the Hair.* Baltimore, University Park Press, 1976, pp 231–245.
80. Imperato-McGinley J: Sexual differentiation: Normal and abnormal. In Martini L, James VGT (eds): *Current Topics in Experimental Endocrinology.* vol. 5. New York, Academic Press, 1983, pp 231–307.
81. Rittmaster RS et al.: The effects of N,N-diethyl-4-methyl-3-oxo-4-aza-5 alpha-androstane-17 beta-carboxamide, a 5 alpha-reductase inhibitor and anti-androgen, on the development of baldness in the stumptail macaque. J Clin Endocrinol Metab 65:188–193, 1987.
82. Diani AR et al.: Hair growth effects of oral administration of finasteride, a steroid 5 alpha-reductase inhibitor, alone and in combination with topical minoxidil in the balding stumptail macaque. J Clin Endocrinol Metab 74:345–350, 1992.
83. Takayasu S, Adachi K: The conversion of testosterone to 17 beta-hydroxy-5 alpha-androstan-3-one (dihydrotestosterone) by human hair follicles. J Clin Endocrinol Metab 34:1098–1101, 1972.
84. Schweikert HU, Wilson JD: Androgen metabolism in isolated human hair roots. In Orfanos CE, Montagna W, Stuttgen G (eds): *Hair Research.* Berlin, Springer-Verlag, 1981, pp 210–214.
85. Sawaya ME, Penneys NS: Immunohistochemical distribution of aromatase and 3B-hydroxysteroid dehydrogenase in human hair follicle and sebaceous gland. J Cutan Pathol 19:309–314, 1991.
86. Schweikert HU, Milewich L, Wilson JD: Aromatization of androstenedione by isolated human hairs. J Clin Endocrinol Metab 40:413–417, 1975.
87. Van Scott E, Ekel TM: Geometric relationships between the matrix of the hair bulb and its dermal papilla in normal and alopecic scalp. J Invest Dermatol 31:281–287, 1958.
88. Ibrahim L, Wright EA: A quantitative study of hair growth using mouse and rat vibrissal follicles: I. Dermal papilla volume determines hair volume. J Embryol Exp Morphol 72:209–224, 1982.
89. Lasnitzki I, Mizuno T: Prostatic induction: Interaction of epithelium and mesenchyme from normal wild-type mice and androgen insensitive mice with testicular feminization. J Endocrinol 85:423–428, 1980.
90. Cuhna GR, Lung B: The possible influence of temporal factors in androgenic responsiveness of urogenital tissue recombinants from wild type and androgen insensitive (TFM) mice. J Exp Zool 205:181–194, 1978.
91. Cooke PS, Young P, Cunha GR: Androgen receptor expression in developing male reproductive organs. Endocrinology 128:2867–2873, 1991.

92. Choudhry R et al.: Localization of androgen receptors in human skin by immunohistochemistry: Implications for the hormonal regulation of hair growth, sebaceous glands and sweat glands. J Endocrinol 133(3):467–475, 1992.
93. Randall VA, Thornton MJ, Messenger AG: Cultured dermal papilla cells from androgen-dependent human hair follicles (e.g., beard) contain more androgen receptors than those from non-balding areas of scalp. J Endocrinol 133:141–147, 1992.
94. Randall VA et al.: Androgens and the hair follicle: Cultured human dermal papilla cells as a model system. Ann NY Acad Sci 642:355, 1991.
95. Itami S, Kurata S, Takayasu S: 5 alpha-reductase activity in cultured human dermal papilla cells from beard compared with reticular dermal fibroblasts. J Invest Dermatol 94:150–152, 1990.
96. Randall VA, Thornton MJ, Hamada K, Messenger AG: Mechanism of androgen action in cultured dermal papilla cells derived from human hair follicles with varying responses to androgens *in vivo.* J Invest Dermatol 98:86S–91S, 1992.
97. Itami S, Kurata S, Sonoda T, Takayasu S: Mechanism of action of androgen in dermal papilla cells. Ann NY Acad Sci 642:385–395, 1991.
98. Cui J, Shen L-Y, Wang G-C: Role of hair follicles in the repigmentation of vitiligo. J Invest Dermatol 97:410–416, 1991.
99. Cesarini JP: Hair melanin and hair color. In Orfanos CE, Happle R (eds): *Hair and Hair Diseases.* Berlin, Springer-Verlag, 1990, pp 165–197.
100. Sugiyama S, Kukita A: Melanocyte reservoir in the hair follicles during the hair growth cycle: An electron microscopic study. In Toda K, Ishibashi Y, Yori Y, Morikawa F (eds): *Biology and Disease of the Hair.* Baltimore, University Park Press, 1976, pp 181–200.
101. Kukita A: Changes in tyrosinase activity during melanocyte proliferation in the hair growth cycle. J Invest Dermatol 28:273–274, 1957.
102. Fitzpatrick TB, Brunet P, Kukita A: The nature of hair pigment. In Montagna W, Ellis RA (eds): *The Biology of Hair Growth.* New York, Academic Press, 1958, pp 255–303.
103. Montagna W, Parakkal PF: *The Structure and Function of Skin.* New York, Academic Press, 1974.
104. Jackson IJ: Mouse coat colour mutations: A molecular genetic resource which spans the centuries. BioEssays 13:439–446, 1991.
105. Nishikawa S et al.: *In utero* manipulation of coat colour formation by a monoclonal anti-c-kit antibody: Two distinct waves of c-kit-dependency during melanocyte development. Embo J 10:2111–2118, 1991.
106. Jimbow K et al.: Combined chemical and electron microscopic studies of pheomelanosomes in human red hair. J Invest Dermatol 81:506–511, 1983.
107. Burchill SA, Thody AJ: Melanocyte stimulating hormone and the regulation of tyrosinase activity. J Endocrinol 111:225–232, 1986.
108. Burchill SA, Virden R, Thody AJ: Regulation of tyrosinase synthesis and its processing in the hair follicular melanocytes of the mouse during eumelanogenesis and pheomelanogenesis. J Invest Dermatol 93:236–240, 1989.
109. Levine N et al.: Stimulation of follicular melanogenesis in the mouse by topical and injected melanotropins. J Invest Dermatol 89:269–273, 1987.
110. Burchill SA, Ito S, Thody AJ: Tyrosinase expression and its relationship to eumelanin and pheomelanin synthesis in human hair follicles. J Dermatol Sci 2:281–286, 1991.
111. Weatherhead B: The pineal gland and pigmentation. In Jarrett A (ed): *The Physiology and Pathophysiology of the Skin,* vol 7. London, Academic Press, 1982, pp 2165–2179.
112. Bloch B: Uber die Entwicklung des Haut-und Haarpigmentes beim menslichen Embryo und uber das Erloschen der Pigmentbildung im ergrauenden Haar (Ursache der Canities). Arch Dermatol Syph (Berlin) 135:77–108, 1921.
113. Nanninga PB et al.: Evidence for alpha-MSH binding sites on human scalp hair follicles. Pigment Cell Res 4:193–198, 1991.
114. Fitzpatrick TB, Szabo G, Mitchell RE: Age changes in the human melanocyte system. In Montagna W (ed): *Advances in Biology of Skin,* vol 6. Oxford, Pergamon Press, 1965, pp 35–50.
115. Herzberg J, Gusek W: Das ergrauen des kopfhaares. Arch Klin Exp Dermatol 236:368–384, 1970.
116. Sato S, Kukita A, Jimbow K: Electron microscopic studies of dendritic cells in the human gray and white hair matrix during anagen. Pigment Cell 1:20–26, 1973. In: McGovern VJ, Russel P (eds): *Pigment Cell,* vol 1. Basel Karger, 1973, pp 20–27.
117. Comaish S: White scalp hairs turning black—An unusual reversal of the aging process. Br J Dermatol 86:513–514, 1972.
118. Verbov J: Erosive candidiasis of the scalp, followed by the reappearance of black hair after 40 years. Br J Dermatol 105:595–598, 1981.

Chapter

4

CLINICAL TOOLS FOR ASSESSING HAIR LOSS

Elise A. Olsen

INTRODUCTION

Physicians often find it problematic to manage patients with hair loss because of both the difficulty in making a specific diagnosis and the small therapeutic armamentarium currently available. However, many hair loss problems *can* be treated effectively with existing measures, and mechanistic and therapeutic advances are occurring at a rapid pace. The key to proper management is correct diagnosis, which can be accomplished in an outpatient visit with the clinical tools of a thorough history, a limited physical examination, microscopic analysis of the hair, and, in some cases, a scalp biopsy. Each of these important components of the evaluation of a patient with hair loss will be discussed in this chapter.

SCALP EXAMINATION

As with other medical disorders, the diagnosis of hair loss is best approached by first developing a differential diagnosis and then performing a directed history and physical examination and appropriate ancillary tests. Perhaps the easiest way to immediately focus and narrow the differential is to determine if the hair loss is (1) diffuse or focal and (2) scarring or nonscarring. These two physical aspects of the hair loss, which can be easily determined by a quick inspection of the scalp, will determine how to effectively approach the workup of the patient. Hence, to expedite matters, the evaluation of a new patient with hair loss should begin with an examination of the scalp.

Diffuse hair loss, according to this definition, implies a more or less even distribution of hair loss. If there is a question as to whether the hair loss is truly diffuse or variably affects different areas of the scalp (focal), parting the hair in various sections of the scalp and comparing the part width may be helpful. For example, in most women with androgenetic alopecia, the hair density will be greater and the part width narrower in the occiput than on the top of the head

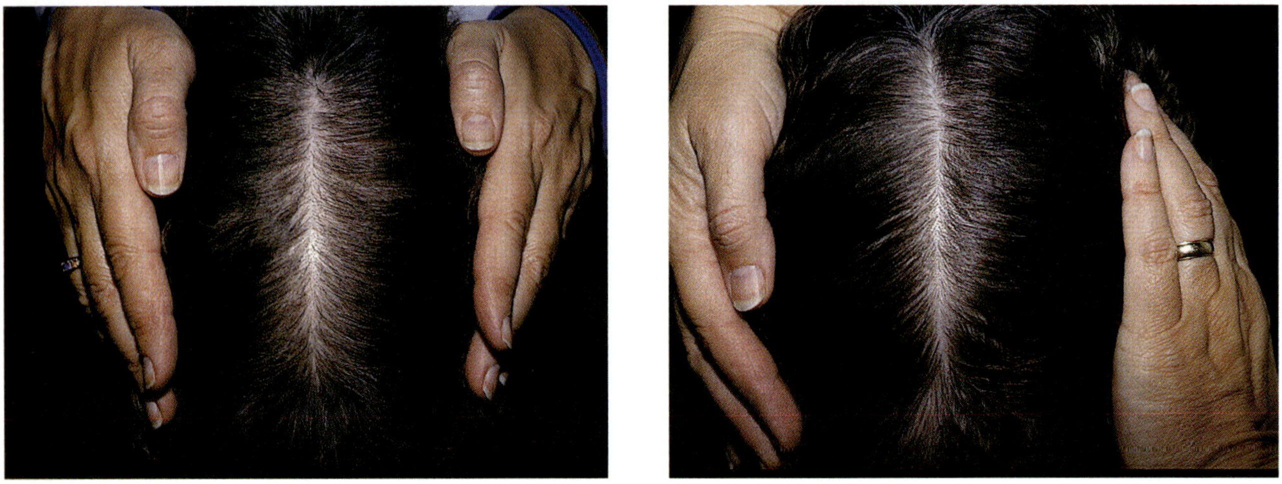

A B

Figure 4-1 Woman with early androgenetic alopecia demonstrating differential hair density on the top of the scalp (*A*) vs. occiput (*B*).

(Fig. 4-1*A* and *B*). *Focal* hair loss may be either unifocal or multifocal and either limited or widespread.

Scarring (or *permanent*) vs. *nonscarring* alopecia depends on whether there has been permanent destruction of the hair follicle or temporary cessation of hair growth. In the former, the bulge area and sebaceous gland are affected and the upper follicular duct generally is obliterated. Hence, the overlying skin is relatively smooth and devoid of pores in scarring alopecia (Fig. 4-2*A* and *B*). Occasionally, however, it is difficult to determine this clinically, and one must resort to a biopsy to determine if scarring is present.

Once the physician has determined these two simple physical features, diffuse versus focal loss and scarring versus nonscarring, the schema shown in Table 4-1 can be used to direct further evaluation. There are obvious problems in trying to pigeonhole some disorders such as alopecia areata, which can assume many different guises, but this schema works well in most situations. It is important to note that the history, physical examination, and hair analysis will be the most important determinants of the etiology of non-

Figure 4-2 Close-up of scalp demonstrating scarring (*A*) vs. nonscarring (*B*) alopecia.

A B

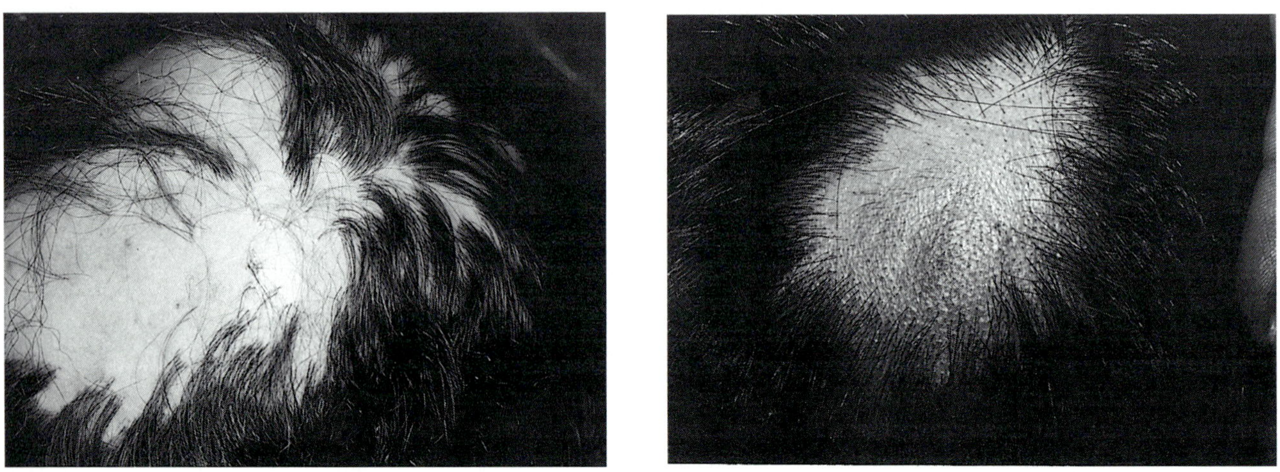

Table 4-1
DIFFERENTIAL DIAGNOSIS OF HAIR LOSS

Nonscarring hair loss
Diffuse
Breakage
Anagen effluvium
Hair shaft disorder
Physical or chemical processing
Telogen effluvium
Androgenetic alopecia (women)
Alopecia totalis or universalis
Loose anagen syndrome
Failure of or abnormal production
Focal
Infection
Traumatic
Alopecia areata
Hair breakage
Androgenetic alopecia (men and women)
Developmental
Scarring hair loss
See Chapter 12, Table 12-2

scarring loss, whether focal or diffuse, whereas a scalp biopsy is the *only* way to determine the etiology of a scarring alopecia. Each of the causes of hair loss will be discussed thoroughly in subsequent chapters.

Diffuse Hair Loss

In the case of diffuse hair loss, one would want to determine if the loss is (1) active, stable, or resolving; (2) secondary to hair breakage or to damage or transformation of the hair root; and (3) predominantly anagen or telogen loss. Sometimes it is difficult to determine from mere visual inspection that hair loss has even occurred. This is particularly true in patients who normally have very thick (dense) hair, who can lose up to 50 percent of their hair without it being obvious to people unfamiliar with the patient.

THE HAIR PULL

There are two ways to corroborate that abnormal hair loss is actively occurring. First and simplest is the *hair pull.* In this procedure, the physician grasps the base of a clump of 50 to 100 hairs between thumb and forefinger and gently pulls on the hair proximally to distally. This is repeated in various sections of the scalp, six to eight times total. Normally, a total of 2 to 5 telogen hairs will be obtained in this manner, depending on when the hair was last shampooed and styled. The latter situations will, of course, have removed many of the readily shed telogen hairs so that the longer the time period since shampooing, the more telogen hairs obtained in a hair pull. An active telogen effluvium is generally easy to recognize since, in this situation, the number of hairs in a hair pull will be at least three to four times normal, with 1 to 5 hairs shed *per clump* of hair examined. Disorders such as androgenetic alopecia or a resolving telogen effluvium may have a slight to moderate increase in hairs shed in a hair pull but generally fewer than that seen in an active telogen effluvium.

QUANTITATIVE ANALYSIS OF HAIR SHEDDING

Determining the actual number of hairs shed per day can be helpful to corroborate the loss, or to reassure the patient that the process is either stable or resolving. Because shampooing and grooming practices vary from day to day and each affects hair shedding, averaging the daily hair shedding over at least a week's span is important. Patients are asked to collect all hairs shed in the shower, sink, brush, and on the counter, pillow, etc. daily for 7 days in individual plastic bags and then to count and average these. Normally, the daily loss is 50 to 100 hairs per day[1]: the 100 hairs per day quoted widely in the literature[2] appears in practice to be far more than the average young, healthy person loses. The hair shedding can be several hundred per day in an active telogen effluvium, which is to be expected if the telogen percentage increases from a normal of 10 percent to 30 to 40 percent. Performing a hair count is tedious and time-consuming for the patient but is often reassuring. In addition, it is a simple tool that patients can use at home to follow the progress of their hair loss or regrowth.

MICROSCOPIC HAIR ANALYSIS

The proximal end of those hairs obtained on a hair pull should be evaluated microscopically. The proximal ends are placed on a glass slide on which a drop of cyanoacrylic glue (example: Acrytol, Surgipath Medical Industries, Inc., Grayslake, IL) has been placed. This not only serves to facilitate the correct orientation and placement of the hair on the slide, but once a coverslip is placed over this, it provides a permanent record of the hair in question. A fine-tipped marker (such as a Sharpie) can be used to write the patient's name, date, and identifying number directly on the slide for permanent record keeping. The distal excess hair can be cut off but should be kept initially, in case the entire shaft warrants inspection. The proximal hairs are then evaluated under light microscopy at low (×10) power.

One of three findings will be evident on examination of the proximal hairs: normal telogen bulbs, broken hairs, or abnormal anagen hairs. In the vast majority of cases, one will see only normal telogen bulbs: this is what you would see on examination of a normal scalp, in androgenetic alopecia, in telogen effluvium, or in late anagen effluvium when all the anagen hairs have already been shed. The telogen hair bulb is easy to recognize. To the naked eye, it appears to have a dry, rounded-up, bulbous white end which, on microscopic exam, looks like a "club." There is no terminal hair shaft pigment and no keratogenous zone.[3] There is no attached inner or outer root sheath (Fig. 4-3).

If examination of the proximal ends of the hairs obtained on a hair pull reveals anagen hair(s), one is almost certainly dealing with an anagen effluvium or loose anagen syndrome. Normal anagen hairs cannot be dislodged by the degree of traction generated by a simple hair pull but rather require forcible plucking with a forceps, hemostat, or needle holder. Pulling on anagen hairs will generally cause breakage before extraction of the entire hair shaft occurs. Therefore, any number of anagen hairs present on a hair pull is abnormal.

Clinically, an extracted anagen hair has a moist, pigmented hair bulb compared with the

Figure 4-3 Telogen hair obtained by hair pull. (× 10)

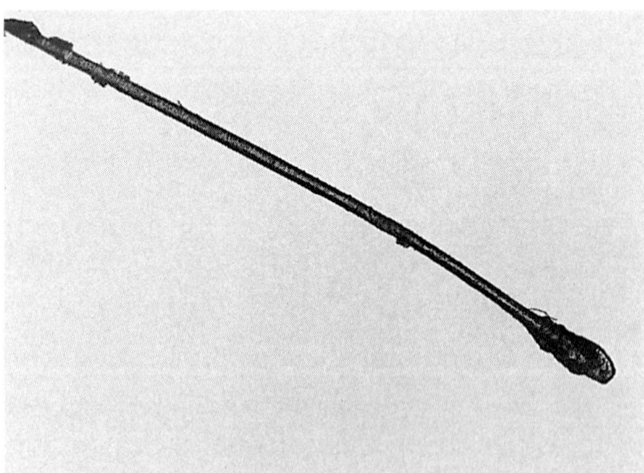

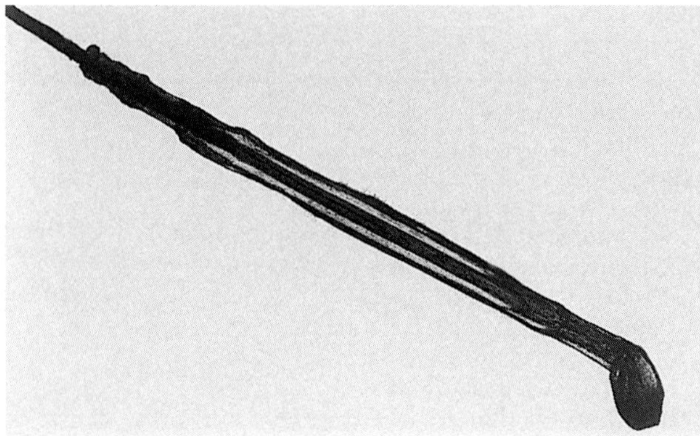

Figure 4-4 Normal anagen hair obtained by plucking. Note dark keratogenous zone, medulla, inner root sheath, outer root sheath. (× 10)

hard, dry, unpigmented bulb of a telogen hair. On light microscopy, normal anagen hairs have a somewhat pyramidal-shaped bulb with attached inner and outer root sheaths (Fig. 4-4). The latter can be documented by staining with 4-dimethyl-amino-cinnamaldehyde (DACA), which selectively stains the citrulline-rich inner root sheath[4] (see Fig. 9-3*B*). The shed anagen hair of the loose anagen syndrome is distinct for the poor attachment of the cuticle to the shaft[5] and, hence, a "floppy-sock" appearance (Fig. 4-5). If intact anagen hairs are obtained on a hair pull in an anagen effluvium, the hair bulbs are typically distorted in appearance. The proximal anagen roots of hairs at the periphery of an area of alopecia areata may be tapered or, rarely, arrowhead-shaped (Fig. 4-6).

In an anagen effluvium, in cases of endogenous or exogenous hair shaft abnormalities, and

Figure 4-5 Abnormal anagen hair of loose anagen syndrome. Note ruffled cuticle. (× 10)

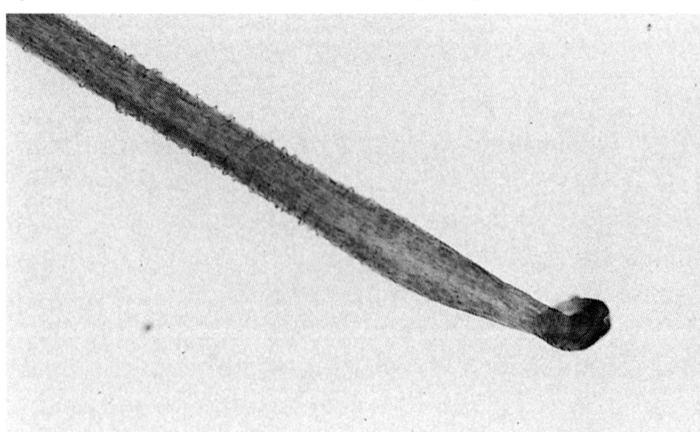

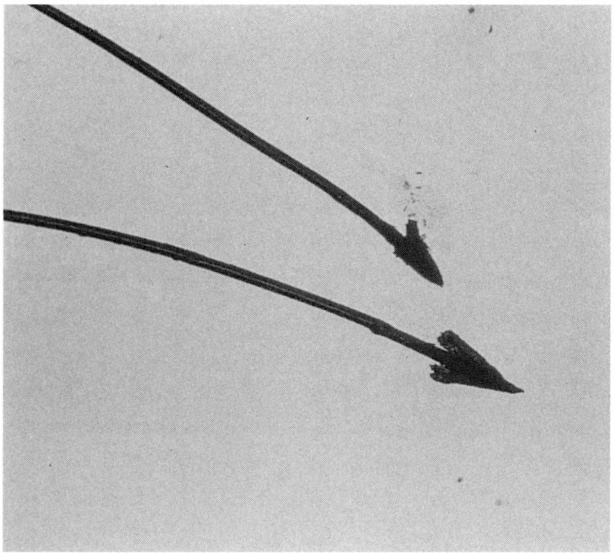

Figure 4-6 Arrowhead-shaped proximal anagen hairs in alopecia areata. (*Courtesy of Dr. David Pariser; reprinted with permission from Pariser DM, Caserio RJ, Eaglstein WH:* Techniques for Diagnosing Skin and Hair Disease, *New York, Thieme Inc., 1986.*)

in the exclamation-point hairs of alopecia areata, at least some of the proximal hairs will demonstrate breakage. In cases of presumed hair breakage or fragility, one will also need to examine cut hairs not subjected to the trauma of pulling or plucking. A group of 10 to 20 hairs should be grasped at the base and cut with scissors close to the scalp. The hairs should be mounted on a slide in which cyanoacrylic glue has been placed (as noted earlier): this slide preparation is easy to do and causes little artifact. One should keep the cut ends together and all the hairs oriented in the same direction to facilitate the microscopic examination. Distal hairs that protrude from the edge of the slide can be clipped and similarly placed on a second slide for separate evaluation. Other methods of slide preparation have been suggested, including placing hairs between two slides and taping closed,[6] placing double-sided sticky tape on a slide and placing the hair on this,[7] or placing the hair in a petri dish with water.[8] All of these can then be examined by light microscopy under low power. The entire shaft should be evaluated for areas of potential hair fragility. Examination of the distal ends may confirm hair breakage, but often it is evaluation of the proximal ends that demonstrates the diagnostic pathology. Looking at the distal ends of the hair in areas where patients complain that the hair does not grow, however, can be extremely useful. If the distal ends are blunt and artificially flat, they are almost certainly cut, suggesting factitial disease.

Besides hair breakage, microscopic hair shaft analysis may be useful in assessing the relative diameter of the hairs. In a normal scalp, terminal hairs are of variable diameter.[9] In women with androgenetic alopecia, this variability is exaggerated in involved areas, exhibiting a mosaic of miniaturized and normal-sized terminal hair shafts.[10]

In some cases of fragile hair, light-microscopic examination may suggest, but not confirm, the diagnosis. In these cases, one may wish to do an examination by polarized light microscopy or scanning electron microscopy (SEM). Although a special polarizing microscope is ideal, one can modify an ordinary microscope to perform this function. One plastic polarizing lens is placed between the light source and the microscope stage, and the second lens is placed in the body or the eyepiece of the microscope or over the slide on the microscope stage. The top lens is then rotated until the background becomes completely dark. Use of polarized light microscopy is particularly useful in cases where one sees trichoschisis and/or trichorrhexis nodosa on light microscopy in a clinical setting of a child with diffuse fragile, short hair. A diagnosis of trichothiodystrophy would then be suggested and would be confirmed under polarized microscopy by the presence of zigzag alternating light and dark transverse bands on the affected hairs.[11]

No special preparation of the hair needs to be performed prior to SEM. Some selectivity should be used when choosing representative sections of hair (confirmed by light microscopy) to be evaluated by SEM. The hairs are then mounted on aluminum stubs with double-sided tape and coated with 200 Å of gold-palladium. Certain abnormalities, such as the longitudinal furrows of spun-glass hair, may be apparent with SEM but not with light microscopy.

HAIR PLUCK

In cases where one wishes to establish an anagen-telogen ratio or to evaluate whether any catagen hairs are present, a hair pluck should be performed. As originally described, a hair pluck involved grasping about 50 hairs with a needle holder or hemostat at the base of the hairs and extracting them with a quick, forceful pull.[8] The tips of the hemostat could be covered with rubber tips (those from needle covers for injectable medications may be used) to facilitate grasping.[12] In practice, this method is too painful and causes too much distortion of the anagen bulbs to be useful. Instead, a rapid hair pluck of only 15 to 20 hairs will produce a tolerable brief discomfort and will minimize distortion because tension is more evenly distributed on all hairs. This can be repeated to obtain the total number of hairs desired for evaluation. The proximal hairs are then mounted on a slide as for routine hair analysis and an anagen-telogen ratio determined. With this procedure, one may see an occasional catagen root which has a club-shaped keratinized tip like a telogen hair, but with an attached inner and outer root sheath. A slow pluck can artifactually cause a normal anagen hair to appear dystrophic, resembling the bulb seen in loose anagen syndrome.[13] There is little reason to do a hair pluck in the face of the information that can be obtained by analyzing hairs obtained by the painless hair pull. One can clearly establish an anagen or telogen effluvium by a hair pull alone. Where one needs to evaluate the roots of short or broken hairs, individual hairs can be epilated.

Whatever the findings, the combination of a scalp examination, hair pull, and microscopic evaluation of hair from this pull can narrow the differential diagnosis of diffuse hair loss to telogen effluvium, a hair shaft abnormality, anagen effluvium, or loose anagen syndrome (Fig. 4-13).

Focal Hair Loss

Focal hair loss can be localized to certain sections of the scalp that assume an easily recognizable pattern (e.g., androgenetic alopecia) or can be present in single or multiple foci on the scalp. Although some types of "focal" hair loss can be quite widespread (e.g., alopecia areata; Fig. 4-7), none of these conditions assumes the more or less uniform diminution in hair density seen in the conditions arbitrarily classified under "diffuse" hair loss. In focal hair loss, aside from androgenetic alopecia, one generally finds diagnostic short or broken hairs. In alopecia areata, short (< 4 mm) hairs with the distal tip larger than the proximal end take on the appearance of "exclamation-point" hairs. These are classic for active alopecia areata[14] (Fig. 4-8).

Fungal infections of the hair affect the structural integrity of the hair shaft. Clinically, affected hairs are either broken off at various points above the scalp surface or fill, but do not come out from, the follicular opening ("black-dot" ringworm). To establish a diagnosis of tinea capitis, broken hairs should be plucked, placed on a slide with potassium hydroxide (KOH), and examined microscopically. In a positive KOH preparation, one sees spores in or on the hair shaft. A negative KOH preparation does not rule out the diagnosis, since many more tinea capitis infections are KOH-negative than are culture-negative.[15] Broken hairs should be planted on Sabouraud's agar with added chlorhexidine and an antibiotic. There are no nonpathogenic fungi that can cause hair loss analogous to nail dystrophy, and only fungal cultures of dermatophytes are clinically important.

As previously discussed, normal anagen hairs

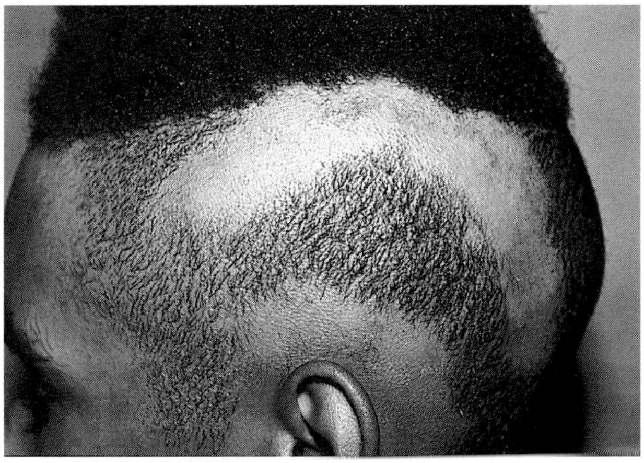

Figure 4-7 Widespread alopecia areata.

Figure 4-8 Exclamation-point hairs.

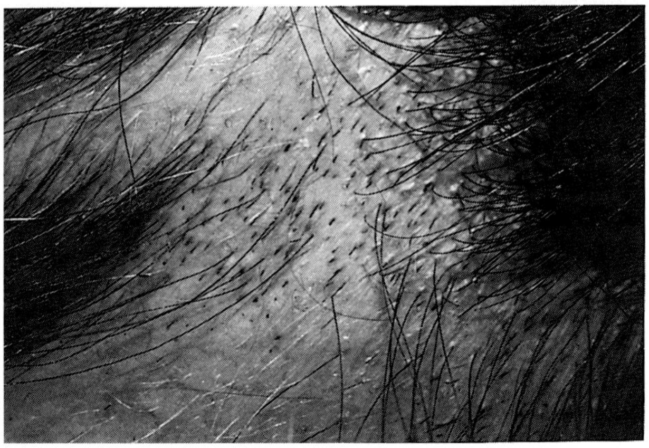

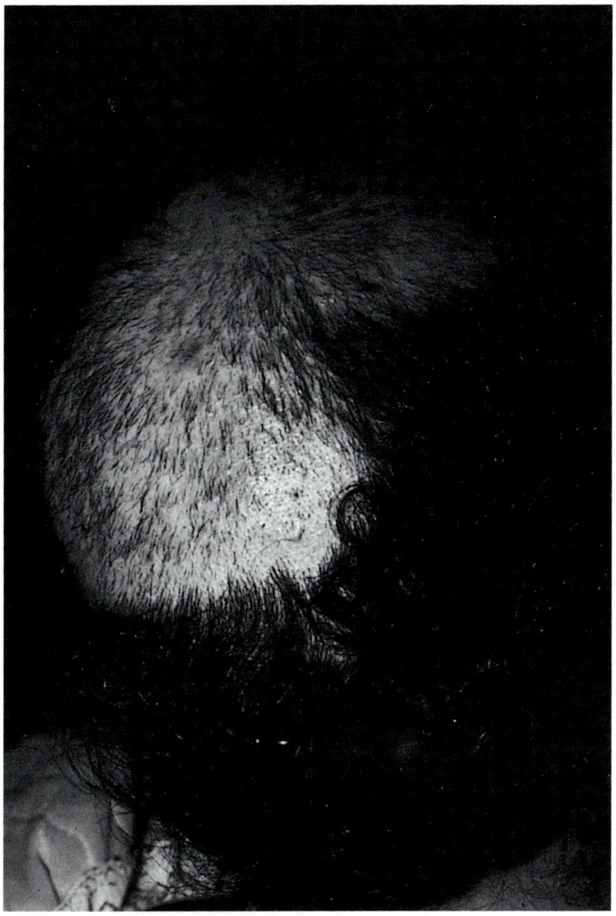

Figure 4-9 Trichotillomania.

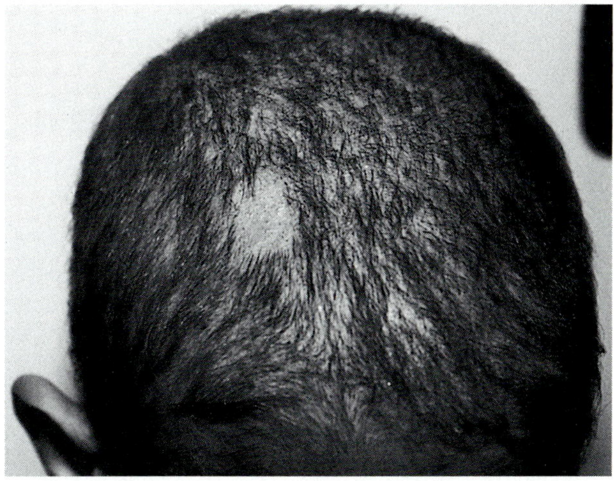

Figure 4-10 Trichotillomania, diffuse involvement. Note hair window.

cannot be pulled out by simply grasping and pulling with the fingers, but rather usually break off. In trichotillomania, the clinical hallmark is multiple broken-off hairs of variable length[16] (Fig. 4-9). The hair loss is generally focal but can be diffuse (Fig. 4-10). Patients with trichotillomania may also secretly cut rather than pull out their hair. Trichotillomania can look similar to tinea capitis, but microscopic evaluation of the short hairs shows either broken or cut (blunt) ends and normal hair shafts.

One would want to pluck and evaluate microscopically both the short hairs and surrounding longer hairs in areas of suspected physical damage from chemicals and/or heat. One usually sees early hair shaft abnormalities in some of the longer hairs that will explain the hair breakage seen in the shorter hairs.

HAIR WINDOW

Occasionally, one will see a patient who states categorically that the hair will not grow in a given area. Typically, these patients have sparse hair of variable length in the area in question and a negative KOH and hair shaft analysis of involved hairs. Trichotillomania is commonly suspected but usually unproven. Either a "hair window" or a scalp biopsy can provide valuable objective corroborative evidence. A hair window is produced by clipping or shaving a small area of the scalp and observing the hair growth after a period of days to weeks. To eliminate any potential confusion with a naturally occurring spot of hair loss, a square or rectangular area at least one square inch in area is preferred. Since most hair windows are done in patients with suspected trichotillomania, it is preferable to choose a site on the back of the head or where the patient cannot easily reach. Some physicians may wish to place something over the site to keep patients from potentially manipulating the area: a small piece of Duoderm cut to fit within the margins of the hair window can do this effectively and will not prevent hair growth. Since scalp hair normally grows approximately 1 cm per month,[17] the patient should be expected to have proportional hair growth when evaluated 2 to 4 weeks later (Fig. 4-11*A*, *B*).

HISTORY

Each patient with hair loss should have a thorough, directed history taken. Diffuse scalp hair loss implies an insult to the anagen hair population, which makes up 85 to 90 percent of the

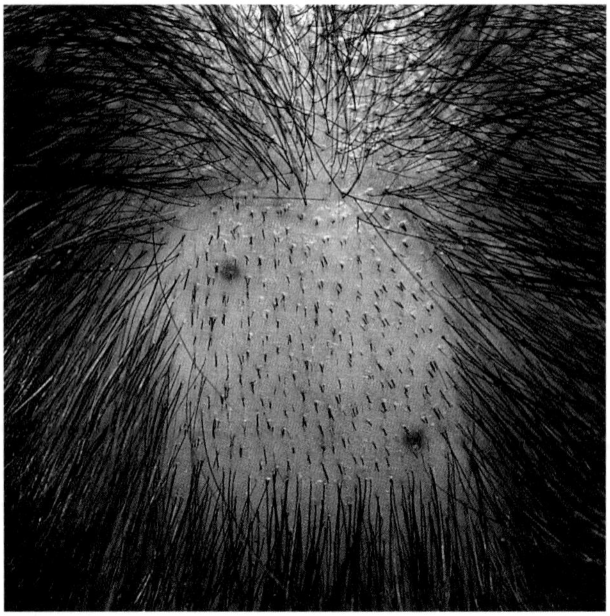
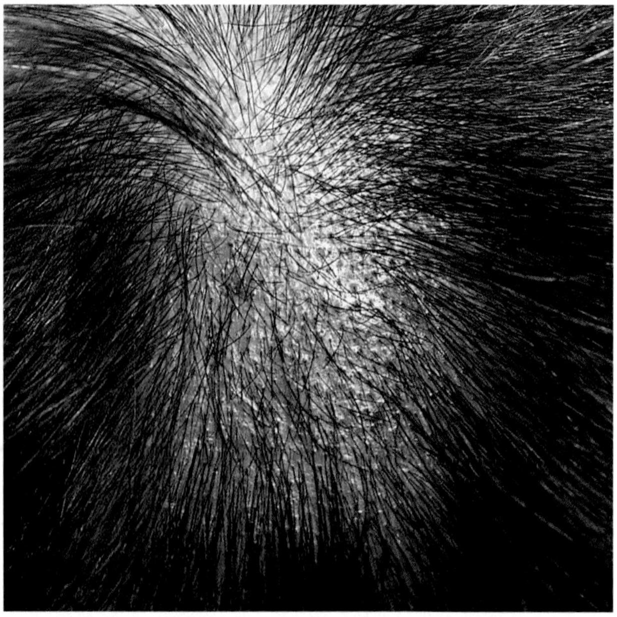

A B

Figure 4-11 Hair window at baseline (*A*) and 2 weeks (*B*). The tattoos were placed as part of a study but serve to demonstrate the identical location of the target area.

scalp hair.[2,17] Any generalized physical insult, whether it be illness, nutritional deprivation, or toxicity from a drug, can affect the rapidly dividing matrix cells. There are two potential responses of the hair to this insult: (1) to prematurely terminate anagen and move into telogen, or (2) to temporarily interrupt or slow the normal cell division and differentiation of matrix cells in anagen. The first response results clinically in the common condition termed *telogen effluvium.* Telogen scalp hair loss has an obligatory delay of 3 to 4 months from the time of the insult because of the time required for conversion of the hair from anagen to telogen, an obligatory passage in telogen, and, finally, dislodgement of the telogen hair once anagen begins again.[18] Thus, the history of a patient with telogen hair loss must commence some months prior to the time when telogen hair shedding is first noticed.

The second response noted earlier, the interruption rather than cessation of anagen production, will lead to a weakened hair shaft that continues to grow. Scalp hair normally grows at the rate of 1 cm per month,[17] and since anagen hair bulbs are located in the subcutaneous tissue approximately 0.4 mm from the scalp surface,[10] it takes about 2 weeks from the time of the insult for the section of damaged anagen hair to reach the scalp surface. Once free of the supporting follicular duct, the damaged hair will generally break off at the point of the weakened shaft. In a patient with anagen hair breakage, the pertinent history will focus primarily on events in the past 4 to 6 weeks.

A clue to the chronicity of the insult (if there is one) can be gleaned from observing in what body sites the hair loss is occurring. As previously noted, most scalp hair is in anagen, so an insult will readily become apparent in this region. Other areas of the body have quite varied percentages of anagen hairs: moustache 55 to 75 percent,[19] axillary hair 40 to 50 percent,[20] pubic hair approximately 50 percent,[20] and arm hair 25 to 45 percent.[19,21] The duration of anagen and telogen also varies widely between different body areas (e.g., scalp hair: 2–6 years anagen, 3–4 months telogen; arm hair: 1–2 months anagen, 3–4 months telogen).[18,21] Areas other than the scalp will uncommonly manifest prominent hair loss unless the inciting insult is long-standing and thus has involved a high proportion of the anagen population. If the primary hair is vellus, the loss may also go unnoticed. Some hairs (beard, axillary, pubic) are under androgen control and may be lost preferentially secondary to interruption of androgen support. Patients generally seek medical advice for scalp, not body, hair loss, but determining the extent of the loss outside the scalp will help elucidate the duration of the problem as well as point to a systemic versus local disorder.

In the case of chronic hair loss (> 6 months), it is important to ascertain the age of onset, family history, and any relationship to hormonal changes (puberty, pregnancy, menopause, exogenous hormones). Hair loss that begins in infancy or childhood (discussed in Chapter 7) is often of an inherited nature and may be but one component of a genetic syndrome. Although children are potentially subject to the same causes of hair loss as adults, the early onset of some of the hormone-related disorders (e.g., androgenetic alopecia) may signal precocious puberty or a different prognosis. Family history typically is incomplete, as the patient may not be aware of or have taken notice of a limited or transient hair loss in other family members.

The importance of the temporal relationship of hair loss to hormonal changes cannot be emphasized enough—this gives valuable clues as to the etiology of the problem and leads one to primarily investigate the organ systems responsible for steroid production: the gonads, adrenals, and pituitary-hypothalamus. In a woman with hair loss, one must ask questions probing for potential androgen excess: these include the regularity of menses; the presence of acne, hirsutism, or virilization; and the presence of women family members with hirsutism.

A medical history in those with diffuse hair loss must include any chronic illnesses, recent surgeries, recent new physical complaints, and medications within the past 6 months. Many chronic illnesses, especially connective tissue disease, bowel disorders involving malabsorption, endocrine abnormalities, and cancer (without chemotherapy) are associated with hair loss and may be otherwise unsuspected. Additional unexplained physical signs or symptoms should especially lead one to consider one of the preceding diseases. Surgery as a cause of hair loss includes not only the actual repair or removal of a damaged organ but the stress of anesthesia and postoperative complications which, in themselves, can trigger hair loss.

Perhaps the most overlooked cause of hair loss is the omnipresent use of prescribed or over-the-counter drugs or "vitamins." There are certain drugs that carry a high incidence of hair loss as a side effect (Chapters 9 and 10), but anyone familiar with the *Physicians' Desk Reference* (PDR) will realize that hair loss is a common potential side effect of many drugs. It should be recognized, however, that drug companies are obliged to include in their package insert any "possible" or "probable" drug-related side effect that occurred during a clinical trial of a drug. Since most study investigators fail to distinguish hair loss secondary to alopecia areata, androgenetic alopecia, or other non-drug-related etiologies that occurs during a drug trial from that secondary to a potentially drug-related telogen or anagen effluvium, information on hair loss in the PDR is notoriously unreliable. Nevertheless, just as any drug can cause a drug "rash" in a susceptible individual, so can any drug potentially cause hair loss. Certain vitamins can cause hair loss if given in superphysiologic doses (e.g., vitamin A)[22] or if adulterated during manufacture or processing (e.g., L-tryptophan).[23,24] Patients may not think of over-the-counter products or vitamins as medications and must be questioned specifically about their use.

SCALP BIOPSY

In cases where the alopecia appears to be a scarring process, a scalp biopsy is necessary to establish a diagnosis. A biopsy also yields important information in cases of questionable alopecia areata or trichotillomania, in unexplained diffuse and/or dramatic hair loss, and in situations where the potential for regrowth is in question.

The site of biopsy is very important. In cases of scarring alopecia, one should perform a biopsy not from the center of a bald area but from the periphery, where some hairs still remain. In the case of potential alopecia areata, the biopsy can be either from the center of the bald area or at the periphery, since the peribulbar infiltrate is equally present at both locations. If any clinical inflammation is present, then the biopsy should sample an area that shows this.

A scalp biopsy should be a minimum of 3 mm and preferably 4 to 6 mm in diameter. Extrapolating from data on the number of hairs observed clinically in a 1-inch-diameter area of a normal adult occipital scalp,[25] there should be approximately 30 terminal hairs per each 4-mm biopsy from normal scalp. This corresponds to the average of 35 terminal hairs seen on transverse sections of a 4-mm punch biopsy.[26] Biopsies smaller than 4 mm reduce the total number of follicles available for examination, and since follicles are not usually uniformly affected by the disease and some are lost in a given disease process, a smaller biopsy diminishes the probability of making a definitive diagnosis.

The biopsy will need to include the entire follicular unit: the depth of the biopsy must include the subcutaneous tissue in order to capture anagen hair bulbs. A punch biopsy used for hair transplants, such as an Orentreich punch, is preferred by the author for two reasons over the disposable punch generally used for routine skin biopsies: it tends to be sharper and the unguarded section of the punch is longer, hence facilitating a deeper biopsy. The punch should, as in hair transplants, be directed in the direction of hair growth so as not to cut through follicles. Clipping the hair in the area to approximately 2 to 3 mm in length and taping down the surrounding hair prevents extraneous hairs from getting caught in the punch or in the process of suturing. The biopsy site can be closed with no. 4–0 nylon or Proline sutures left in for 7 to 10 days. Special stains may be helpful, including a periodic acid–Schiff stain for potential fungal infection or an elastin stain in cases of scarring alopecia. A biopsy for immunofluorescence should be performed in addition to one for hematoxylin and eosin staining whenever lupus, lichen planus, or one of the blistering diseases is a possible diagnosis. The same principles of location and size apply as with the hematoxylin and eosin biopsy.

At the present time, it is often difficult to establish the etiology of hair loss by histopathologic examination of a scalp biopsy. Having an experienced histopathologist review the biopsies is paramount. Whether the sections should be oriented horizontally or vertically is still uncertain. Traditionally, biopsies are cut vertically, which gives immediate information about the integrity of the follicles, abnormalities of the overlying epidermis, and the location of any inflammatory infiltrate. However, horizontal sections offer the advantages of evaluating large numbers of follicular structures simultaneously and of determining hair density and anagen-telogen ratio.[27] Some changes, such as those typical of the follicular degeneration syndrome, may be apparent only on horizontal sectioning of biopsies. The major disadvantages with horizontal sections are the inability to visualize the overlying epidermis[27] and the unfamiliarity of most pathologists with hair pathology presented in this manner. In most practices, the histopathologist of record will determine the type of sections to be performed, and most will choose to do vertical sections.

CONCLUDING REMARKS

Hair loss is common, and the psychological stress it causes means that physician visits for this problem are frequent. Through the use of directed physical examination, history, microscopic hair analysis, and scalp biopsy, most causes of hair loss can be established and appropriate therapy initiated.

REFERENCES

1. Orentreich N: Scalp hair replacement in man. In Montagna W, Dobson RL (eds): *Advances in Biology of the Skin,* vol. 9. Oxford, Pergamon Press, 1967, pp 99–108.
2. Van Scott EJ: Keratinization and hair growth. Annu Rev Med 19:337–350, 1968.
3. Van Scott EJ: Response of hair roots to chemical and physical influence. In Montagna W, Ellis R (eds): *The Biology of Hair Growth.* New York, Academic Press, 1958, pp 441–449.
4. Baden HP, Kubilus J, Baden L: A stain for plucked anagen hairs. J Am Acad Dermatol 1:121–122, 1979.
5. Price VH, Gummer CL: Loose anagen syndrome. J Am Acad Dermatol 20:249–256, 1989.
6. Caserio RJ: Diagnostic techniques for hair disorders: II. Microscopic examination of hair bulbs, tips, and casts. Cutis 40:321–325, 1987.
7. Shelley WB: Hair examination using double-stick tape. J Am Acad Dermatol 8:430–431, 1983.
8. Van Scott EJ, Reinertson RP, Steinmuller R: The growing hair roots of the human scalp and morphologic changes therein following amethopterin therapy. J Invest Dermatol 29:197–204, 1957.
9. Montagna W: A review of hair and hair growth. In Camacho F, Montagna W (eds): *Trichology.* Proceedings of the Symposium on Trichology, Granada, Spain, February 9, 1980. Madrid, EGRAF, S.A., 1982.
10. Jackson D, Church RE, Ebling FJ: Hair diameter in female baldness. Br J Dermatol 87:361–367, 1972.
11. Price VH et al.: Trichothiodystrophy. Arch Dermatol 116:1375–1384, 1980.
12. Caserio RJ: Diagnostic techniques for hair disorders: III. Clinical hair manipulations and clinical findings. Cutis 40:442–448, 1987.

13. Maguire HC Jr, Kligman AM: Hair plucking as a diagnostic tool. J Invest Dermatol 43:77–79, 1964.
14. Eckert J, Church RE, Ebling FJ: The pathogenesis of alopecia areata. Br J Dermatol 80:203–210, 1968.
15. Gan VN, Petruska M, Ginsburg CM: Epidemiology and treatment of tinea capitis: Ketoconazole vs. griseofulvin. Pediatr Infect Dis J 6:46–49, 1987.
16. Mehregan AH: Trichotillomania. Arch Dermatol 102: 129–133, 1970.
17. Barman JM, Astore I, Pecoraro V: The normal trichogram of the adult. J Invest Dermatol 44:233–236, 1965.
18. Braun-Falco O, Heilgemeir GP: The trichogram. Semin Dermatol 4:40–51, 1985.
19. Saitoh M, Uzuka M, Sakamoto M: Human hair cycle. J Invest Dermatol 54:65–81, 1970.
20. Trotter M: The life cycles of hair in selected regions of the body. Am J Phys Anthropol 7(4):427–437, 1924.
21. Seago SV, Ebling FJG: The hair cycle on the human thigh and upper arm. Br J Dermatol 113:9–16, 1985.
22. Flesch P: Inhibition of keratinizing structures by systemic drugs. Pharmacol Rev 15:653–671, 1963.
23. Kaufman LD, Seidman RJ, Phillips ME, Gruber BL: Cutaneous manifestations of the L-tryptophan-associated eosinophilia-myalgia syndrome: A spectrum of sclerodermatous skin disease. J Am Acad Dermatol 23:1063–1069, 1990.
24. Culpepper RC et al.: Natural history of the eosinophilia-myalgia syndrome. Ann Intern Med 115:437–442, 1991.
25. Olsen EA, Pinnell SR, Weiner MS, DeLong E: Reply: Letter to the editor. J Am Acad Dermatol 14(5):850–851, 1986.
26. Whiting DA: The diagnostic and predictive value of horizontal sections of scalp biopsies in male pattern androgenetic alopecia. J Am Acad Dermatol 28(5):755–763, 1993.
27. Whiting DA: The value of horizontal sections of scalp biopsies. J Cutaneous Aging & Cosmetic Dermatol 1(3):165–173, 1990.

Chapter

5

INFECTIOUS, PHYSICAL, AND INFLAMMATORY CAUSES OF HAIR AND SCALP ABNORMALITIES

Richard L. DeVillez

INTRODUCTION

In this chapter, infectious and physical causes of temporary and/or permanent alopecia are discussed. The alopecia resulting from these conditions usually is of a focal (unifocal or multifocal) nature and commonly is associated with scalp inflammation. Although inflammation is generally seen with scalp psoriasis and seborrheic dermatitis, associated hair loss is uncommon except in severe cases. Pityriasis amiantacea has overlapping clinical features with seborrheic dermatitis and psoriasis but can be associated with both transient and permanent hair loss. Acne miliaris necrotica may present with a clinical picture that can cause confusion with a dermatophyte or bacterial infection. The diagnostic techniques and current treatment of each of these disorders will be discussed here.

INFECTIOUS CAUSES OF HAIR LOSS

Dermatophyte

EPIDEMIOLOGY

Various species of dermatophytes from two of the three genera, *Microsporum* and *Trichophyton,* may cause tinea capitis. *Epidermophyton* spp. do not invade hair. The predominant organism(s) causing tinea capitis in a given area of the world depends on the dermatophyte species that are endogenous to the people, soil, or animals of that particular area. The organism causing tinea capitis in a group of immigrants may reflect the organisms endemic in their native vs. their adoptive country. For example, in the Netherlands, *Microsporum canis* is the predominant dermatophyte causing tinea capitis in the native population, while *Trichophyton violaceum* is the most common cause in immigrants from Morocco.[1] In addition, the predominant dermatophyte causing a particular kind of infection may change over time. Prior to 1950, *Microsporum audouini* was the main causative agent of tinea capitis in the United States and Europe, being replaced by *M. canis* in the 1960s.[2,3] By the early 1970s, *Trichophyton tonsurans* had become the usual causative agent of tinea capitis in the United States.[4]

It has generally been recognized that tinea capitis caused by both *Microsporum* and *Trichophyton* organisms occurs most frequently in prepubertal children.[3] Surface lipids inhibit the growth of certain fungi; this may account for the spontaneous remissions which occur at puberty and for the adult resistance to these infections. Although scalp ringworm in adults is not a common occurrence, it must be considered, especially when patients present with atypical chronic lesions resistant to the usual forms of therapy.[5–7] This is particularly important in the elderly, since 50 percent of the cases of tinea capitis in patients over the age of 20 occur in individuals older than 60 years of age. Whether this relative increase in frequency in the elderly is secondary to qualitative and/or quantitative differences in the sebum is speculative.[8]

Tinea capitis caused by *Microsporum* organisms is transmitted primarily from animal to man, with frequent spontaneous resolution in humans. *T. tonsurans* is transmitted from person to person and is contagious.[9] The latter infection can be passed by adults to successive generations of children by transfer of organisms from combs, brushes, caps, and linens.[10] Day-care centers[11] and boarding schools[12] are potential sources of epidemics and deserve close attention when an infection is noted in a child. Organisms have been cultured from pillow slips, floors, and curtains in the bedrooms of infected children.[12]

Presently, *T. tonsurans* accounts for more than 90 percent of the cases of tinea capitis in the United States.[13] In urban clinics, *T. tonsurans* is more commonly found in black patients and may exist in an asymptomatic state.[13,14] The vast majority of *T. tonsurans* infections occur in black children. The cultural practice of tight braiding and dressing of hair with oils in young black girls may contribute to the problem: the braiding may expose the stratum corneum of the scalp to easier contact with the infective spores, and petrolatum or other oils may facilitate adherence of the spores to the hair until the fungus generates a penetrating hypha.[13] A suggestion to reduce the use of braids and oils may help decrease susceptibility to infection.

CLINICAL FEATURES

Scalp ringworm presents in two main forms differentiated by the type of hair invasion that occurs. Ectothrix infections are caused most frequently by the *Microsporum* spp. On microscopic examination, they characteristically show hyphae that emerge through the hair surface, destroy the cuticle, and fragment into masses of spores predominantly outside of the hair shaft (Fig. 5-1). The infected hair grows upward and breaks off a few millimeters above the scalp surface. The stumps are twisted, brittle, and frequently grayish white in color (Fig. 5-2). The individual patch of affected hair seldom exceeds 5 cm in diameter but may become confluent with neighboring patches, forming large areas of hair loss. The small spore ectothrix of the *Microsporum* genera give a yellow-green fluorescence under Wood's light (320–400 nm) examination. The responsible fluorescent substance is formed only when the keratin of the hair is invaded, and thus its presence under Wood's light examination is dependent upon the degree to which the hairs are infected. It is important to remember that when performing a Wood's light examination, the scalp must first be cleaned of any ointment or cream that would interfere with the procedure. The

Figure 5-1 Ectothrix infection with *M. canis* spores surrounding and within hair shaft.

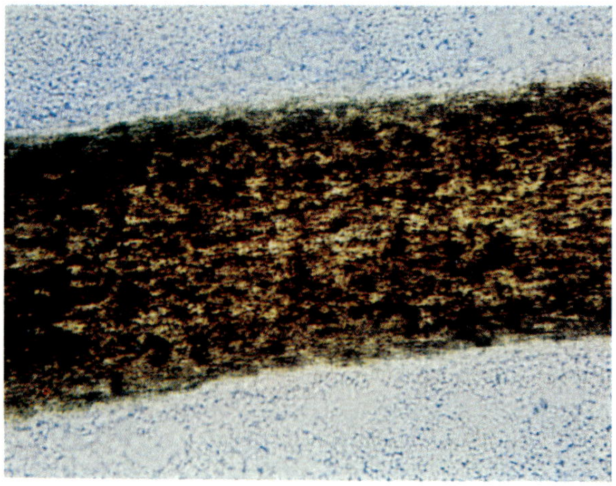

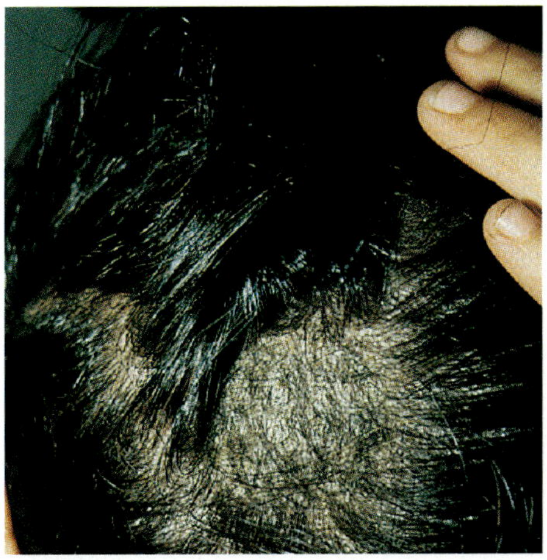

Figure 5-2 Ectothrix infection with *M. canis.*

most common cause of a fluorescent ectothrix tinea capitis in the United States is *M. canis.*

Endothrix infections are caused by fungi that invade and fill the cortex of the hair with masses of spores but remain confined within the cuticle of the hair shaft (Fig. 5-3*A* and *B*). The hairs are so damaged that they usually break off at the surface of the scalp. The most common organism to invade the hair in this way is *T. tonsurans,* specifically the subspecies *sulfureum.*[15] The population at highest risk comes from the lower socioeconomic scale, particularly inner-city black children.[7,13] These patients present with "black dots" on the scalp which represent the hair shafts broken off flush with the scalp (Fig. 5-4). Hair loss may be minimal, however, and often other clinical findings are meager, with only mild scaling and little inflammation. *T. tonsurans* scalp infection can also present as folliculitis[7] or is often dismissed as seborrheic or atopic dermatitis[13] (Fig. 5-5). This organism does not fluoresce under Wood's light.

Favus is a specific type of tinea capitis characterized by scutula, which are sulfuric-yellow concretions of hyphae and skin debris at the orifices of hair follicles.[15] The fungal organism invades the hair in the center of the scutula. Favus is usually caused by *Trichophyton schoenleini.* The microscopic appearance of infected hairs is distinctive for arthrocondia, hyphae, and air spaces within the hair shaft. Favus, left untreated, can progress to scarring alopecia.[16] Favus is an uncommon type of tinea capitis in the industrialized world.

M. canis and other zoophilic organisms, as well as the anthropophilic *T. tonsurans,*[17] may cause a severe inflammatory lesion, known as a *kerion,* in a localized area of the scalp. In one series of tinea capitis infections seen over a period of 20 years at Cook County Hospital in Chicago, 60 percent of all tinea capitis and 34 percent of tinea capitis caused by *T. tonsurans* were keri-

Figure 5-3 Endothrix infection caused by *T. tonsurans.* (*A*) Spores within hair shaft on microscopic examination. (*B*) Spores and hyphae within hair cortex in horizontal section of scalp biopsy. (Light micrograph ×400) (*Courtesy of Dr. David A. Whiting.*)

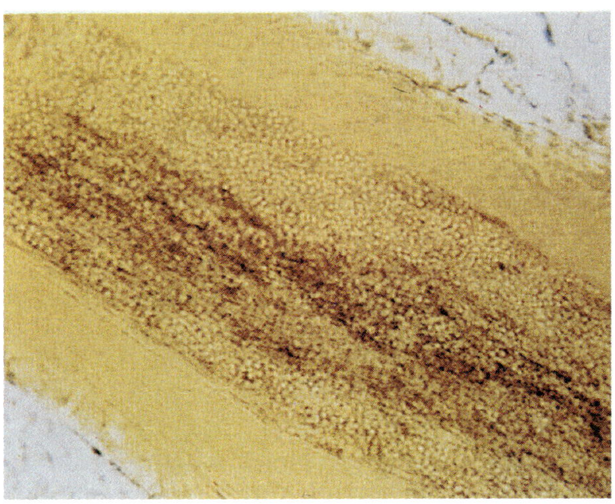

A

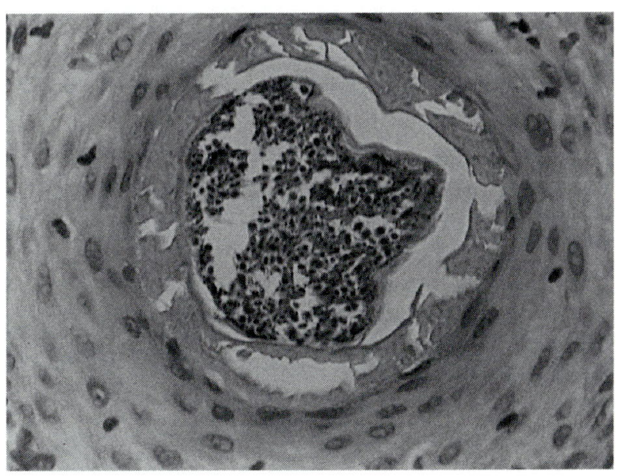

B

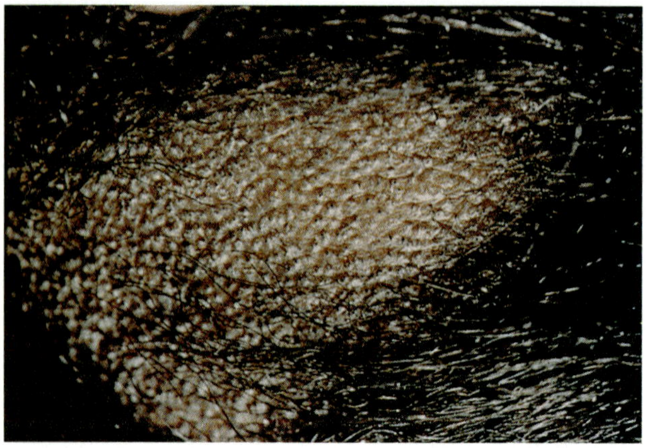

Figure 5-4 Endothrix infection caused by *T. tonsurans.* Note "black dots" of broken, infected hairs within follicular canals.

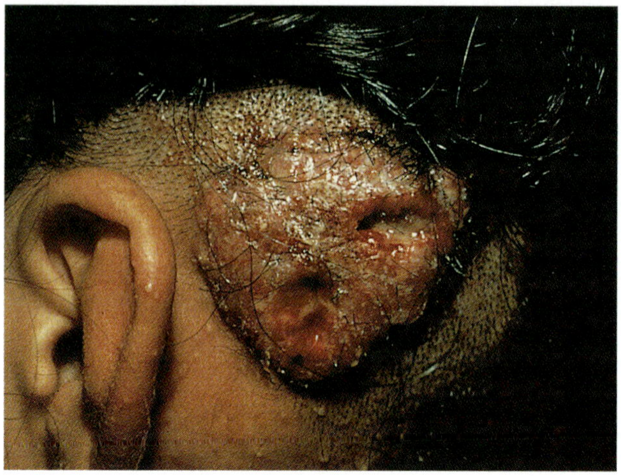

Figure 5-6 Kerion caused by *T. tonsurans.*

Figure 5-5 Endothrix infection with *T. tonsurans* presenting as seborrheic dermatitis. (*Courtesy of Dr. Elise A. Olsen.*)

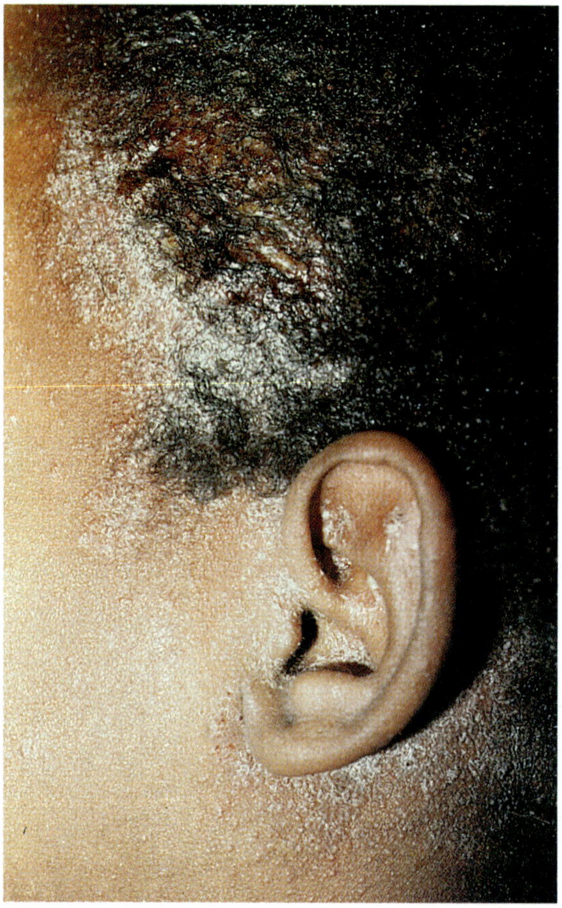

ons.[7] Infections manifesting as kerions have marked inflammatory changes from the first appearance of the lesions; following an interval of about 10 days, severe pustulation usually develops. There is rapid development of a plaque of erythema, which becomes edematous and studded with large follicular pustules and presents as a raised, boggy mass (Fig. 5-6). This represents an immune reaction to the fungus and is not a bacterial suprainfection.[18,19] The results of skin testing in children with *T. tonsurans* tinea capitis support the hypothesis that those with cell-mediated immunity to the organism develop a kerion while those without immunity to *Trichophyton* develop the "black-dot" pattern.[10,20] Spontaneous healing with a kerion is the rule. Some scarring is inevitable, but the degree of hair regrowth is often greater than the severity of the reaction would lead one to expect.

DIAGNOSTIC PROCEDURES

The diagnosis of tinea capitis can be made in several ways. Clinically, the presence of alopecia, scaling, follicular inflammation, posterior auricular or posterior cervical adenopathy, or a kerion may herald scalp infections with a dermatophyte. The discovery of a classic ringworm lesion on other areas of the body should prompt careful examination of the scalp. Confirmation of infection is possible utilizing a potassium hydroxide (KOH) preparation and a culture of the scalp scale and broken hairs. The KOH preparation should include scraping the scalp scales directly onto a slide and obtaining broken-off hairs for microscopic examination. When the patient is infected with *T. tonsurans,* the hairs are frequently broken off at the level of the scalp, giving the appearance of black dots. These tiny hairs can be plucked with tweezers, loosened with a large bore needle, or rubbed off with a moist piece of gauze. This last method usually allows several hairs to be obtained quickly and without frightening the patient.[21] The presence of the tiny hairs on the gauze will invariably yield a positive KOH preparation, identifying either an ectothrix or an endothrix infection of the hair (Figs. 5-1 and 5-3).

Cultures of the scalp can be obtained by a variety of approaches. The scales may be collected by scraping the scalp with a glass slide, surgical blade, piece of gauze,[14] toothbrush,[6] hairbrush,[22] or a sterile cotton swab moistened with tap water.[23] The sterile swab can be used to rub several areas of the scalp and directly inoculate a plate of Sabouraud's agar. Sabouraud's agar with chloramphenicol to inhibit bacterial growth and cycloheximide to inhibit certain saprophytic and pathogenic fungi (Mycosel's medium) will make overgrowth with a contaminant less likely.

M. canis cultured on Sabouraud's agar at room temperature for 1 to 2 weeks reveals a white top growth with a bright-yellow underside pigment (Fig. 5-7). The microscopic features are large, thick-walled, rough spores containing more than six septae (Fig. 5-8). *T. tonsurans* cultured on Sabouraud's agar for 2 weeks at room temperature demonstrates a powdery white to yellow to brown wrinkled colony on the surface of the culture medium with a red-brown undersurface (Fig. 5-9). The yellow variant is the *sulfureum* variety.

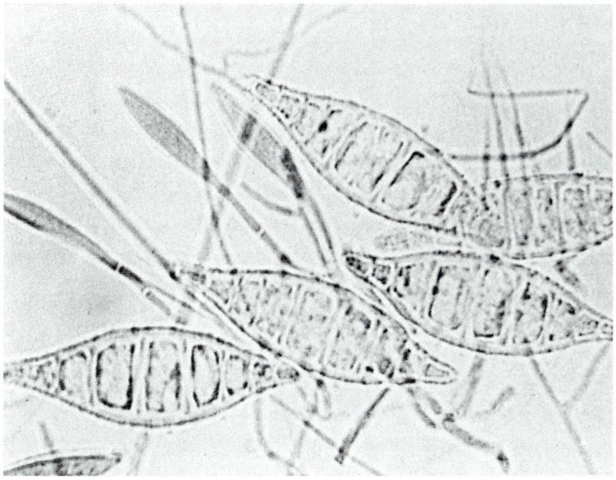

Figure 5-8 Microscopic examination of *M. canis* culture.

The microscopic features of this organism demonstrate many small, club-shaped spores, often enlarging to resemble small balloons (Fig. 5-10).

Dermatophyte test medium (DTM) containing a phenol red indicator and cycloheximide is an alternative fungal culture medium.[24] Dermatophytes produce an alkaline condition when grown on this glucose-peptone medium, permitting the indicator, phenol red, to change the color of the medium from yellow to red (Fig. 5-11). The cultures are stored at room temperature for 14 days and give better than a 90 percent specificity for dermatophyte identification based on color change alone. The growth of certain contaminants, such as the black molds, *Penicil-*

Figure 5-7 Colony growth of *M. canis.*

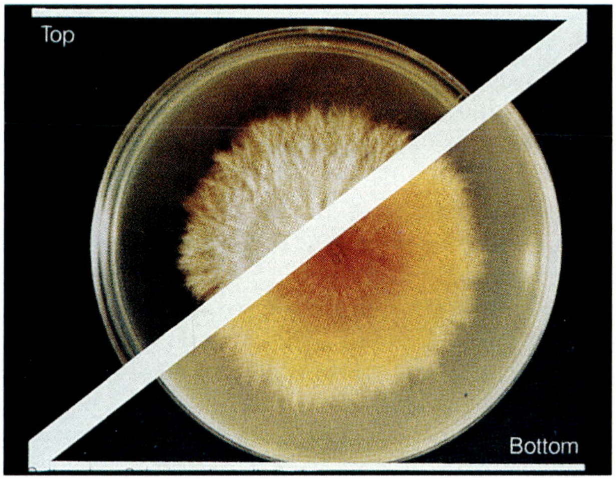

Figure 5-9 Colony growth of *T. tonsurans.*

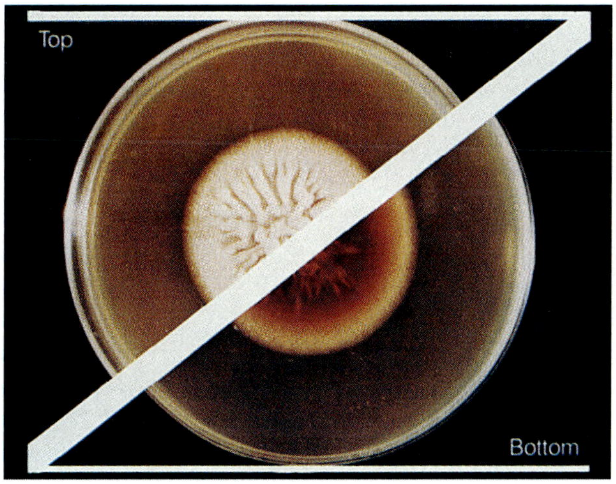

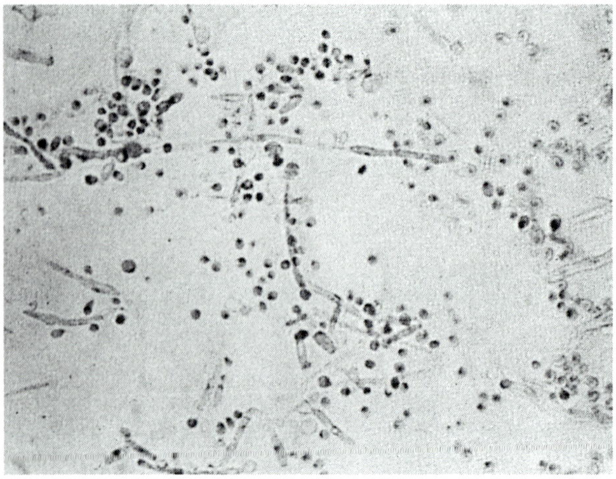

Figure 5-10 Microscopic examination of *T. tonsurans* culture.

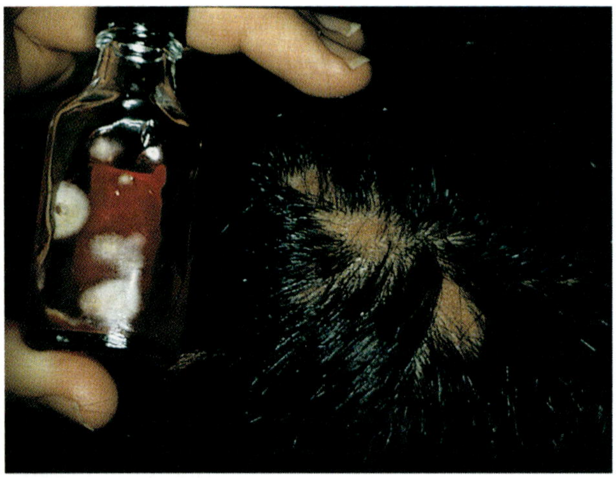

Figure 5-11 Color change in positive DTM fungal culture.

lium and *Aspergillus*, may turn the DTM medium red within 2 weeks but are not generally confused with a culture of a dermatophyte.[24] However, subculturing from DTM is difficult due to the phenol red, so that if species identification is necessary, this is probably not the medium to use. Species identification from cultural and microscopic characteristics is more precise when the organism is grown on Sabouraud's agar.

The correlation between the clinical characteristics of the lesion and the results of the KOH-treated hair samples reveals that the more inflammatory the lesion, the less reliable the KOH interpretation.[25] In a study of 80 children with tinea capitis, 66 percent of patients with patchy hair loss and minimal inflammation were KOH-positive, compared with 29 percent of those with marked erythema and a purulent, crusted exudate.[25] Cultures, however, were positive in 96 percent and 86 percent of these two patient groups. Clearly, fungal culture is superior to KOH in documenting a suspected tinea capitis. This also has important implications for the clinician, who should treat not only to complete clearing of the obvious scalp infection but until a mycological cure is obtained. A negative culture vs. negative KOH will be the best indicator of eradication of the infection.

TREATMENT

With the advent of oral griseofulvin therapy in the late 1950s, the use of x-ray or thallium for epilation treatment of tinea capitis became obsolete. Even though it has been recognized by many investigators that the inflammatory lesions of *M. canis* and kerions undergo spontaneous remission without antifungal therapy, it has long been the practice to treat all forms of tinea capitis with systemic antimycotic therapy because of the disability involved. Moreover, when *T. tonsorans* infection is confirmed, all family members should be evaluated and scalp cultures performed.[9,26] Failure to treat all affected family members increases the risk of recurrent infection.

Oral griseofulvin at a dose of 10 to 20 mg/kg per day of the microsize product (5–10 mg/kg per day of the ultra microsize form) is the treatment of choice for tinea capitis.[25] The absorption of the drug is increased if taken with a fatty meal. Griseofulvin is recognized as relatively safe and effective in children as well as adults provided it is given to individuals who are not sensitive to the drug. A treatment interval of 6 to 8 weeks generally suffices, but a culture of the affected area should be taken after 4 weeks of therapy and every 2 weeks thereafter until a negative culture is obtained.[6] If cultures are positive beyond 6 to 8 weeks, medication should be continued until cultures are negative. A 2.5% selenium sulfide shampoo used two to three times per week is an important adjunctive therapy to reduce the period of active spore shedding:[27] the spores may remain viable even after 8 weeks of therapy with griseofulvin alone. Those treated with selenium sulfide twice weekly plus griseofulvin daily generally become culture-negative after 2 weeks of therapy.[27] Selenium sulfide shampoo has also been used prophylactically on those in close contact with affected patients. There has been no benefit noted to using topical clotrimazole twice daily to the infected area in conjunction with oral griseofulvin.[27] Ketoconazole shampoo has not been evaluated as an adjuvant in the treatment of tinea capitis.

The potential adverse effects from griseofulvin include nausea, vomiting, diarrhea, blurred vision, dizziness, and mental confusion. The incidence of headache may be as high as 15 percent.[28] Griseofulvin induces hepatic microsomal enzymes which increase the rate of metabolism of warfarin, reduce the efficacy of oral contraceptives, and augment the effect of alcohol. Barbiturates increase the metabolic clearance of griseofulvin.[28]

Kerion formation, thought to be a local immune response by the host, has been treated with griseofulvin in conjunction with intralesional steroids such as triamcinolone acetonide (10 mg/ml) or orally administered prednisone (0.5–1.0 mg/kg per day) for 3 to 4 weeks in a gradually tapering dose.[29] The purpose of the added steroid was ostensibly to prevent scarring and permit quicker regrowth of hair. However, it has been shown that intralesional steroids in conjunction with griseofulvin are no better than griseofulvin alone for the treatment of kerion: there are no significant differences in regard to new hair growth, time of scalp clearing, or permanent alopecia.[30] Intralesional corticosteroids are not recommended for the treatment of kerion. Griseofulvin (15 mg/kg per day of the microsize variety) administered once daily with a glass of whole milk and biweekly use of selenium sulfide shampoos is the treatment of choice for a kerion.

In the 1980s, a new oral imidazole antifungal agent, ketoconazole (Nizoral), was found to be effective for dermatophyte infections.[31] In several studies comparing griseofulvin with ketoconazole for tinea capitis infection, ketoconazole has been shown to be less effective than griseofulvin.[25,32] In one study of 80 children with tinea capitis, fungal cultures were sterile in 69 percent and 29 percent of patients treated with griseofulvin and ketoconazole for 1 month, respectively.[25] After 8 weeks, the cure rates were 92 percent and 59 percent, respectively, with griseofulvin and ketoconazole.[25] In a second study of 68 evaluable children with tinea capitis who were treated with either griseofulvin or ketoconazole for 12 weeks, treatment was successful in 96 percent of the griseofulvin-treated patients and 73 percent of the ketoconazole-treated patients.[32] Ketoconazole should not replace griseofulvin as a first-line therapy for tinea capitis but has a role in the treatment of patients who are unable to take griseofulvin or for those who demonstrate a griseofulvin-resistant dermatophyte infection.[33] The dose for administration of ketoconazole in tinea capitis is 200 to 400 mg daily or 3.3 to 6.6 mg/kg per day for several weeks.

Side effects from ketoconazole include nausea, vomiting, and anorexia in 20 percent of patients receiving 400 mg daily. An allergic rash occurs in 4 percent and pruritus in 2 percent of patients.[28] Ketoconazole inhibits the cytochrome P_{450} enzyme system, and its use with other drugs whose metabolism is through the P_{450} system, such as terfenadine, astemizole, erythromycin, and cyclosporine, can lead to toxicity from these other agents. Approximately 10 percent of females report menstrual irregularities, and a variable number of men report gynecomastia and decreased libido with ketoconazole use. Patients receiving rifampin or isoniazid concurrently with ketoconazole may experience a marked drop in their serum concentration of ketoconazole.[32] Asymptomatic hepatic dysfunction may be seen in 5 to 10 percent of patients.[28] Hepatitis is rare but potentially fatal:[29] it has occurred in less than 1 per 10,000 cases of patients treated for dermatophyte infection.[28]

Itraconazole (Sporonox) is a new triazole antifungal drug which has been evaluated for the treatment of tinea capitis.[34] At a dose of 100 mg per day for 5 weeks in 50 patients with tinea capitis, 94 percent responded clinically to therapy and 38 of 42 evaluable patients were culture-negative at the end of treatment. In one Italian study of 20 patients with *M. canis* tinea capitis treated with itraconazole for 30 days, clinical and mycological improvement continued for at least 2 to 4 weeks off drug.[34] This latter phenomenon may be secondary to the persistent levels of itraconazole in the scalp and/or hair.[34] These studies were uncontrolled, and further data on both the effectiveness and the safety of itraconazole in tinea capitis are needed.

Approximately 10 to 15 percent of patients taking itraconazole complain of nausea or vomiting. Rash, pruritus, weakness, dizziness, vertigo, paresthesia, impotence, and loss of libido have been reported occasionally.[28] Itraconazole interferes with the cytochrome P_{450} enzyme system and carries the same precautions as ketoconazole with respect to concomitant use of terfenadine, astemizole, erythromycin, and cyclosporine.[28]

Fluconazole (Diflucan) is a fluorinated bis-triazole which has less hepatotoxicity and may prove a useful alternative to ketoconazole; however, its safety and effectiveness in tinea capitis have yet to be determined.[28]

Terbinafine (Lamisil) is a member of a new class of antifungals called *allylamines.* It is fungicidal in nature, has superior penetration into the epidermis, and is concentrated in hair and sebum.[35] Few studies have been published on its use in tinea capitis, but preliminary results show comparable efficacy of 4 weeks of terbinafine with 8 weeks of griseofulvin.[35,36] Larger controlled trials are needed to definitively determine the efficacy and safety of terbinafine in tinea capitis when compared with griseofulvin and the other newer antifungal agents.

Syphilis

EPIDEMIOLOGY

In 1990, the incidence of syphilis in 26 of the 50 U.S. states was greater than 7 per 100,000 persons. The current syphilis epidemic began in 1986 and parallels the epidemic use of crack cocaine.[37] Despite the increase in the incidence of secondary syphilis, there has not been a substantial increase in the number of patients noted with hair loss as part of the clinical presentation of their disease. Acute hair loss is probably a common manifestation of secondary syphilis, but it tends to be overlooked by both the patient and the physician. Careful inspection of a group of patients with secondary syphilis revealed that 48 percent had acute hair loss at the time of presentation.[38]

CLINICAL PRESENTATION

Scalp hair loss does not occur in primary syphilis unless a primary lesion is in the scalp. Hair loss is not uncommon in the secondary and tertiary stages of syphilis. In its classic form, the hair loss in secondary syphilis is an irregular "moth-eaten" loss of hair scattered throughout the scalp, resembling in some cases a diffuse, patchy alopecia areata (Fig. 5-12). The eyebrows may be shed, and there may be a patchy alopecia noted

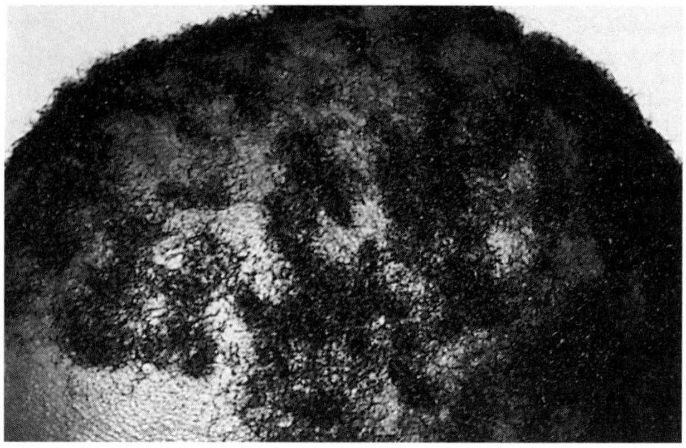

Figure 5-12 Syphilitic patchy alopecia: "moth-eaten" alopecia.

in the beard and other hair-bearing areas of the body. A second presentation in secondary syphilis is a diffuse hair loss resembling that seen in telogen effluvium. A third form of hair loss is that associated with the noduloulcerative cutaneous lesions found in patients with lues maligna.[39,40] This noduloulcerative presentation of secondary syphilis may affect the scalp as well as other areas of the body. It presents as a papular eruption, becomes generalized, and develops numerous cutaneous ulcerations. Histologically it is a necrotizing vasculitis.[41] The pleomorphic lesions may be pustular or ulcerative and occur more frequently in immunocompromised hosts. There seems to be a correlation between the papulopustular type and the development of neurosyphilis.[42,43] In tertiary syphilis, hair loss occurs in the area overlying a gumma.

The diagnosis of secondary syphilis is usually made by a positive rapid plasma reagin (RPR) titer.[40] An RPR may be negative in active secondary syphilis due to an extremely high antibody titer (prozone reaction), but this can be detected by quantitation and serial dilution of the patient's serum. The antibody response in patients infected with human immunodeficiency virus (HIV), particularly in the later stages of acquired immunodeficiency syndrome (AIDS), may be compromised and thus the diagnosis obscured.[44,45]

HISTOLOGY

Microscopic examination of an area of patchy or diffuse alopecia in a patient with syphilis reveals an inflammatory, nonscarring alopecia. The follicular changes include a decrease in anagen follicles and an increase in catagen and telogen follicles with the presence of peribulbar inflammation and fibrous tract formation. There tends to be a sparse, predominantly lymphocytic, superficial perivascular infiltrate with scattered plasma cells. In most cases, even when using special stains, spirochetes are rarely demonstrated in the tissue. This is in contrast to the histology of the scalp alopecia in the noduloulcerative form of syphilis. In the latter specimens, the entire dermis shows a perivascular lymphohistiocytic infiltrate with epithelioid histiocytic granulomata. In the center of the dermis, there is a zone of degenerated collagen and an infiltrate consisting of lymphocytes, histocytes, neutrophils, and fragmented nuclear particles. This pattern follows vessels that show varying degrees of degeneration and necrosis of vessel walls. Throughout the whole inflammatory reaction, plasma cells are predominant and many spirochetes are demonstrated by the Warthin-Starry stain.[40,46]

TREATMENT

The current Centers for Disease Control (CDC) treatment recommendation for secondary syphilis is an intramuscular injection of benzathine penicillin G of 2.4 million units weekly for 2 consecutive weeks. For alternative treatments, for patients with AIDS and for those who are allergic to penicillin, consult the CDC brochure on syphilis (Division of Sexually Transmitted Diseases, Centers for Disease Control, Atlanta, GA). The patients with early syphilis who are successfully treated have a characteristic pattern of serological response. The RPR titer declines approximately fourfold in 3 months and eightfold by 6 months. In patients who are immunocompromised due to HIV infection, these titers should be evaluated at 1, 2, 3, 6, and 12 months to assure a continued decline and, therefore, adequate therapeutic response. A Jarisch-Herxheimer reaction often occurs after the treatment of primary and secondary syphilis. This reaction can usually be controlled with corticosteroids or indomethacin.[46]

PHYSICAL CAUSES OF HAIR LOSS

Mechanically Induced Alopecia

In adults and children, an acute or chronic mechanical insult to the scalp may lead to a reversible or irreversible alopecia. If this alopecia persists for a long time, permanent hair loss due to follicular atrophy develops. Mechanically induced alopecias are usually of three types: trauma, pressure, and/or traction.

TRAUMATIC INJURIES

The most frequent form of cicatricial alopecia of the scalp develops from traumatic injury. It is interesting that minimal, as well as severe, injuries to the head may cause alopecia. The alopecia usually presents as a fine streak of hair loss, but if the wound borders undergo contusion and destruction, this may result in irregular and large patches of hair loss. Traumatic birth-induced cicatricial alopecia is infrequent: causes include mechanical extractor marks, tears or contusions, and infections thereof. The localization of the cicatricial alopecia depends on the position of the child's head at the time of application of the extraction instrument. In the differential diagnosis, only aplasia cutis might be considered; however, the history and clinical picture make the two causes easily distinguishable. If the defect is large in traumatic alopecia, this can be corrected surgically.

PRESSURE INJURIES

Pressure injuries occur if the patient is unconscious and lies completely immobile for a sufficient length of time to permit his or her body weight to lead to ischemia of the skin with subsequent necrosis, ulceration, and scar formation.[47] This may occur with drug overdose or during anesthesia for an operative procedure.[48] In most patients, there is a slow and sparse regrowth of hair after several months, but if pressure caused necrosis of the hair follicles, the alopecia will be permanent.

TRACTION INJURIES

Chronic traction of the hair may lead to a transient alopecia which, if continued over a period of time, may cause the follicles to atrophy, thus leading to a permanent alopecia. This form of alopecia commonly presents as short broken hairs, follicular inflammation, and focal scarring in circumscribed patches at the scalp margin (Fig. 5-13). The location on the scalp and the etiology of this type of alopecia are commonly dependent upon ethnic practices. Frontal and parietal traction alopecia occurs in young Sikh boys

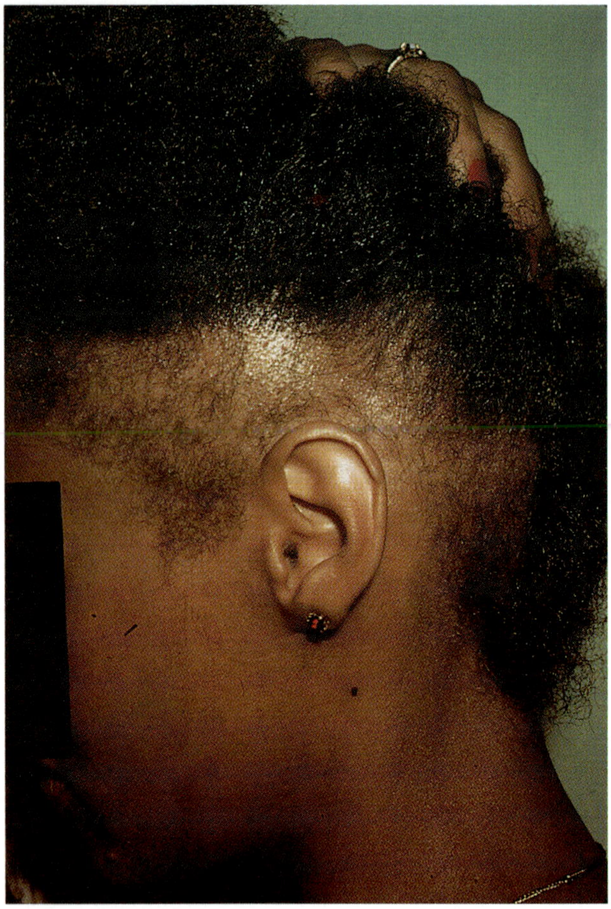

Figure 5-13 Traction alopecia. (*Courtesy of Dr. Dirk M. Elston.*)

as a result of twisting their uncut hair tightly on top of the head.[49] Tight braiding produces a traction alopecia in central areas of the scalp in Sudanese women, and young Zande males develop a frontal hairline traction alopecia secondary to hardwood combs thrust horizontally back in the scalp.[50] Afro-Caribbean hairstyles with tight braiding of the hair in rows known as "cornrows" or "cane rows" or braids may cause marginal alopecia or central alopecia with widening of the hair parts. Brush-roller alopecia from vigorously attached rollers may produce irregular areas of alopecia on the scalp.[51] Patchy traction alopecia has been noted in patients who use the weaving procedure to camouflage common baldness.[51] The process of hair weaving involves the attachment of sections of artificial hair to the existing hair by means of weaving the two together. If too much traction is applied to the normal hair, patchy alopecia ensues.[52]

TREATMENT

The diagnosis of mechanical alopecia is not difficult provided the possibility is considered. The cause is rarely recognized by the patient, and often the patient has trouble accepting the physician's diagnosis. In the case of traction alopecia, the treatment involves educating the patient as to the advantages of an alternate hairstyle or method of styling. In those patients with cicatricial alopecia from either pressure, traction, or trauma, hair transplantation or other appropriate surgical procedures may be necessary to help cover the defect.

Trichotillomania

Trichotillomania is a form of traction alopecia characterized by an irresistible urge to pluck one's hair. This disorder, inappropriately classified as a "mania," is a disturbance of impulse control, with an estimated incidence of up to 1 million Americans.[53] Two types of trichotillomania are recognized: a temporary, localized childhood pattern (Fig. 5-14) and a severe form typically occurring in adult women[54] (Fig. 5-15). Trichotillomania has been linked with other habit tics and is classified under the psychiatric association list of disorders as an impulse-control disorder.[55] It is attributed to a variety of psychodynamic conflicts, but the ultimate cause re-

Figure 5-14 Trichotillomania: localized area. (*Courtesy of Dr. Elise A. Olsen.*)

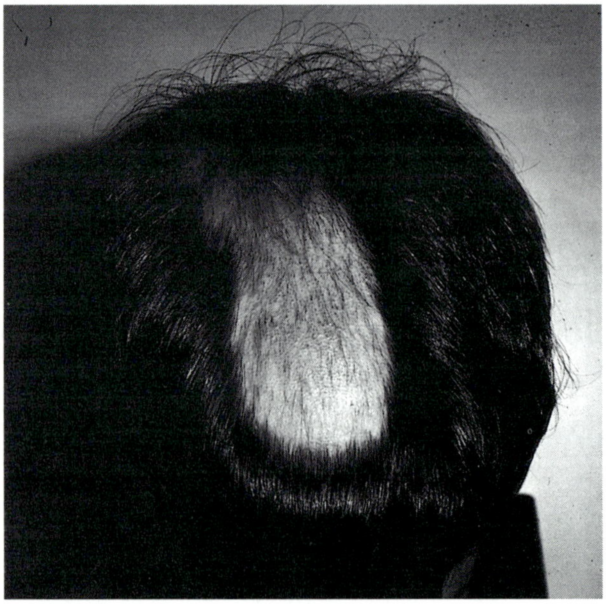

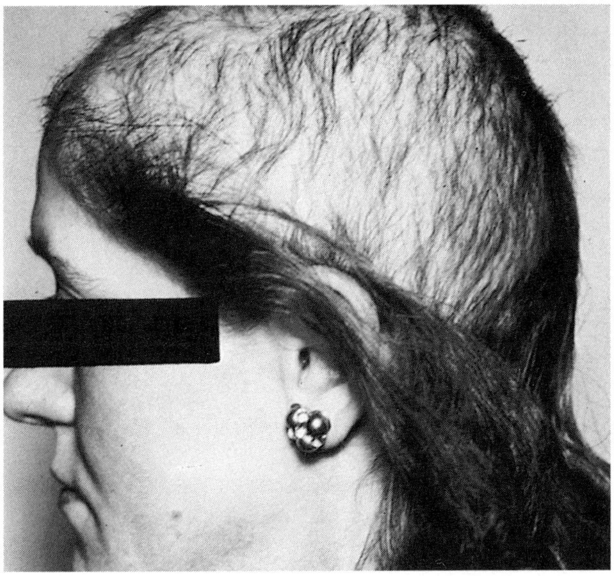

Figure 5-15 Trichotillomania: diffuse involvement. (*Courtesy of Dr. Dirk M. Elston.*)

mains unclear. Two-thirds of affected patients are children, adolescents, and young adults: boys outnumber girls by 3 to 2, but there is a marked predominance of females in the older age-groups.[55,56]

CLINICAL FEATURES

Single or multiple areas of the scalp, especially in the frontal, parietal, or occipital regions, are commonly involved in trichotillomania. The patches of alopecia are of variable size and are usually irregular, oval, or asymmetrical. Telogen hairs in the involved areas are pulled out, and anagen hairs are characteristically twisted and broken at various lengths from the otherwise normal, noninflammatory scalp. The texture and color of the broken hairs remain unaffected. Although pruritus is uncommon, some patients do complain of itching and may have excoriations.

In the more severe form of trichotillomania, patients consistently deny touching their hair. These patients are usually teenagers or adults. In some cases, patients complain that uncomfortable sensations are relieved by plucking their hair.[54] In those in whom the condition has lasted for several years, there may be signs of scarring. Involvement of eyebrows and eyelashes may be seen in as many as one-fourth of affected patients.

Clinically, trichotillomania can be distinguished from other causes of patchy nonscarring hair loss by the incomplete nature of the hair loss and the absence of underlying scalp inflammation or scale. The broken hairs do not resemble the "exclamation-point" hairs of alopecia areata, and the sparseness of hair in the involved area is unusual for a hair shaft disorder. Usually, no hairs are obtained in a hair pull in the involved areas secondary to all the telogen hair population having already been pulled or plucked out by the patient. Examination of the distal ends of plucked hairs reveals either broken hairs, straight ends (from the not-uncommon process of cutting the hair by these patients), or tapered ends of new anagen growth. KOH examination and fungal culture are negative. In cases where the patient or family member insists that the hair "just won't grow," a "hair window" with occlusion of the clipped area should be performed. The hair window should be done in an area that the patient cannot see. Removal of the occlusion in 1 to 3 weeks should show the proportional 1 cm per month hair growth typical for the normal scalp.

HISTOLOGY

Biopsy from an involved area of the scalp reveals a decreased number of telogen follicles and an increased number of catagen follicles.[56] Because catagen hairs make up only approximately 1 percent of the scalp hairs, finding two to three catagen hairs is suggestive of the diagnosis (Fig. 5-16*A*). Characteristically, normal follicles are found among involuted, damaged, or empty follicles.[57] Although inflammation of the hair bulb is generally absent, mild lymphocytic folliculitis may occasionally be noted. A characteristic feature found in approximately 60 percent of biopsies of affected scalp is the presence of pigmented casts, usually in the isthmus or infundibular area of the follicle, representing clumps of melanin and keratinaceous debris (Fig. 5-16*B*). Trichomalacia, evidenced by clumped, plicated, amorphous, corkscrew terminal hairs, is uncommon but is thought to be specific for trichotillomania. Rarely, in advanced cases, a fibrotic-type reaction localized to the hair papillae has been noted in the deep dermis and subcutis.[56]

TREATMENT

Patients with trichotillomania and their families usually do not readily admit to the self-induced nature of this hair loss. Frequently, scalp biopsies

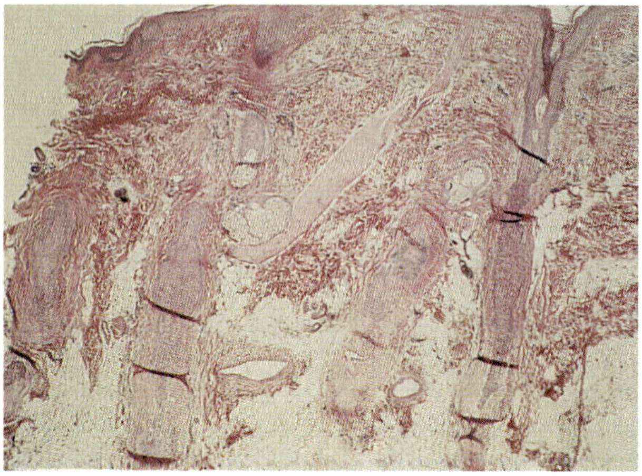

A

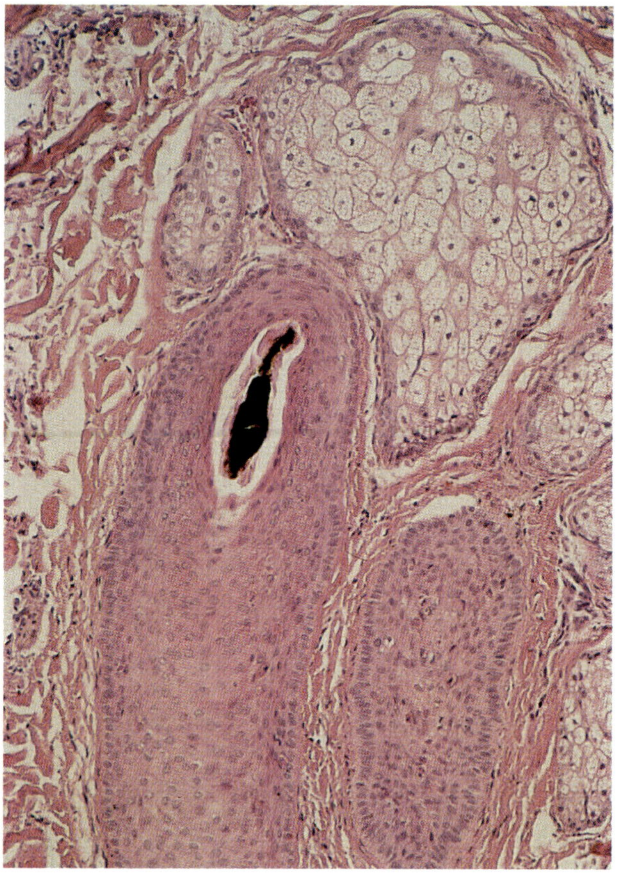

B

Figure 5-16 Trichotillomania. (*A*) Note four normal-appearing catagen hairs. (Hematoxylin and eosin stain; ×64) (*B*) Note solid, oval melanin cast in upper isthmus (Hematoxylin and eosin stain; ×115) (*Both photographs courtesy of Dr. Sigfrid A. Muller. Reprinted with permission from Muller.*[56])

do help convince the parents of children with this disorder of the nature of the problem. Children, much more than adults, with trichotillomania are more cooperative and accepting of the diagnosis thereafter. In some instances, the patient is relieved to know that a serious disorder is not present and that the hair loss is a sign of excessive manipulation of the hair.

The author prefers to discuss the problem frankly with the parents of an affected child, and some young children do stop plucking their hairs when it is explained to them in a straightforward manner that they are causing their hair loss. Unfortunately, in most patients this approach will not solve the problem. The explanation does, however, relieve a certain amount of anxiety in the family. Frequently, regrowth of affected hair under a protected hair window will reassure the family of the reversible nature of the hair loss. Psychiatric consultation should be arranged when there is a suspicion of a serious psychological disorder: failure to do so usually results in the patient endlessly seeking yet another opinion.

Treatments for trichotillomania have included psychotherapy, behavior-modification therapy, and antidepressant medications. The disorder in the older patient is generally resistant to treatment, and relapse is common. Psychoanalysis and intensive psychotherapy have been reported to be helpful in some cases.[58] Treatments using desipramine, clomipramine, or fluoxetine have all been reported to be effective in the short term; however, treatment should be carried out under psychiatric guidance.[59] Desipramine is a tricyclic antidepressant. Clomipramine and fluoxetine are selective inhibitors of the neuronal uptake of 5-hydroxytryptamine. Clomipramine seems to exert a specific effect on the obsessive-impulsive tendencies of trichotillomania separate from its antidepressive qualities.[53,55] Clomipramine, desipramine, and fluoxetine have significant side effects with an incidence of up to 5 percent. The most frequent reactions include antimuscarinic effects, cerebral intoxication, cardiac toxicity, and orthostatic hypotension.[60] Extreme care must be used when prescribing these medications.

INFLAMMATORY SCALP CONDITIONS

Seborrheic Dermatitis

CLINICAL FEATURES

Seborrheic dermatitis is an inflammatory condition that presents as areas of erythema covered by large, yellow, greasy scales which diffusely involve the scalp (Fig. 5-17). This may be associated with a transient alopecia.[61] Seborrheic dermatitis frequently extends beyond the margins of the hair onto the forehead and behind the ears and posterior neck. A crusted fissure in the retroauricular region with dull, red scale extending into the scalp and to the back of the pinna is common. Scaling and redness may be seen in the beard, the external auditory canal, nasolabial folds, anterior chest, and groin. Secondary infection may produce an eczematization with exudate and crusting.

The cause of seborrheic dermatitis is unknown but appears dependent on androgen production. It occurs in the infant under the influence of maternal androgens and reappears later in the adolescent and adult when sebaceous activity has been reestablished. It has been noted that the incidence of seborrheic dermatitis is increased in patients with Parkinson's disease, who have abnormally high sebum excretion rates: this is improved by levodopa therapy, which reduces the rate of sebum excretion.[62] However, there is a large variation in the level of sebum production in normal adults. There does not appear to be a correlation between the amount of sebum production and the presence or absence of seborrheic dermatitis.

Recent literature suggests that *Pityrosporon ovale* may contribute to the pathogenesis of seborrheic dermatitis.[63–66] Others speculate that epidermal scale provides a nutrient source for the *P. ovale* and that the increased presence of *P. ovale* in seborrheic dermatitis is a secondary and not a primary phenomenon.[67] The density of *P. ovale* organisms has been correlated with the clinical severity of seborrheic dermatitis. Using scrapings of stratum corneum, Heng et al. showed that mild disease was associated with fewer than 200 yeast cells per high-powered field, whereas moderate to severe disease was associated with more than 200 yeast cells per high-powered field.[65] The same finding was noted in AIDS patients with seborrheic dermatitis. In the latter patients, the seborrheic dermatitis was often explosive and yeast spores were seen in large numbers. It has been suggested that the lipase activity of *P. ovale* causes the generation of free fatty acids, which could contribute to the inflammatory process.[64]

Figure 5-17 Seborrheic dermatitis in a patient after chemotherapy epilation.

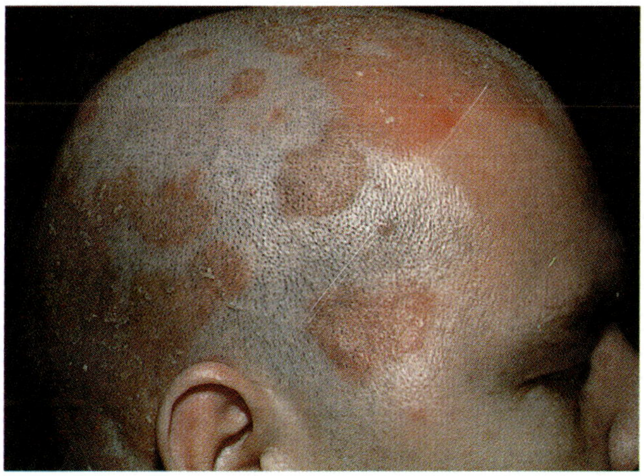

HISTOPATHOLOGY

The histological changes of seborrheic dermatitis lie somewhere between that of chronic eczema and psoriasis. The epidermis shows moderate acanthosis and slight to moderate spongiosis with exocytosis of mononuclear cells in the areas of spongiosis. The horny layer shows focal areas of parakeratosis. In the dermis, there is a mild, chronic inflammatory infiltrate. In patients with AIDS, the histology shows keratinocyte necrosis, leukoexocytosis, a superficial perivascular mixed plasma cell and neutrophil infiltrate with occasional leukocytoclasis. In most biopsies of seborrheic dermatitis, yeast forms of *Pityrosporon* are noted in the stratum corneum, but they are present in much larger numbers in patients with AIDS than in normal hosts.[64]

TREATMENT

Treatment of seborrheic dermatitis is directed at reducing both the scale and the inflammation.

Ideally, the scalp should be shampooed daily or, at the very least, every other day until the dermatitis is under control. Tar shampoo sharply inhibits epidermal proliferation and scale formation.[63] It may also stain gray or white hair an unsightly yellow color. Zinc pyrithione, salicylic acid, sulfur, and selenium sulfide shampoos are also effective agents secondary to their antimitotic activity. Certainly, alternating medicated shampoos in the daily shampooing regimen may prevent tachyphylaxis from developing with continued use of one medicated shampoo. Alternating a tar shampoo with another medicated shampoo that more effectively decreases the number of yeast organisms on the scalp (e.g., one containing ketoconazole or selenium sulfide) may be useful. Oral ketoconazole has also been used to treat seborrheic dermatitis.[68]

The amount of time the medicated shampoo stays on the scalp is less important than the frequency of shampooing. Patients should be told, however, that it is the scalp and not the hair that needs to be treated. The adjunctive use of nonmedicated shampoos and/or conditioners to improve the condition of the hair will not adversely affect the treatment. Following the shampoo application, a topical fluorinated corticosteroid lotion or solution is recommended. Available topical steroid solutions range in potency from class II to class V. The more potent topical steroid can be used every other day vs. daily until the erythema has subsided, thus minimizing the potential for steroid-induced atrophy of the scalp. If secondary infection is present, a topical antibiotic should be used; if the infection is severe, systemic antibiotics are preferred. Once the dermatitis is under control, regular shampooing and alternating the types of shampoo are important to maintain a remission. The treatment of African Americans with seborrheic dermatitis of the scalp will differ from the general recommendations noted above secondary to different grooming practices, especially a decreased frequency of shampooing. This is discussed further in Chapter 17.

Psoriasis

Psoriasis affects as many as 2 to 3 percent of the world population, and the scalp is a site of predilection. Typical lesions of psoriasis are characteristically located elsewhere on the body and help in distinguishing psoriasis from other scalp conditions. Psoriasis of the scalp may be prominent in AIDS patients and extremely difficult to manage.[69] The presence of large numbers of *P. ovale* organisms in the scalp may be adequate to provoke a psoriatic (Koebner) reaction in susceptible persons.[70] *P. ovale* organisms have the ability to activate complement to initiate inflammation in cutaneous lesions.[71]

CLINICAL FEATURES

Psoriasis of the scalp is present in approximately 50 percent of all psoriatics and begins as small, erythematous papules which usually collect to form lesions with thick, silvery scales that may eventually cover the entire scalp (Fig. 5-18). Not uncommonly, the psoriatic plaque will extend 1 to 3 cm below the hairline, with an elevated erythematous border. The thick scales may cause the hairs to be funneled together to form the "tepee sign" of scalp psoriasis (Fig. 5-19). The shafts of scalp hairs in psoriasis appear lusterless, are dry, and break easily. There is increased shedding of telogen hairs and a reduction of hair density in the common plaques of psoriasis. There may be extensive hair loss in the erythrodermic forms of psoriasis. The latter type of hair loss represents a telogen effluvium due to the disease process.[72]

The increased labeling index typical of the epidermis in psoriasis has been noted only in the upper part of the external root sheath and not the hair bulb. Clinically, this fits with the fact that the rate of hair growth is not increased in psoriasis.[72] Any associated hair loss is generally reversible unless there is chronic secondary folliculitis or another traumatic influence that may cause a scarring alopecia.

Figure 5-18 Psoriasis of scalp.

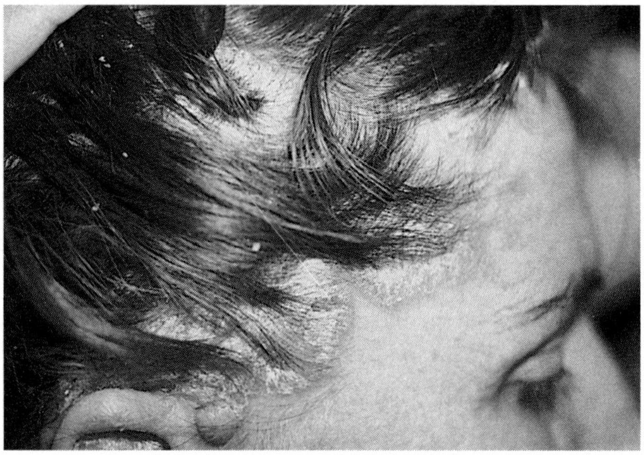

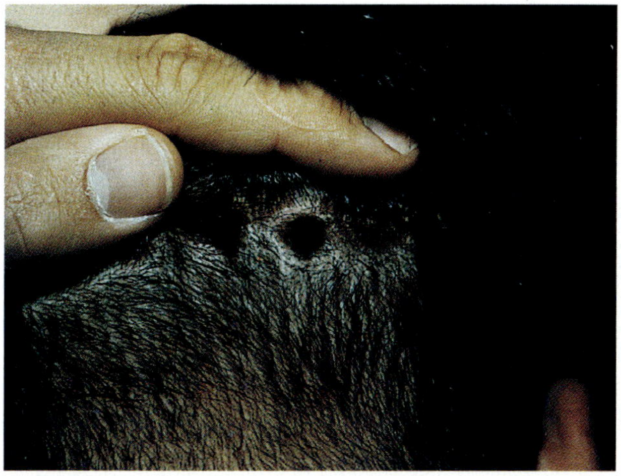

Figure 5-19 "Tepee sign" of psoriasis.

HISTOLOGY

In general, three histological features are most characteristic of psoriasis of the scalp: early involvement of the hair follicles with follicular plugging, enlargement of the follicular ostium, and follicular parakeratosis. Otherwise, only mild acanthosis with irregular hyperkeratosis and foci of hypogranulosis are seen, with Munro microabscesses rarely present.[73] Sebaceous gland atrophy, which is frequently noted in the psoriatic scalp lesions, is felt to be concomitant with reduction in the size of the hair follicle and thinner shafts.[74]

TREATMENT

An important part of the treatment of psoriasis of the scalp is to educate the patient about the condition, explaining that at the present time it cannot be eradicated, that exacerbations may be controlled, and that long-term remissions are possible. Most scalp psoriasis will respond well to systemic agents alone plus or minus use of a medicated shampoo. However, with the typical, topical approach to body psoriasis, various topical medications are used on the scalp. The failure of most treatment regimens of scalp psoriasis is related to the patient's inability to understand the necessity for carrying out the prescribed regimen.

First, the scalp should be cleansed with a medicated shampoo. Patients should alternate their shampoos for more effective control, from a tar shampoo to a nontar shampoo, and should shampoo daily. The scales in the involved scalp are usually thick, and shampooing alone will not suffice in most cases. It is usually necessary to apply a keratolytic substance, such as one containing phenol and/or salicylic acid, overnight under a bathing or shower cap to enhance the penetration of the medication. After the removal of the excess scales by the medicated shampoo, one should apply a fluorinated topical corticosteroid lotion or spray to the erythematous, indurated, and pruritic area(s). Midpotency, group IV to V preparations are best over the long term and generally do not cause atrophy of the scalp skin. Mometasone furoate lotion, triamcinolone acetonide spray, and betamethasone dipropionate lotion are three preparations that can be used carefully over a long time period. Scalp psoriasis needs frequent follow-up, and patients need encouragement to continue the complex treatment regimens often necessary to control the disease.[75]

Treating psoriasis with oral ketoconazole, 200 mg daily, has been advocated by those who consider *P. ovale* to be an incipient cause for the disease.[76] Shampoos containing ketoconazole also have been used as an adjunct to therapy of scalp psoriasis.[77] The effectiveness of these therapies in psoriatic scalp disease has not been thoroughly studied in controlled trials.

Pityriasis Amiantacea

Pityriasis amiantacea is a scalp condition with an uncertain etiology. It may complicate seborrheic dermatitis, psoriasis, tinea infections of the scalp, or neurodermatitis, or it may represent poor hygiene. It is a rare phenomenon in today's society, which prides itself on having healthy hair and scalp.[78,79]

CLINICAL FEATURES

Pityriasis amiantacea is a cutaneous disease affecting the scalp with local areas of characteristic asbestoslike sticky scales and temporary hair loss.[78] These masses of silvery scales overlap like tiles of a roof, adhere to the scalp, and attach in layers to the shafts of the hair which they surround (Fig. 5-20*A*). The scalp may be red and moist. Pityriasis amiantacea is most commonly seen in young girls presenting with chronic fissuring behind one or both ears and scales extending some distance into the neighboring scalp. It is usually confined to small areas of scalp but

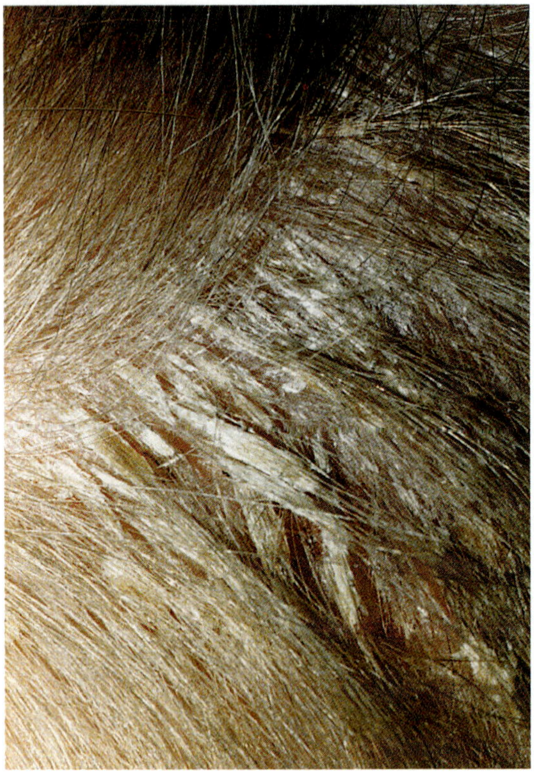

A

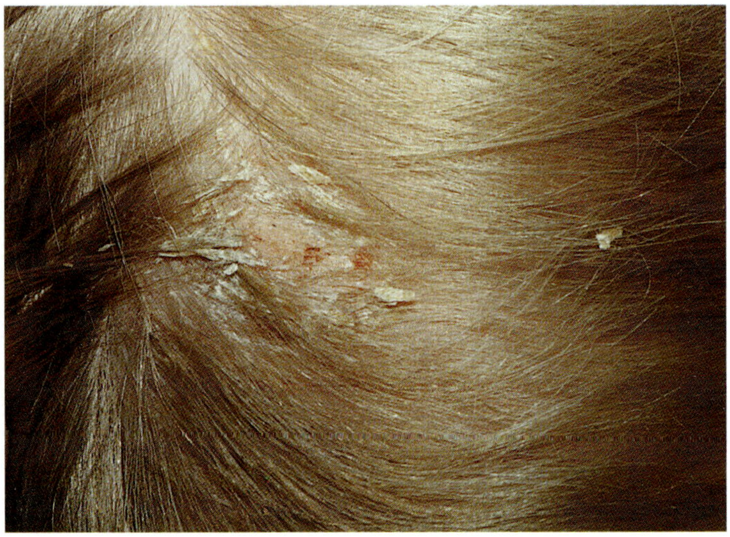

B

Figure 5-20 Pityriasis amiantacea (*A* and *B*). Note area of patchy alopecia after manual removal of scale (*B*). (*Both photographs courtesy of Dr. Elise A. Olsen.*)

may be extensive. Temporary hair loss due to a local physical removal of the scale and adherent hairs is often present (Fig. 5-20*B*), but a scarring hair loss can develop.[80]

HISTOPATHOLOGY

The most consistent finding histologically is the presence of spongiosis, parakeratosis, and migration of lymphocytes into the epidermis with a variable degree of acanthosis. There is no migration of polymorphonuclear leukocytes into the epidermis, and there are no Munro microabscesses in the stratum corneum. The stratum corneum is adherent to the hair in the follicular canal and remains so as it grows out from the follicular sheath, causing a funnel-shaped enlargement of the follicular opening.[79]

TREATMENT

Frequent shampooing, alternating between a tar and a nontar shampoo, is effective. A phenol and salicylic acid solution or a topical 5% crude coal tar mixed with 2% salicylic acid in soft yellow paraffin applied to the scalp 4 to 5 hours prior to shampooing will loosen and remove the scales. Any potential underlying disease, be it psoriasis, seborrheic dermatitis, or tinea capitis, needs to be investigated. Regular shampooing prevents recurrence of the disease and usually permits regrowth of the lost hair.

Acne Miliaris Necrotica

Acne miliaris necrotica is a clinical syndrome with a multiplicity of redundant synonyms. The clinical varieties of acne frontalis, acne pilaris, acne varioliformis, and acne miliaris necrotica all represent the same pathophysiologic entity.[81]

CLINICAL FEATURES

The primary lesion in acne miliaris necrotica is an erythematous follicular papule that undergoes central necrosis (Fig. 5-21). The early lesion is edematous, becomes umbilicated, and subsequently develops a central adherent crust that is shed to leave a localized depressed varioliform scar.[82] Lesions are described as being painful and are often very pruritic. They occur characteristi-

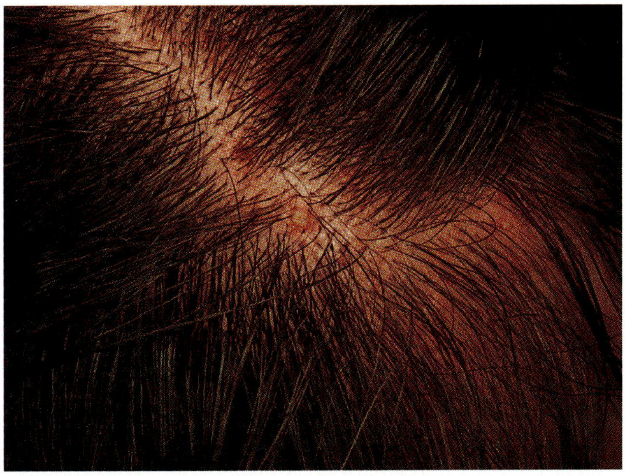

Figure 5-21 Excoriated papule of acne miliaris necrotica.

cally along the frontal hair line and parietal area of the scalp but may have associated lesions on the cheek, neck, or chest. The condition is protracted, and usually only a small number of active lesions are present at any one time. New lesions continue to develop at irregular intervals, and the pruritus seems to be disproportionately severe relative to the size of the lesion. Patients admit to being anxious or nervous, describing exacerbations of the disease during times of stress.[83]

Although bacterial cultures have revealed a variety of organisms, it is postulated that the initial lesion of acne miliaris necrotica is a folliculitis with *Propionibacterium acnes* as the microbiological agent. A Gram stain from an early lesion demonstrates gram-positive pleomorphic rods compatible with the organism *P. acnes*.[84] The patient subsequently manipulates and excoriates the initial lesion, which probably accounts for the common misdiagnosis of staphylococcal folliculitis. The lesion may progress to a crusting, necrotic eschar with ultimately multiple minute scarred areas on the scalp.[83] The lesions appear more frequently in men than in women; in most cases, the patients are between 30 and 50 years of age.

Differential diagnosis would include staphylococcal/streptococcal folliculitis and tinea capitis. In infants, recurrent scalp pustules should lead one to consider scabies as well as eosinophilic pustulosis or acropustulosis of infancy. The latter two would both show eosinophils on microscopic examination of pustule contents and a negative culture, but distribution of lesions and histology would separate these out.[85]

HISTOLOGY

Histological features of an early lesion of acne miliaris necrotica demonstrate a lymphocytic infiltrate centered around a central follicle, with extensive individual cell necrosis of keratinocytes within the external root sheath and surrounding epidermis. There is subepidermal and perifollicular edema. In a late lesion, there is a lymphocytic perivascular and perifollicular infiltrate and a mixed inflammatory infiltrate including plasma cells in the resolving destructive acute folliculitis.[84]

TREATMENT

The acute lymphocytic folliculitis of acne miliaris necrotica may well be triggered by *P. acnes*. Acne miliaris necrotica responds to treatment with a broad-spectrum antibiotic such as tetracycline at doses of 250 mg twice a day. In patients who are anxious or nervous, doxepin, 50 mg per day, in addition to the antibiotic, improves the response to therapy. Topical therapy using 1% clindamycin in an alcohol solution twice daily may be a beneficial adjunct to the systemic therapy.

Miscellaneous Conditions Presenting with Scalp Alopecia

SYRINGOLYMPHOID HYPERPLASIA WITH ALOPECIA

There have been a few case reports of patients who presented with focal alopecia associated with reticular erythema, reddish-brown papules, and follicular hyperkeratosis in involved areas[86,87] (Fig. 5-22). Anhidrosis plus or minus diminished sensation with ulceration were also present in the hairless areas, which were distributed on the extremities, chest, and/or scalp. Histologically, these areas showed a dense lymphohistiocytic infiltrate in the dermis and around the hair follicles. Occasional foreign-body giant cells were present. A lymphocytic infiltrate surrounded hyperplastic dermal sweat ducts and coils. Some cases had histological evidence of vasculitis and chest x-ray findings suggestive of lymphomatoid granulomatosis. It has been proposed that, in the absence of the latter two fea-

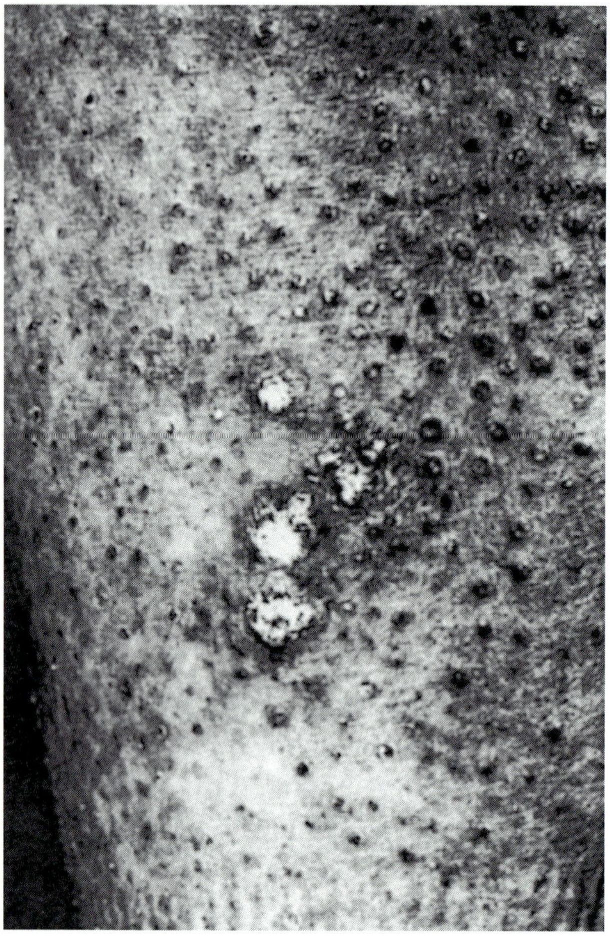

Figure 5-22 Syringolymphoid hyperplasia. (*Reprinted with permission from Vakilzadeh and Bröcker.*[86])

tures, this condition be called *syringolymphoid hyperplasia with alopecia.*

CONCLUDING REMARKS

Infectious and physical causes of alopecia are frequently in the same differential diagnosis list as both generally cause a focal, nonscarring alopecia. There are exceptions to this, of course, as trichotillomania can involve the entire scalp and tinea capitis can lead to permanent hair loss (kerion). At times, infectious and physical causes of alopecia may overlap in presentation with inflammatory scalp conditions: e.g., tinea capitis caused by *T. tonsurans* may mimic seborrheic dermatitis. Pityriasis amiantacea is a common cause of scalp scaling and focal hair loss in children, but the diagnosis is often overlooked or misdiagnosed as atypical psoriasis.

A specific diagnosis can be made, however, by using physical clues, the microscopic hair examination and applicable lab tests including VDRL or fungal culture. Although newer treatments offer promise for a reduction in side effects or enhanced efficacy, current therapy can control or eradicate these disorders.

REFERENCES

1. Vander Willigen AH, Oranje AP, de Wurdt van Ameijden S, Wagenvoort JHT: Tinea capitis in the Netherlands (Rotterdam area). Mycoses 33:46–50, 1990.
2. Clayton YM: Scalp ringworm in superficial fungal infections: New clinical applications. In Verbov J (ed): *Dermatology.* Lancaster, England, MTP Press Ltd, 1986, p 12.
3. Seale ER, Richardson JB: Trichophyton tonsurans. Arch Dermatol 81:125–132, 1960.
4. Prevost E: Nonfluorescent tinea capitis in Charleston SC: A diagnostic problem. JAMA 242:1765–1768, 1974.
5. Sinski JT, Flouras K: A survey of dermatophytes isolated from human patients in the United States from 1979 to 1981 with chronological listings of worldwide incidence of five dermatophytes often isolated in the United States. Mycopathologia 85:97–120, 1984.
6. Krowchuk DP, Lucky AW, Primmer SI, McGuire J: Current status of the identification and management of tinea capitis. Pediatrics 72:625–631, 1983.
7. Bronson DM, Desai DR, Barsky S, Foley SM: An epidemic of infection with Trichophyton tonsurans revealed in a 20-year survey of fungal infections in Chicago. J Am Acad Dermatol 8:322–330, 1983.
8. Terragni L, Lasagni A, Oriani A: Tinea capitis in adults. Mycoses 32:482–486, 1989.
9. Hebert AA, Head ES, MacDonald EM: Tinea capitis caused by Trichophyton tonsurans. Pediatr Dermatol 2:219–223, 1985.
10. Pipkin JL: Tinea capitis in the adult and adolescent. Arch Dermatol 66:9–40, 1952.
11. Snowden MS, Loder L, Alexander WJ: Infectious alopecia in a child day-care center (letter to the editor). JAMA 254:3038, 1985.
12. Mackenzie DWR: The extra-human occurrence of Trichophyton tonsurans var. sulfureum in a residential school. Sabouraudia 1:58–64, 1961–1962.
13. Sharma V et al.: Scalp colonization by Trichophyton tonsurans in an urban pediatric clinic. Arch Dermatol 124:1511–1513, 1988.
14. Ravits MS, Himmelstein R: Tinea capitis in the New York City area. Arch Dermatol 119:532–533, 1983.
15. Hebert AA: Tinea capitis. Arch Dermatol 124:1554–1557, 1988.
16. Elewski BE: Superficial mycoses, dermatophytoses, and selected dermatomycoses. In Elewski BE (ed): *Cutaneous Fungal Infections.* New York, Igaku-Shoin, 1992, p 48.
17. Blank F, Mann SJ, Reale RA: Distribution of dermatophytosis according to age, ethnic group and sex. Sabouraudia 12:352–361, 1974.

18. Even-Paz Z, Raubitschek F: Epidemics of tinea capitis due to Trichophyton verrucosum contracted from cattle or sheep. Dermatologica 120:74–76, 1960.
19. Jones HE, Reinhardt JH, Rinaldi M: A clinical, mycological and immunological survey for dermatophytosis. Arch Dermatol 108:61–65, 1973.
20. Rasmussen JE, Ahmed AR: Trichophyton reactions in children with tinea capitis. Arch Dermatol 114:371–372, 1978.
21. Borchers SW: Moistened gauze technic to aid in diagnosis of tinea capitis (letter to the editor). J Am Acad Dermatol 13:672–673, 1985.
22. Mackenzie DWR: "Hairbrush diagnosis" in detection and eradication of non-fluorescent scalp ringworm. Br Med J 2:363–365, 1963.
23. Head ES, Henry JC, MacDonald EM: The cotton swab technic for the culture of dermatophyte infections: Its efficacy and merit. J Am Acad Dermatol 11:797–801, 1984.
24. Sinski JT, Swanson JR, Kelley LM: Dermatophyte test medium: Clinical and quantitative appraisal. J Invest Dermatol 58:405–411, 1972.
25. Gan VN, Petruska M, Ginsburg CM: Epidemiology and treatment of tinea capitis: Ketoconazole vs. griseofulvin. Pediatr Infect Dis J 6:46–49, 1987.
26. Babel DE, Baugham SA: Evaluation of the adult carrier state in juvenile tinea capitis caused by Trichophyton tonsurans. J Am Acad Dermatol 21:1209–1212, 1989.
27. Allen HB, Honig PJ, Leyden JJ, McGinley KJ: Selenium sulfide: Adjunctive therapy for tinea capitis. Pediatrics 69:81–83, 1982.
28. Bennett JE: Antifungal agents. In Gilman AG, Rall TW, Nies AS, Taylor P (eds): *The Pharmacological Basis of Therapeutics.* 8th ed. New York, Pergamon Press, 1990, pp 1170–1174.
29. Leyden JJ: Clinical features and host response. In Special symposia: Tinea capitis: Current concepts. Pediatr Dermatol 2:233–234, 1985.
30. Ginsburg CM, Gan VN, Petruska M: Randomized controlled trial of intralesional corticosteroid and griseofulvin vs. griseofulvin alone for treatment of kerion. Pediatr Infect Dis J 6:1084–1087, 1987.
31. Cox FW et al.: Oral ketoconazole for dermatophyte infections. J Am Acad Dermatol 6:455–462, 1982.
32. Tanz RR, Hebert AA, Esterly NB: Treating tinea capitis: Should ketoconazole replace griseofulvin? J Pediatr 112:987–991, 1988.
33. Robertson MH et al.: Ketoconazole in griseofulvin-resistant dermatophytosis. J Am Acad Dermatol 6:224–229, 1982.
34. Legendre R, Esola-Macre J: Itraconazole in the treatment of tinea capitis. J Am Acad Dermatol 23:559–560, 1990.
35. Haroon TS et al.: An open clinical pilot study of the efficacy and safety of oral terbinafine in dry non-inflammatory tinea capitis. Br J Dermatol 126 (suppl 39):47–50, 1992.
36. Haroon TS et al.: A randomized, double-blind, comparative study of terbinafine vs. griseofulvin in tinea capitis. J Dermatol Treat 3 (suppl 1):25–27, 1992.
37. From the Centers for Disease Control: Primary, secondary syphilis: U.S., 1981–1990. JAMA 265:2940, 1991.
38. Lee Y-YJ, Hsu M-L: Alopecia syphilitica, a simulator of alopecia areata: Histopathology and differential diagnosis. J Cutan Pathol 12:87–92, 1991.
39. Parisu H: Precocious noduloulcerative cutaneous syphilis. Arch Dermatol 111:76–77, 1975.
40. Shulkin D, Tripoli L, Akell E: Lues maligna in a patient with human immunodeficiency virus infection. Am J Med 85:425–427, 1988.
41. Petrozzi JW, Lockskin NA, Berger BJ: Malignant syphilis. Arch Dermatol 109:387–389, 1974.
42. Stokes JH, Beerman H, Ingraham NR: *Modern Clinical Syphilology,* 3d ed. Philadelphia, WB Saunders Co., 1944, p 250.
43. Mikhail GR, Chapel TA: Follicular papulopustular syphilid. Arch Dermatol 100:471–473, 1969.
44. Tramont EC: Syphilis in the AIDS era. N Engl J Med 316(2):1600–1601, 1987.
45. Hicks CB et al.: Seronegative secondary syphilis in a patient infected with the human immunodeficiency virus (HIV) with Kaposi sarcoma: A diagnostic dilemma. Ann Intern Med 107:492–494, 1987.
46. Skeetal S, Weatherhead L: Extensive nodular secondary syphilis. Arch Dermatol 125:1666–1669, 1989.
47. Goerz G, Ippen H: Hautschaden bei Bewubtlosen Patienten. Med Klin 63:2047–2049, 1968.
48. Abel RR, Lewis GM: Postoperative (pressure) alopecia. Arch Dermatol 81:34–42, 1960.
49. Singh G: Traction alopecia in Sikh boys. Br J Dermatol 92:232–235, 1975.
50. Morgan HV: Traction alopecia. Br Med J 2(1):115–117, 1960.
51. Lipnik MJ: Traumatic alopecia from brush rollers. Arch Dermatol 84:493–495, 1961.
52. Pearlstein HH: Traction alopecia due to hair weaving. Cutis 5:440, 1969.
53. Swedo SE et al.: A double-blind comparison of clomipramine and desipramine in the treatment of trichotillomania (hair pulling). N Engl J Med 321:497–501, 1989.
54. Dawber R: Self-induced hair loss. Semin Dermatol 4:53–57, 1985.
55. Christenson GA, Mackenzie TB, Mitchell JE: Characteristics of 60 adult chronic hair pullers. Am J Psychiatry 148:365–370, 1991.
56. Muller SA: Trichotillomania: A histopathologic study in sixty-six patients. J Am Acad Dermatol 23:56–62, 1990.
57. Mehregan AH: Trichotillomania, a clinicopathologic study. Arch Dermatol 102:129–133, 1970.
58. Krishnan KRR, Davidson JRT, Guajardo C: Trichotillomania—A review. Compr Psychiatry 26:123–128, 1985.
59. Alexander RC: Fluoxetine treatment of trichotillomania. J Clin Psychiatry 52:88, 1991.
60. Baldessarini RJ: Drugs and the treatment of psychiatric disorders. In Gilman AC, Rall TW, Nies AS, Taylor P (eds): *The Pharmacological Basis of Therapeutics,* 8th ed. New York, Pergamon Press, 1990, pp 404–414.
61. Apache PG.: Eczematous dermatitis of the scalp. In Ziuak C (ed): *The Science of Hair Care.* New York, Marcel Dekker, 1986, pp 513–521.
62. Parish LC: L-dopa for seborrheic dermatitis. N Engl J Med 283:879, 1970.
63. Stratigos JD et al.: Ketoconazole 2% cream versus hydrocortisone 1% cream in the treatment of seborrheic dermatitis: A double-blind comparative study. J Am Acad Dermatol 19:850–853, 1988.
64. Groisser D, Bottone EJ, Lebwohl M: Association of Pityrosporum orbiculare (Malassezia furfur) with seborrheic

dermatitis in patients with acquired immunodeficiency syndrome (AIDS). J Am Acad Dermatol 20:770–773, 1989.
65. Heng MC et al.: Correlation of Pityrosporum ovale density with clinical severity of seborrheic dermatitis as assessed by a simplified technique. J Am Acad Dermatol 23:82–86, 1990.
66. Senff H et al.: Studies on yeast flora in patients suffering from psoriasis capillitii on seborrheic dermatitis of the scalp. Mycoses 33:29–32, 1990.
67. Leyden JJ, McGinley KJ, Kligman AM: Role of microorganisms in dandruff. Arch Dermatol 112:333–338, 1976.
68. Faergemann J.: Treatment of seborrheic dermatitis with bifonazole. Mycoses 32:309–311, 1989.
69. Skinner RB et al.: Seborrheic dermatitis and AIDS. J Am Acad Dermatol 14:147–148, 1986.
70. Rosenberg EW, Belew PW: Microbial factors in psoriasis. Arch Dermatol 118:143, 1982.
71. Sohnle PG, Collins-Lech C: Activation of complement by Pityrosporum orbiculare. J Invest Dermatol 80:93–97, 1983.
72. Comaish S: Autoradiographic studies of hair growth in various dermatoses: Investigation of a possible circadian rhythm in normal hair growth. Br J Dermatol 81:283–285, 1969.
73. Stadler R, Schaumburg-Lever G, Orfanos CE: Histology. In Mier PD, van de Kerkhof PCM (eds): *Textbook of Psoriasis.* Edinburgh, Churchill Livingstone, 1986, pp 40–54.
74. Headington JT et al.: A morphometric and histologic study of the scalp in psoriasis. Arch Dermatol 125: 639–641, 1989.
75. Dawber R: Aspects of treatment of scalp psoriasis. J Dermatol Treat 1:1–8, 1989.
76. Rosenberg EW, Belew PW: Improvement of psoriasis of the scalp with ketoconazole (letter to the editor). Arch Dermatol 118:370–371, 1982.
77. Rosenberg EW, Noah PW, Skinner RB: Treatment of psoriasis with antimicrobial agents. In Roenigk HH, Maibach HI (eds): *Psoriasis.* New York, Marcel Dekker, 1985, pp 505–511.
78. Hersle K, Lindholm A, Mobacken H, Sandberg L: Relationship of pityriasis amiantacea to psoriasis. Dermatologica 159:245–250, 1979.
79. Knight AG.: Pityriasis amiantacea: A clinical and histopathological investigation. Clin Exp Dermatol 2:137–143, 1977.
80. Langtry JAA, Ive FA: Pityriasis amiantacea, an unrecognized cause of scarring alopecia, described in four patients. Acta Derm Venereol (Stockh) 71:352–353, 1991.
81. Rook A, Dawber R: Acne necrotica. In *Diseases of the Hair and Scalp.* Oxford, Blackwell Scientific Publications, 1982, pp 476–477.
82. Kossard S, Collins A, McCrossin I: Necrotizing lymphocytic folliculitis: The early lesion of acne necrotica (varioliformis). J Am Acad Dermatol 16:1007–1014, 1987.
83. Fisher DA: Acne necroticans (varioliformis) and Staphylococcus aureus. J Am Acad Dermatol 18:1136–1137, 1988.
84. Maibach HI: Scalp pustules due to corynebacterium acnes. Arch Dermatol 96:453–455, 1967.
85. Taïeb A, Bassan-Andrieu L, Maleville J: Eosinophilic pustulosis of the scalp in childhood. J Am Acad Dermatol 27:55–60, 1992.
86. Vakilzadeh F, Bröcker EB: Syringolymphoid hyperplasia with alopecia. Br J Dermatol 110:95–101, 1984.
87. Sarkany I: Patchy alopecia, anhidrosis, eccrine gland wall hypertrophy and vasculitis. Proc R Soc Med 62:157–158, 1969.

Chapter

6

HAIR SHAFT DEFECTS

David A. Whiting

OVERVIEW

Hair shaft defects are common and can sometimes lead to obvious and severe hair loss.[1] Usually the clinical changes are more subtle, comprising changes in hair form, texture, diameter, color, or varying degrees of hair damage caused by minor trauma to injury-prone hair.[2] Defects of the hair shaft can be inherited or acquired and can be useful indicators of underlying disease.[3–5]

In the clinical evaluation of a patient complaining of hair loss or abnormal hair texture, a full history of the hair disorder itself and a detailed, systematic family and drug history should be taken. On examination, hypothyroidism and other endocrine disorders, iron deficiency, malnutrition, metabolic disorders, exposure to drugs or toxic chemicals, collagen diseases, infections such as syphilis, and widespread skin disease should be ruled out.[1] The hair and scalp should be carefully examined to exclude local disease.

Hair samples can be examined in the office setting by light microscopy. Hair shafts are easily mounted in parallel on glass slides previously coated with double-stick clear tape[6] or with two fresh bands of mounting medium such as Accumount (Baxter Scientific Products, McGaw Park, IL) synthetic resin. A permanent slide preparation free of optical distortion can be made by applying several drops of the resin to a large coverslip or to the slide.[7,8] Hair shaft abnormalities must be found consistently in samples from different areas of the scalp if they are to be considered significant.

A reliable diagnosis of a hair shaft abnormality can only be made with an appreciation of the wide structural variations found in normal hair. Shaft diameter, cross section, cuticular pattern, length, and color can differ considerably in the same individual.[9,10] Most hair shaft abnormalities, with notable exceptions such as pili multigemini, pili annulati, and monilethrix, can be seen sporadically in normal hair. Normal hair forms should also be taken into account; these

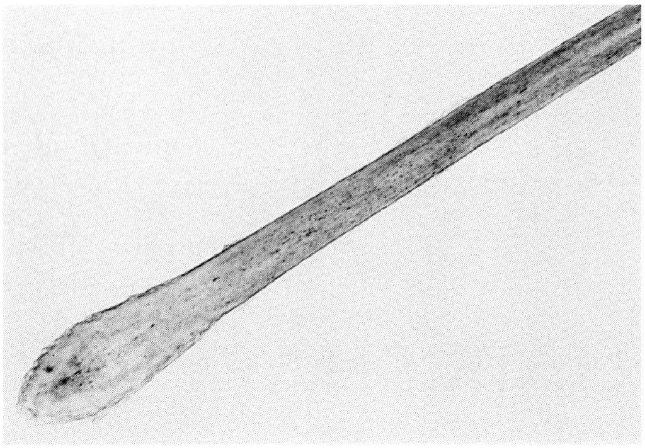

Figure 6-1 Telogen hair bulb: pale color, absent root sheath. (Light micrograph ×100)

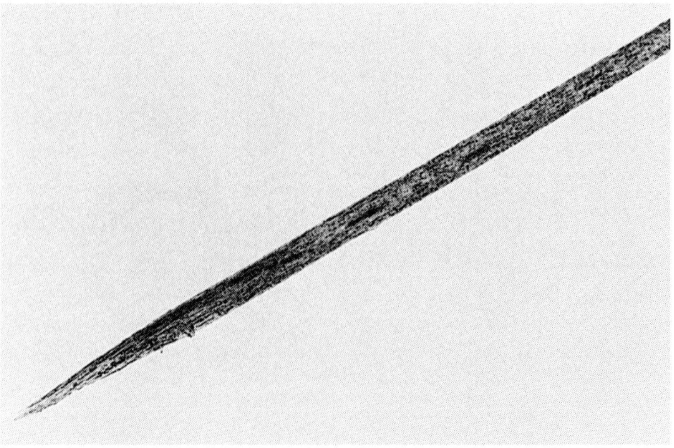

Figure 6-2 Proximal tapering of hair shaft in anagen effluvium. (Light micrograph ×40)

include straight, wavy, curly, woolly, or peppercorn.[11,12] Straight and wavy hair forms are easy to identify; curly hair is spiraled, forming spiral locks; woolly hair, seen commonly in blacks and some whites, occurs as tightly coiled spirals that do not form locks or lie flat; peppercorn hair, seen exclusively in blacks, curls so tightly that little knobs are formed and the scalp is visible between the knobs.

The normal hair shaft is constant in diameter throughout its length and is round or oval in cross section. The anatomy of the normal cuticle, cortex, and medulla is described in Chapter 1. The variations in the anatomy of the hair root during the hair growth cycle must also be recognized and are discussed in detail in Chapter 1. Telogen hairs have short, white, club-shaped roots and no root sheaths, with pigment lacking in the hair shaft adjacent to the root (Fig. 6-1). They constitute 5 to 10 percent of normal, terminal scalp hairs; are increased in telogen effluvium;[13,14] and are easy to detach with pull tests. Anagen hairs have indented, elongated roots and pigmented adjacent shafts; they are covered by long, intact outer and inner root sheaths, and are difficult to detach with pull tests. Anagen and telogen hairs can often be distinguished from one another with the naked eye, and light microscopy will resolve any doubts.[1] Both anagen and telogen hairs are suitable for hair shaft analysis. Abnormalities of the shaft are independent of the hair growth cycle except for the tapered fractures associated with anagen effluvium (Fig. 6-2).[15,16]

An important phenomenon in both normal and abnormal hair is *weathering.* Weathering represents the wear and tear that mainly affects the free end of the hair, causing damage to cuticle and cortex.[2,17] Abnormal hairs with inherited weaknesses are susceptible to excessive weathering.[18] Weathering is exaggerated by excessive hairstyling, washing, friction, sun, wind, swimming, and so forth.[18a] Various physical and chemical factors, both environmental and cosmetic, can cause progressive damage to the hair cuticle. The margins of the cuticular cells are gradually eroded and broken away, especially in the distal shaft, where they are less adherent. Localized areas of cuticle loss lead to longitudinal fissures. The cuticle may be totally lost at the hair tip, with fraying of the underlying cortex (Fig. 6-3). Without the splinting effect of an in-

Figure 6-3 Weathering: distal loss of cuticle with fraying of cortex. (Light micrograph ×100)

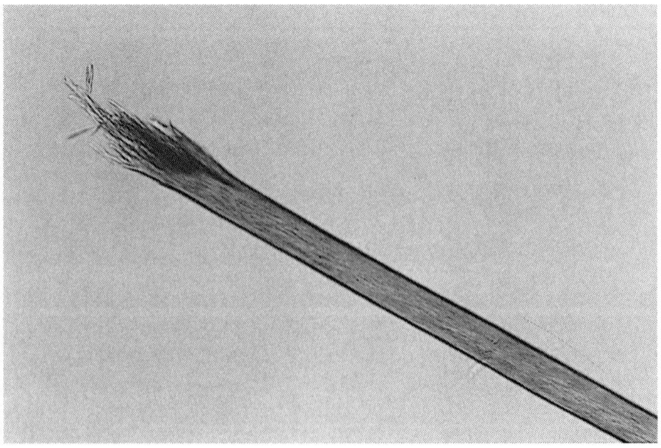

tact cuticle, the underlying fibers fray and separate longitudinally, causing split ends, which in severe cases resemble the nodular fractures of trichorrhexis nodosa. Weathering is less marked near the hair root.[19,20] When evaluating a potential hair shaft abnormality, the proximal 1 or 2 cm of a hair shaft adjacent to the scalp should be examined in order to exclude the effects of weathering.

CLASSIFICATION OF HAIR SHAFT DEFECTS

The evaluation and diagnosis of hair shaft defects depend on both clinical features and microscopic appearances. A useful clinical distinction is based on *hair fragility*.[7,8,21] If the hair is fragile, fractures easily, and leads to obvious alopecia, the following conditions should be considered: trichorrhexis nodosa, pili torti, Menkes' disease, monilethrix, pseudo monilethrix, trichorrhexis invaginata, trichothiodystrophy, and intermittent hair follicle dystrophy. Other conditions causing hair shaft defects do not display inherently fragile hair. However, diagnostic difficulties can arise in the latter group in that clinically apparent hair fragility, usually due to repeated trauma, can be seen in cases of anagen effluvium, bubble hair, traction alopecia, trichonodosis, trichorrhexis nodosa occurring in normal hair, trichotillomania, uncombable hair syndrome, and woolly hair nevus.

Another useful clinical distinction is that of *unruly hair*.[22] Congenital unruly hair, with no apparent associated hair shaft abnormality, arises in the newborn and does not persist beyond infancy. It may occur in normal infants or be associated with defects in early brain development, microcephaly, de Lange's syndrome, or Down's syndrome.[22,23] Congenital unruly hair, associated with a hair shaft abnormality, arises after 3 months of age. Causes of fragile unruly hair include all forms of pili torti. Causes of nonfragile unruly hair include all forms of woolly hair and uncombable hair. Acquired unruly hair is caused by acquired pili torti, acquired progressive kinking, drug-induced kinking, and whisker hair, and is not usually associated with undue hair fragility. The causes of unruly hair are listed in Table 6-1.

Precise diagnosis of the structural abnormality of the hair shaft often depends on the microscopic appearance. The great majority of these abnormalities can be diagnosed by light microscopy in the office, often aided by the use of polarizing sheets. Possible exceptions to this include the uncombable hair syndrome and other causes of longitudinal grooving such as congenital hypotrichosis (Marie Unna). By light microscopy, hair shaft abnormalities can be classified by appearance as fractures, hair shaft coiling and twisting, irregularities, and extraneous (artifactual) matter on the hair shaft (Table 6-2).[1] In this system, most of the defects with hair fragility are included in the fracture group; the remainder are pili torti from the coiling and twisting group, and monilethrix, pseudo monilethrix, and intermittent hair follicle dystrophy from the irregularity group. Unruly hair falls largely into the coiling and twisting group, with the exception of uncombable hair in the irregularity group. The *microscopic classification*, in which hair fragility is also indicated, is listed in Table 6-2. Individual hair shaft defects will be discussed in the order shown in this microscopic classification.

FRACTURES OF THE HAIR SHAFT

Transverse Fractures

TRICHORRHEXIS NODOSA

Trichorrhexis nodosa is the most common defect of the hair shaft.[2,8] Trichorrhexis nodosa appears along the hair shaft as beaded swellings associated with loss of cuticle. The expanded areas are composed of frayed cortical fibers through which the hair readily fractures (Fig. 6-4). The designation trichorrhexis nodosa should be used only when the typical nodular defect occurs along the hair shaft and should not be applied to the brush-like fringe at the distal free end of a hair which occurs as the result of weathering.[8]

The basic cause of trichorrhexis nodosa is mechanical or chemical trauma.[24,25] A contributory factor is an inherent weakness of the hair shaft.

Figure 6-4 Trichorrhexis nodosa: cuticular loss, cortical fraying, expanded fracture.

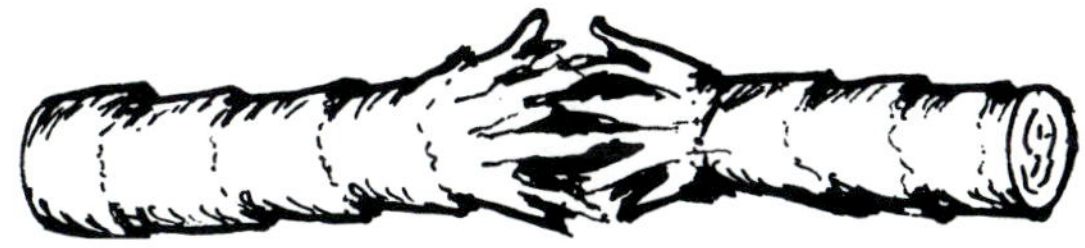

Table 6-1
CAUSES OF UNRULY HAIR

		References
1. CONGENITAL OR INHERITED UNRULY HAIR		
A. No Association with Defined Hair Shaft Abnormality:		
Onset: Neonatal period	Duration: Infancy	
Associations: None or mental retardation		22
(microcephaly, de Lange's syndrome, Down's syndrome)		23
B. Associated with Defined Hair Shaft Abnormality:		
Onset: Infancy to late teens	Duration: Limited or indefinite	
1. Increased hair fragility:		
Congenital pili torti:		
Prepubertal pili torti:		
Classic pili torti (Ronchese)		116
Björnstad's syndrome		121
Crandall's syndrome		124
Familial acne conglobata with pili torti		127
Bazex's syndrome		128
Hypohidrotic ectodermal dysplasia		130
Corkscrew hair		126
Menkes' syndrome		44
Postpubertal pili torti:		
Beare's syndrome		133
Sporadic pili torti:		
Miscellaneous hair shaft defects—		
monilethrix, pseudo monilethrix,		151,152
woolly hair, longitudinal grooving,		153,154
trichorrhexis nodosa,		24
trichorrhexis invaginata		99
Citrullinemia		43
2. No increased hair fragility:		
Woolly hair:	Hereditary woolly hair	153
	Familial woolly hair	153
	Woolly hair nevus	167
Uncombable hair:	(Pili trianguli et canaliculi	211
	or spun-glass hair)	208
2. ACQUIRED UNRULY HAIR		
Acquired pili torti:	Cicatricial alopecia—localized	120
	Drug-induced: oral retinoids	56
Acquired kinking:	Acquired progressive kinking	183
	Drug-induced kinking and twisting: oral retinoids	153
	X-ray–induced kinking and twisting	185
Whisker hair:	(Pubic hair nevus)	186
Matting or felting of hair:	Caused by mechanical trauma, detergent shampoos	51

Source: Modified from Mortimer.[22]

Common examples of physical trauma damaging to hair shafts are excessive brushing, back combing, stressed hairstyles such as tight braids or ponytails, hair weaving, the application of heat, and prolonged ultraviolet exposure.[1] Mechanical causes of shearing and rotational stresses of the hair shaft include head rolling and banging, habit tics, trichotillomania, and the scratching and pulling associated with pruritic dermatoses such as seborrheic dermatitis, lichen simplex, and pediculosis capitis.[1] Chemical trauma can be caused by excessive shampooing, setting, perming, and dyeing of the hair, as well as by excessive exposure to salt water.[1]

Trichorrhexis nodosa should be regarded as a distinctive response of the hair shaft to injury. If the frequency and/or degree of the injury is sufficient, it can be, and often is, induced in normal hair. However, if the hair is abnormally brittle with underlying structural weakness, trichor-

Table 6-2
CLASSIFICATION OF HAIR SHAFT DEFECTS

Fractures of the Hair Shaft
- Transverse
  - Trichorrhexis nodosa, congenital* and acquired
  - Trichoclasis
  - Trichoschisis, including trichothiodystrophy*
  - Trichorrhexis invaginata, including bamboo hair*
- Oblique
  - Tapered fracture*
- Longitudinal
  - Trichoptilosis

Hair-Shaft Coiling and Twisting
- Pili torti, including corkscrew hair and Menkes' syndrome*
- Woolly hair, including acquired progressive kinking, therapy-induced kinking, and whisker hair
- Trichonodosis (knotted hair)
- Circle hairs

Irregularities of the Hair Shaft
- Longitudinal ridging and grooving, including loose anagen syndrome and congenital hypotrichosis
- Uncombable hair or pili trianguli et canaliculi or spun glass hair, including straight hair nevus
- Pili multigemini and pili bifurcati
- Trichostasis spinulosa
- Pili annulati
- Pseudo pili annulati
- Pilar melanin clumps, in Chédiak-Higashi syndrome
- Monilethrix*
- Pseudo monilethrix*
- Tapered hairs*, including Pohl-Pinkus mark, bayonet hairs, tapered newly growing anagen hairs, and trichomalacia
- Bubble hairs
- Intermittent hair-follicle dystrophy*
- Acquired eyelash trichomegaly

Extraneous Matter on the Hair Shaft
- Fungi
  - Tinea capitis
  - Piedra
- Bacteria
  - Trichomycosis axillaris
- Pediculosis
  - Nits
- Peripilar casts
  - Pseudonits
- Deposits
  - Lacquer, paint, glue

*Associated with hair fragility.

rhexis nodosa may follow relatively trivial injury. This is seen in alopecia areata, in which dystrophic anagen hairs fracture readily at the skin surface with a trichorrhexis nodosa–like fracture and are later extruded a few millimeters in the telogen phase as "exclamation-point" hairs.[26] Defined structural hair shaft abnormalities associated with increased fragility, and subject to trichorrhexis nodosa as a secondary event, include trichorrhexis invaginata (bamboo hair), monilethrix, pseudo monilethrix, intermittent hair follicle dystrophy, and pili torti. Brittle hairs susceptible to trichorrhexis nodosa also include those weakened by metabolic abnormalities of keratin formation, among which are the low sulfur content found in trichothiodystrophy, the amino acid abnormalities in argininosuccinicaciduria, and the copper defects in Menkes' syndrome. Pili annulati is sometimes associated with trichorrhexis nodosa.[2]

In the pathogenesis of trichorrhexis nodosa, the earliest observed change is a localized loss of cuticle cells.[24,27,28] The exposed cortical fibers later separate and fray, causing a nodular

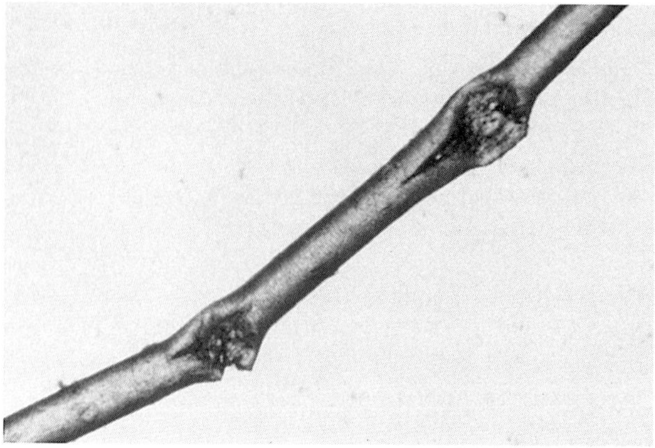

Figure 6-5 Trichorrhexis nodosa: expanded fractures. (Light micrograph ×100)

swelling of the hair shaft (Fig. 6-4). Individual cortical fibers start to fracture, producing the appearance of two paintbrushes thrust into one another. Before complete breakage, the typical expanded fracture is seen (Fig. 6-5).

On clinical inspection, one or more nodes may be found as gray-white or yellow specks on the affected hair shafts.[8] They commonly involve the distal portion of the hair shaft but may occur proximally. Because hairs tend to fracture at the site of the nodes, patchy or diffuse alopecia may result, depending on the severity and extent of the trichorrhexis nodosa. The condition is usually seen on the scalp hair but under certain circumstances can involve the pubic hair[24] or even the body hair, the eyebrows, or the eyelashes.

Figure 6-6 Normal and alternative pathways of waste nitrogen excretion: AL = arginosuccinate lyase or argininosuccinase; arg = arginine; AS = argininosuccinic synthetase; asa = argininosuccinic acid (which is normally split by AL into arg and fumaric acid); cp = carbamylphosphate; CPS = carbamylphosphate synthetase; ha = hippuric acid; OTC = ornithine transcarbamylase; pa = phenylacetic acid; pag = phenylacetylglutamine; sb = sodium benzoate. (*Reprinted from Batshaw, Thomas, and Brusilow.*[34])

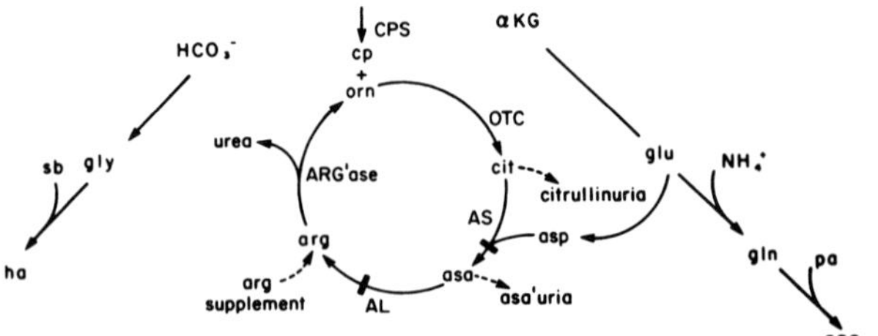

CONGENITAL TRICHORRHEXIS NODOSA

Congenital trichorrhexis nodosa exclusive of underlying metabolic defects, or trichorrhexis congenita, is rare. Both familial and sporadic cases have been seen. Initially the hair may be normal-appearing, but within a few months of life the formation of nodes with resultant fractures is induced by slight trauma. Congenital trichorrhexis nodosa has been described as occurring alone[29] and also has been associated with defective teeth and nails in a few familial cases.[30] The association of follicular hyperkeratosis has also been described in some cases.[31] No abnormal laboratory findings have been reported in these patients.

Congenital trichorrhexis nodosa may occur with underlying metabolic defects such as some, but not all, cases of *argininosuccinicaciduria,* an inborn error of urea synthesis.[32] Inherited defects in the urea cycle are characterized by an inability to synthesize and excrete waste nitrogen in the form of urea[33] (Fig. 6-6).[34] This allows nitrogenous precursors to accumulate and cause organ toxicity. In the rare condition of argininosuccinicaciduria, argininosuccinic acid increases because of the inborn absence of the cleavage enzyme argininosuccinase, which normally splits it into arginine and fumaric acid.[35,36] The associated arginine deficiency in hair has been postulated to lead to abnormal keratin formation and structural weakness of the hair, although this has been disputed by finding that the hair defect may improve despite persistence of the same high level of argininosuccinic acid.[37]

There are three clinical forms of argininosuccinicaciduria.[38] In the first form, symptoms of lethargy, seizures, and respiratory distress begin at birth, with death following within 2 weeks. In the second, or subacute, form, there is a gradual onset of physical and mental retardation and hepatomegaly during the first few months of life. The third form begins from the second year onward and manifests with psychomotor retardation and episodes of ataxia. In most of these children, the hair is dry, dull, brittle, lusterless, and matted; the hair changes can appear in infancy and early childhood.[39] There is a stubbly appearance of the hair due to characteristic fractures of trichorrhexis nodosa.

Diagnosis of an inborn error of urea synthesis is suspected by finding acidosis and hyperammonemia, normal serum organic acids, and low serum arginine.[34] Argininosuccinase deficiency is diagnosed by additionally finding elevated serum and urine citrulline and argininosuccinic acid.[34] Both citrulline and argininosuccinic acid may serve as waste nitrogen products, although less efficient than urea, as they contain nitrogen normally destined for urea synthesis.[33,34] Their synthesis and excretion are enhanced by arginine supplementation.[33] Dietary restriction of protein to reduce waste nitrogen excretion as urea, together with supplementation with arginine, allows adequate synthesis of argininosuccinic acid to meet waste nitrogen excretion; this may help prevent further intellectual impairment.[34,39] The administration of sodium benzoate can further divert ammonium nitrogen from the defective urea cycle to hippurate synthesis.[33]

It should be noted that citrulline, which occurs only in the hair medulla and internal root sheath, is the normal precursor of argininosuccinic acid in the urea cycle. The rare inborn deficiency of argininosuccinic acid synthetase causes *citrullinemia,* along with a resultant low plasma arginine level.[40] This condition can lead to atrophic hair bulbs, hair weakness, trichorrhexis nodosa,[41,42] pili torti,[43] and irregular hair shaft banding.[3] A scaly skin eruption can occur; it may be widespread and exfoliative, with dry or moist red patches and plaques that predominate in the perioral and diaper regions.[40]

Another rare metabolic disorder associated with trichorrhexis nodosa is *Menkes' syndrome,* in which defective copper metabolism is present.[44,45] Copper is required for proper keratin formation, and the resultant keratinization defect leads to pili torti and trichorrhexis nodosa. In this disease, the entire hair shaft is abnormal, except for the proximal 0.5 to 1 cm. Menkes' kinky hair syndrome is discussed further in the etiology of pili torti.

A number of cases of trichothiodystrophy, which is discussed later, have been reported in which brittle hair was associated with a low sulfur content.[46] With trauma, the hair fractures easily. The classic fracture seen in these cases is *trichoschisis,* in which a localized absence of cuticle cells is associated with a straight break across the hair shaft. However, the nodular fractures of trichorrhexis nodosa are often seen. Presumably, a low cystine content accounts for the weakness in the keratin of the hair cuticle and cortex. A patient with hair low in cystine has been described with generalized trichorrhexis nodosa affecting all body hair.[47] Electron microscopy and histochemical studies showed both a disorder in the formation of alpha protein chains within the globular matrix of the cortex with respect to cystine and multiple vacuoles in the endocuticle. These intrinsic defects evidently allowed relatively trivial trauma to cause trichorrhexis nodosa.

ACQUIRED TRICHORRHEXIS NODOSA

Acquired proximal trichorrhexis nodosa is common in blacks, usually after years of hair straightening with hot combs or permanent waves.[7] The lesions of trichorrhexis nodosa develop abruptly in the proximal hair shaft, with subsequent breakage and resultant alopecia in areas subject to friction from brushing, combing, or sleeping.[8] These patients complain that the scalp hairs do not grow longer than a few inches, break readily, are extremely brittle, and look as if they have been cut. Microscopic examination of the easily detached hair shafts shows trichorrhexis nodosa and the longitudinal splitting of the hair shaft known as *trichoptilosis.*

The treatment is to minimize trauma, i.e., stop the hot-combing and permanent waving. For unknown reasons, this condition may take 2 to 4 years to clear, and cure is perhaps dependent on the formation of new anagen hairs.[8]

Acquired distal trichorrhexis nodosa is seen mostly in whites and Orientals.[5] The nodes appear on the distal few inches of hair, which is the older and therefore more weathered portion (Fig. 6-7). The hair looks dull and uneven, and shows drying, thinning, and splitting. A history of excessive brushing, back combing, chemical processing, and other hairstyling is common.[8] The

Figure 6-7 Trichorrhexis nodosa: distal type in Caucasian hair from constant brushing. (*Reprinted from Whiting.*[1])

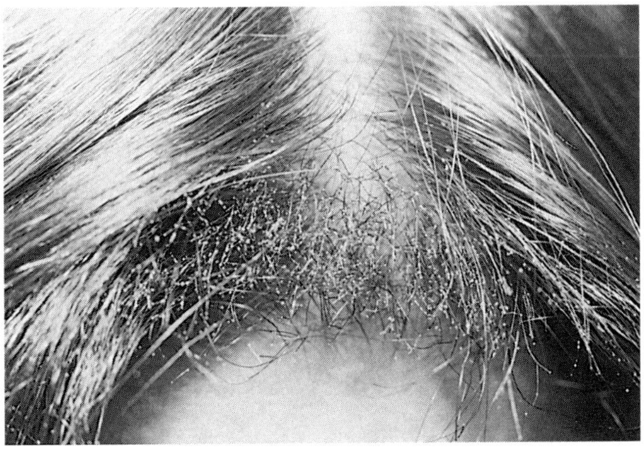

cuticular cells are lost at the sites of nodules, probably secondary to weathering.[48] There is concomitant reduction in cystine at the prenodule and postnodule sites that may reflect not only a decrease in the cuticle but a decrease in the underlying cortex as well.[48] Distal trichorrhexis nodosa can be reversed by gentle hair care.

Acquired localized trichorrhexis nodosa is found in patches of trichotillomania, lichen simplex chronicus, and other pruritic dermatoses[49,50] but occasionally appears spontaneously in the scalp, the beard, or the moustache in circumscribed patches 3 to 4 cm in diameter. The hair is faded, lighter than normal, and lacks luster. The condition may eventually resolve spontaneously but may persist in some cases.

In general, the correct treatment for patients with trichorrhexis nodosa or other causes of fragile hair is to minimize trauma. Shampooing should always be gentle, and mild detergent shampoos should be used. The use of cream rinse conditioners is advised to prevent matting of hair.[51] Hairbrushes should be avoided. Only styling brushes with rounded prongs or wide-toothed combs should be used, and their use should be restricted to the minimum possible. Back combing, tight ponytails, and tight braids should be avoided. All affected hair should be cut short. The use of permanent waves, hair straighteners, hair dyes, and treatment involving heat such as hot combs, hot curlers, and curling irons should be restricted in all cases of hair fragility.

TRICHOCLASIS

Trichoclasis is the common "greenstick" fracture of the hair shaft.[52] It consists of a transverse fracture of the shaft which is splinted partly or wholly by intact cuticle (Fig. 6-8). There is no constant abnormality of cuticle, cortex, or sulfur content.

Trichoclasis does not indicate any specific underlying disease. It can be associated with congenital hair shaft abnormalities in which cuticles remain intact, such as pili torti or pseudo monilethrix, or it can occur in normal hair. It is caused by physical trauma, such as that produced by overzealous hair care, or chemical trauma and can be associated with trichoptilosis and trichorrhexis nodosa. It is usually sporadic and occurs in patchy rather than widespread fashion. It also indicates the need for gentle hair care.

Stankler and coworkers recently reported a peculiar type of hair shaft abnormality in two siblings who had unexplained diarrhea, unusual facies, and failure to thrive.[53] Budlike projections were found in multiple sites arising from the convex surface of a kinked hair. The condition was named *trichorrhexis blastysis*. Affected sites of the hair had some cuticular interruption with loss of architecture, and fracturing. The published scanning electron micrograph suggests a type of trichoclasis, hence the inclusion of this condition here. However, longitudinal fractures and kinked and twisted hairs were also described in this condition.

TRICHOSCHISIS

Trichoschisis is a clean transverse fracture across the hair shaft through the cuticle and cortex. The fracture is associated with a localized absence of cuticle cells (Fig. 6-9).[54] Trichoschisis can occur sporadically in otherwise normal hair as an isolated finding.[1] However, it is usually seen in the congenitally brittle, low-sulfur hair which characterizes trichothiodystrophy, and affects many hairs. It should be noted that causes of low cystine in hair, other than trichothiodystrophy, include cold-waving solution, depilatories, hair bleaches and dyes,[55] different types of ichthyosis,[56] Clouston's ectodermal dysplasia,[57] and kwashiorkor.[58] There is a single case report of a patient with trichoschisis and brittle, low-sulfur hair with no other signs of cutaneous or systemic involvement.[54]

The term *trichothiodystrophy* has been applied to neuroectodermal abnormalities caused by a mutation of a regulatory gene or genes and includes the abnormal hair that serves as an important marker for this condition.[46] Other vari-

Figure 6-8 Trichoclasis: greenstick fracture of shaft with one side of cuticle intact.

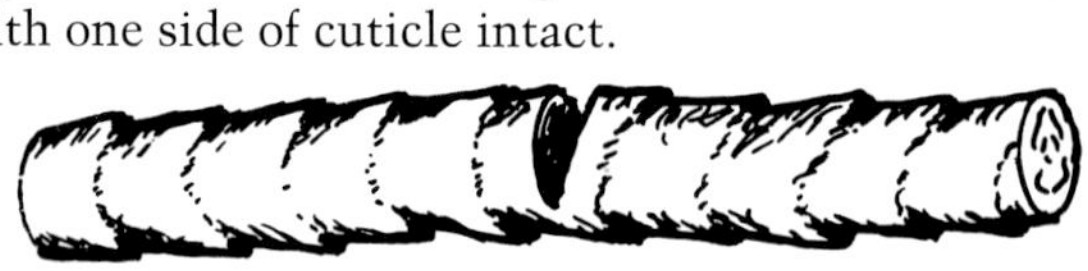

Figure 6-9 Trichoschisis: localized absence of cuticle, clean transverse fracture.

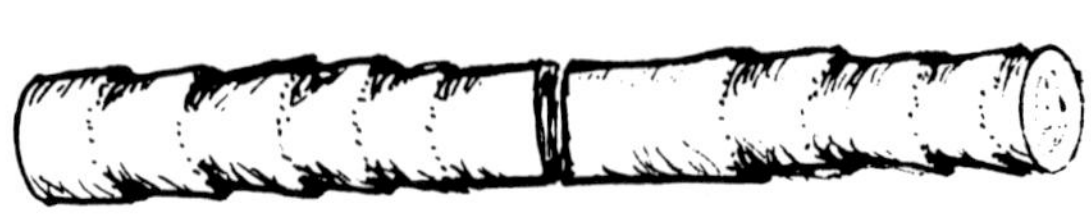

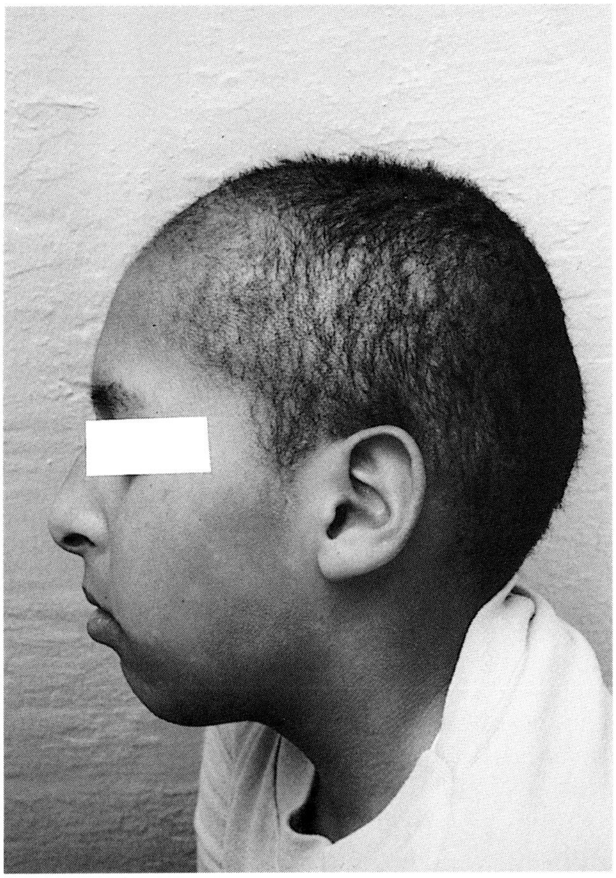

Figure 6-10 Trichothiodystrophy: short, sparse hair. (*Courtesy of Dr. Vera H. Price.*)

able features of trichothiodystrophy include mental retardation, short stature, ichthyosis (lamellar), nail dystrophy, congenital cataracts, dental caries, neurological defects, decreased fertility, photosensitivity, and neutropenia.[8,46,59–61] It is not yet certain whether the different syndromes, of which brittle hair with low sulfur content is a constant feature, represent a single entity or multiple entities.[8,59,60] The hair abnormality is the key to identifying these patients. Clinically, there is persistent alopecia of the scalp, eyebrows, and eyelashes caused by the extremely brittle, short, flattened hairs (Fig. 6-10). Hairs may also be affected elsewhere on the body, particularly after puberty.

On light microscopy, the hair shaft is often flattened and folded over in a ribbonlike fashion, and its outline tends to be undulating and irregular, with a wavy pattern of melanin granules.[46] Due to the brittle nature of the hair shaft, most fractures on light microscopy show the clean

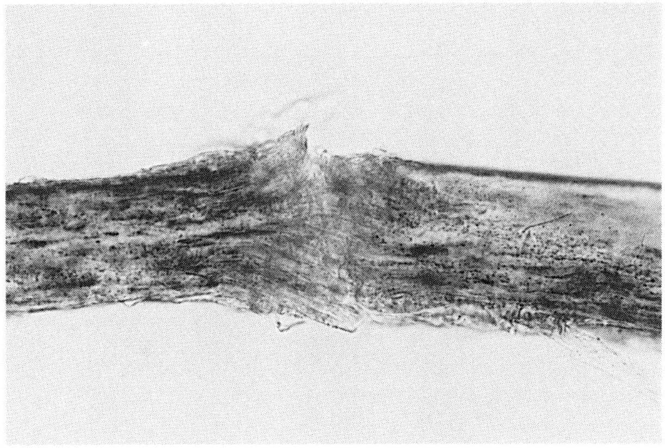

Figure 6-11 Trichoschisis: transverse fracture. (Light micrograph ×400)

breaks of trichoschisis (Fig. 6-11), but some have the expanded appearance of trichorrhexis nodosa. Examination of the affected hair shafts under polarized light shows the characteristic "tiger tail" or "zigzag" pattern of alternating bright and dark diagonal bands (Fig. 6-12*A* and *B*), which can be reversed by turning the crossed polarizer. The original terminology of alternating birefringence was incorrectly applied to these hairs, since no fixed angle of light splitting is detectable and all regions of the hairs are birefringent.[60,62] The structural abnormality that causes the alternate transverse bands is not known, although an alternating sulfur content along the long axis of the hair has been found by x-ray microanalysis.[63]

Scanning electron microscopy reveals increased weathering, with localized areas in which cuticle cells are lost. Fractures occur, as well as significant ridging and fluting of the shaft.[64] Transmission electron microscopy with histochemical methods has shown that the cuticular weathering and hair shaft weakening are due to discontinuity or complete absence of the cuticular A layer.[65] The cuticle A region, which is rich in cystine and consequently in high-energy disulfide bonds, occurs on the outer aspect of the cuticle cell. In addition, a disorderly arrangement of microfibrils has been demonstrated in the keratogenous zone of the abnormal hairs.[62,66]

The sulfur content of the hair associated with trichothiodystrophy is generally reduced to 50 percent of its normal value, as is the level of the amino acid cystine, in both the cuticle and the cortex.[65] Electrophoretic patterns of the high-sulfur proteins in trichothiodystrophic hair differ

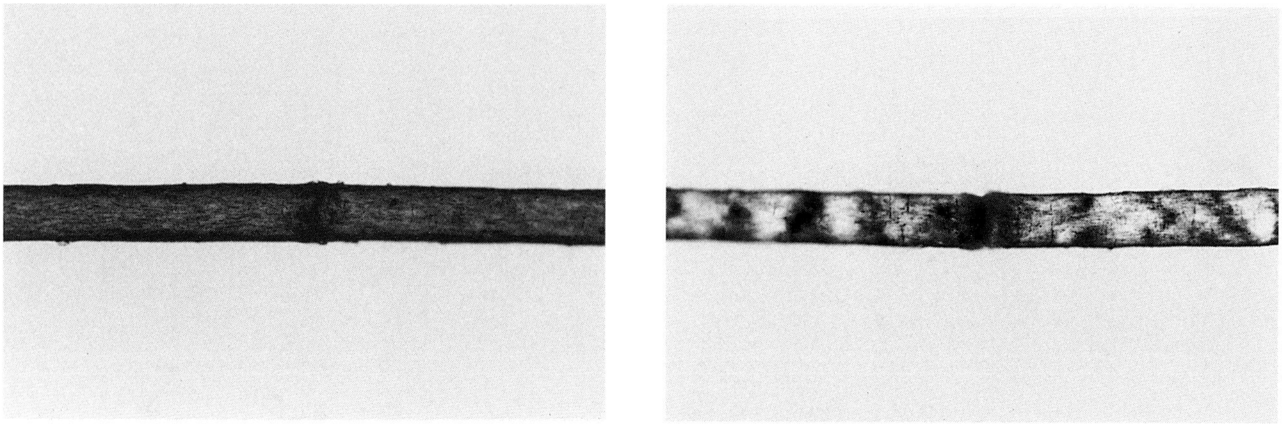

A B

Figure 6-12 Trichothiodystrophy. (*A*) Hair shaft with trichoschisis without polarization. (Light micrograph ×100) (*B*) Hair shaft with trichoschisis with polarization showing alternating light and dark bands. (Light micrograph ×100)

from those in normal hair, the most obvious difference being absence of most of the ultrahigh-sulfur proteins and a lower cystine content of the remaining high-sulfur proteins.[67,68] Low-sulfur protein content is generally higher than normal.[46] This has led to the hypothesis that the basic defect in trichothiodystrophy may be an altered regulatory gene which suppresses synthesis of some high-sulfur proteins and enhances synthesis of other proteins.[67]

Patients with trichothiodystrophy may have impaired DNA repair with or without photosensitivity.[69–73] Although some cases of trichothiodystrophy have the same molecular defects in response to ultraviolet light as xeroderma pigmentosum cases, the former have no increased incidence of skin cancers.

The wide spectrum of associated abnormalities suggests that trichothiodystrophy is heterogeneous.[60] The association of various other neuroectodermal abnormalities is extremely variable and, thus far, has been reported under various eponyms or acronyms. Patients with trichothiodystrophy have been categorized into seven subgroups; these, together with the related Marinesco-Sjögren's syndrome, are listed in Table 6-3.[74–85]

For definitive diagnosis of trichothiodystrophy, hair mounts, polarizing microscopy, total sulfur content, or amino acid analysis of hair is necessary. A positive diagnosis depends upon the presence of low-sulfur hair and either trichoschisis or alternating light and dark bands by polarizing microscopy, or severe cuticular damage by scanning electron microscopy.[60] Light-sensitive patients should be tested with medium-wave ultraviolet (UVB) rays for phototoxicity.[59] All patients should be tested for their cellular responses to ultraviolet radiation, which can be done by in vitro radiation of peripheral blood lymphocytes or cultured skin fibroblasts.[71,76] Coexisting xeroderma pigmentosum may be responsible for low levels of DNA repair.[71] It would appear that a possible but not obligatory link exists between trichothiodystrophy and xeroderma pigmentosum.

No treatment is available, but early prevention of sun-induced skin damage is necessary in photosensitive patients. Dietary cystine supplementation for the milder cases has been suggested, but its value is unproven.[8]

TRICHORRHEXIS INVAGINATA, OR BAMBOO HAIR

Trichorrhexis invaginata, or "bamboo hair," is a nodular expansion of the hair shaft in which a ball-and-socket joint is formed. The club-shaped distal hair fragment is surrounded by a cuplike expansion of the proximal hair shaft (Figs. 6-13 and 6-14*A* and *B*). On clinical inspection, multiple small nodules or concretions are seen spaced along the shaft at irregular intervals. The hair is usually short, thin, and friable (Fig. 6-15).[86]

Isolated lesions of trichorrhexis invaginata can occur sporadically from trauma in normal hair, or in congenital hair shaft abnormalities. Wide-

Table 6-3
SYNDROMES ASSOCIATED WITH TRICHOTHIODYSTROPHY

Group	*Brittle Hair*	*Brittle Nails*	*Intellectual Impairment*	*Decreased Fertility*	*Short Stature*	*Ichthyosis*	*Photosensitivity*	*Neutropenia*	*Other Findings*	*Acronym/ Eponym*	*References*
A. Isolated hair defect	+									Trichoschisis	54
B. Hair and nail dystrophy	+	+								Trichoschisis / onychodystrophy	59, 46
C. Above and mental retardation, infertility	+	+	+	+					Astigmatism, pale optic discs, retinopathy	Sabinas syndrome	77, 78
D. Above and growth retardation	+	+	+	+	+				Quadriplegia, seizures, microcephaly	BIDS, Amish brittle hair syndrome	62, 79
E. Above and ichthyosis	+	+	+	+	+	+			Abnormal teeth, tongue plaques, cataract, V.S.D.	IBIDS, Tay syndrome, Pollitt syndrome	80,81, 82, 83, 84
F. Above and photo-sensitivity	+	+	+	+	+	+	+		Xeroderma pigmentosum	PIBIDS	85, 70,75, 76
G. Most of above and chronic neutropenia	+	+	+		+	+		+	Recurrent infections, folliculitis, conjunctivitis	ONMR, Onychotricho-dysplasia, neutro-penia, mental retardation	61, 62
H. Marinesco-Sjögren syndrome	+	+	+		+				Ataxia, dysarthia, cataracts, abnormal teeth (primarily nonectodermal)	Marinesco-Sjögren syndrome	41, 62, 74, 60

V.S.D. = ventricular septal defect.
Source: Modified from Van Neste, Miller, and Bohnert[59] and Itin and Pittelkow.[60]

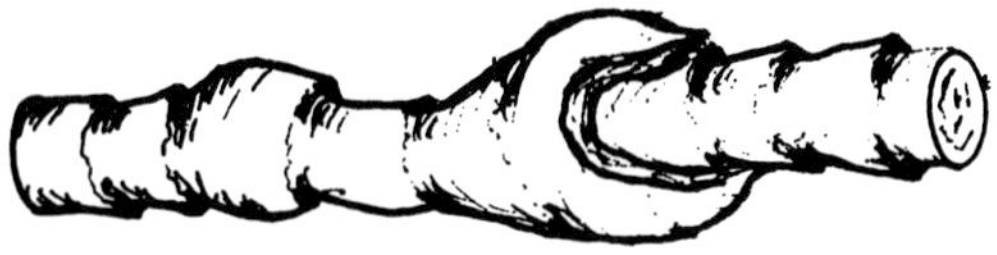

Figure 6-13 Trichorrhexis invaginata: bamboo hair. Cup-shaped proximal hair fragment surrounds distal club-shaped fragment.

spread involvement is associated with *Netherton's syndrome,* a triad of ichthyosiform dermatosis, multiple defects of the hair shaft, and an atopic diathesis.[87–90] Most cases of Netherton's syndrome are associated with ichthyosis linearis circumflexa,[91,92] but others show nonbullous congenital ichthyosiform erythroderma (lamellar ichthyosis).[90] This hair abnormality has also been reported to occur in isolated cases of ichthyosis vulgaris and sex-linked ichthyosis.[93] Generalized scaling and erythema are present from birth or in the first 10 days of life,[94] but the degree, extent, and persistence of the erythema are highly variable. One aspect that has not been emphasized is the remarkable erythroderma that follows any infection.[94] On the trunk and limbs, ichthyosis linearis circumflexa develops as a polycyclic and serpiginous scaling eruption which is constantly changing in pattern. The advancing borders of these lesions have a characteristic, double-edged scale (Fig. 6-16). Atopy is present in 75 percent of cases and was part of Wilkinson's original description of Netherton's syndrome;[88] thus, lichenification and dry skin are common. Aminoaciduria has been described in some 25 percent of cases and can be intermittent;[95] glycine, serine, and histidine were found in the urine in one case.[88] It has been suggested that the reported aminoaciduria was artifactual due to transient renal tubular impairment as a result of excess absorption of locally applied corticosteroids.[90] Recurrent infections, short stature,[96] and mental defects are rare. This syndrome is seen more often in girls than in boys and is probably due to an autosomal recessive gene of variable expressivity.[90] There are two reports of Netherton's syndrome affecting two sisters.[97,98]

The hair defect appears in infancy and may affect all hair to some degree.[87] The scalp hair is dry and lusterless. Its fragility is such that the shortness of the hair is directly proportional to the degree of trauma to which the scalp hair is subjected. Body hair is also affected. The dull and brittle hair cannot grow to a normal length. In addition to the bamboo nodes of trichorrhexis invaginata, associated hair shaft abnormalities include pili torti, trichorrhexis nodosa, and torsion nodes, in which the two former abnormalities are combined to produce a fusiform swelling of the hair shaft traversed by several oblique spiral invaginations running parallel to one another (Fig. 6-17).[99,100] One or more nodes of trichorrhexis invaginata may occur along the hair shaft; the nodes occur irregularly, with no periodicity. In some nodes the cuplike proximal portion is expanded into a tuliplike form. Should

Figure 6-14 Trichorrhexis invaginata: Netherton's syndrome. (*A*) Bamboo hair. (Light micrograph ×100) (*B*) Bamboo hair. (Light micrograph ×400)

A

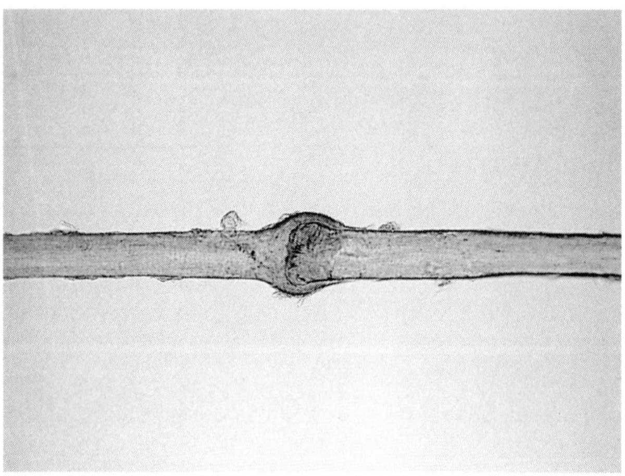

B

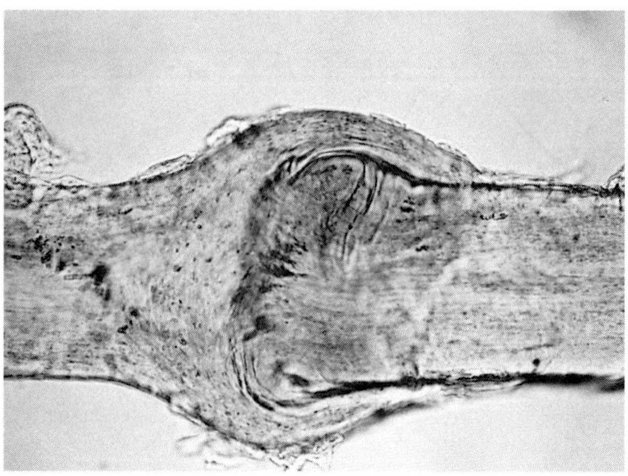

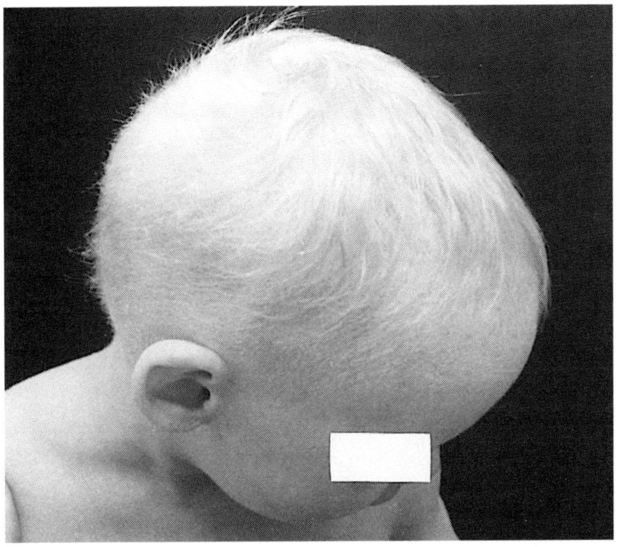

Figure 6-15 Trichorrhexis invaginata: Netherton's syndrome. Scalp hair is short and thin. (*Courtesy of Dr. Vera H. Price.*)

the distal club-shaped fragment be detached, only the proximal fragment remains, the so-called golf-tee hairs of Netherton's syndrome

Figure 6-16 Trichorrhexis invaginata: Netherton's syndrome. Skin with ichthyosis linearis circumflexa. (*Courtesy of Dr. Vera H. Price.*)

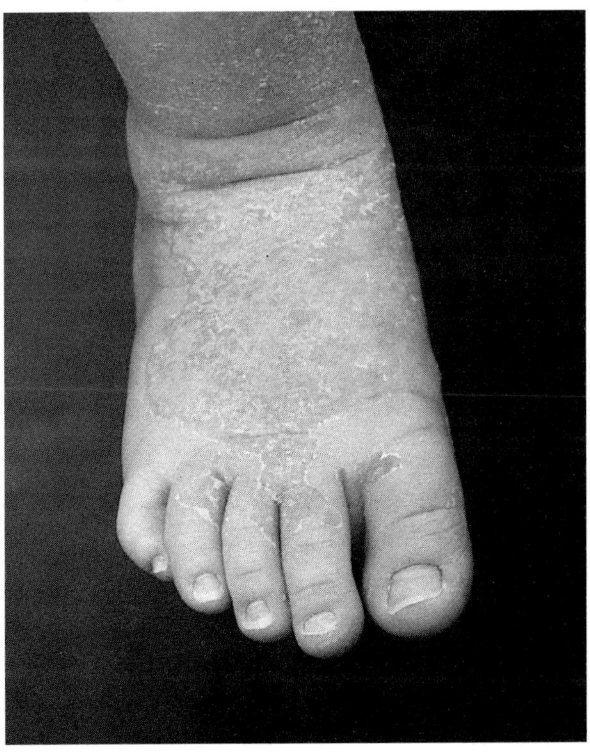

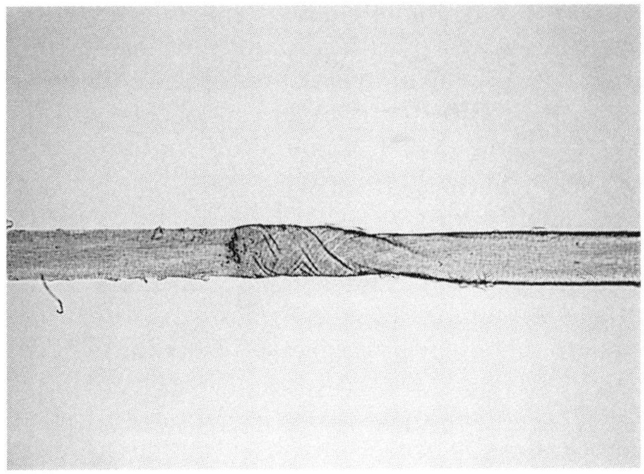

Figure 6-17 Trichorrhexis invaginata: Netherton's syndrome: Torsion node (Light micrograph ×100).

(Fig. 6-18).[101] Not all hairs are involved, and sometimes more vellus than terminal scalp hairs are affected.[102]

The presence of a transient defect of keratinization in the keratogenous zone has been suggested by scanning and transmission electron-microscopic studies of plucked hairs.[100,103] The defect occurs at a level where the internal root sheath is fully keratinized but the shaft is not. The softness of the hair cortex in the keratogenous zone may result from an incomplete conversion of sulfhydryl groups into disulfide bonds in cortical fibers.[100] The tonofilaments in the hair cortex show a remarkable zigzag pattern.[100] The distal keratinized portion of the hair shaft may then readily intussuscept into the

Figure 6-18 Trichorrhexis invaginata: Netherton's syndrome: Golf-tee hair—expanded proximal hair fragment. (Light micrograph × 100)

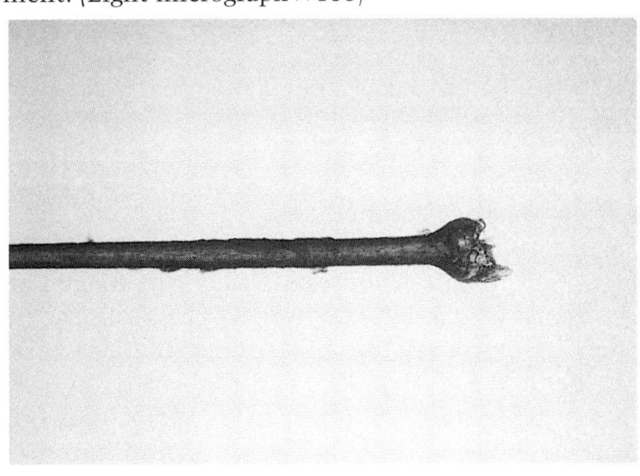

proximal soft, incompletely keratinized portion, which envelops it with a cuplike expansion compressed by the firm internal root sheath.[104] Possibly the cuticles of the inner root sheath and the shaft become detached and allow more mobility between shaft and sheath. It is not clear whether this abnormality is caused by an intermittent disorder of keratinization or whether there is a continuous defect which is only accentuated by transient trauma.

The histological changes of the skin rash are not diagnostic. Psoriasiform changes are often present on histological examination of the affected skin.[105] An eosinophilic degeneration of cells in the upper malpighian layers has been described in the figurate lesions.[106,107] This material is probably a glycolipoprotein and has also been seen in the overlying, parakeratotic, horny layer. A localized disturbance of keratinization has been confirmed by electron microscopy.[108]

There is no specific treatment for trichorrhexis invaginata, but the hair does tend to improve spontaneously as the patient ages. Some improvement of the hair and skin has been reported from the use of systemic retinoids,[109,110] but another patient did not benefit.[90] The protection of the hair from physical and chemical trauma can be of considerable cosmetic benefit. Various remedies used for the ichthyosis include vitamin A and topical corticosteroids, antibiotics, emollients, and keratolytic agents. Topical 12% ammonium lactate solution has shown promise.[97] Photochemotherapy has also been helpful.[111]

Oblique Fractures

TAPERED FRACTURE

Fractures of the hair which resemble pencil points are due to inhibition of nucleic acid and protein synthesis, and therefore of mitosis, in the hair root during anagen.[52] Progressive narrowing of the emerging hair shaft may lead to a fracture near the skin surface, resulting in a detached hair with a *tapered* proximal end.

Widespread fractures of tapered hairs or complete failure of hair formation occur in anagen effluvium, caused, for example, by the systemic effect of a cytostatic drug. Many fragmented hairs are detached easily all over the scalp on pull tests, and examination of the proximal portions of these hairs will often reveal tapered fractures

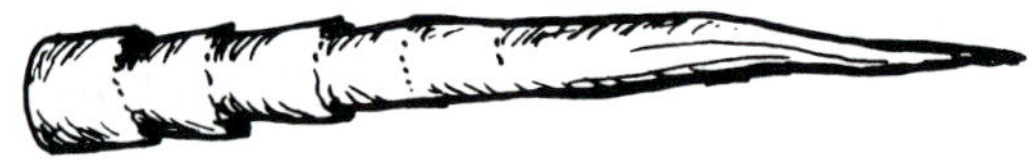

Figure 6-19 Tapered hair: loss of cuticle and tapered cortex.

(Fig. 6-2). Whereas a gentle pull test is usually diagnostic, forcible extraction of hair in advanced cases of anagen effluvium can be misleading in that telogen hairs may be all that remain. Hair growth resumes after withdrawal of the drug, and the hair thickens up again, resulting in an attached hair with distal tapering (Fig. 6-19). This phenomenon can also be seen in localized areas following radiotherapy, as well as in alopecia areata. In alopecia areata, following fracture at the site of constriction, some anagen hairs may resume growth and emerge as short, pigmented dystrophic hairs with a tapered distal end which lacks a cuticle.[1] This contrasts with the nodular fracture seen in the classic exclamation-point hair of alopecia areata, which has a trichorrhexis nodosa–like fracture at the distal end and proximal depigmentation of the hair shaft adjacent to a telogen root.[26,112] Tapered hairs may also occur in severe protein-calorie malnutrition, such as marasmus or kwashiorkor.

Longitudinal Fractures

TRICHOPTILOSIS

Trichoptilosis is a longitudinal splitting of the distal end of the hair.[52] Following cuticular loss from weathering, the cortical fibers separate like the frayed end of a rope, giving rise to the common "split ends" or "frizzies" (Fig. 6-20).[7] Central trichoptilosis is sometimes seen when the longitudinal split does not involve the free end of the hair (Fig. 6-21*A* and *B*).[113]

Trichoptilosis is a common fracture caused by trauma, which is easy to see clinically. It can occur in normal hair from weathering or more

Figure 6-20 Trichoptilosis: cuticular loss, and splits in cortex.

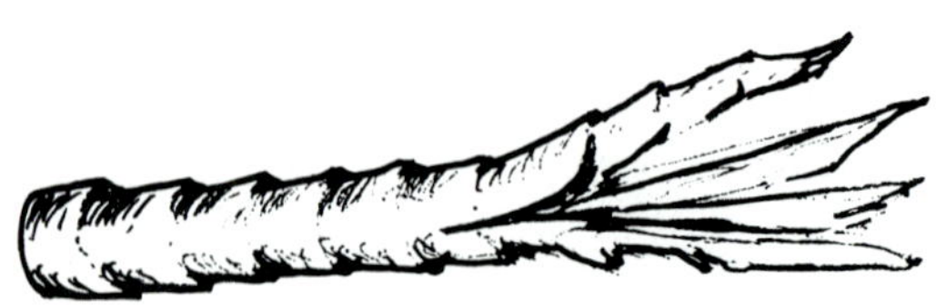

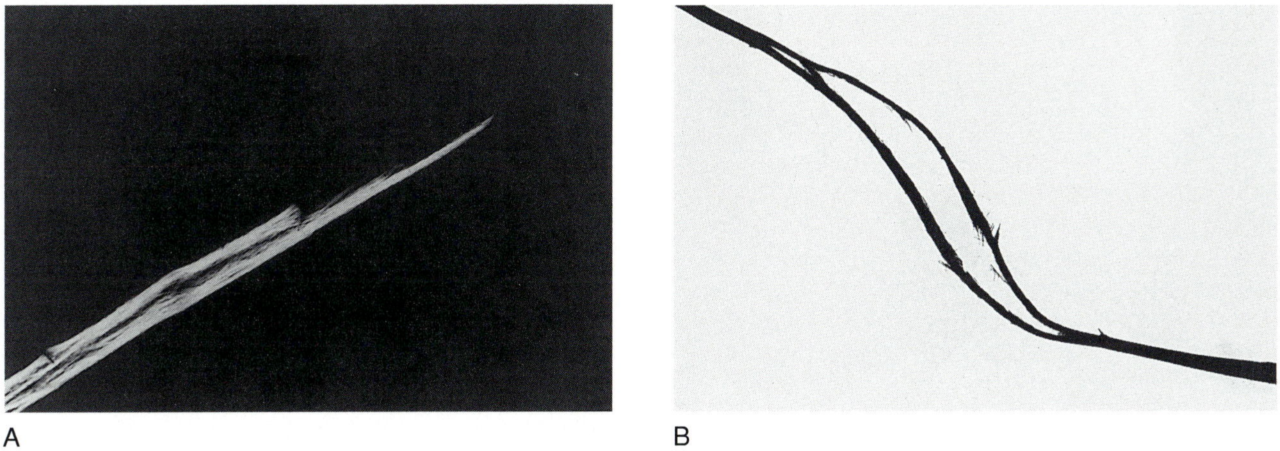

Figure 6-21 Trichoptilosis. (*A*) Terminal: cortical splits at end of hair. (Light micrograph ×100 polarized) (*B*) Central: cortical split in hair shaft, not affecting free end of hair. (Light micrograph ×100)

commonly from the excessive damage caused by trichotillomania, pruritic dermatoses, or excessive hairstyling. It is frequently seen in the congenitally brittle hair found in pili torti, monilethrix, trichothiodystrophy, and trichorrhexis invaginata.[1] Gentle hair care is needed to control trichoptilosis.

HAIR SHAFT COILING AND TWISTING

Pili Torti

In pili torti, the affected hair shaft is flattened and twisted on its own axis, usually through an angle of 180 degrees (Fig. 6-22),[114] with a range of 90 to 360 degrees. Typically, four or five twists are found at irregular intervals along an otherwise straight hair shaft with an intact cuticle, giving it a spangled or beaded appearance (Fig. 6-23*A* and *B*). The affected hairs are brittle, break easily, and fail to attain normal length. They poorly resist stretching and tend to fracture within the twists, where the shaft is oval.[115] The hair follicles show no histological changes except for some curvature and twisting. The hairs themselves show a normal alpha keratin pattern on x-ray diffraction.[114]

Figure 6-22 Pili torti: 180-degree twists in hair shaft.

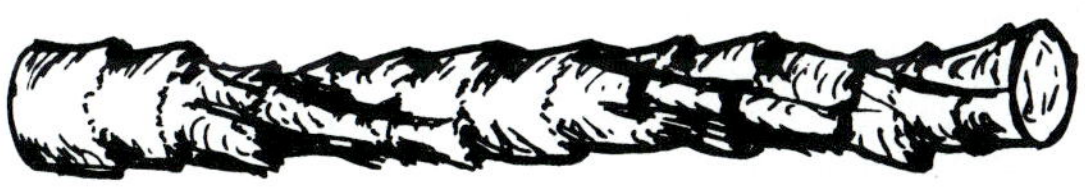

It is important to remember that twisted hairs are commonly seen in normal scalps, and to a minor degree are associated with many other conditions of the scalp and the scalp hair.[116,117] Twisted hairs need to be present in sufficient numbers and density, and to occur over an appreciable area, in order to be classified as a true pili torti. Note that pubic and axillary hairs are normally twisted. Pili torti is usually congenital but is sometimes acquired. On light microscopy, true pili torti usually shows narrow twists in groups of 3 to 10 on a flattened shaft. These are more numerous than the occasional twists seen as a result of other structural abnormalities or from trauma or artifact in normal hairs. Pili torti is also easy to distinguish from the longer and coarser spirals seen in curly hair.

CONGENITAL PILI TORTI

Congenital pili torti may occur as an isolated phenomenon or may occur in association with other abnormalities.

CLASSIC PILI TORTI (RONCHESE)

The classic type of pili torti as described by Ronchese is a diffuse abnormality usually found in association with thin, blond hair.[116] It may occur alone or as part of an ectodermal dysplasia syndrome in association with widely spaced teeth and enamel hypoplasia,[116,118] nail dystrophy,[119] corneal opacities,[120] keratosis pilaris, and

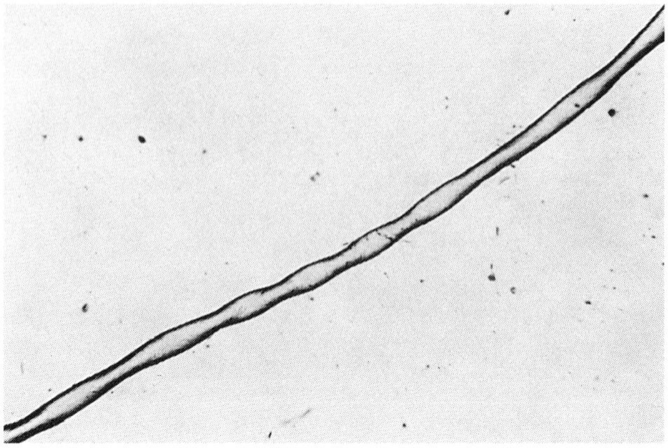

A

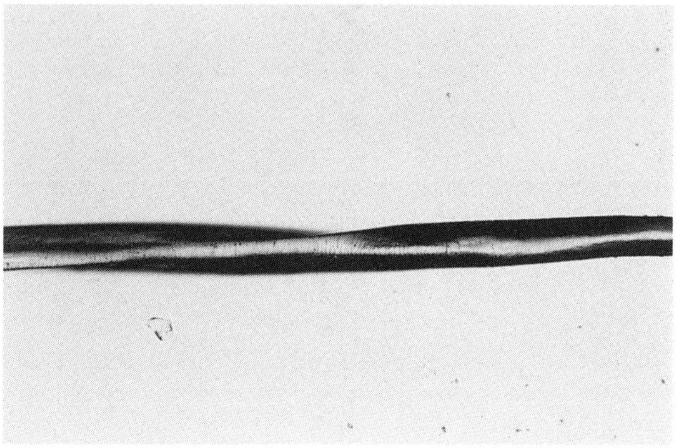

B

Figure 6-23 Pili torti. (*A*) Irregularly spaced 180-degree twists in shaft. (Light micrograph ×40) (*B*) 180-degree twist, intact cuticle. (Light micrograph ×100)

ichthyosis.[89,105,120] Sensorineural deafness of the cochlear type has now been described in a number of children with pili torti of the prepubertal type.[121–124] Early auditory testing is therefore mandatory in pili torti. Intelligence is usually normal. Inheritance is usually autosomal dominant in cases of pili torti[114] but may be autosomal recessive[120] or sporadic.[125] Females are predominantly affected, suggesting that the gene might often be lethal in males.[126]

Scalp hair in the classic type of pili torti may be abnormal at birth, or the abnormality may develop within the first 2 years of life.[114] Normal scalp hairs are replaced by brittle, spangled hairs, especially in the occipital (Fig. 6-24) and temporal regions. The eyebrows and eyelashes may also be involved. The clinical picture, which varies with the degree of hair fragility, ranges from patchy alopecia through coarse stubble to longer hairs of 5 cm or more. Pili multigemini, which consist of two to eight hairs arising from separate papillae and matrices but emerging through one pilary canal, is sometimes present.[116] Pili torti may improve after puberty or persist throughout life.

OTHER SYNDROMES ASSOCIATED WITH PILI TORTI

There are many cases of pili torti which have been described in association with other defects, some of which fall into recognizable syndromes. Most of these cases were described with an onset before puberty, as seen in familial acne conglobata,[127] Bazex's syndrome,[128] Rapp-Hodgkin hypohidrotic ectodermal dysplasia,[129–131] corkscrew hair,[126,132] and Menkes' syndrome.[44] Other cases of pili torti manifesting after puberty have been described by Beare,[133] Ullmo,[134] and Kurwa and Abdel-Aziz[120] (Table 6-4).

Other combinations of abnormalities can be expected with pili torti, such as the facial deformities, syndactyly of digits, and mental retardation reported recently.[135] Not all cases reported as pili torti can be regarded as genuine examples of the anomaly. For example, the hair abnormalities seen in the ectodermal dysplasias are poorly characterized and need reevaluation.

Corkscrew Hair. A unique type of pili torti in which many hairs are twisted in a double spiral has been described as *corkscrew hair* (Fig. 6-25), occurring in association with widely spaced teeth and syndactyly of fingers and toes.[126] This

Figure 6-24 Pili torti: twisted hairs in lower, occipital region.

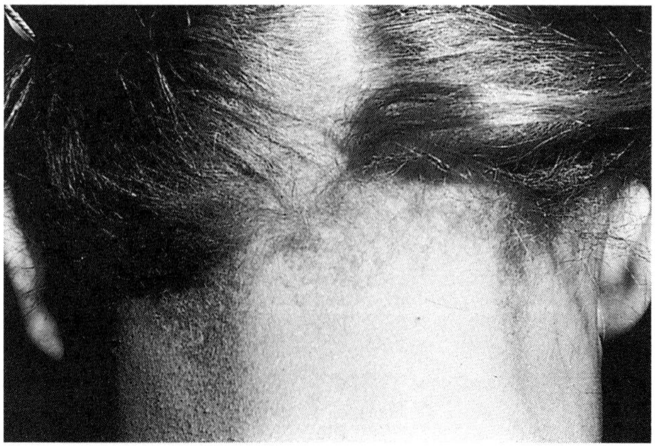

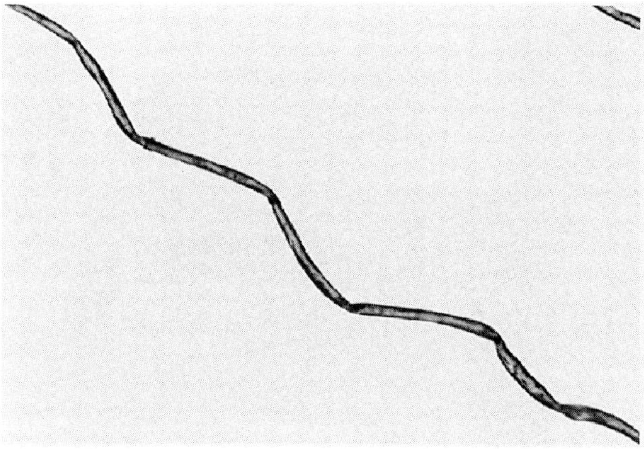

Figure 6-25 Corkscrew hair: double twist. (Light micrograph ×40)

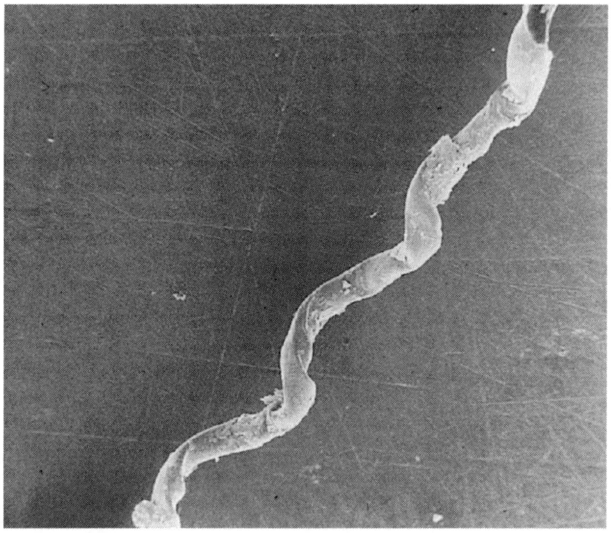

Figure 6-27 Corkscrew hair: double twist. (Scanning electron micrograph)

was originally described in one female patient with severe alopecia (Fig. 6-26), but a large group of similar cases has recently been described[132] (Table 6-4). Scanning electron microscopy showed ordinary pili torti in many thin scalp hairs, but a number of thick, dark hairs were coiled uniquely into a double spiral that resembled a corkscrew (Fig. 6-27).

Menkes' Syndrome. Pili torti occurs in combination with trichorrhexis nodosa in Menkes' kinky hair syndrome, also called *steely hair syndrome* or *trichopoliodystrophy* (Table 6-4).[44,136,137] The condition, which generally begins in infancy, is associated with depigmented hair; mental retardation; degeneration of cerebral, cerebellar, bone, and connective tissue; and hypothermia.[136,138] Low serum concentrations of copper and ceruloplasmin are diagnostic. The hair is normal at birth but when shed is replaced by sparse, short, brittle, depigmented hair which stands on end and looks and feels like steel wool (Fig. 6-28).[136,139] The face is characteristically expres-

Figure 6-26 Corkscrew hair: severe alopecia. (*Reprinted from Whiting, Jenkins, and Whitcomb.*[126])

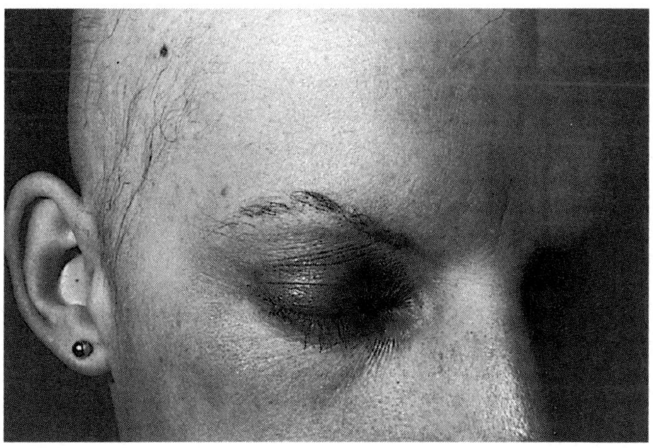

Figure 6-28 Menkes' disease: sparse hair. (*Courtesy of Dr. Mary K. Spraker.*)

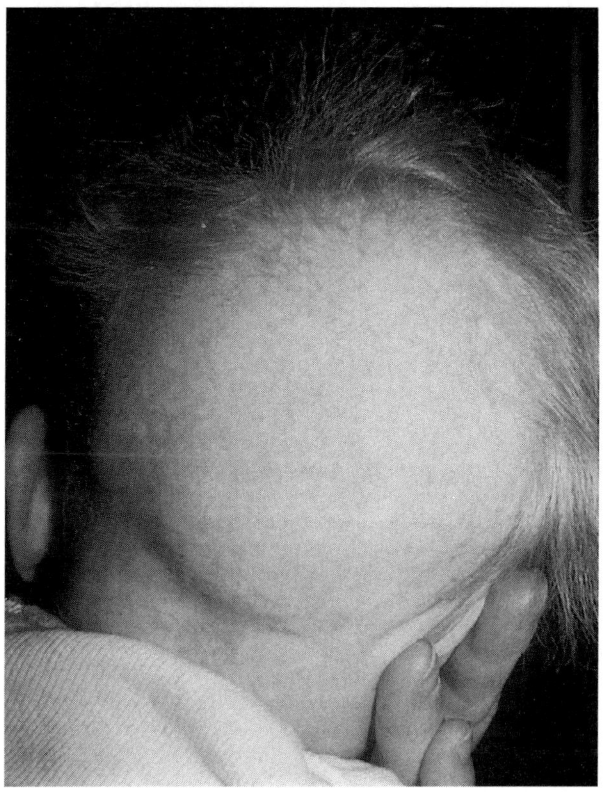

Table 6-4
CONDITIONS ASSOCIATED WITH PILI TORTI

Syndrome With Pili Torti	*Inheritance*	*Abnormal Hair*	*Abnormal Nails*	*Abnormal Teeth*	*Abnormal Skin*	*Miscellaneous Abnormalities*	*References*
I. Congenital							
A. Early onset (prepubertal)							
1. Classic (Ronchese)	AR, AD, or S	Usually blond, spangled, fragile, twisted hairs	+/– Leukonychia, nail dystrophy	+/–Hypoplastic enamel, widely spaced teeth	+/– Keratosis pilaris, ichthyosis	+/–Corneal opacities, +/–sensorineural deafness	114,116,120 122 123
2. Björnstad's syndrome	AD	Twisted hairs				Sensorineural deafness	121
3. Crandall's syndrome	SR	Twisted hairs				Sensorineural deafness, hypogonadism	124
4. Familial acne conglobata	AD	Twisted hairs			Acne conglobata, hidradenitis suppurativa	Cataracts	127
5. Bazex's syndrome	?AD	Congenital hypotrichosis scalp, face, body; twisted hairs			Follicular atrophoderma, milia, basal cell carcinomas	Hypohidrosis	128
6. Rapp-Hodgkin hypohidrotic ectodermal dysplasia	AD	Twisted hairs		Dental defects	Palmar keratoderma	Characteristic facies	129 130 131
7. Corkscrew hair	?AD	Twisted hairs in double spiral		Conical, widely spaced teeth		Webbing of fingers and toes	126 132
8. Menkes' syndrome	XR	Hair normal at birth; at 3 months becomes fair and twisted, and later depigmented, stubby, and sparse. Horizontal and twisted eyebrows. Pili torti in female carriers.			Skin pallor, plump cheeks, lack of facial expression	Retarded growth, focal cerebral, cerebellar, and arterial degeneration. Hypothermia. Focal or generalized seizures. Low serum copper and ceruloplasmin levels.	44 136 139

Table 6-4 (cont.)
CONDITIONS ASSOCIATED WITH PILI TORTI

Syndrome With Pili Torti	*Inheritance*	*Abnormal Hair*	*Abnormal Nails*	*Abnormal Teeth*	*Abnormal Skin*	*Miscellaneous Abnormalities*	*References*
B. Late onset (postpubertal)							
1. Beare's syndrome	AD	Black scalp hair, patchy alopecia, scanty facial and body hair, twisted hairs. Eyebrows and eyelashes are lost in childhood.				+/–Mental deficiency	133 134 120
II. Sporadic							
A. Miscellaneous hair shaft defects	AD AD AD, AR, S	Twisted hairs with monilethrix, pseudo monilethrix, woolly hair, longitudinal grooving, *T. nodosa*, or *T. invaginata*			+/–	+/–	151 152 153 154 24
B. Citrullinemia	? AR	Brittle, stubbly hair, *T. nodosa*, twisted hairs			Scaly skin rash	Mental retardation	43
III. Acquired							
A. Cicatricial alopecia		Twisted hairs in scarred areas				Possible associated signs of the disease causing cicatricial alopecia	120
B. Oral retinoids		Twisted hairs			Dry skin		156

AD = autosomal dominant; AR = autosomal recessive; S = sporadic; SR = sex-linked recessive; XR = X-linked recessive.

sionless, with pale, lax skin, plump cheeks, and horizontal twisted eyebrows. Other congenital malformations may include micrognathia, arched palate, pectus excavatum, club feet, and urinary tract abnormalities.[140,141] From approximately the third month of life, the child fails to thrive, becomes drowsy and lethargic, and may have convulsions and impaired vision. Most patients die by the age of 3 years.

In Menkes' kinky hair syndrome, a partial block in the intestinal absorption of copper leads to a gross copper deficiency with markedly decreased copper levels in the brain, liver, serum, and hair of affected patients.[140,142,143] The symptoms have been attributed to copper deficiency, since copper is known to have a role in the formation of myelin, keratin, melanin, elastin, and collagen. Copper is also essential for ascorbic acid metabolism as well as electron transport.[138] Paradoxically, a significant cellular affinity for copper can be shown in many tissues, including cultured fibroblasts and red blood cells, and may provide a genetic marker for this disease.[138,143–145] Excess copper in cultured cells and tissue is accumulated in metallothioneins, which are small cysteine-rich proteins that chelate copper.[143] In Menkes' syndrome patients, but not in normal persons, low serum copper is able to induce metallothionein messenger RNA synthesis.[143] This X-linked recessive disorder was thought to affect male infants exclusively, but three cases have been reported recently in females.[146] Furthermore, female heterozygotes may have pili torti.[139]

There are no structural differences between the twisted hair in Menkes' syndrome and that found in classic pili torti, although irregular left- and right-hand twists may be found in the same hair in Menkes' disease.[147] A ninefold excess of free-sulfhydryl groups is present in hair secondary to the impaired formation of disulfide cross-links in the keratin molecules.[144] Treatment with parenteral copper has not halted neurodegeneration in Menkes' disease,[148] but copper histidinate may be more effective in this regard.[149]

SPORADIC PILI TORTI

Sporadic cases of pili torti have been reported; in one, pili torti persisted in adult life, although affected hairs became longer, darker, and stronger.[125,150] Twisted hairs are sometimes found in association with other genetic abnormalities of the hair shaft, such as monilethrix,[151] pseudo monilethrix,[152] woolly hair,[153] longitudinal grooves,[154] trichorrhexis nodosa,[24] and trichorrhexis invaginata.[99] Pili torti has also been reported in citrullinemia (Table 6-4).[43]

ACQUIRED PILI TORTI

Pili torti can also be acquired, but the abnormality is localized or patchy rather than diffuse.[120,155] It is usually associated with some form of trauma to the hair or with some sort of scarring process in the scalp itself (Table 6-3).[120] Cases of localized pili torti have been reported in association with cicatricial alopecia resulting from systemic lupus erythematosus, pseudopelade, congenital erythropoietic porphyria, systemic sclerosis,[120] and infected insect bites.[155] In all cases, there were a few short, wiry hairs within the scarred area. Presumably, the perifollicular fibrosis creates rotational forces which distort the hair follicle and produce twisted hair.[120] Two patients with epidermolytic hyperkeratosis have been reported to have acquired pili torti after treatment with oral isotretinoin (Table 6-4).[156] The mechanism causing pili torti in these cases is speculative but must be similar to that causing the acquired progressive kinking reported in patients treated with etretinate.[157] Presumably, a fault in the inner root sheath impairs the molding of the developing hair shaft and leads to twisting, but why such a fault should be common to the diverse conditions causing pili torti is unknown.

There is no effective treatment for pili torti, but the hair may grow longer if trauma from hairstyling is minimized.

Woolly Hair

Woolly hair is normal in most blacks.[12] The clinical syndromes of which woolly hair is a feature occur in persons not of Negro origin.[2] Woolly hair is unruly and difficult to style because it does not lie flat or form normal locks. It is tightly coiled, with an average curl diameter of approximately 0.5 cm (Fig. 6-29).[153] It is easily distinguished from straight and wavy hair, and from curly hair, which forms longer spiral locks. The hair shafts show a variable number of 180-degree axial twists, in two forms.[153] The first occurs when hairs adopt a wave rather than a spiral form, and a gradual twist extending over several millimeters is situated between the maximum

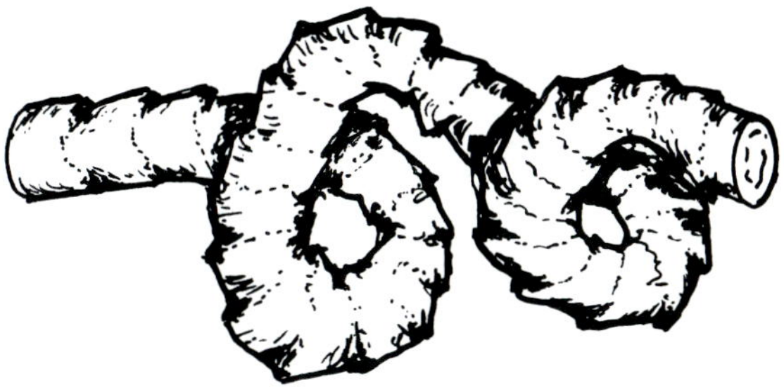

Figure 6-29 Woolly hair: tightly coiled hair shaft.

and minimum points of the wave; it should be regarded as pseudo pili torti, occurs in all forms of woolly hair, and can also be seen in curly hair. The second form occurs in three to six twists situated over a much shorter length of hair and unrelated to a wave form; it represents true pili torti and is rare in woolly hair. The hairs are usually ovoid rather than round in cross section. The shaft diameter is less than that of normal controls in some cases of familial woolly hair and in woolly hair nevus.[153] The hair may be fragile, and trichorrhexis nodosa is common. Pili annulati, which shows alternating light and dark bands on light microscopy, may also occur.[153] The anagen-to-telogen ratio is normal, but the anagen root is commonly dystrophic and often lacks root sheaths.[153] The hair growth rate is normal.

There are three major groups of woolly hair—hereditary dominant woolly hair, familial recessive and sporadic woolly hair, and a localized nevoid form called *woolly hair nevus.* The onset of woolly hair occurs at or soon after birth, with maximum severity occurring during childhood. Some improvement in woolly hair can be expected in adult life. Lesser-known forms of woolly hair include acquired progressive kinking, drug-induced kinking, and whisker hair.

HEREDITARY DOMINANT WOOLLY HAIR

Hereditary dominant woolly hair is initially seen at birth or in the first few months of life.[153,158,159] It affects the scalp hair diffusely. Tight curls remain throughout childhood but may be replaced by highly waved hair in adulthood. Woolly hair has also been called curly, bushy, twisted, and frizzled, although some describe it as Negroid. There is a great variability in hair color, which ranges from dark to very fair in different cases.[153] The growth rate is apparently normal, but at least in some cases there may be an inability to grow long hairs, perhaps due to increased fragility. Hair diameter is normal or somewhat reduced. Severity is variable, and the hair usually improves in adult life. Hairs on sites other than the scalp are usually not affected. Associated abnormalities are usually absent, but pili torti and pili annulati,[153] enamel hypoplasia,[160] ocular defects,[161,162] congenital perceptive deafness and dominant ichthyosis vulgaris,[163] keratosis pilaris atrophicans,[164] and Noonan's syndrome have been reported.[165]

A family with six individuals affected by diffuse partial woolly hair has been reported.[166] Two individuals complained of hair thinning, and the other four had not noticed abnormalities. The condition is characterized by shorter, finer, kinky hairs interspersed with normal hair throughout the scalp.[166] It presents in early adult life and appears to be inherited as an autosomal dominant trait.

FAMILIAL SPORADIC RECESSIVE WOOLLY HAIR

This type of woolly hair presents at birth and is brittle, tightly curled, and fine with a white-blond color.[153] The growth rate of the hair is probably normal, but the hair may not grow beyond the length of a few centimeters, probably because of a shortened anagen time rather than hair breakage. The vellus hair, in particular, is short and difficult to see, and the lateral portions of the eyebrows may be sparse. There is a reduction in the diameter of the hair. Some cuticular wear and tear may occur, but trichorrhexis nodosa is not obvious.[153]

WOOLLY HAIR NEVUS

Woolly hair nevus is a rare nonhereditary condition which appears at birth or within the first 2 years of life and involves a circumscribed area of the scalp.[167,168] The affected hair is usually finer and lighter than the surrounding normal hairs (Fig. 6-30).[2] One case has been reported with onset during adolescence, a biopsy of which showed a curved hair follicle.[168] About 50 percent of cases are associated with either a verrucous or epidermal linear nevus, or a pigmented nevus, usually on the neck or arms.[169,170] One reported case had a linear epidermal nevus beneath the woolly hair nevus, associated with bone growth retardation, delayed speech, and a dental

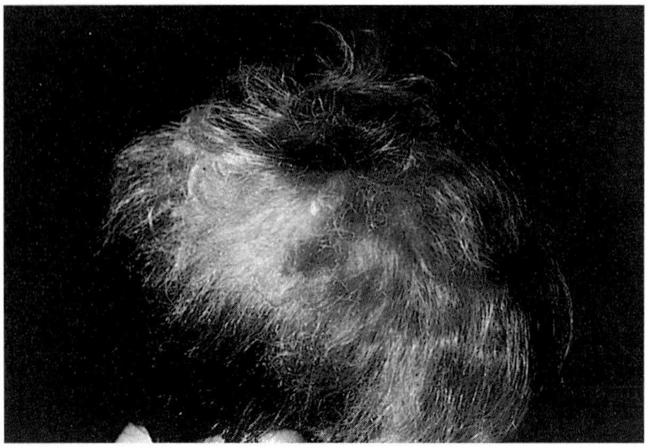

Figure 6-30 Woolly hair nevus: fair, woolly hair surrounded by normal dark hairs. (*Reprinted from Whiting.*[1])

anomaly, for which the name *woolly hair nevus syndrome* was proposed.[171] Ocular involvement may occur as an associated feature, including a persistent pupillary membrane and patchy loss of retinal pigment epithelium.[161,172]

The hairs may show other abnormalities besides the expected coiling, and, in one case, marked hair shaft tapering with cortical vacuolation and loss of cuticle was observed (Fig. 6-31);[1] in this case both normal and woolly hairs from the same patient showed a normal alpha keratin pattern on x-ray diffraction. Other hair shaft abnormalities found with scanning electron microscopy include absence of cuticle with trichorrhexis nodosa,[173] triangular hairs with longitudinal grooves,[174] and flattening and twisting of the shaft.[175]

Figure 6-31 Woolly hair nevus: woolly vs. normal hair. Woolly hair shows loss of cuticle, tapering, and cortical vacuolation. (Scanning electron micrograph) (*Reprinted from Whiting.*[1])

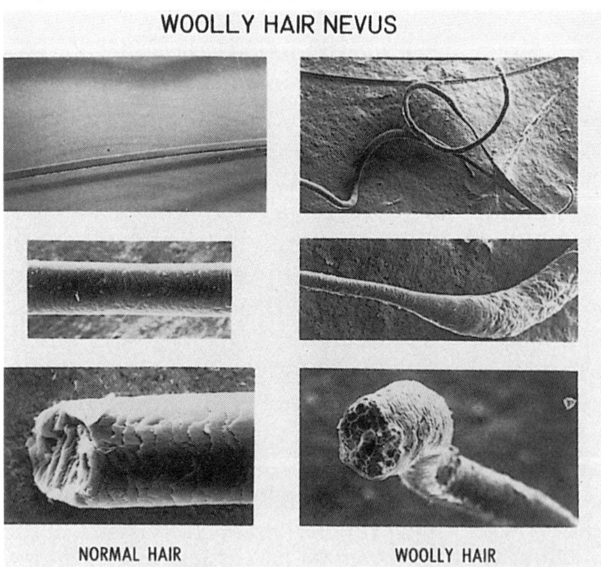

It should be noted that *curly hair,* which is otherwise normal in structure, occurs in two ectodermal dysplasias: In the trichodento-osseous syndrome, all affected children are born with a full head of tightly curled hair, which often straightens in later childhood. Associated abnormalities include small, eroded, widely spaced teeth; frontal bossing; square jaw; and dolichocephaly.[176] In the CHAND syndrome, curly hair, ankyloblepharon, and nail dysplasia are seen.[177]

There is no effective treatment for woolly hair, although spontaneous improvement in the one adolescent-onset case has been noted.[168] Ophthalmoscopic examination may be warranted.[161]

ACQUIRED PROGRESSIVE KINKING

Acquired progressive kinking of the hair is rarely recorded and is largely a male disorder.[178–182] The first case was described in 1932 by Wise and Sulzberger.[183] It appears in the late teens or early twenties, with gradual, symmetrical curling and darkening of the hair in the frontal, temporal, auricular, and vertex areas (Fig. 6-32). The patient gradually becomes aware that the hair in one region of the scalp is becoming kinky and rarely requires cutting.[178] On examination, the hair in one or more regions of the scalp is dry, lusterless,

Figure 6-32 Acquired progressive kinking: symmetrical curling of frontal hair.

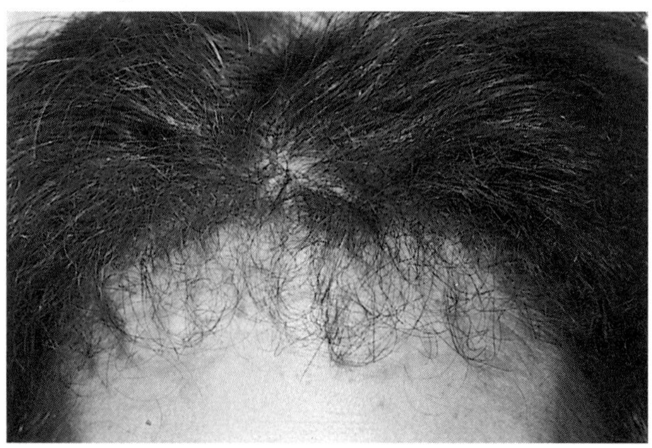

unruly, wiry, and kinky, resembling pubic hair. There are no sharply defined boundaries between the normal and abnormal hairs.

Under light microscopy, most of the affected hairs are shorter than normal, with finely tapered tips, probably caused by a shortened anagen phase. Hair shafts may be finer or thicker than normal and have kinks and half twists.[178] Additional changes include longitudinal grooving, spindle-shaped broadening of the shafts, and occasional fractures.[181,182] Scalp biopsies have shown no abnormalities.[179]

Male patients with acquired progressive kinking of the hair generally have had associated progressive hair loss in a pattern typical of androgenetic alopecia,[179] but alopecia does not eventuate in all cases.[184] A case of acquired nonprogressive kinking of the hair has been described, in which the hair anomaly remained static over a long period of time.[181]

THERAPY-INDUCED KINKING

Three patients developed a dose-dependent, reversible kinking of the hair while receiving etretinate therapy, possibly due to the drug's effect on the inner root sheath of the hair.[153] Another patient with straight hair was given radiotherapy to one side of the scalp for metastatic breast cancer, and the resultant hair loss was replaced by a heavy growth of curly hair.[185]

WHISKER HAIR

Norwood has described whisker hair as short, curly, dark hair that grows anterior to, above, and behind the ears in men aged 18 to 25 (Fig. 6-33), in whom severe androgenetic alopecia eventually develops.[186,187] It was named whisker hair by laypersons because of its proximity and resemblance to the beard. Whisker hair was described in 1955 by Knierer as allotrichia circumscripta symmetrica capillitii, or pubic hair nevus,[188] and has even been described elsewhere as a woolly hair nevus,[189] despite the fact that it is bilateral, symmetrical, and common. Whisker hair is not seen in older people, and Norwood speculates that whisker hair goes into a permanent telogen phase and, when combined with senile alopecia, eventuates in complete periauricular and occipital alopecia. Whisker hair, however, does resemble woolly hair and has been classified as such. Whisker hair is probably a variant of acquired progressive kinking.

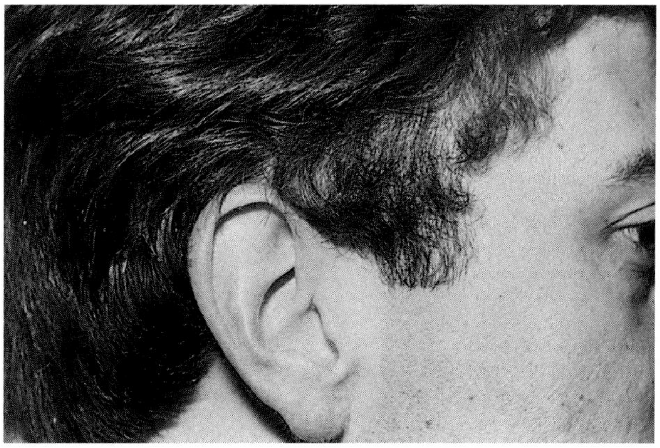

Figure 6-33 Whisker hair: short curly hair around ear.

Trichonodosis (Knotted Hair)

In trichonodosis, a single (Figs. 6-34 and 6-35), or sometimes a double, knot occurs in the hair shaft.[1] No underlying abnormalities are present, and the changes that are seen occur in the vicinity of the knot and are secondary to it. A localized loss of cuticle cells secondary to longitudinal fissuring and exposure of the underlying cortical fibers is common.[190] Similar cuticular changes can be produced by knotting and tightening of normal hairs.

Many slack knots may be produced by friction on pillows and by various cosmetic procedures. Combing may tighten the knots and even pull out hair in the anagen phase or cause a fracture of the hair shaft at the site of the knot. Reports of trichonodosis are not common in dermatologic literature,[191] but Dawber noted that the condition is not rare. In an examination of 80 normal women, he found the condition in 5 of 20 blacks with short, tightly curled hair and in 3 of 20 whites with short, curly hair; knotting had occurred in 1 of 20 white patients with long,

Figure 6-34 Trichonodosis: single knot, normal cuticle.

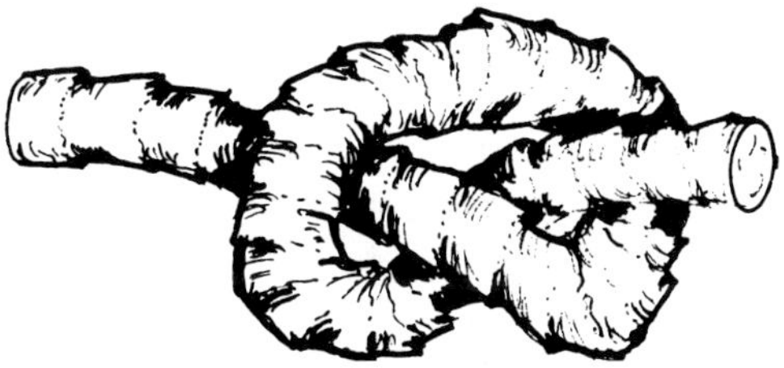

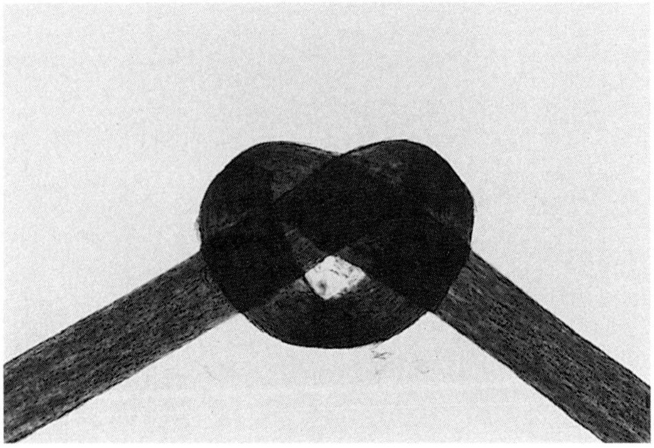

Figure 6-35 Trichonodosis: single knot in hair shaft. (Light micrograph ×100)

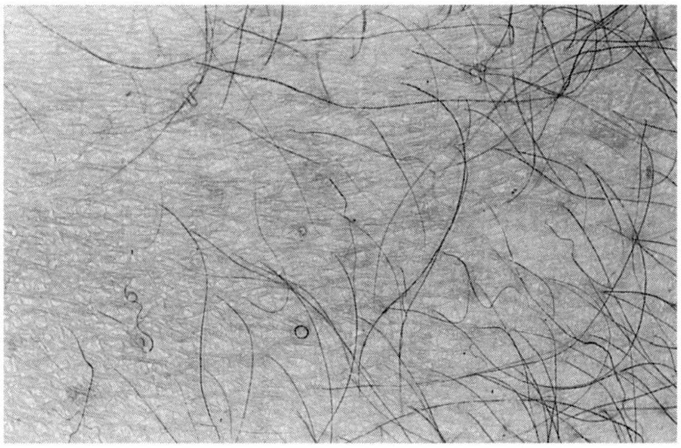

Figure 6-37 Circle hair: small-diameter coils in hairs.

curly hair, but in no white patients with long, straight hair.[190] It can be deduced that short, curly hair of Negroid or Caucasoid type is particularly predisposed to knotting, and that straight hair is much less likely to be affected, despite a recent report to the contrary.[192] Associated defects have not been recorded.

Knotting mainly affects the scalp hair but can occur in pubic[193] and other body hairs. It is usually an incidental finding and therefore does not require treatment. Because it is due to trauma, hair care should be as gentle as possible.

Circle Hairs

Circle (Fig. 6-36) and spiral hairs occur as small, dark circles next to hair follicles on the back, abdomen, and thighs in middle-aged men (Fig. 6-37).[194,195] These hairs, which are not associated with follicular abnormalities, represent an unusual form of ingrown hair, but no inflammation is present. The tightly coiled hair, which lies in a circular track just below the stratum corneum, is easily extracted. It can be unrolled into a length of up to 2.5 cm but retains its recoil ability (Fig. 6-38).

The dark, annular discoloration produced by circle hairs has led to concern about early melanoma in more than one patient known to the author. The correct diagnosis is quickly made by removing the hair that springs back into a perfect circle. The appearance of the hair and the lack of any follicular abnormality readily distinguish circle hairs from the rolled hairs of keratosis pilaris[196] or the looped, "corkscrew" hairs of scurvy, both of which are associated with follicular, keratin plugs.

Figure 6-36 Circle hair: tightly coiled hair, normal cuticle.

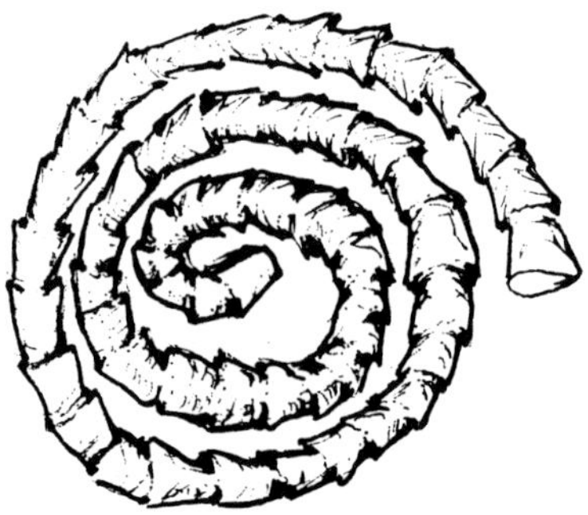

Figure 6-38 Circle hair: extracted hair retains recoil ability.

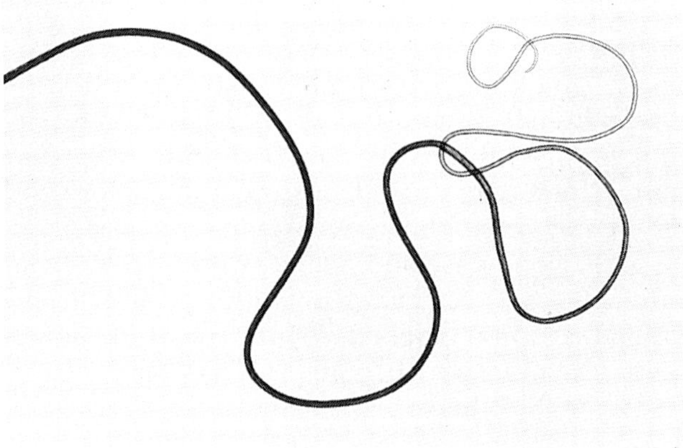

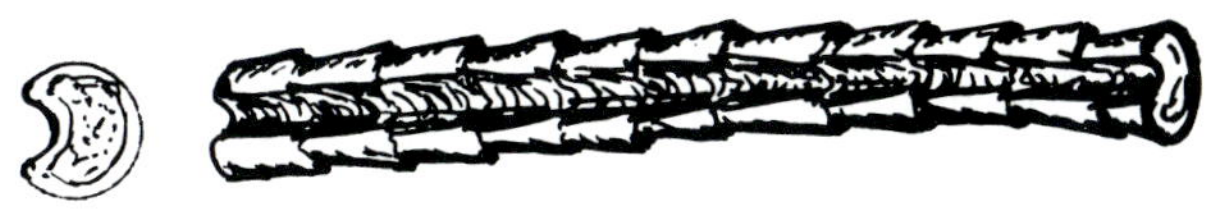

Figure 6-39 Longitudinal grooving: vertical grooving, intact cuticle.

IRREGULARITIES OF THE HAIR SHAFT

Longitudinal Ridging and Grooving

One or more longitudinal grooves can occur along the hair shaft (Fig. 6-39). Usually the overlying cuticle is intact, unless subjected to undue weathering (Fig. 6-40). Multiple finer grooves or fluting is sometimes present.[1]

Longitudinal grooving is probably the most common hair shaft irregularity. It is frequently seen in normal hair, where it appears as a sporadic phenomenon in isolated hairs. It is more significant if it occurs diffusely. Widespread grooving is commonly seen in congenital hypotrichosis of the Marie Unna type[154] (Fig. 6-41) or in related syndromes and in some forms of ectodermal dysplasia. It has also been seen in pili torti,[123] pili bifurcati,[197] uncombable hair syndrome,[198,199] acquired progressive kinking,[181,182] and trichothiodystrophy.[46,80]

Longitudinal grooving has also been seen in the recently described loose anagen syndrome, in which misshapen anagen hairs with ruffled cuticles (Fig. 6-42*A* and *B*), lacking external root sheaths, and with normal tensile strength are easily pulled from the scalp of affected patients.[200–202] Handfuls of hair may inadvertently be detached by other children during play (Fig. 6-43). Most of these patients are blond girls aged 2 to 5. Histological examination of affected hairs may show premature keratinization of Huxley's and Henle's layers of the inner root sheath; longitudinal grooving is common in these hairs (Fig. 6-42*A*). Vertical grooves traverse the internodes in monilethrix, and fine fluting may be seen in pili annulati.[27] Hair grooving is also seen in progeria.[203] Longitudinal grooving does not cause increased hair fragility and has little practical importance except as a nonspecific marker of some congenital abnormalities of the hair shaft.

Figure 6-40 Longitudinal grooving: vertical grooving, intact cuticle. (Light micrograph ×400)

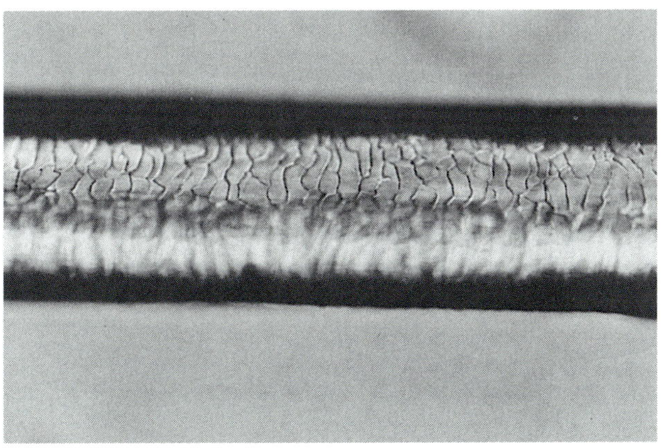

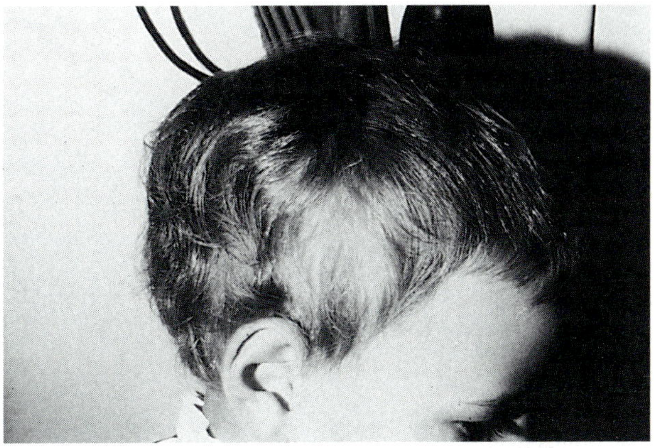

Figure 6-41 Congenital hypotrichosis: sparse, fine hairs.

Uncombable Hair Syndrome

Uncombable hair syndrome is characterized by hair shafts that are mainly triangular in cross section. They are sometimes flattened, irregular, or kidney-shaped, and longitudinal grooves are present (Fig. 6-44). The descriptive term for this condition is *pili trianguli et canaliculi.*[204] The entire hair shaft is involved, but the cuticle is intact, and twists or bends are unusual. Uncombable hair may represent a diffuse form of a straight hair nevus.

Sulfur levels are usually normal in the affected hairs, and no significant physical or chemical abnormalities have been found.[198,205] However, one electron-histochemical study indicated that the stiffness of the uncombable hair might be due to increased high-sulfur protein in the

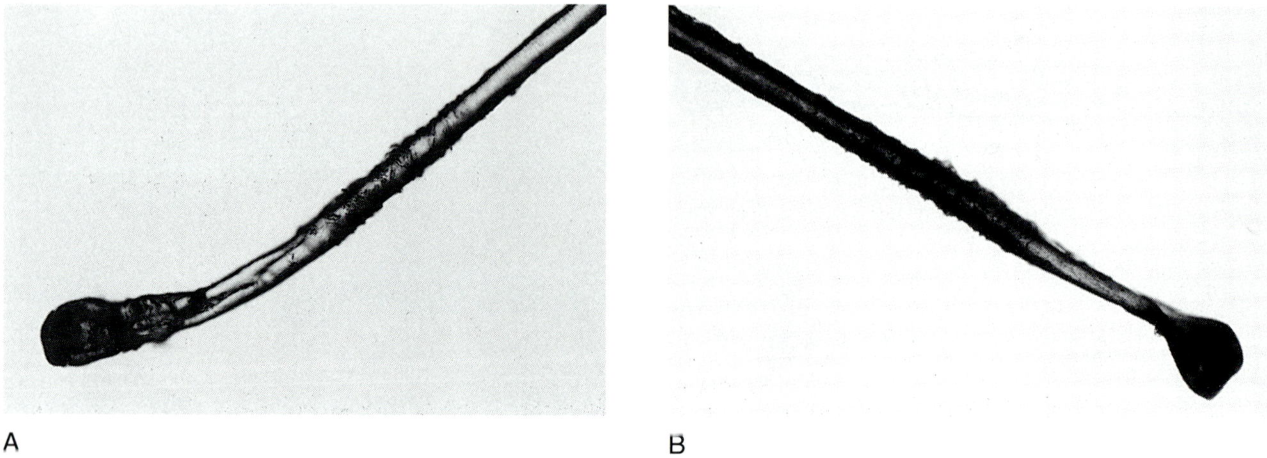

Figure 6-42 Loose anagen syndrome. (*A*) Anagen hair, with vertical grooving and no root sheath. (Light micrograph ×100) (*B*) Anagen hair with ruffled cuticle and no root sheath. (Light micrograph ×100)

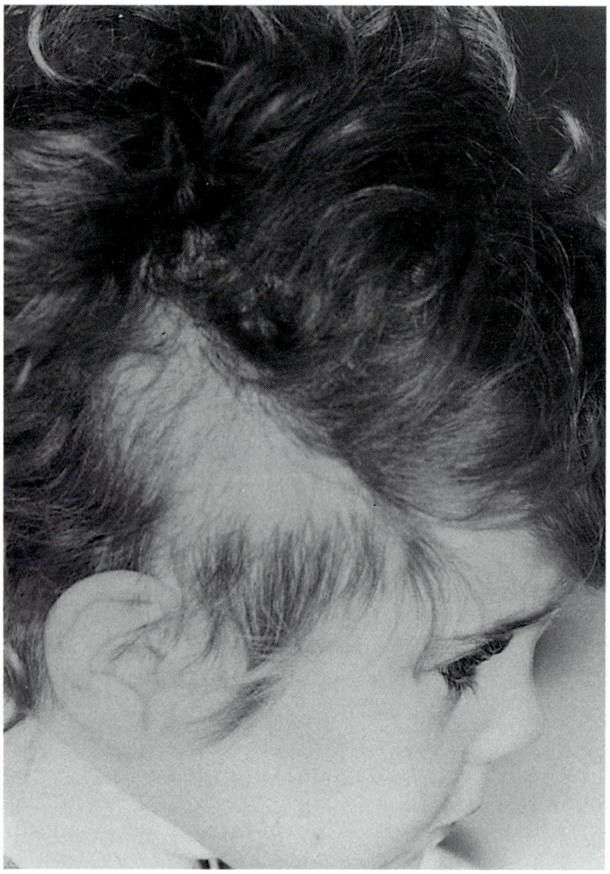

Figure 6-43 Loose anagen syndrome: fair-haired child with bare patch from which hair was pulled out painlessly on school playground.

exocuticle.[206] Abnormal fibrous protein patterns have been demonstrated in some cases.[205,207] The condition may result from premature keratinization of the inner root sheath, which forms an irregular, rigid tube that then alters the shape of the emerging hair shaft.[208] Serial transverse sections of a scalp biopsy have revealed that, in addition to varying cross-sectional shapes, the inner root sheath conforms in configuration to the abnormal outline of the hair shaft.[208] This is considered to represent a failure in normal complementation of the inner root sheath, which in usual circumstances will average out differences in cross-sectional shape of the hair shaft, with the sheath itself presenting an overall round or oval configuration.[209] Van Neste et al. have suggested that the abnormally shaped dermal papilla alters the internal root sheath into a triangular tube which then hardens, molding the growing hair into a similar shape which is perpetuated when the ascending hair shaft keratinizes.[206] Stone et al. described focal atrophy of the hair bulb in a single Japanese patient with uncomb-

Figure 6-44 Uncombable hair: grooved shaft with triangular cross section.

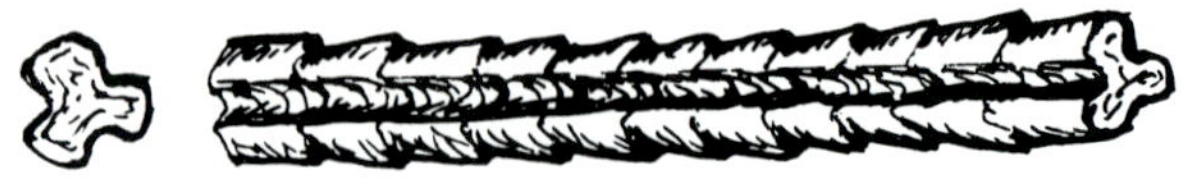

able hair syndrome and hypothesized that a matrix defect caused the longitudinal grooves; previous hair biopsy specimens have been reported to show normal hair bulbs.[210] The glittering, spangled appearance of the affected hairs may be due to reflection and refraction of incident light by the differently angulated hair shafts.

Uncombable hair syndrome was first described in the French literature by Dupre et al. in 1973[211] and in the U.S. literature by Stroud and Mehregan in 1974; the latter named it *spun-glass hair.*[208] The hair usually has a characteristic silvery-blond color or can be straw-colored.[204,208] It stands out from the scalp, is disorderly, and cannot be combed flat (Fig. 6-45). Uncombable hair syndrome, which is sometimes noticed in young infants or as late as age 12,[212] is usually seen in patients at about 3 years of age and may persist for some time, although spontaneous improvement has occurred in later childhood. The hairs grow slowly and may or may not be brittle. Familial cases occur and show autosomal dominant inheritance with both complete and incomplete penetrance.[199,213,214] Associated features of ectodermal dysplasia such as craniofacial abnormalities and cleft palate have been reported in some cases,[198] and in one patient a crystalline cataract was associated with the uncombable hair.[215]

The diagnosis of uncombable hair syndrome is difficult to make with a light microscope, although the hair shaft has a characteristic homogeneous band on one edge under polarized light caused by the shadow thrown as light passes over the pili canaliculi.[214,216,217] Examination of cross sections of hairs embedded in paraffin can be helpful.[218] Scanning electron microscopy may be necessary to confirm the diagnosis (Fig. 6-46).[198,219,220] Treatment is usually unsuccessful, although a positive response to biotin has been reported in one case.[198,221]

STRAIGHT HAIR NEVUS

Straight hair nevus may be a limited form of uncombable hair. It occurs as a localized area of straight hairs in the scalp of blacks. The affected hair shafts are round in cross section. The affected hairs are about one-half the normal diameter, and cuticular cells are small and disorganized. The condition may be associated with an epidermal nevus.[222,223] In one case, the straight hair regrew from an area of alopecia that had previously been covered with normally kinked hair, and the hair remained straight thereafter.[224]

Unilateral, straight hair has been described in a child with congenital Horner's syndrome caused by a tumor of the stellate ganglion.[225] Localized or diffuse straight hair has also been seen in patients with the acquired immunodeficiency syndrome (AIDS). One report described four black patients with AIDS who developed diffuse straightening of the hair, associated with lengthening, lightening, and softening.[226] Such cases are not uncommon and should be distinguished from the dry, brittle hair which often occurs in patients with AIDS. Scalp biopsies, seen personally, from two AIDS patients with localized

Figure 6-45 Uncombable fair hair. (*Courtesy of Dr. Vera H. Price.*)

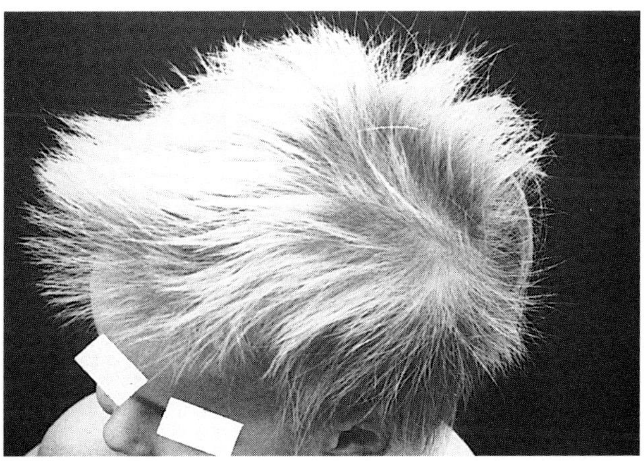

Figure 6-46 Longitudinal grooving: deep grooving, intact cuticle. (Scanning electron micrograph)

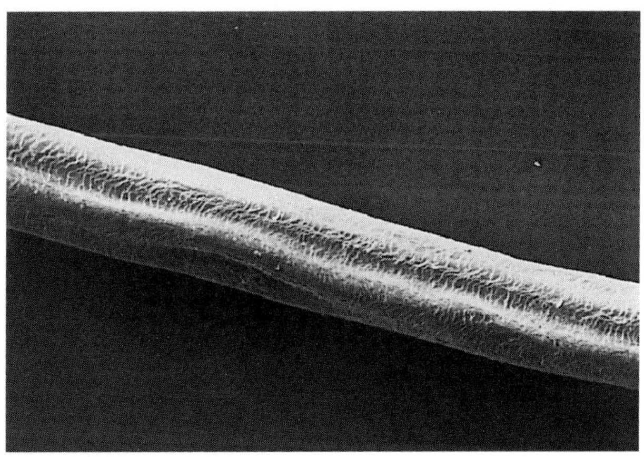

straight hair, have shown perifollicular, lymphohistiocytic infiltrates and fibrosis, around the upper and mid follicle.

Pili Multigemini and Pili Bifurcati

In pili multigemini, hairs are formed from two to eight hair papillae and matrices (Fig. 6-47).[227] The hairs are surrounded by a common outer root sheath, but each hair has its own inner root sheath. These hairs emerge from one follicular canal; are flattened, triangular, or ovoid in cross section; and may show longitudinal grooves. In the follicular canal, adjacent hairs may adhere, bifurcate, and then readhere. They usually emerge as a tuft of individual hairs. Pili multigemini needs to be differentiated from compound follicles, in which two different hair follicles with separate roots and lower follicles emerge through a single infundibulum, and from trichostasis spinulosa, in which many short vellus hairs are retained in the hyperkeratotic follicles.

In adults, pili multigemini is usually found in the beard area.[228] In children, the condition is usually reported on the scalp; many affected follicles have been described in classic pili torti (Ronchese)[116] and also in cleidocranial dysostosis.[228] The author has seen a biopsy specimen from a patient with many lesions of pili multigemini of the beard area following a course of oral isotretinoin. There is no specific treatment for this condition, which tends to be persistent. The abnormal hairs regrow after plucking.

Pili bifurcati was described by Weary et al. in

Figure 6-47 Pili multigemini: three hair shafts arising from a common root system. (Light micrograph ×40)

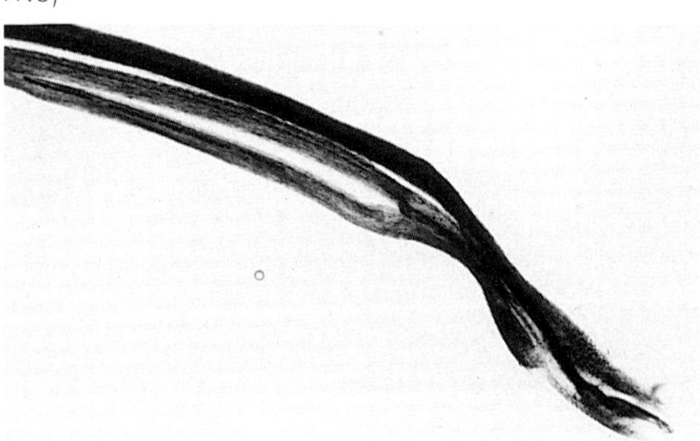

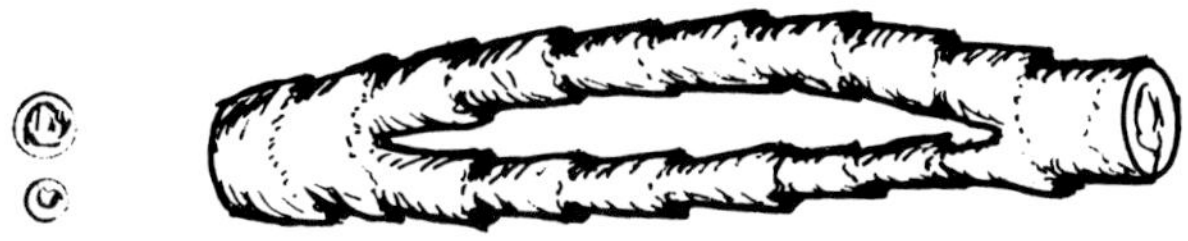

Figure 6-48 Pili bifurcati: a single hair divides into two separate hair shafts with their own cuticles with subsequent readherence.

a 3-year-old boy.[197] It was an isolated abnormality occurring on the scalp. The hairs arise from a single papilla and then divide into two separate shafts, each invested by its own cuticle. These shafts are reunited proximally (Fig. 6-48). The affected hairs emerge from a single pilosebaceous canal. This splitting and fusing of a single hair may be caused by the same mechanism as proposed by Pinkus in pili multigemini, in which a single papilla splits into a number of tips. Each tip gives rise to a separate hair shaft surrounded by its own root sheath.[227] However, the papilla changes shape repeatedly during anagen, so that the papillary tips may reunite later on and form a single composite shaft. Pili bifurcati may also occur as an isolated defect in normal follicles. It appears to represent a restricted form of pili multigemini, occurring on the scalp rather than on the beard area.

Trichostasis Spinulosa

Trichostasis spinulosa is another condition in which multiple hairs may be present in one follicular canal.[2] From 5 to 50 normal clubbed, vellus hairs are embedded in a large comedo (Fig. 6-49). There is only one hair matrix and papilla at the base of the follicle. Trichostasis is now regarded by some authors as a normal, age-related process in which extruded telogen hairs are retained in sebaceous follicles.[229] It has been regarded as a variant of a comedo,[230] but its etiology is unknown. It occurs at all ages and mainly affects the chest and back, especially the scapular area, and is less common on the abdomen, face, and neck. It presents as horny, spinous plugs which vary in number, sometimes show tufts of hair, and are easily removed.[231] It is readily distinguished from keratosis pilaris, which affects all ages and mainly involves the extensor surface of arms, thighs, and buttocks; the follicular papules are easy to remove, and each contains a single, coiled vellus hair. Trichostasis spinu-

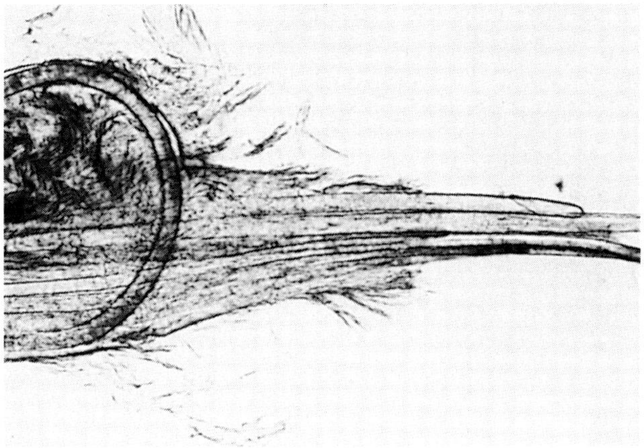

Figure 6-49 Trichostasis spinulosa: multiple vellus hairs are embedded in a large comedo. (Light micrograph ×40) (*Reprinted from Young MC et al.*[231])

losa is sometimes confused with eruptive vellus hair cysts, which most commonly affect the sternal area and abdomen in young people; these lesions present as soft, umbilicated, nonpigmented papules which resist removal due to their dermal location.[231]

Topical retinoic acid is the most effective treatment for trichostasis spinulosa.

Pili Annulati

Pili annulati, or ringed hairs, have characteristic alternating light and dark bands in the hair shafts (Fig. 6-50). These can be seen both clinically and under the light microscope (Fig. 6-51). The colors of the bands are reversed when viewed by reflected light.

Clinically the hair shows a ringed appearance which is clinically detectable only in blond or lightly pigmented hair.[8] In dark hair, the additional pigment absorbs most of the incident light and obscures the banding which would be expected from the underlying cortical cavities. In a hair mount, the cavities, seen as bright regions with reflected light, appear as dark patches with transmitted light.

Ringed hair can be present at the time of the patient's birth or can appear during infancy. It is a rare keratinization abnormality which can be familial, usually with autosomal-dominant inheritance,[232,233] or sporadic.[234] The hair grows normally and is usually not brittle. The axillary hair is occasionally affected.[235] The hair growth rate was measured in one case and found to be half that of normal.[233]

Figure 6-50 Pili annulati: alternate light and dark bands in hair shaft with intact cuticle.

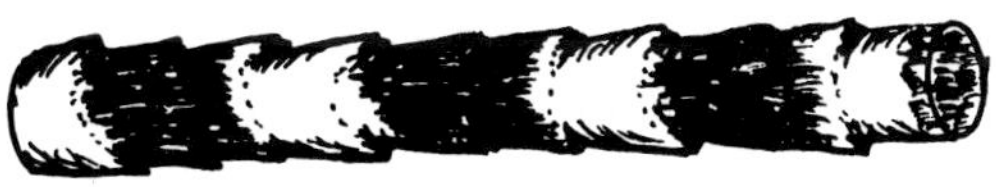

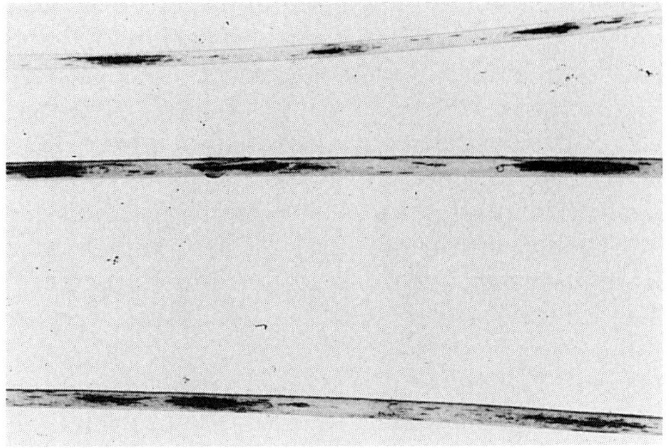

Figure 6-51 Pili annulati: ringed hairs. (Light micrograph ×40)

The underlying hair abnormalities are in the cortex,[234] in which both small and large spaces are found within cortical cells, between the macrofibrillar units of each cell. These air-filled spaces scatter reflected light.[234] A defect in the formation of the microfibril matrix complex is the most likely cause.[236] The hairs themselves are not usually fragile, but when they fracture they do tend to fracture within the abnormal bands.[233]

Figure 6-52 Pili annulati: delicate longitudinal fluting on hair shaft. (Scanning electron micrograph) (*Reprinted from Whiting.*[1])

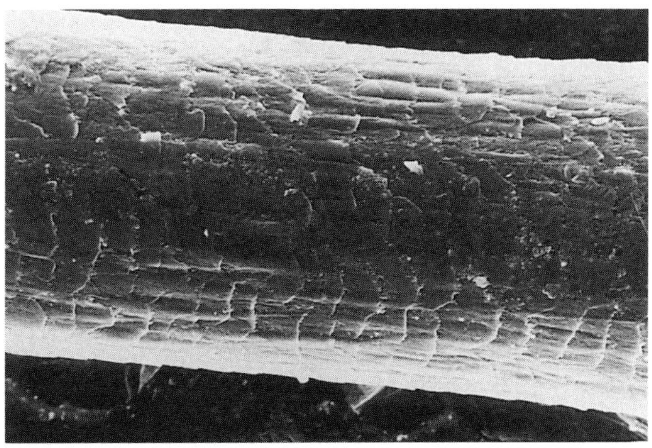

On examination by scanning electron microscopy, the cuticle appears cobblestoned[233] and can also have a fluted appearance (Fig. 6-52).[1] Electron-histochemical studies have shown that the cuticular cells are thrown into folds.[237] On transmission electron microscopy, a large number of abnormal holes of varying shapes and sizes are visible within the cortex. They range in size from less than 1 μmm to 10 μmm in diameter.[234] The cavities can readily be filled with various liquids such as water, ethanol, and xylene.[234] Dawber has claimed that the cystine content of hair from pili annulati is lower than normal, although the amino acid analysis is normal.[233] Total sulfur content of the hair is normal.

There are usually no associated abnormalities. However, alopecia areata is not infrequently found in patients with pili annulati,[8] and the association of pili annulati with woolly hair has been noted.[153] Pili annulati has also been reported with blue nevi.[233]

The spangled appearance is attractive, and no treatment is necessary, although hairstyling should be gentle.

Pseudo Pili Annulati

Pseudo pili annulati is a normal variant in which light and dark bands are found under reflected light. There is no hair shaft abnormality in this condition.[238] There are no internal defects of the hair shaft, and amino acid analysis is normal. The hair is not brittle. The appearance is due to a flattened hair shaft that is elliptic in cross section and partially twisted every 1 to 2 mm. The successive, flattened surfaces on the shaft act as mirrors and reflect light as periodic bright bands.[238]

The hair is blond, strong, and entirely normal apart from the unusual and attractive banded appearance.[238] This bright banding is conspicuous only in blond hair because brunet hair, even if twisted, absorbs most of the incident light. The sporadic bright highlights seen in all normal blond hair are probably due to the same phenomenon.

In pseudo pili annulati, the banded appearance is seen with transverse illumination only if the light strikes the hair at right angles to the hair's long axis. In pili annulati, the banding is obvious regardless of which direction the light strikes the hairs. The banding is seen in pseudo pili annulati only when the fiber is rotated into certain positions, but in others it is not visible. In pili annulati, the banding is seen whatever way the fiber is oriented. Periodic dark patches in the hair of pili annulati are not seen in pseudo pili annulati.[8]

Pilar Melanin Clumps in the Chédiak-Higashi Syndrome

The hair shafts in the Chédiak-Higashi syndrome can vary in color but usually have a characteristic silvery sheen.[239] Light microscopy shows a transparent hair shaft containing characteristic large clumps of melanin (Fig. 6-53).[239] These represent abnormal melanin aggregation into giant melanosomes rather than any absence of melanin.[240]

The Chédiak-Higashi syndrome is an autosomal-recessive disorder. It is characterized by oculocutaneous hypopigmentation, and neurological and hematologic abnormalities.[239] Massive intracellular inclusions are present in all white blood cells, and most patients die by the age of 10 years from recurrent infections.

Monilethrix

Monilethrix hair shafts show characteristic elliptic nodes, 0.7 to 1 mm apart, with intervening, tapered constrictions that are nonmedullated (Fig. 6-54). The nodes occur at seemingly regular intervals, and the intervening hair shaft is not twisted (Fig. 6-55). The beading may be gross and obvious on clinical inspection, or so subtle that the diagnosis is missed.[241] Weathering may lead to a loss of cuticle cells over the nodes, which are exposed to maximal trauma.[115] The cuticular cells are nonetheless intact over the internodes. Longitudinal ridges are often present over the internodes (Fig. 6-56)[2,27] and are progressive as the internodes move away from the scalp.[18]

Monilethrix is characterized clinically by fragile, beaded hair and baldness. It usually appears in early childhood but can occur as late as the second decade of life,[242] mostly affecting the hair

Figure 6-53 Chédiak-Higashi syndrome: pilar melanin clumps.

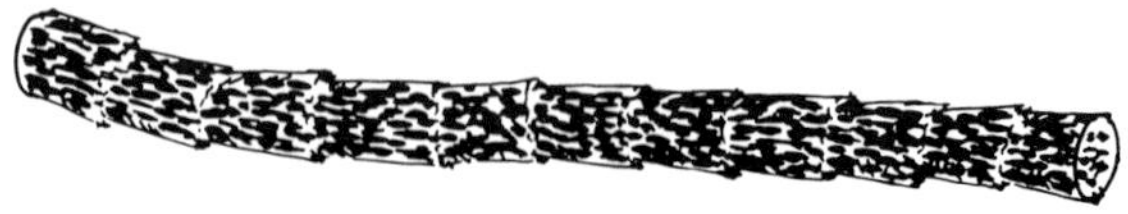

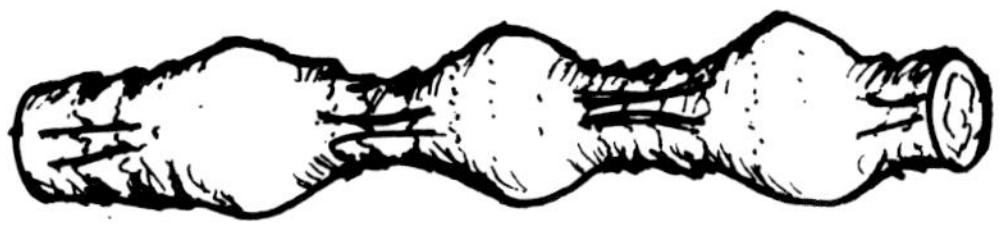

Figure 6-54 Monilethrix: repetitive beading of shaft with longitudinal grooving over internodes and absent cuticle over nodes.

on the nape of the neck and on the occiput. However, it can affect hairs on the entire scalp and even the facial, axillary, pubic, and body hair.[242] Brittle, beaded hairs emerge from keratotic, follicular papules and rarely grow more than 1 to 2 cm long (Fig. 6-57). The follicular keratosis is not directly related to the beading, since either can precede the other, or the keratosis may be absent.[2] The hair fractures easily, and the resultant alopecia can be severe.

On light microscopy, the regular, dark beads are seen alternating with the pale constrictions of the internodes. Fractures are seen to occur at the internodes. With electron microscopy, structural abnormalities are found in the cortex and cuticle and arise in the zone of keratinization in the follicles. The cell membranes of the deeper, cuticular cells are thrown into folds, particularly over the internodes, where breakages actually occur.[243] Abnormalities are also present in the adjacent inner root sheath. X-ray diffraction of monilethrix hairs reveals that they have a less well accentuated alpha keratin pattern than do normal hairs.[244]

There are considerable variations in the beading configuration in monilethrix, both in single

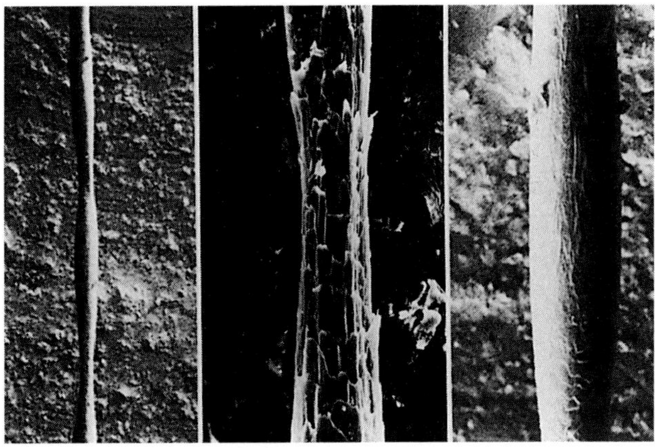

Figure 6-56 Monilethrix: beading of shaft, grooved internodes, absent cuticle over nodes. (Scanning electron micrograph) (*Reprinted from Whiting.*[1])

hairs and in hairs from the same scalp. These hairs show no mutual coordination of beading configuration. Also, the beading does not correlate with diurnal cycles or with any other obvious coordinating influences. In monilethrix there appears to be substantial follicular autonomy in allowing marked variations in the amplitude and frequency of beading.[241,245] The diagnosis is made by careful examination of the hairs under the light microscope to confirm the regular beading and the lack of twisting.

Inheritance of monilethrix is usually autosomal dominant and penetrance is high, but expressivity is variable.[151] Contrary to some previous reports, evidence does not support an association of monilethrix with argininosuccin-

Figure 6-55 Monilethrix: repetitive beading on hair shaft (often visible with naked eye). (Light micrograph ×40)

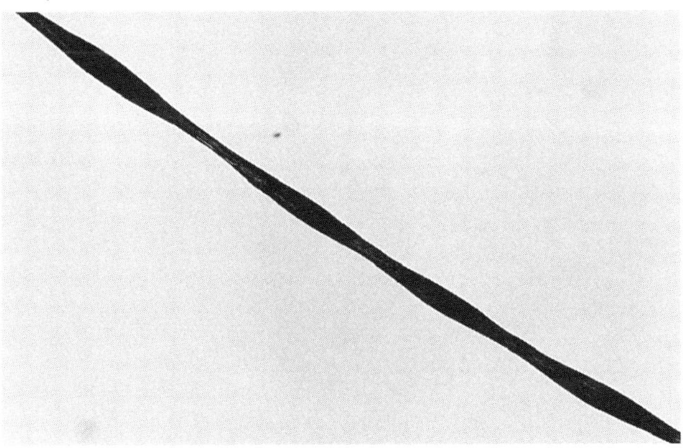

Figure 6-57 Monilethrix: scalp shows follicular plugging with severe alopecia.

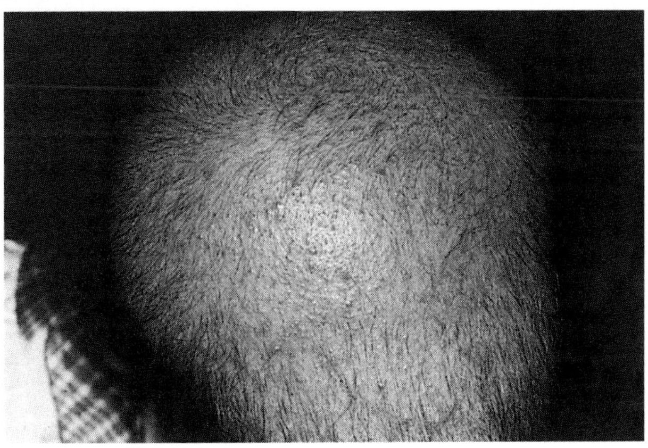

icaciduria[246] or with any other metabolic abnormality. Keratosis pilaris is frequently associated with monilethrix but does not always coincide with the distribution of normal hair. It has been reported to occur either alone or in association with other abnormalities such as physical retardation, syndactyly, juvenile cataracts, defects of nails, such as koilonychia, and of teeth,[247] and other hair defects, including trichorrhexis nodosa and, probably erroneously, pili torti.

The course of monilethrix is variable and seasonal, and improvement may occur during the summer. Temporary improvement has occurred during pregnancy.[151] Some cases improve in adult life and others deteriorate.[242] There is no specific treatment for monilethrix, although gentle hair care is advisable. Oral etretinate has been reported to improve hair growth,[248,249] as has topical minoxidil.[250]

Pseudo Monilethrix

In pseudo monilethrix, irregular beading is present along the hair shaft, as opposed to the regularity seen with monilethrix.[152] The beaded appearance is actually produced by expansion of the normal hair shaft due to indentation and flattening. The cuticle cells are intact over the nodes and internodes, and no longitudinal grooves are present over the internodes (Fig. 6-58*A* and *B*). There is no recurrent twisting of the hair shaft. The nodes in pseudo monilethrix are likely to be transient and may be absent on subsequent review of the same slide.[1] It is highly probable that these nodes are artifactual and may be produced by trauma of various kinds, including compression by tweezers or forceps.[1] Some of the changes can be produced in normal hairs by compressing overlapping hairs between two glass slides, where the indentation in one shaft caused by another overlying hair exactly mimics the appearance described in pseudo monilethrix.[1,251] It requires less pressure to produce the artifact in thin hair than in thick hair, and more pressure when more than two overlapping hairs are on the slide.[252] The artifact is more easily seen in light hair than in dark hair, but its magnitude is unrelated to hair color.[252] It has been stated that hair fragility from hair shaft dysplasias or cosmetic damage can lead to easy compressibility of hair, in which pseudo monilethrix is more easily produced than in normal hair.[253] This concept may account for reports of pseudo monilethrix occurring in acquired progressive kinking, acrodermatitis enteropathica, bubble hair, monilethrix, trichorrhexis nodosa, uncombable hair, and

Figure 6-58 Pseudo monilethrix. (*A*) Beading is caused by flattening of shaft. (Scanning electron micrograph) (*B*) Cuticular cells are present over beaded node. (Scanning electron micrograph)

A

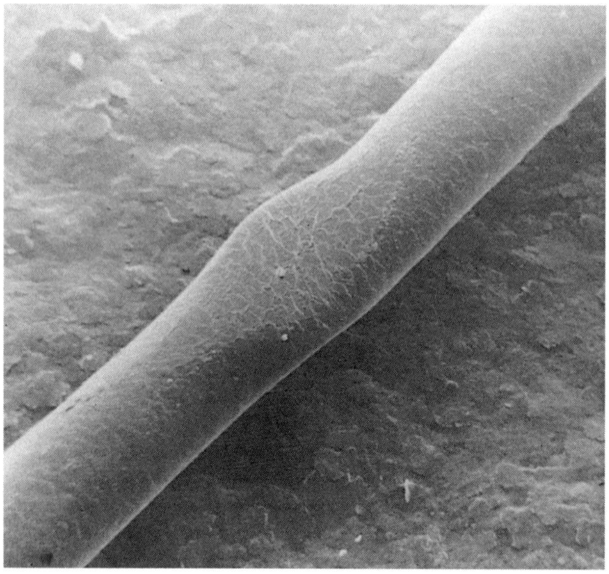

B

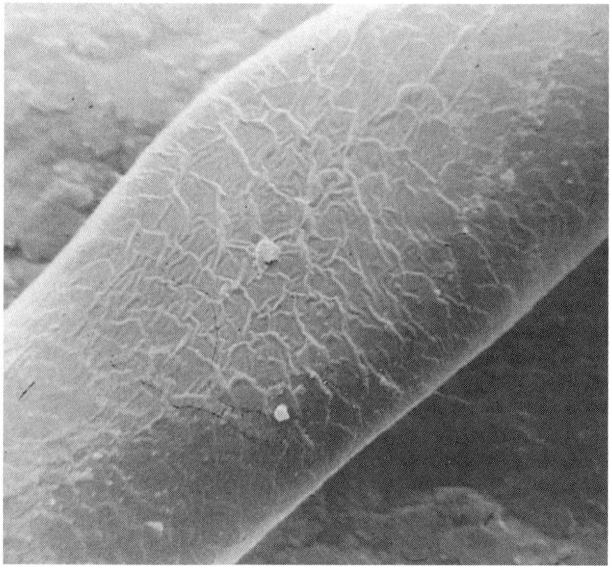

woolly hair, as well as in a familial syndrome of easily compressible hair.[254]

Since the status of pseudo monilethrix is controversial, the following classification is suggested: *familial pseudo monilethrix,* in which families with fragile, easily compressible hair exhibit the artifact; *acquired dysplastic pseudo monilethrix,* in which individuals with demonstrable hair dysplasia may show the artifact; and *acquired traumatic pseudo monilethrix,* in which the artifact occurs sporadically in normal hair (F. Camacho, J. Ferrando, and A. Rodriguez-Pichardo, personal communication).

Familial pseudo monilethrix is the name applied to a hair shaft abnormality present in four large families of Dutch, German, British, and Indian origin.[152,255] It is an autosomal dominant condition with equal sex incidence and variable penetrance. The irregular nodes found along the hair shaft may be associated with trichorrhexis nodosa and pili torti, and possibly with prepubertal hair thinning. Only the scalp hair is affected, and the hair color remains normal. The onset of hair thinning, if it occurs, is between age 8 and puberty. There is no increased incidence of pattern alopecia. Keratosis pilaris is not present. A history of excessive trauma due to combing, brushing, back combing, and massaging is always present. The possibility of an inherited weakness of the hair shaft that renders it susceptible to distortions from trauma has not been disputed.[252–254,256] No underlying chemical abnormalities or associated defects have been found.

Treatment consists of reassurance and gentle hair care with minimum manipulation. The hair responds to this and grows out normally in due course.

Tapered Hairs

Tapered hairs can be seen in association with many other structural abnormalities of the hair shaft. In one patient with woolly hair nevus, substantial tapering of some affected hairs was noticed.[1]

Tapered hairs can also arise in the same way as tapered fractures. If mitosis is temporarily inhibited in the hair matrix by an adverse influence, cell turnover is diminished and inadequate formation of the hair shaft results, with loss of cuticle and narrowing of the cortex.[52] The degree of constriction is proportional to the severity of the metabolic upset. If the adverse metabolic influence is removed before a fracture occurs, the shaft gradually rethickens with continued hair growth, leaving a dumbbell-like constriction in the shaft. Such constrictions weaken the hair shaft and allow for easy kinking, the so-called coudability or angulated bending described by Shuster as a diagnostic sign of alopecia areata.[112]

POHL-PINKUS CONSTRICTION

A constrictive phenomenon of the hair shaft, of the preceding type, was described by Pohl-Pinkus in 1894 (Fig. 6-59). In such cases the appearance of a zone of decreased shaft diameter coincides with a significant surgical operation or illness. More recently the disorder has been associated with antimitotic drugs. It seems likely that hairs in the early anagen phase of the hair cycle are more susceptible to a period of hypoproteinemia or disturbed protein synthesis.[2] These constrictions have been considered analogous to Beau's lines in the fingernails, although one patient has been described in whom Beau's lines were accompanied by periodic expansions of the hair shaft. The most prominent hair constrictions have been described following hemorrhage from a duodenal ulcer.[257] Repetitive, wider constrictions have been seen following intermittent doses of cytotoxic drugs, which were not large enough to cause actual fracturing of the hairs.

BAYONET HAIRS

Bayonet hairs were described by Pinkus in 1910. They are characterized by a 2- to 3-mm spindle-shaped, hyperpigmented expansion of the hair cortex just proximal to a tapered tip (Figs. 6-60 and 6-61). These hairs can occur in normal subjects but have also been seen following a febrile illness[258] and in patients with seborrheic dermatitis, ichthyosis,[259] and Hodgkin's disease treated with x-ray therapy and cytostatics.[52] This abnormality has been hypothesized to occur secondary to a transient decrease in cortical mitotic activity followed by overcompensation.[260]

The affected hairs occur mainly on the scalp

Figure 6-59 Pohl-Pinkus mark: dumbbell constriction with absent cuticle.

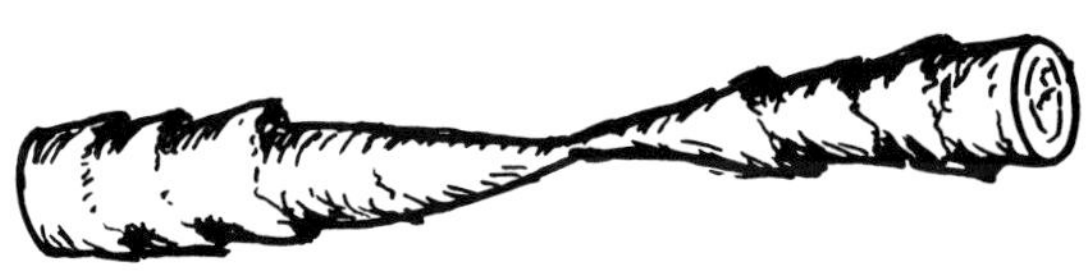

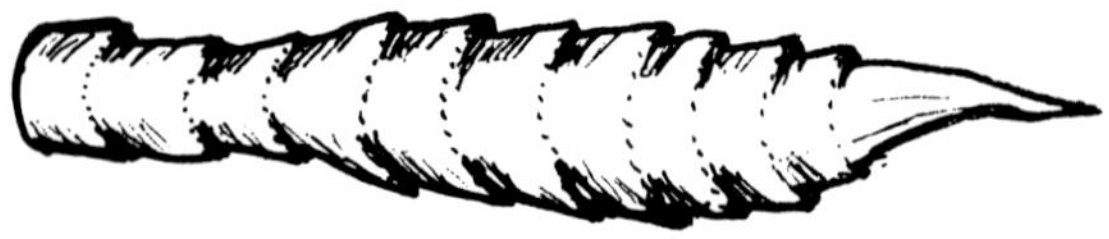

Figure 6-60 Bayonet hair: tapered tip with proximal expansion of shaft.

but have been found in the eyebrows or on the face and lower limbs. They are noticeably shorter than normal hair, seldom exceeding 8 cm in length. These hairs are potentially more fragile, but breakages are infrequently noted, perhaps due to short hairstyles in which the affected ends are trimmed off.[8] If present, the broken ends are often fibrillar, or sometimes rounded.[260]

TAPERED NEWLY GROWING ANAGEN HAIRS

Tapered newly growing anagen hairs are short hairs with intact cuticles and tapered, hypopigmented tips. They normally represent some 5 percent of scalp hair and, being firmly rooted, are more difficult to grasp and pull out than telogen hairs. In trichotillomania, most of the short hairs present within the patches of hair thinning are tapered, newly growing anagen hairs.[261] This is caused by the continual plucking of graspable hairs more than 2 to 3 cm long. This picture contrasts with the pigmented, broken-off hairs that make up the irregular stubble usually found in more acute lesions. Short anagen hairs are therefore a useful diagnostic marker of chronic trichotillomania, especially if associated with a total lack of telogen hairs.[15]

Figure 6-61 Bayonet hair: tapered tip with proximal broadening of shaft. (Light micrograph ×100)

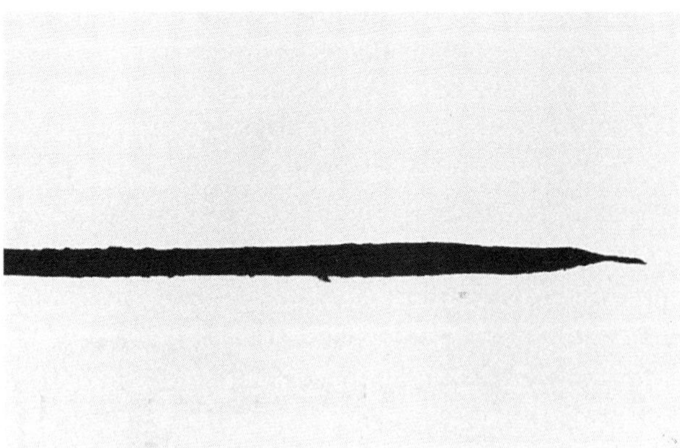

A preponderance of short, finely tapered, new anagen hairs has also been described in association with acquired progressive kinking[178] and is also seen when hair regrows in alopecia areata.[1]

TRICHOMALACIA

Trichomalacia represents the damage inflicted on the underlying anagen hair root in trichotillomania by repeated attempts at plucking.[1,262] This is best seen on microscopic examination of a scalp biopsy specimen. The partially plucked hair bulb is deformed and twisted, and clefts occur between the hair matrix cells and between the hair bulb and connective tissue sheath. The affected hair shaft is misshapen and twisted, and irregular melanin deposits are present.[1] There is no inflammatory reaction. High proportions of catagen and telogen hairs are present. The histological changes of trichomalacia are usually diagnostic of trichotillomania, but similar changes can result from other forms of severe traction alopecia; a reliable clinical history is needed before a correct diagnosis of the underlying cause can be made. In chronic traction alopecia, such as that seen with hair weaves where large amounts of additional hair are woven into existing hair, trichomalacia is infrequent, but abnormally large proportions of catagen and telogen hairs are present.

Bubble Hairs

Bubble hairs are characterized by the appearance of rows of bubbles within the hair shaft (Fig. 6-62). No obvious abnormality of the hair cuticle is present. In the original case, bubble hairs were found in a localized area of brittle hairs on the scalp of a 16-year-old girl who was otherwise healthy.[263] The probable cause was trauma, and the condition resolved spontaneously 10 months after onset. Two other cases of bubble hair have recently been described.[264] In these cases, hair fibers demonstrated a boomerang deformity containing small and large bubbles (Fig. 6-63*A* and *B*). Electron microscopy showed a loss of cortical cells and medulla at these sites. A reticulated Swiss-cheese-like loss of cells was seen on cross section. One of the two recent cases appeared to be related to recent highlighting of the patient's hair. In both cases, the involved tufts of wiry hair (Fig. 6-64) eventually grew out normally with gentle hair care. A fourth patient has now been described with bubble hair caused by an

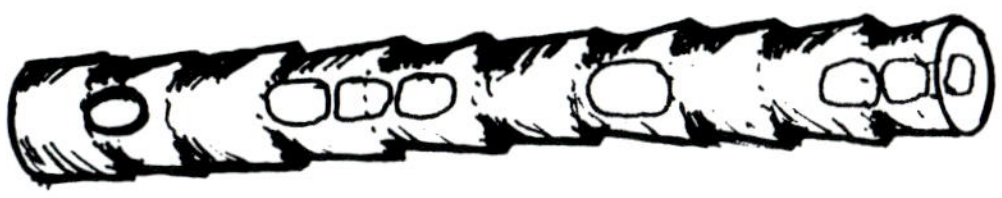

Figure 6-62 Bubble hair: a row of bubbles is present in hair shaft.

overheating hair dryer; the application of sufficient heat to unaffected hairs from the patient and from 16 human volunteers produced gaseous bubbles in all cases.[264a]

Intermittent Hair Follicle Dystrophy

In intermittent hair follicle dystrophy, hair shafts are brittle and broken off, and under scanning electron microscopy they show irregular loss of cuticle with transverse and longitudinal cracks and longitudinal ridges. Intermittent hair follicle dystrophy has been described in a 6-year-old girl with extensive hair loss and periods of partial remission.[265] Increased hair fragility was present secondary to abnormalities of keratinization in the hair shaft. The abnormal keratinization of cortex and medulla was most marked in the suprabulbar region of the hair shaft but also occurred in isthmic and infundibular portions of the follicle. The abnormal hair shafts were composed of polygonal keratinocytes, forming expansile masses which compressed surrounding follicular epithelium.[265] The most consistent change seen by transmission electron microscopy was intercellular edema of the outer root sheath, although Henle's and Huxley's layers were variably involved. The disease was localized to the scalp, the eyebrows and eyelashes were spared, and a clinical pattern of exacerbations and remissions was present.

Acquired Eyelash Trichomegaly

Acquired eyelash trichomegaly has recently been described in patients with AIDS.[266,267] The abnormality is quite striking, in that the eyelashes become considerably longer and more curly than normal, and may even double in length. Some hypertrichosis of eyebrows may also occur. Anecdotal evidence suggests that eyelash trichomegaly is not uncommon in AIDS patients. Eyelash trichomegaly has also been described in patients receiving interferon[268] and cyclosporine,[269] perhaps suggesting that immune dysregulation may be responsible for this unusual phenomenon.[267]

EXTRANEOUS MATTER ON THE HAIR SHAFT

Fungi

TINEA CAPITIS

Tinea capitis is caused by dermatophytes that invade and weaken the hair, leading to breakage.[270,271] It is discussed in detail in Chapter 5. Note that hairs with ectothrix infections have a gray, lusterless appearance and break off a few

Figure 6-63 Bubble hair. (*A*) Row of adjacent bubbles in shaft. (Light micrograph ×100) (*B*) Double row of bubbles in shaft. (Light micrograph ×400)

A

B

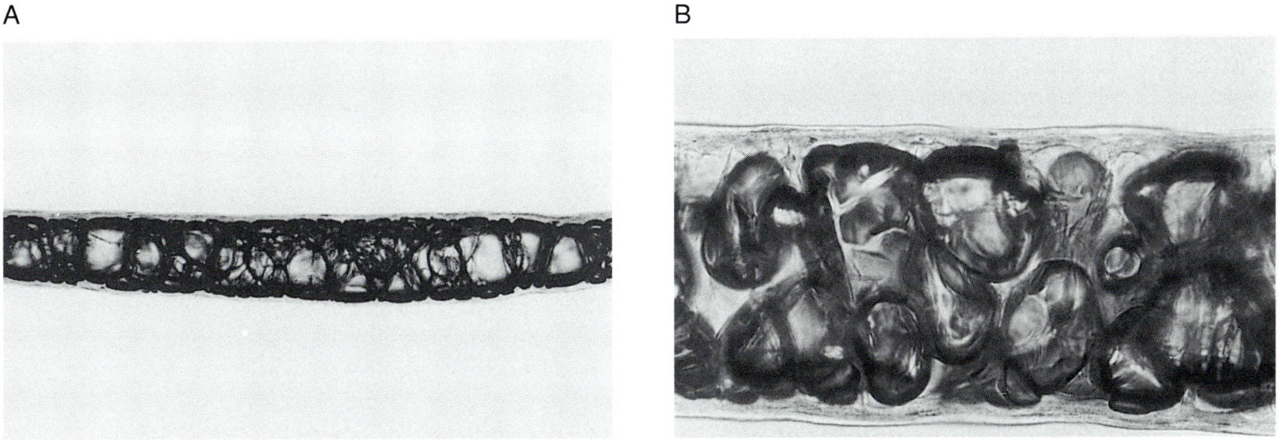

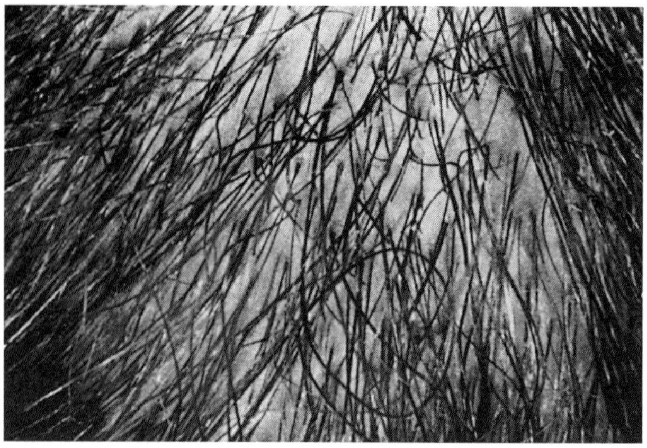

Figure 6-64 Bubble hair: affected hairs are kinked or broken off short. (*Reprinted from Elston et al.*[264])

millimeters away from the skin surface.[272] Hairs with endothrix infections are enlarged, coiled, and black, and break off flush with the scalp, producing a "black-dot" appearance.[273] Favic hairs appear dull and gray and break off much farther away from the scalp. Favus is caused by an endothrix infection in which characteristic air spaces resembling Swiss cheese are seen in the hair cortex, with many hyphae but few arthrospores.[274] The microscopic demonstration of spores and septate hyphae involving the hair shaft, in a potassium hydroxide (KOH) preparation or in a biopsy, is diagnostic of a dermatophytic infection. Culture of hairs or skin scrapings is necessary for identification of the fungal species.

BLACK PIEDRA

Black piedra, caused by *Piedraia hortae,* is characterized by the presence of adherent, gritty, black, often multiple nodules on the scalp, the beard, the moustache, and even the body hair. The fungi penetrate the cuticle, grow into the shaft, proliferate, and subsequently escape to surround the hair shaft with hyphae, asci, and ascospores.[272] Fractures can occur in the infected hair shaft. For treatment to be effective, all affected hairs must be cut off. Daily washing may help to minimize recurrences.

WHITE PIEDRA

White piedra, caused by *Trichosporon beigelii,* affects mainly the pubic hairs but can involve the beard, the moustache, and the scalp hairs as well. Soft, spongy, whitish nodules which are easily detachable develop on the hair shaft (Fig. 6-65). They can also invade the hair shaft and cause fractures. The nodular masses that occur are full of fungal spores. White piedra is now known to be common, endemic to Houston, Texas, and possibly to much of the United States, is linked to poor hygiene, and is more frequent in blacks.[275] Recent studies of these patients have indicated that white piedra is a mixed infection caused by a synergistic action between *T. beigelii* and a specific but unidentified coryneform bacteria.[276] The diagnosis is established by microscopic examination and by fungal and bacterial culture.

The primary treatment is to cut off the affected hairs and to institute daily washing.[272] Topical amphotericin B solution has been used successfully in one case of white piedra.[277] *T. beigelii* has been found to be sensitive to imidazole compounds in vitro,[278] and combination therapy with topical 1% econazole nitrate and oral ketoconazole may produce the best clinical results.[275] Other topical antifungal preparations, such as naftifine, can be tried.

Bacteria

TRICHOMYCOSIS AXILLARIS

Trichomycosis axillaris is a superficial infection of axillary or pubic hair by one of several species of *Corynebacterium tenuis.*[279–281] Adherent yellow, black, or red nodules are found, the latter two in the tropics.[282] The hairs become brittle and are easily broken. On scanning electron microscopy, the bacteria are seen to penetrate the

Figure 6-65 White piedra: irregular nodules on hair shaft. (Light micrograph ×100)

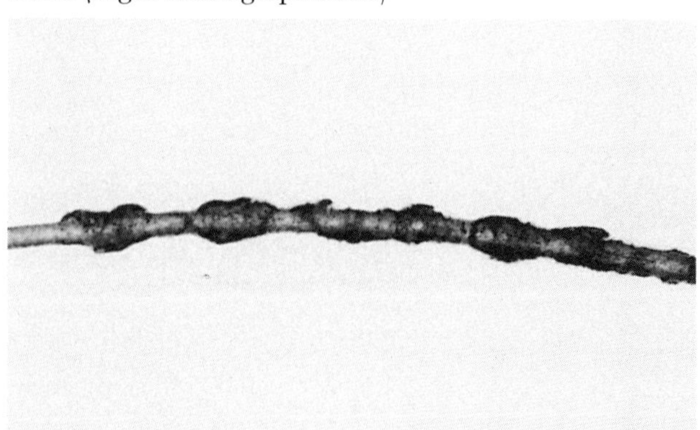

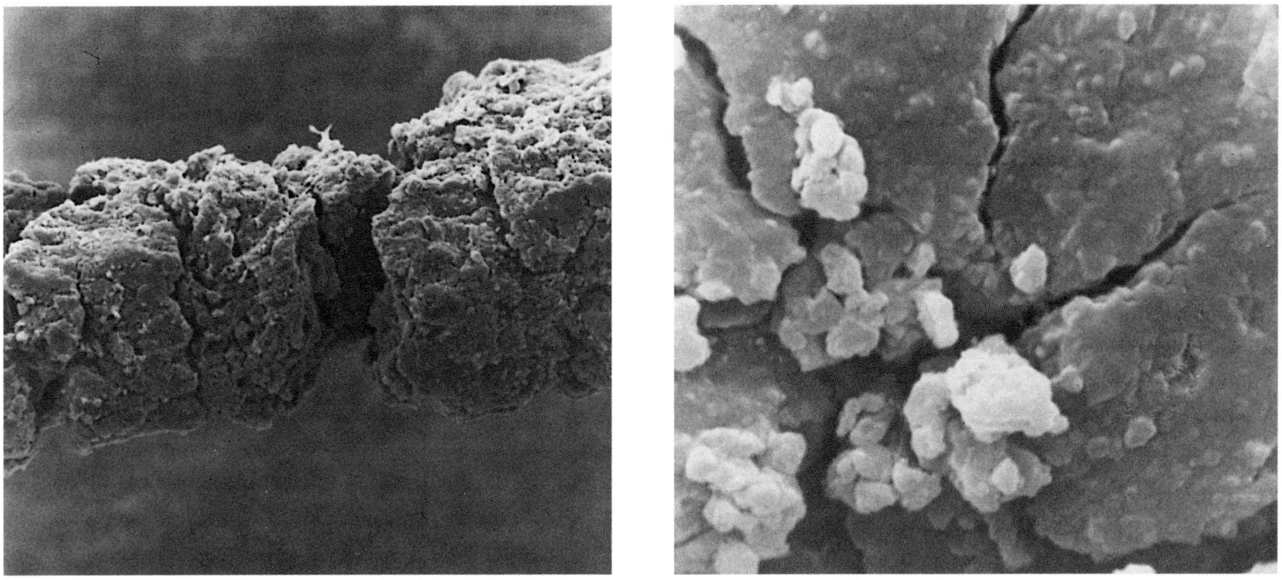

A B

Figure 6-66 Trichomycosis axillaris. (*A*) Nodules around hair shaft. (Scanning electron micrograph) (*B*) Organisms of *Corynebacterium tenuis* perforating hair cuticle. (Scanning electron micrograph)

hair cuticle and destroy the underlying cortex (Fig. 6-66*A* and *B*).[283] Myriads of the diphtheroid bacteria around the hair shaft are seen to be embedded in an insoluble cement substance, recently suggested to be dried apocrine sweat.[284]

The diagnosis can be confirmed by microscopic examination. Cultures must be done in a bacterial rather than a fungal medium, such as sheep blood agar. Growth from contaminants should be reduced by dipping affected hairs in 70% alcohol for 1 second before inoculation into the culture medium.[280] The condition is treated by cutting off all affected hairs and beginning regular washing.[272] Topical 1% clindamycin may be effective.[282]

Pediculosis Capitis: Nits

The true nit is ovoid, lies to one side of the hair shaft, and is anchored to it proximally by a sheath that envelops both the nit and the shaft.[1] The distal end of the nit points toward the free end of the hair and is covered by a lid, or operculum. A plane of cleavage is visible between the egg case and the lid. The operculum is capped by a central dome that contains air holes to allow the developing larva to breathe (Fig. 6-67).

Clinically the nits appear as small, ovoid structures that attach to the hair and that cannot be moved along the hair shaft (Fig. 6-68). Their color varies from whitish to brownish and depends on the color of the developing louse and whether or not it has hatched (Fig. 6-69). Nits appear on the scalp and beard hair with pediculosis capitis, and *Phthirus pubis* attaches nits to pubic, abdominal, thoracic, axillary, eyelash, eyebrow, and even scalp hair.[272] Nits are often easier to find than adult lice (Fig. 6-70). On the scalp, both nits and lice are most numerous behind the ears and on the occiput. Pruritus is invariable and leads to excoriations, secondary infection, and lymphadenopathy. The diagnosis of pediculosis is easily confirmed by microscopic examination of an affected hair. The characteristic oval egg case and lid lying to one side of the hair shaft and attached to it by an enveloping sheath are easy to recognize. The egg case may or may not contain a louse.

The treatment of choice, after shampooing and rinsing the hair, is to apply 1% permethrin, a pyrethroid, to the hair and scalp for 10 minutes, followed by a clean water rinse. An alternative therapy is to apply 1% lindane shampoo to the dry scalp, add water until a lather forms, and

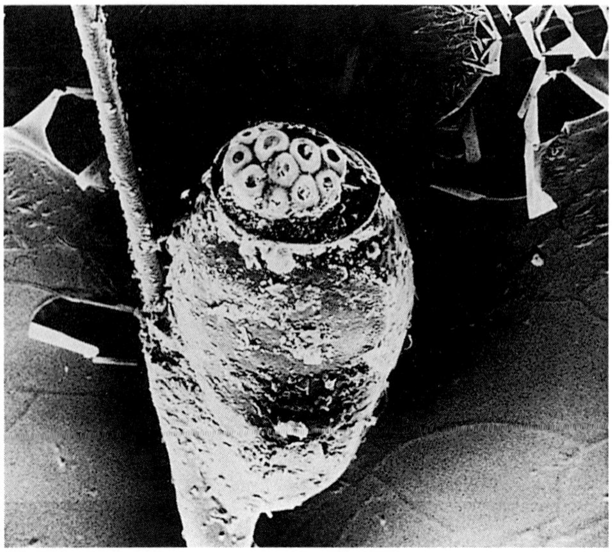

Figure 6-67 Pediculosis capitis: nit attached securely to one side of hair shaft by sheath, capped with operculum containing air holes. (Scanning electron micrograph)

leave in place for 4 minutes before rinsing. These treatments can be repeated weekly if necessary. All contacts should be checked for symptoms and signs of infection and treated if indicated. The most effective ovicide is 0.5% malathion, which is not currently available in the United States.[285]

Peripilar Casts: Pseudo nits

Peripilar casts are tubular masses of amorphous material of varied length and diameter. They are

Figure 6-68 Pediculosis capitis: multiple nits are attached to scalp hairs.

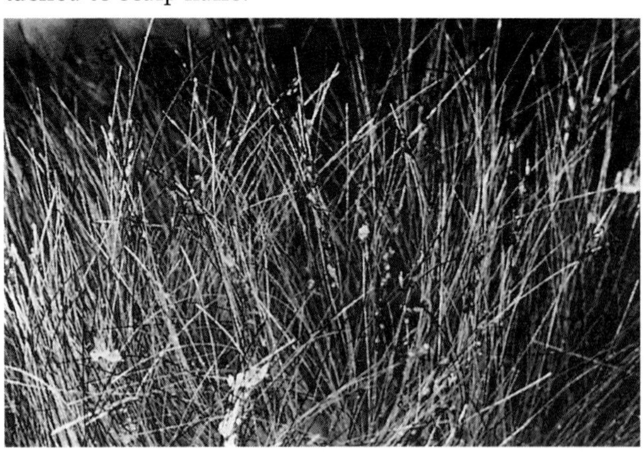

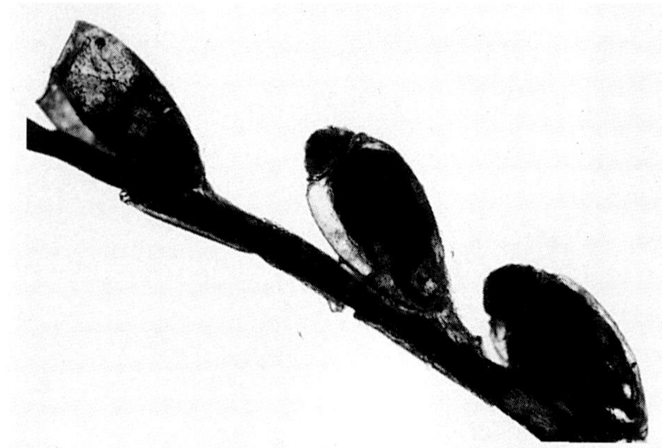

Figure 6-69 Pediculosis capitis: three nits are attached to hair shaft; distal nit empty. (Light micrograph ×100)

conical proximally and are perforated centrally by the hair shaft. The distal end of the cast may taper or, in the case of larger casts, may expand into a funnel shape. The shape of the cast may depend on the site of origin in the pilary canal, or infundibulum, or both. Peripilar casts, or so-called pseudo nits, are commonly found in normal hair in children and adults of either sex. They are whitish or yellowish and can be moved up and down the hair shaft. Pseudo nits are distinguished from true nits by their mobility and because they uniformly surround a central hair.

There are two types of hair casts.[286] The common type is the parakeratotic hair cast which is found frequently in children and adults, associ-

Figure 6-70 Phthirus pubis: adult louse removed from eyelash. (Light micrograph ×30)

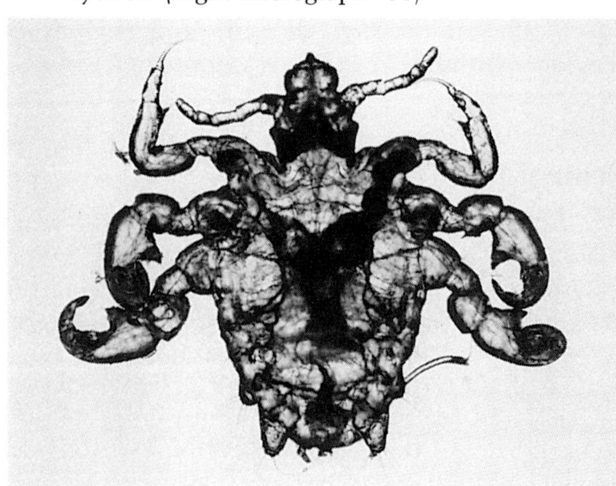

ated with the active lesions of parakeratotic scalp diseases such as psoriasis, seborrheic dermatitis, and tinea (or pityriasis) amiantacea.[287,288] Before they separate, these casts may bulge out from follicular openings, and they were originally described as parakeratotic comedones.[289] The cast is often large and irregular; it is composed of parakeratotic squamous cells from the follicular infundibulum and adjacent skin, and may sometimes contain external root sheath.[290] It can be moved along the hair shaft but is easily broken.[290]

The uncommon type of hair cast is the peripilar keratin cast, which is usually seen as a diffuse abnormality in girls aged 2 to 8, without associated scalp disease. The cast is often translucent and cylindrical, and fully invests the hair shaft, along which it can easily be moved without breakage.[286] It is commonly composed of external root sheath, sometimes composed of both external and internal root sheaths, and infrequently composed of internal root sheath alone (Fig. 6-71).[290] These differences can be distinguished by staining with either 4-dimethylaminocinnamaldehyde dissolved in 0.5N hydrochloric acid (1% DACA, Delasco, Council Bluffs, IA), an anagen hair marker which reacts with the citrulline in the inner root sheath to produce a reddish color,[291] or toluidine blue, which stains the inner root sheath intensely blue.[292] Peripilar keratin casts are usually idiopathic but are sometimes found on scalp margins or vertex associated with chronic traction from ponytails or pigtails.[293,294] The diagnosis is easily confirmed by light microscopy of the affected hair and cast, which bears little resemblance to a true nit.

Figure 6-71 Peripilar cast: sleevelike tubular structure loosely investing the hair shaft, composed of external root sheath. (Light micrograph ×100)

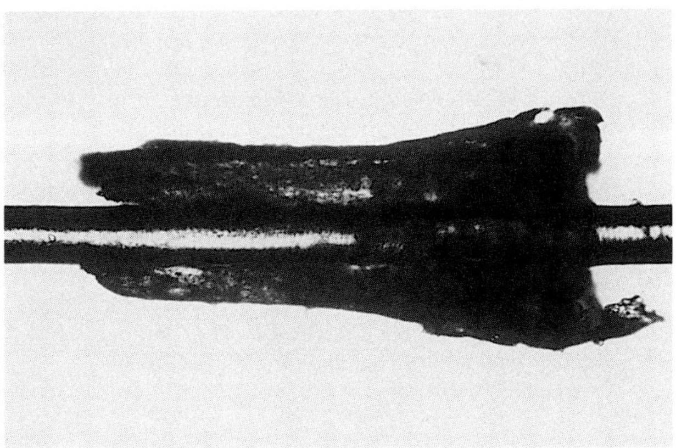

Treatment by mechanical removal of casts is tedious. Some success with the use of tretinoin lotion has been reported.[289] The major importance of this condition lies in distinguishing it from true nits.

Deposits: Lacquer, Paint, and Glue

Deposits of extraneous material from many sources can adhere to hair shafts and cause diagnostic difficulties.[1] These particles are not usually generalized throughout the scalp but are localized to areas of contact with paint, hair spray, lacquer, glue, and so forth. Unlike peripilar casts, the deposits cannot easily be moved up and down the hair shaft (Fig. 6-72).

The diagnosis can usually be made by clinical examination together with information obtained from the patient's history. Careful evaluation under the microscope will establish that the deposits are not inherent parts of the hair shaft.

Widespread coating of the hair with viscous fluid can, in rare cases, produce sudden and irreversible effects. Severe matting of the hair, or "bird's nest" hair, has been described following repeated shampoos with 2% cetrimide, a cationic detergent.[295] The main factor causing matting is thought to be the physical phenomenon of felting, which results from the tangling of imbricated hair by friction.[51] The process is potentiated by mechanical trauma, a fluid medium, and detergents which lead to electrostatic attraction between adjacent hair shafts.[51] An additional factor in the matting process induced by cetrimide was the viscous fluid "welding" of points of contact between hairs, which was

Figure 6-72 Lacquer: two beads of hair lacquer attached to hair shaft. (Light micrograph ×40)

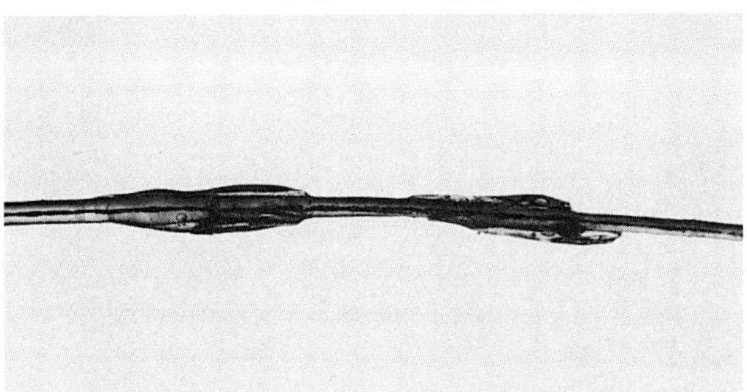

demonstrated by scanning electron microscopy.[295] The matted hair could not be freed, and was cut off.[295] Milder shampoos and the use of conditioners are indicated in such patients, as is the avoidance of excessive bleaching, permanent waving, and straightening procedures.[296]

CONCLUDING REMARKS

The evaluation and diagnosis of hair shaft defects must take into account both clinical features and the microscopic appearance of the affected hairs. Clinically, hair shaft defects usually cause hair fragility or hair unruliness. By light microscopy, hair shaft abnormalities may be classified according to whether fractures, coiling or twisting, or irregularities in or on the shaft are present. Diagnosis may ultimately depend on further evaluation including polaroscopic examination or scanning electron microscopic examination of hairs, amino acid analysis of hair or urine, or analysis of hair sulfur content. Unfortunately, an accurate diagnosis, while giving valuable prognostic information, generally does not suggest effective therapy for most of these conditions. Further delineation of the basic genetic and molecular causes of these hair shaft defects is necessary before normalization of hair growth can be a realistic goal.

ACKNOWLEDGMENTS

Illustrations of hair shafts were drawn by F. Lester Howsden, M.D., Dallas, Texas.

REFERENCES

1. Whiting DA: Structural abnormalities of the hair shaft. J Am Acad Dermatol 16:1–25, 1987.
2. Rook A, Dawber R: *Diseases of the Hair and Scalp,* 2d ed. Oxford, Blackwell Scientific Publications, 1991, pp 200–255.
3. Porter PS, Lobitz WC: Human hair: A genetic marker. Br J Dermatol 83:225–241, 1970.
4. Aoyagi T, Porter PS: Genetic disorders of hair growth: Pathogenesis of human hair defects. In Kobori T, Montagna W, Toda K (eds): *Biology and Disease of the Hair.* Baltimore, University Park Press, 1976, pp 473–487.
5. Muller S: Alopecia: Syndromes of genetic significance. J Invest Dermatol 60:475–492, 1973.
6. Shelley WB: Hair examination using double-stick tape (letter). J Am Acad Dermatol 8:430–431, 1983.
7. Price VH: Office diagnosis of structural hair anomalies. Cutis 15:231–240, 1975.
8. Price VH: Structural anomalies of the hair shaft. In Orfanos CE, Happle R (eds): *Hair and Hair Diseases.* Berlin, Springer-Verlag, 1990, pp 363–422.
9. Montagna W, Parakkal PF: *The Structure and Function of Skin,* 3d ed. New York, Academic Press, 1974, pp 172–182.
10. Wyatt EH, Riggott JM: Scanning electron microscopy of hair: Observations on surface morphology with respect to site, sex and age in man. Br J Dermatol 96:627–633, 1977.
11. Hrdy D: Quantitative hair form variation in seven populations. Am J Phys Anthropol 39:7–18, 1973.
12. Lantis SDH, Pepper MC: Woolly hair nevus. Two case reports and a discussion of unruly hair forms. Arch Dermatol 114:233–238, 1978.
13. Kligman AM: Pathologic dynamics of human hair loss: 1. Telogen effluvium. Arch Dermatol 83:175–198, 1961.
14. Steck WD: Telogen effluvium: A clinically useful concept, with traction alopecia as an example. Cutis 21:543–548, 1978.
15. Steck WD: The clinical evaluation of pathologic hair loss with a diagnostic sign in trichotillomania. Cutis 24:293–301, 1979.
16. Rook A, Dawber R: *Diseases of the Hair and Scalp,* 2d ed. Oxford, Blackwell Scientific Publications, 1991, pp 154–156.
17. Rook A: Review: The clinical importance of "weathering" in human hair. Br J Dermatol 95:111–112, 1976.
18. Dawber RPR: Weathering of hair in some genetic hair dystrophies. In Brown AC, Crounse RG (eds): *Hair, Trace Elements and Human Illness.* New York, Praeger, 1980, pp 273–280.
18a. Swift JA, Brown AC: The critical determination of fine changes in the surface architecture of human hair due to cosmetic treatment. J Soc Cosmet Chem 23:695–702, 1972.
19. Montagna W, Parakkal PF: *The Structure and Function of Skin,* 3d ed. New York, Academic Press, 1974, pp 178–179.
20. Swift JA, Brown AC: Scanning electron microscopy observations of human hair weathering. In Brown AC (ed): *The First Human Hair Symposium.* New York, Medcom Press, 1974, pp 332–345.
21. Price VH: Disorders of the hair in children. Pediatr Clin North Am 25:305–320, 1978.
22. Mortimer PS: Unruly hair. Br J Dermatol 113:467–473, 1985.
23. Smith DW, Greely MJ: Unruly scalp hair in infancy: Its nature and relevance to problems of brain morphogenesis. Pediatrics 61:783–785, 1978.
24. Chernosky ME, Owens DW: Trichorrhexis nodosa: Clinical and investigative studies. Arch Dermatol 94:577–585, 1966.
25. Owens DW, Chernosky ME: Trichorrhexis nodosa: *In vitro* reproduction. Arch Dermatol 94:586–588, 1966.
26. Eckert J, Church RE, Ebling FJ: The pathogenesis of alopecia areata. Br J Dermatol 80:203–210, 1968.
27. Dawber RPR, Comaish S: Scanning electron microscopy

of normal and abnormal hair shafts. Arch Dermatol 101:316–322, 1970.
28. Papa CM, Mills OH, Hanshaw W: Seasonal trichorrhexis nodosa: Role of cumulative damage in frayed hair. Arch Dermatol 106:888–892, 1972.
29. Wolff HH, Vigl E, Braun-Falco O: Trichorrhexis congenita. Hautarzt 26:576–580, 1975.
30. Rousset MJ: Genodermatose difficilement classable (trichorrhexis nodosa) predominant chez les males dans quatre generations. Bull Soc Fr Dermatol Syphiligr 59:298–300, 1952.
31. Munro DD: Disorders affecting the skin appendages. In Fitzpatrick TB et al. (eds): *Dermatology in Genral Medicine.* New York, McGraw-Hill, 1971, pp 297–331.
32. Brenton DP et al.: Argininosuccinicaciduria: Clinical, metabolic and dietary study. J Ment Defic Res 18:1–13, 1974.
33. Batshaw ML et al.: Treatment of inborn errors of urea synthesis: Activation of alternative pathways of waste nitrogen synthesis and excretion. N Engl J Med 306:1387–1392, 1982.
34. Batshaw ML, Thomas GH, Brusilow SW: New approaches to the diagnosis and treatment of inborn errors of urea synthesis. Pediatrics 68:290–297, 1981.
35. Allan JD, Cusworth DE, Dent CE, Wilson VK: A disease, probably hereditary, characterized by severe mental deficiency and a constant gross abnormality of amino acid metabolism. Lancet 1:182–187, 1958.
36. Levin B, Mackay HMM, Oberholzer VG: Argininosuccinic aciduria, an inborn error of amino acid metabolism. Arch Dis Child 36:622–632, 1961.
37. Potter JL, Timmons GD, Silvidi AA: Argininosuccinicaciduria: The hair abnormality revisited. Am J Dis Child 134:1095–1096, 1980.
38. Shih VE: Early dietary management in an infant with argininosuccinase deficiency: Preliminary report. J Pediatr 80:645–648, 1972.
39. Rauschkolb EW, Chernosky ME, Knox JM, Owens DW: Trichorrhexis nodosa—An error of amino acid metabolism? J Invest Dermatol 48:260–263, 1967.
40. Goldblum OM, Brusilow SW, Maldonado YA, Farmer ER: Neonatal citrullinemia associated with cutaneous manifestations and arginine deficiency. J Am Acad Dermatol 14:321–326, 1986.
41. Porter PS: The genetics of human hair growth. In Bergsma D (ed): *Birth Defects, Original Article Series.* Baltimore, Williams and Wilkins, The National Foundation—March of Dimes, 1972, pp 69–85.
42. Danks DM, Tippett P, Zentner G: Severe neonatal citrullinemia. Arch Dis Child 49:579–581, 1974.
43. Patel HP, Unis ME: Pili torti in association with citrullinemia. J Am Acad Dermatol 12:203–206, 1985.
44. Menkes JH et al.: A sex-linked recessive disorder with retardation of growth, peculiar hair and focal cerebral and cerebellar degeneration. Pediatrics 29:764–779, 1962.
45. Menkes JH: Kinky hair disease. Pediatrics 50:181–183, 1972.
46. Price VH, Odom RB, Ward WH, Jones FT: Trichothiodystrophy: Sulfur-deficient brittle hair as a marker for a neuroectodermal symptom complex. Arch Dermatol 116:1375–1384, 1980.
47. Leonard JN, Gummer CL, Dawber RPR: Generalized trichorrhexis nodosa. Br J Dermatol 103:85–90, 1980.
48. Rushton DH, Norris MJ, James KC: Amino acid composition in trichorrhexis nodosa. Clin Exp Dermatol 15:24–28, 1990.
49. Camacho-Martinez F: Localized trichorrhexis nodosa. J Am Acad Dermatol 20:696–697, 1989.
50. Camacho-Martinez F, Ferrando J: Hair shaft dysplasias. Int J Dermatol 27:71–80, 1988.
51. Bogaty H, Dunlap FE: Matting of hair. Arch Dermatol 101:348–351, 1970.
52. Brown AC: Congenital hair defects. In Bergsma D (ed): *Birth Defects, Original Article Series.* Baltimore, Williams and Wilkins, The National Foundation—March of Dimes, 1972, pp 52–68.
53. Stankler L et al.: Unexplained diarrhea and failure to thrive in 2 siblings with unusual facies and abnormal scalp hair shafts: A new syndrome. Arch Dis Child 57:212–216, 1982.
54. Brown AC, Belser RB, Crounse RG, Wehr RF: A congenital hair defect: Trichoschisis and alternating birefringence and low sulfur content. J Invest Dermatol 54:496–509, 1970.
55. Miyazawa F, Tamura T, Nozaki F: Alteration of amino acid composition and keratinolysis of hair due to chemical damage. In Kobori T, Montagna W (eds): *Biology and Disease of the Hair.* Baltimore, University Park Press, 1976, pp 659–667.
56. Morganti P et al.: Abnormal amino acid changes in human hair associated with rare congenital syndromes. In Orfanos CE, Montagna W, Stuttgen G (eds): *Hair Research: Status and Future Aspects.* Berlin, Springer-Verlag, 1981, pp 442–445.
57. Gold RJM, Scriver CR: The characterization of hereditary abnormalities of keratin: Clouston's ectodermal dysplasia. Birth Defects 7:91–95, 1971.
58. Gillespie JM: The dietary regulation of the synthesis of hair keratin. In Crewther WG (ed): *Symposium on Fibrous Proteins.* London, Butterworths, 1968, pp 362–363.
59. Van Neste D, Miller X, Bohnert E: Clinical symptoms associated with trichothiodystrophy: A review of the literature with special emphasis on light sensitivity and the association with xeroderma pigmentosum (complementation group D). In Van Neste D, Lachapelle JM, Antoine JL (eds): *Trends in Human Hair Growth and Alopecia Research.* Dordrecht, Kluwer Academic Publishers, 1989, pp 183–193.
60. Itin PH, Pittelkow MR: Trichothiodystrophy: Review of sulfur-deficient brittle hair syndromes and association with ectodermal dysplasias. J Am Acad Dermatol 22:705–717, 1990.
61. Itin PH, Pittelkow MR: Trichothiodystrophy with chronic neutropenia and mild mental retardation. J Am Acad Dermatol 24:356–358, 1991.
62. Baden HP et al.: The physicochemical properties of hair in the BIDS syndrome. Am J Hum Genet 28:514–521, 1976.
63. Calvieri S, Zampetti M, Corbo A: Preliminary results using a microanalysis system on the hair of patients af-

fected with trichothiodystrophy (abstract). Clin Exp Dermatol 14:404, 1989.
64. Venning VA, Dawber RPR, Ferguson DJP, Kanan MW: Weathering of hair in trichothiodystrophy. Br J Dermatol 114:591–595, 1986.
65. Gummer CL, Dawber RPR, Price VH: Trichothiodystrophy: An electron-histochemical study of the hair shaft. Br J Dermatol 110:439–449, 1984.
66. Gummer CL, Dawber RPR: Trichothiodystrophy: An ultrastructural study of the hair follicle. Br J Dermatol 113:273–280, 1985.
67. Gillespie JM, Marshall RC: A comparison of the proteins of normal and trichothiodystrophic human hair. J Invest Dermatol 80:195–202, 1983.
68. Gillespie JM, Marshall RC: Effect of mutations on the proteins of wool and hair. In Rogers GE et al. (eds): *The Biology of Wool and Hair.* London, Chapman & Hall, 1989, pp 257–273.
69. Crovato F, Borrone C, Rebora A: The Tay syndrome (congenital ichthyosis with trichothiodystrophy). Eur J Pediatr 142:233–234, 1984.
70. Crovato F, Rebora A: PIBI(D)S syndrome: A new entity with defect of the deoxyribonucleic acid excision repair system. J Am Acad Dermatol 13:683–685, 1985.
71. Van Neste D, Caulier B, Thomas P, Vasseur F: Tay's syndrome and xeroderma pigmentosum. J Am Acad Dermatol 12:372–373, 1985.
72. Lehmann AR: Cockayne's syndrome and trichothiodystrophy: Defective repair without cancer. Cancer Rev 7:82–103, 1987.
73. Lehmann AR et al.: Trichothiodystrophy, a human DNA repair disorder with heterogeneity in the cellular response to ultraviolet light. Cancer Res 48:6090–6096, 1988.
74. Norwood WF: The Marinesco-Sjögren syndrome. J Pediatr 65:431–437, 1964.
75. Lucky PA, Kirsch N, Lucky AW, Carter DM: Low-sulfur hair syndrome associated with UVB photosensitivity and testicular failure. J Am Acad Dermatol 11:340–346, 1984.
76. Rebora A, Guarrera M, Crovato F: Amino-acid analysis in hair from PIBI(D)S syndrome. J Am Acad Dermatol 15:109–111, 1986.
77. Arbisser AI et al.: A syndrome manifested by brittle hair with morphologic and biochemical abnormalities, developmental delay and normal stature. Birth Defects 12:219–228, 1976.
78. Howell RR et al.: The Sabinas brittle hair syndrome. In Brown AC, Crounse RG (eds): *Hair, Trace Elements and Human Illness.* New York, Praeger, 1980, pp 210–219.
79. Jackson CE, Weiss L, Watson JHL: "Brittle" hair with short stature, intellectual impairment and decreased fertility: An autosomal recessive syndrome in an Amish kindred. Pediatrics 54:201–207, 1974.
80. Jorizzo JL, Crounse RG, Wheeler CE Jr: Lamellar ichthyosis, dwarfism, mental retardation and hair shaft abnormalities: A link between the ichthyosis-associated and BIDS syndromes. J Am Acad Dermatol 2:309–317, 1980.
81. Jorizzo JL, Atherton DJ, Crounse RG, Wells RS: Ichthyosis, brittle hair, impaired intelligence, decreased fertility and short stature (IBIDS syndrome). Br J Dermatol 106:705–710, 1982.
82. Tay CH: Ichthyosiform erythroderma, hair shaft abnormalities, and mental and growth retardation: A new recessive disorder. Arch Dermatol 104:4–13, 1971.
83. Happle R, Traupe H, Grobe H, Bonsmann G: The Tay syndrome (congenital ichthyosis with trichothiodystrophy). Eur J Pediatr 141:147–152, 1984.
84. Pollitt RJ, Jenner FA, Davies M: Sibs with mental and physical retardation and trichorrhexis nodosa with abnormal amino acid composition of the hair. Arch Dis Child 43:211–216, 1968.
85. Crovato F, Borrone C, Rebora A: Trichothiodystrophy—BIDS, IBIDS and PIBIDS? Br J Dermatol 108:247–251, 1983.
86. Brodin MB, Porter PS: Netherton's syndrome. Cutis 26:185–191, 1980.
87. Netherton EW: A unique case of trichorrhexis nodosa—"Bamboo hairs." Arch Dermatol 78:483–487, 1958
88. Wilkinson RD, Curtis GH, Hawk WA: Netherton's disease. Arch Dermatol 89:106–113, 1964.
89. Marshall J, Brede HD: Black piedra in a child with pili torti, bamboo hair and congenital ichthyosiform erythroderma. S Afr Med J 35:221–225, 1961.
90. Greene SL, Muller SA: Netherton's syndrome. J Am Acad Dermatol 13:329–337, 1985.
91. Comel M: Ichthyosis linearis circumflexa. Dermatologica 98:133–136, 1949.
92. Mevorah B, Frenk E, Brooke EM: Ichthyosis linearis circumflexa comel: A clinico-statistical approach to its relationship with Netherton's syndrome. Dermatologica 149:201–209, 1974.
93. Hurwitz S, Kirsch N, McGuire J: Reevaluation of ichthyosis and hair shaft abnormalities. Arch Dermatol 103:266–271, 1971.
94. Krafchik BR: Netherton syndrome. Pediatr Dermatol 9:158–160, 1992.
95. Hersle K: Netherton's disease and ichthyosis linearis circumflexa: Report of a case and review of the literature. Acta Derm Venereol (Stockh) 52:298–302, 1972.
96. Greig D, Wishart J: Growth abnormality in Netherton's syndrome. Aust J Dermatol 23:27–30, 1982.
97. Kassis V et al.: Familial Netherton's disease. Cutis 38:175–178, 1986.
98. Stankler L, Cochrane T: Netherton's disease in two sisters. Br J Dermatol 79:187–196, 1967.
99. Stevanovic DV: Multiple defects of the hair shaft in Netherton's disease: Association with ichthyosis linearis circumflexa. Br J Dermatol 81:851–857, 1969.
100. Ito M, Ito K, Hashimoto K: Pathogenesis in trichorrhexis invaginata (bamboo hair). J Invest Dermatol 83:1–6, 1984.
101. De Berker D, Paige D, Harper J, Dawber RPR: Golf tee hairs: A new sign in Netherton's syndrome. Br J Dermatol 127(suppl 40):30, 1992.
102. Menne T, Weisman K: Canestick lesion of vellus hair in Netherton's syndrome. Arch Dermatol 121:451, 1985.
103. Orfanos CE, Mahrle G, Salamon T: Netherton-Syndrom. Ichthyosiforme Hautveranderungen und Trichorrhexis invaginata, Nachweis eines krankhaft veranderten Cortexkeratins im Haar. Hautarzt 22:397–409, 1971.
104. Pinkus H: Discussion. In Wilkinson RD, Curtis GH, Hawk WA: Netherton's disease. Arch Dermatol 89:46–54, 1964.

105. Altman J, Stroud J: Netherton's syndrome and ichthyosis linearis circumflexa: Psoriasiform ichthyosis. Arch Dermatol 100:550–558, 1969.
106. Mevorah B, Frenk E: Ichthyosis linearis circumflexa comel with trichorrhexis invaginata (Netherton's syndrome): A light microscopical study of the skin changes. Dermatologica 149:193–200, 1974.
107. Thorne EG et al.: Netherton's syndrome: An electron-microscopic study. Arch Dermatol Forsch 253:177–183, 1975.
108. Frenk E, Mevorah B: Ichthyosis linearis circumflexa comel with trichorrhexis invaginata (Netherton's syndrome): An ultrastructural study of the skin changes. Arch Dermatol Forsch 245:42–49, 1972.
109. Hausser I, Anton-Lamprecht I, Hartschuh W, Petzoldt D: Netherton's syndrome: Ultrastructure of the active lesion under retinoid therapy. Arch Dermatol Res 281:165–172, 1989.
110. Happle R, Traupe H: Etretinat bei Genodermatosen und verschiedenen entzundlichen Hautkrankheiten. In Bauer RH, Gollnick H (eds): *Retinoide in der Praxis.* Berlin, Grosse, 1984, pp 35–49.
111. Nagata T: Netherton's syndrome which responded to photochemotherapy. Dermatologica 161:51–56, 1980.
112. Shuster S: "Coudability": A new physical sign of alopecia areata. Br J Dermatol 111:629, 1984.
113. Burkhart CG, Huttner JJ, Bruner J: Central trichoptilosis (letter). J Am Acad Dermatol 5:703–705, 1981.
114. Hellier RR, Astbury WT, Bell FO: A case of pili torti. Br J Dermatol Syph 52:173–182, 1940.
115. Dawber RPR: Weathering of hair in monilethrix and pili torti. Clin Exp Dermatol 2:271–277, 1977.
116. Ronchese F: Twisted hairs (pili torti). Arch Dermatol Syph 26:98–109, 1932.
117. Danforth CH: Studies on hair with special reference to hypertrichosis: IV. Regional characteristics of human hair. Arch Dermatol Syphilol (Chicago) 12:76–94, 1925.
118. Appel B, Messina SJ: Pili torti hereditaria. N Engl J Med 226:912–915, 1942.
119. Calzavara-Pinton P, Carlino A, Benetti A, De Panfilis G: Pili torti and onychodysplasia: Report of a previously undescribed hidrotic ectodermal dysplasia. Dermatologica 182:184–187, 1991.
120. Kurwa AR, Abdel-Aziz AM: Pili torti—Congenital and acquired. Acta Derm Venereol (Stockh) 53:385–392, 1973.
121. Björnstad R: Pili torti and sensory-neural loss of hearing. Proceedings, 17th meeting of the Fennoscandinavian Association of Dermatologists, Copenhagen, 1965, p 3.
122. Reed WB, Stone VM, Boder E, Ziprkowski L: Hereditary syndromes with auditory and dermatological manifestations. Arch Dermatol 95:456–461, 1967.
123. Robinson GC, Johnston MM: Pili torti and sensory neural hearing loss. J Pediatr 70:621–623, 1967.
124. Crandall BG, Samec L, Sparkes RS, Wright SW: A familial syndrome of deafness, alopecia and hypogonadism. J Pediatr 82:461–465, 1973.
125. Lyon JB, Dawber RPR: A sporadic case of dystrophic pili torti. Br J Dermatol 96:197–198, 1977.
126. Whiting DA, Jenkins T, Whitcomb MJ: Corkscrew hair—A unique type of congenital alopecia in pili torti. In Brown AC, Crounse RG (eds): *Hair, Trace Elements, and Human Illness.* New York, Praeger, 1980, pp 228–239.
127. Gold SC, Delaney TJ: Familial acne conglobata, hidradenitis suppurativa, pili torti and cataracts. Br J Dermatol 91(suppl 10):54–57, 1974.
128. Plosila M, Kiistala R, Niemi K-M: The Bazex syndrome: Follicular atrophoderma with multiple basal cell carcinomas, hypotrichosis and hypohidrosis. Clin Exp Dermatol 6:31–41, 1981.
129. Silengo MC et al.: Distinctive hair changes (pili torti) in Rapp-Hodgkin ectodermal dysplasia syndrome. Clin Genet 21:297–300, 1982.
130. Lavrijsen APM, Breslau-Siderius EJ: Pili torti as a marker of Rapp-Hodgkin ectodermal dysplasia syndrome in three generations. Br J Dermatol 121:812–813, 1989.
131. O'Donnell BP, James WD: Rapp-Hodgkin ectodermal dysplasia. J Am Acad Dermatol 27:323–326, 1992.
132. Abramovits-Ackerman W et al.: Cutaneous findings in a new syndrome of autosomal recessive ectodermal dysplasia with corkscrew hairs. J Am Acad Dermatol 27:917–921, 1992.
133. Beare JM: Congenital pilar defect showing features of pili torti. Br J Dermatol 64:366–372, 1952.
134. Ullmo A: Un nouveau type d'agenesie et de dystrophie pilaire familiale et hereditaire. Dermotologica 90:75–79, 1944.
135. Zlotogora J, Zilberman Y, Tenenbaum A, Wexler MR: Cleft lip and palate, pili torti, malformed ears, partial syndactyly of fingers and toes, and mental retardation: A new syndrome? J Med Genet 24:291–293, 1987.
136. Danks DM et al.: Menkes' kinky hair syndrome. An inherited defect in copper absorption with widespread effects. Pediatrics 50:188–201, 1972.
137. French JH et al.: Trichopoliodystrophy. Arch Neurol 26:229–244, 1972.
138. Goka TJ, Stevenson RE, Hefferan PM, Howell RR: Menkes' disease: A biochemical abnormality in cultured human fibroblasts. Proc Natl Acad Sci USA 73:604–606, 1976.
139. Collie WR, Moore CM, Goka TJ, Howell RR: Pili torti as marker for carriers of Menkes' disease. Lancet 1:607–608, 1978.
140. Singh S, Bresnan MJ: Menkes' kinky-hair syndrome (trichopoliodystrophy). Am J Dis Child 125:572–578, 1973.
141. Wheeler EM, Roberts PF: Menkes' steely hair syndrome. Arch Dis Child 51:269–274, 1976.
142. Lott IT et al.: Copper metabolism in the steely-hair syndrome. N Engl J Med 292:197–199, 1975.
143. Leone A, Pavlakis GN, Hamer DH: Menkes' disease: Abnormal metallothionein gene regulation in response to copper. Cell 40:301–309, 1985.
144. Danks DM et al.: Menkes' kinky hair syndrome. Lancet 1:1100–1103, 1972.
145. Horn N: Copper incorporation studies on cultured cells for prenatal diagnosis of Menkes' disease. Lancet 1:1156–1158, 1976.
146. Gerdes AM et al.: Clinical expression of Menkes' syndrome in females. Clin Genet 38:452–459, 1990.
147. Dupre A, Enjobras O: Syndrom de Menkes an Pilotorten alternant. Ann Dermatol Venereol 102:269–271, 1980.
148. Johnsen DE, Coleman L, Poe L: MR of progressive neu-

rodegenerative change in treated Menkes' kinky hair syndrome. Neuroradiology 33(2):181–182, 1991.
149. Sherwood G, Sarkar B, Kortsak AS: Copper histidinate therapy in Menkes' disease: Prevention of progressive neurodegeneration. J Inherited Metab Dis 12(suppl 2):393–396, 1989.
150. Telfer N, Cutler TP, Dawber RPR: The natural history of pili torti. Br J Dermatol 120:323–325, 1989.
151. Summerly R, Donaldson EM: Monilethrix: A family study. Br J Dermatol 74:387–391, 1962.
152. Bentley-Phillips B, Bayles MAH: A previously undescribed hereditary hair anomaly (pseudo-monilethrix). Br J Dermatol 89:159–167, 1973.
153. Hutchinson PE, Cairns RJ, Wells RS: Woolly hair: Clinical and genetic aspects. Trans St John's Hosp Dermatol Soc 60:160–177, 1974.
154. Peachey RDG, Wells RS: Hereditary hypotrichosis (Marie Unna type). Trans St John's Hosp Dermatol Soc 57:157–166, 1971.
155. Scott OLS: Localized pili torti. Proc R Soc Med 43:68, 1950.
156. Hays SB, Camisa C: Acquired pili torti in two patients treated with synthetic retinoids. Cutis 35:466–468, 1985.
157. Graham RM, James MP, Ferguson DJP, Guerrier CW: Acquired kinking of the hair associated with etretinate therapy. Clin Exper Dermatol 10:426–431, 1985.
158. Hoffman E: Uber einen Krauselnevus innerhalb sonst glatten Kopfhaares in Vergleich zum erblichen Kraushaar und zur Lockenbildung nach Rontgenepilation. Dermatologica 197:281–292, 1953.
159. Mohr OL: Woolly hair, a dominant mutant character in man. J Hered 23:345–352, 1932.
160. Robinson GC, Miller JR: Hereditary enamel hypoplasia: Its association with characteristic hair structure. Pediatrics 37:498–502, 1966.
161. Jacobsen KU, Lowes M: Woolly hair nevus with ocular involvement: Report of a case. Dermatologica 151: 249–252, 1975.
162. Taylor AEM: Hereditary woolly hair with ocular involvement. Br J Dermatol 123:523–525, 1990.
163. Verbov J: Woolly hair—Study of a family. Dermatologica 157:42–47, 1978.
164. McHenry PM, Nevin NC, Bingham EA: The association of keratosis pilaris atrophicans with hereditary woolly hair. Pediatr Dermatol 7:202–204, 1990.
165. Neild VS, Pegum JS, Wells RS: The association of keratosis pilaris atrophicans and woolly hair, with and without Noonan's syndrome. Br J Dermatol 110: 357–362, 1984.
166. Ormerod AD, Main RA, Ryder ML, Gregory DW: A family with diffuse partial woolly hair. Br J Dermatol 116:401–405, 1987.
167. Wise F: Woolly Hair Nevus. A peculiar form of birthmark of hair of the scalp, hitherto undescribed, with report of two cases. Med J Rec 125:545–547, 1927.
168. Reda AM, Rogers RS, Peters MS: Woolly hair nevus. J Am Acad Dermatol 22:377–380, 1990.
169. Wright S, Lemoine NR, Leigh IM: Woolly hair naevi with systematized linear epidermal naevus. Clin Exp Dermatol 11:179–182, 1986.
170. Peteiro C, Oliva NP, Zulaica A, Toribio J: Woolly-hair nevus: Report of a case associated with a verrucous epidermal nevus in the same area. Pediatr Dermatol 6:188–190, 1989.
171. Al-Harmozi SA, Mahmoud SF, Ejeckam GC: Woolly hair nevus syndrome. J Am Acad Dermatol 27:259–260, 1992.
172. Grant PW: A case of woolly hair nevus. Arch Dis Child 35:512–514, 1960.
173. Crosti C, Menni S: Woolly hair nevus: Osservazion sutre casi clinici. Minerva Dermatol 114:45–49, 1979.
174. Harper MF, Klokke AH: Woolly hair nevus with triangular hairs (abstract). Br J Dermatol 108:111–113, 1983.
175. Goldin HM, Branson DM, Fretzin DF: Woolly-hair nevus: A case report and study by scanning electron microscopy. Pediatr Dermatol 2:41–44, 1984.
176. Lichtenstein J et al.: The Tricho-dento-osseous (TDO) syndrome. Am J Hum Genet 24:569–582, 1972.
177. Baughman FA: CHANDS: The curly hair–ankyloblepharon–nail dysplasia syndrome. Birth Defects 7:100–102, 1971.
178. Coupe RL, Johnston MM: Acquired progressive kinking of the hair: Structural changes and growth dynamics of affected hairs. Arch Dermatol 100:191–195, 1969.
179. Mortimer PS, Gummer C, English J, Dawber RPR: Acquired progressive kinking of hair: Report of six cases and review of literature. Arch Dermatol 121:1031–1033, 1985.
180. Rebora A, Guarrera M: Acquired progressive kinking of the hair. J Am Acad Dermatol 12:933–936, 1985.
181. Balsa RE, Ingratta SM, Alvarez AG: Acquired kinking of the hair: A methodologic approach. J Am Acad Dermatol 15:1133–1136, 1986.
182. Esterly NB, Lavin MP, Garancis JC: Acquired progressive kinking of the hair. Arch Dermatol 125:813–815, 1989.
183. Wise F, Sulzberger MB: Acquired progressive kinking of the scalp hair accompanied by changes in its pigmentation. Arch Dermatol Syph 25:99–110, 1932.
184. Coupe RL: Acquired progressive kinking of the hair. Arch Dermatol 122:133, 1986.
185. Pfahler DR: Epilation of half the scalp in a patient with straight hair, followed by a regrowth of curly hair. Arch Dermatol Syphilol (Chicago) 15:214, 1927.
186. Norwood OT: Whisker hair. Arch Dermatol 115: 930–931, 1979.
187. Norwood OT: Whisker hair—An update. Cutis 27: 651–652, 1981.
188. Knierer W: Allotrichia Circumscripta Asymmetrica Capillitii (Pubeshaarnaevus). Dermatol Monatsschr 132:794, 1955.
189. Bovenmyer DA: Woolly hair naevus. Cutis 24:322–325, 1979.
190. Dawber RPR: Knotting of scalp hair. Br J Dermatol 91:169–173, 1974.
191. English DT, Jones HE: Trichonodosis. Arch Dermatol 107:77–79, 1973.
192. Laing V, Resnick SD: Trichonodosis in a patient with straight hair. J Am Acad Dermatol 23:756–757, 1990.
193. Scott MJ: Trichonodosis: Report of a case. Arch Dermatol Syph 63:769–771, 1951.
194. Adatto R: Poils en spirale (poils enroules). Dermatologica 127:145–147, 1963.
195. Levit F, Scott MJ Jr: Circle hairs. J Am Acad Dermatol 8:423–425, 1983.

196. Fergusson AG, Derblay PR: Rolled hairs, a possible complication of corticosteroid therapy. Arch Dermatol 127:145–147, 1963.
197. Weary P, Hendricks AA, Warner F, Ajkaonkar G: Pili bifurcati: A new anomaly of hair growth. Arch Dermatol 108:403–407, 1973.
198. Shelley WB, Shelley ED: Uncombable hair syndrome: Observation on response to biotin and occurrence in siblings with ectodermal dysplasia. J Am Acad Dermatol 13:97–102, 1985.
199. Larralde de Luna MM, Robinson R, Gehman de Kohan ZB: Pili trianguli canaliculi: Uncombable hair syndrome in a family with apparent autosomal dominant inheritance. Pediatr Dermatol 2:324–327, 1985.
200. Nodl F, Zaun H, Zinn KH: Gesteigerte Epilierbarkeit von Anagenhaaren bei Kindern a/s Folge eines Reifungsdefekts der Follikel mit gestorter Verhaftung von Haarschaft und Wurzelscheiden. Aktuel Dermatol 12:55–57, 1986.
201. Hamm H, Traupe H: Loose anagen hair of childhood: The phenomenon of easily pluckable hair. J Am Acad Dermatol 20:242–248, 1989.
202. Price VH, Gummer CL: Loose anagen syndrome. J Am Acad Dermatol 20:249–256, 1989.
203. Fleischmajer R, Nedwich A: Progeria (Hutchinson-Gilford). Arch Dermatol 107:253–258, 1973.
204. Dupre A, Bonafe JL, Litoux F, Victor M: Le syndrome des cheveux incoiffables: Pili trianguli et canaliculi. Ann Dermatol Venereol (Paris) 105:627–630, 1978.
205. Baden HP, Schoenfeld RJ, Stroud JD, Happle R: Physicochemical properties of "spun glass" hair. Acta Derm Venereol (Stockh) 61:441–445, 1981.
206. Van Neste D et al.: The uncombable hair syndrome: Four non-familial cases of pili trianguli et canaliculi. Arch Dermatol Res 271:223–227, 1981.
207. Van Neste D, Baden HP: Abnormal fibrous protein patterns in the uncombable hair syndrome. Arch Dermatol Res 277:151–152, 1985.
208. Stroud JD, Mehregan AH: "Spun glass" hair: A clinicopathologic study of an unusual hair defect. In Brown AC (ed): *The First Human Hair Symposium.* New York, Medcom, 1974, pp 103–107.
209. Stroud JD: Complementation of the inner root sheath of human hair. In Brown AC, Crounse RG (eds): *Hair, Trace Elements and Human Illness.* New York, Praeger, 1980, pp 163–168.
210. Stone JL, Reizner GT, Muller SA, Elpern DJ: Hair bulb anomaly in a Japanese girl with uncombable hair. J Am Acad Dermatol 17:841–843, 1987.
211. Dupre A, Rochiccidi P, Bonafe JL: "Cheveux incoiffable": Anomalie congenitale des cheveux. Bull Soc Fr Dermatol Syph 80:111–112, 1973.
212. Ferrando J, Fontarnau R, Gratacos MR, Mascaro JM: Pili canaliculi ("cheveux incoiffables" ou "cheveux en fibre de verre"): Dix nouveaux cas avec etude au microscope electronique a balayage. Ann Dermatol Venereol (Paris) 107:243–248, 1980.
213. Garty B, Metzker A, Mimouni M, Varsano L: Uncombable hair: A condition with autosomal dominant inheritance. Arch Dis Child 57:710–712, 1982.
214. Hebert AA, Charrow J, Esterly NB, Fretzin DF. Uncombable hair (pili trianguli et canaliculi): Evidence for dominant inheritance with complete penetrance based on scanning electron microscopy. Am J Med Genet 28:185–193, 1987.
215. de Jong PT et al.: Crystalline cataract and uncombable hair: Ultrastructural and biochemical findings. Ophthalmology 97:1181–1187, 1990.
216. Dupre A, Bonafe JL: Etude en lumier polarisee des dysplasies pilaires: Essai d'actualisation de la nomenclature. Ann Dermatol Venereol (Paris) 105:921–930, 1978.
217. Matis WL et al.: Uncombable-hair syndrome. Pediatr Dermatol 4:215–219, 1987.
218. Shelley WB, Ohman S: Technique for cross sectioning hair specimens. J Invest Dermatol 52:533–536, 1969.
219. Rest EB, Fretzin DF: Quantitative assessment of scanning electron microscope defects in uncombable-hair syndrome. Pediatr Dermatol 7:93–96, 1990.
220. McCullum N, Sperling LC, Vidmar D: The uncombable hair syndrome. Cutis 46:479–483, 1990.
221. Williams ML, Packman MD, Cowan MJ: Alopecia and periorificial dermatitis in biotin-responsive multiple carboxylase deficiency. J Am Acad Dermatol 9:97–103, 1983.
222. Day TI: Straight-hair nevus, ichthyosis hystrix, leukokeratosis of the tongue. Arch Dermatol 96:606, 1967.
223. Gibbs RC, Berger RA: The straight hair nevus. Int J Dermatol 9:47, 1970.
224. Downham TF, Chapel TA, Lupulescu AP: Straight-hair nevus syndrome: A case with scanning electron microscopic findings of hair morphology. Int J Dermatol 15:438–443, 1976.
225. Shewmon DA: Unilateral straight hair in congenital Horner syndrome due to stellate ganglion tumor. Ann Neurol 13:345–346, 1983.
226. Leonidas J-R: Hair alteration in black patients with the acquired immunodeficiency syndrome. Cutis 39:537–538, 1987.
227. Pinkus H: Multiple hairs (Flemming-Giovannini): Report of two cases of pili multigemini and discussion of some other anomalies of the pilary complex. J Invest Dermatol 17:291–301, 1951.
228. Mehregan AH, Thompson WS: Pili multigemini: Report of a case in association with cleidocranial dysostosis. Br J Dermatol 100:315–322, 1979.
229. Goldschmidt H, Hojyo-Tomoka MT, Kligman AM: Trichostasis spinulosa: A common inapparent follicular disorder of the aged. In Brown AC (ed): *The First Human Hair Symposium.* New York, Medcom Press, 1974, pp 50–60.
230. Ladany E: Trichostasis spinulosa. J Invest Dermatol 23:33–41, 1954.
231. Young MC et al.: Trichostasis spinulosa. Int J Dermatol 24:575–580, 1985.
232. Ashley LM, Jacques RS: Four generations of ringed hair. J Hered 41:82–84, 1950.
233. Dawber R: Investigation of a family with pili annulati associated with blue naevi. Trans St John's Hosp Dermatol Soc 58:51–58, 1972.
234. Price VH, Thomas RS, Jones FT: Pili annulati: Optical and electron microscopic studies. Arch Dermatol 98:640–647, 1968.
235. Montgomery RM, Binder AI: Ringed hair. Arch Dermatol Syph 58:177–179, 1948.
236. Musso LA: Pili annulati. Aust J Dermatol 11:67–75, 1970.

237. Gummer CL, Dawber RPR: Pili annulati: Electron histochemical studies on affected hairs. Br J Dermatol 105:303–309, 1981.
238. Price VH, Thomas RS, Jones FT: Pseudopili annulati: An unusual variant of normal hair. Arch Dermatol 102:354–358, 1970.
239. Anderson LL et al.: Chédiak-Higashi syndrome in a black child. Pediatr Dermatol 9:31–36, 1992.
240. Zeleckson AS, Windhurst DB, White JG, Good RA: The Chédiak-Higashi syndrome: Formation of giant melanosomes and the basis for hypopigmentation. J Invest Dermatol 49:575–581, 1967.
241. de Berker D, Dawber RPR: Monilethrix: Clinical and microscopic findings in 21 cases. Br J Dermatol 125(suppl 38):24, 1991.
242. Gilchrist TC: A case of monilethrix with an unusual distribution. J Cutaneous and Genito-Urinary Diseases 16:157–169, 1898.
243. Gummer CL, Dawber RPR, Swift JA: Monilethrix: An electron microscopic and electron histochemical study. Br J Dermatol 105:529–541, 1981.
244. Malt RA: Keratin in monilethrix. J Invest Dermatol 44:364, 1965.
245. de Berker D, Dawber RPR: Variations in the beading configuration in monilethrix. Pediatr Dermatol 9:19–21, 1992.
246. Efron ML, Hoefnagel D: Argininosuccinic acid in monilethrix. Lancet 1:321–322, 1966.
247. Salamon T, Schnyder UW: Uber die Monilethrix. Arch Klin Exp Dermatol 215:105, 1962.
248. Tamayo L: Monilethrix treated with the oral retinoid RO 10-9359 (Tegison). Clin Exp Dermatol 8:393–396, 1983.
249. de Berker D, Dawber RPR: Monilethrix treated with oral retinoids. Clin Exp Dermatol 16:226–228, 1990.
250. Saxena U, Ramesh V, Misra RS: Topical minoxidil in monilethrix (letter). Dermatologica 182:252–253, 1991.
251. Zitelli JA: Pseudomonilethrix: An artifact. Arch Dermatol 122:688–690, 1986.
252. Zitteli JA: Is pseudomonilethrix a genuine hair disorder (letter). Arch Dermatol 123:564, 1987.
253. Crounse RG: Artifactual production of pseudomonilethrix (letter). Arch Dermatol 123:563, 1987.
254. Ferrando J, Fontarnau R, Haussman G: Is pseudomonilethrix an artifact? Int J Dermatol 29:380–381, 1990.
255. Bentley-Phillips B, Bayles MAH: Pseudo-monilethrix. Br J Dermatol 92:113–115, 1975.
256. Bentley-Phillips B: Is pseudomonilethrix a genuine hair disorder? (letter). Arch Dermatol 123:563–564, 1987.
257. Sims RT: "Beau's lines" in hair: Reduction of hair shaft diameter associated with illness. Br J Dermatol 79:43–49, 1967.
258. Pierard G: Structure du Poil en Baionnette. Arch Belg Dermatol 28:359–362, 1972.
259. Stroud JD: Hair shaft defects. Cutis 5:1375–1382, 1969.
260. Pierard GE: Structure et interpretation pathogenique: Dystrophies acquise du cheveu. Ann Dermatol Syph 102:137–143, 1975.
261. Sanderson KV, Hall-Smith P: Tonsure trichotillomania. Br J Dermatol 82:343–350, 1970.
262. Miescher G, Schmuziger P: Trichomalacie und Trichotillomanie. Dermatologica 114:199–203, 1957.
263. Brown VM, Crounse RG, Abele DC: An unusual new hair shaft abnormality: "Bubble hair." J Am Acad Dermatol 15:1113–1117, 1986.
264. Elston DM et al.: Bubble hair. J Cutan Pathol 19:439–444, 1992.
264a. Detwiler SP, Carson JL, Woosley JT, Gambling TM, and Briggaman RA: Bubble hair: Case caused by an overheating hair dryer and reproducibility in normal hair with heat. J Am Acad Dermatol (in press).
265. Birnbaum PS et al.: Intermittent hair follicle dystrophy: Report of a new disorder. J Am Acad Dermatol 15:54–56, 1986.
266. Casanova JM, Puig T, Rubio M: Hypertrichosis of the eyelashes in acquired immunodeficiency syndrome. Arch Dermatol 123:1599–1601, 1987.
267. Kaplan MH, Sadick NS, Talmar M: Acquired trichomegaly of the eyelashes: A cutaneous marker of acquired immunodeficiency syndrome. J Am Acad Dermatol 25:801–804, 1991.
268. Foon KA, Dougher G: Increased growth of eyelashes in a patient given leukocyte A interferon. N Engl J Med 311:1259, 1984.
269. Weaver DT, Bartley GB: Cyclosporine-induced trichomegaly. Am J Ophthalmol 109:293, 1990.
270. Kligman AM: The pathogenesis of tinea capitis due to *Microsporum audouinii* and *Microsporum canis*. J Invest Dermatol 18:231–246, 1952.
271. Kligman AM: Tinea capitis due to *M. audouinii* and *M. canis*. Arch Dermatol 71:313–357, 1955.
272. Rook A, Dawber R: *Diseases of the Hair and Scalp*, 2d ed. Oxford, Blackwell Scientific Publications, 1991, pp 396–457.
273. Lee JY, Hsu ML: Pathogenesis of hair infection and black dots in tinea capitis caused by *Trichophyton violaceum:* A histopathological study. J Cutan Pathol 19:54–58, 1992.
274. Roberts SOB, Mackenzie DWR: Tinea capitis. In Rook A, Wilkinson DS, Ebling FJG (eds): *Textbook of Dermatology*, vol. 1, 3d ed. Oxford, Blackwell Scientific Publications, 1979, pp 793–798.
275. Kalter DC et al.: Genital white piedra: Epidemiology, microbiology and therapy. J Am Acad Dermatol 14:982–993, 1986.
276. Ellner KM et al.: White piedra: Evidence for a synergistic infection. Br J Dermatol 123:355–363, 1990.
277. Smith JD, Murtishaw WA, McBride ME: White piedra (trichosporosis). Arch Dermatol 107:439–442, 1973.
278. McBride ME, Kalter DC, Wolf JE: Evaluation of methods for *in vitro* sensitivity testing of *Trichosporon beigelii* to imidazole compounds. J Invest Dermatol 86:492, 1986.
279. Freeman RG, McBride ME, Knox JM: Pathogenesis of trichomycosis axillaris. Arch Dermatol 100:90–95, 1969.
280. McBride ME, Freeman RG, Knox JM: The bacteriology of trichomycosis axillaris. Br J Dermatol 80:509–513, 1968.
281. Freeman RG, McBride ME, Duncan WC, Wand C: Pathogenesis of trichomycosis axillaris. South Med J 62:78–80, 1969.
282. White SW, Smith J: Trichomycosis pubis. Arch Dermatol 115:444–445, 1979.

283. Orfanos CE, Schloesser E, Mahrle G: Hair destroying growth of *Corynebacterium tenuis* in the so-called trichomycosis axillaris. Arch Dermatol 103:632–639, 1971.
284. Levit F: Trichomycosis axillaris: A different view. J Am Acad Dermatol 18:778–779, 1988.
285. Meinking TL, Taplin D, Kalter DC, Eberle MW: Comparative efficacy of treatments for pediculosis capitis infestations. Arch Dermatol 122:267–271, 1986.
286. Keipert JA: Hair casts: Review and suggestion regarding nomenclature. Arch Dermatol 122:927–930, 1986.
287. Dawber RPR: Hair casts. Br J Dermatol 100:417–421, 1979.
288. Taieb A, Surleve-Bazeille JE, Maleville J: Hair casts: A clinical and morphologic study. Arch Dermatol 121:1009–1013, 1985.
289. Kligman AM: Hair cast: Parakeratotic comedones of the scalp. Arch Dermatol 75:509–511, 1957.
290. Scott MJ, Roenigk HH Jr: Hair casts: Classification, staining characteristics, and differential diagnosis. J Am Acad Dermatol 8:27–32, 1983.
291. Baden HP, Kubilus J, Baden L: A stain for plucked anagen hairs. J Am Acad Dermatol 1:121–122, 1979.
292. Sperling LC: Hair anatomy for the clinician. J Am Acad Dermatol 25:1–17, 1991.
293. Rollins T: Traction folliculitis with hair casts and alopecia. Am J Dis Child 101:639–640, 1961.
294. Zhu W-Y, Xia M-Y, Wu J-H, Do D-A: Hair casts: A clinical and electron microscopic study. Pediatr Dermatol 7:270–274, 1990.
295. Dawber RPR, Calnan CD: Bird's nest hair: Matting of scalp hair due to shampooing. Clin Exp Dermatol 1:155–158, 1976.
296. Wilson CL, Ferguson DJP, Dawber RPR: Matting of scalp hair during shampooing—A new look. Clin Exp Dermatol 15:139–142, 1990.

Chapter 7

HAIR LOSS IN CHILDHOOD

Elise A. Olsen

INTRODUCTION

Infants and children with hair loss present quite different problems for the clinician than do adults with hair loss. The potential etiologies are expanded, the linkage to a genetic disorder is a much greater probability, the treatments may be different, and the prognosis may be modified for a child vs. an adult with hair loss. The list of differential diagnoses for hair loss in childhood contains all those seen in adults as well as an exhaustive list of uncommon or rare disorders that may include hair loss as one of the signs. The astute clinician may find that microscopic examination of the hair in childhood alopecia yields the definitive clue to an elusive diagnosis, but hair evaluation is often belatedly performed.

The purpose of this chapter is to present an effective approach to the diagnosis of children presenting with hair loss. A working schema of differential diagnoses and tools for narrowing the differential will be provided. This may facilitate the consideration of both common and rare causes of alopecia. Topics that are discussed in detail elsewhere in this book will be mentioned only briefly here, and the reader referred to the other chapter(s) for further information. A review of normal hair growth and loss in the fetus and child will help the reader to recognize abnormalities of hair growth in infancy and childhood.

NORMAL HAIR GROWTH IN THE FETUS, INFANT, AND CHILD

Through a cephalocaudal spread of follicular differentiation, anagen hairs cover the entire scalp by 18 to 20 weeks of gestation.[1] These initial hairs are lanugo, unmedullated hairs. At about the fifth month of gestation, over a period of 7 to 10 days, a wavelike transition of anagen to telogen hairs from the frontal to the parietal area begins.[2] The hairs in the occiput do not change their status at this point. The telogen lanugo hairs in the frontoparietal areas are usually then shed in utero at 7 to 8 months[1] and are replaced by a second wave of anagen vellus hair growth (second pelage) in the frontal to parietal areas.[2] There may, however, be a delay in shedding of the underlying vellus telogen hairs which can make the hair density appear very thick at birth: this more commonly occurs in infants with dark complexion.[2]

The lanugo hairs in the first pelage of the occiput remain in anagen until near term, when they abruptly go into telogen.[2] These occipital telogen hairs are generally shed approximately 8 to 12 weeks later[1] and, until they are replaced by the new emergent anagen hair growth, account for the decreased density of hair normally seen in this area in 2- to 3-month-old infants (the physiological "occipital alopecia") (Fig. 7-1).

During fetal life and for at least the first 7 months postnatally, all scalp hairs are synchronous in growth except, as noted earlier, those in the occiput. Toward the end of the first year, although the time is variable, a mosaic pattern of hair growth emerges which exists throughout the rest of life.[1] No new follicles are formed after birth, but rather the existing ones are spread over a greater body surface area. The density of scalp hair at birth is 1135/cm^2, at 3 to 12 months 795/cm^2, and at age 20 to 30 years 615/cm^2.[3]

During childhood, there is a gradual transition of scalp hairs from vellus to intermediate and finally to terminal hairs,[4,5] although Danforth has estimated that 6 to 25 percent of scalp hairs remain as vellus hairs into adult life.[6] There is a correlation of increasing proportion of medullated hairs with increasing age and increasing hair shaft diameter.[7] The cross-sectional area of the hair shaft increases rapidly over the first 3 to 4 years, then less rapidly over the next 6 years.[7] The prepubertal increase in shaft diameter is proportional to the sequential enlargement of the scalp hair follicles.[1] The color of the scalp hair generally darkens as the child ages.[8]

Pubic and axillary hair will not be present until later in childhood, and body hair is often scant or barely obvious in infancy. However, a normal complement and density of eyelashes and eyebrows should be present from birth.

Figure 7-1 Occipital alopecia. (*Courtesy of Dr. Julian Barth.*)

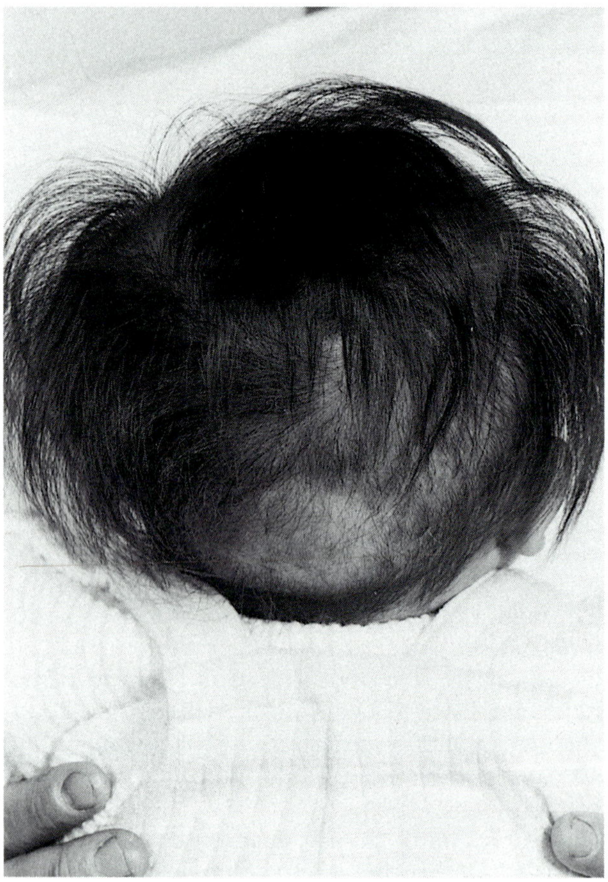

EVALUATION

Newborns may have either a full head of hair or little or no hair: all three presentations are normal variants, but the latter two could be the first sign of abnormal hair growth and development. In normal infants, the scalp pelage will generally thicken and assume normal growth characteristics by the end of the first year of life. Thus, congenital hair growth problems may only become obvious as the hair fails to come in or comes in abnormally during infancy. For this reason, the author has arbitrarily divided the differential diagnoses of childhood hair loss into those presenting (1) in infancy (the first year of life) or (2) after 1 year of age (Table 7-1). Normal-appearing hair covering the scalp at birth does not preclude a hereditary type of hair loss developing later in infancy, childhood, or young adulthood.

The evaluation of a child with hair loss should include a history, physical examination, and microscopic examination of the hair bulb and shaft (Table 7-2).

Table 7-1
ETIOLOGY OF HAIR LOSS IN INFANCY AND CHILDHOOD

- I. Hair loss in infancy
  - A. Diffuse process
    - 1. Near or complete universal atrichia
      - AD, X-linked, or AR inheritance single anomaly
      - Associated with mental retardation
        - Baraitser's syndrome
        - Shokeir's syndrome
        - Moynahan's syndrome
        - Perniola's syndrome
      - Mendes da Costa–van der Valk genodermatosis
      - Atrichia with papular lesions
      - Alopecia areata
    - 2. Hypotrichosis
      - Miscellaneous syndromes
        - Hypomelia-hypotrichosis-facial hemangioma
        - Kallin's syndrome
        - Marie Unna hypotrichosis
        - Jeanselme and Rime hypotrichosis
        - Cartilage-hair hypoplasia
        - Regional choroidal atrophy and alopecia
    - 3. Ectodermal dysplasias (see Table 7-5)
    - 4. Hair shaft defects not clearly part of an ectodermal dysplasia
      - Pili torti
        - Björnstad's dysplasia
        - Salti-Salem syndrome
        - Crandall's syndrome
        - Menkes' kinky hair syndrome
        - Tay's syndrome
        - Conradi-Hünermann chondrodysplasia punctata
        - Bazex's syndrome
        - Citrullinemia
      - Trichorrhexis nodosa
        - Argininosuccinicaciduria
        - Citrullinemia
        - Menkes' kinky hair syndrome
      - Trichoschisis
        - Trichothiodystrophy (see Table 6-2)
      - Trichorrhexis invaginata
        - Netherton's syndrome
    - 5. Nutritional/metabolic disorder
      - Zinc deficiency
      - Essential fatty acid deficiency
      - Biotin deficiency
      - Aminoacidurias
        - Homocystinuria
        - Hartnup disease
      - Protein malnutrition
      - Caloric malnutrition
  - B. Focal hair loss
    - 1. Nonscarring
      - Occipital alopecia of the newborn
      - Sutural alopecia of Hallermann-Streiff
      - Alopecia areata
      - Tinea capitis
    - 2. Scarring
      - Birth trauma
      - Aplasia cutis congenita
        - Single anomaly
        - Associated with other anomalies
          - Associated with limb abnormalities
          - 46XY genotype/gonadal dysgenesis
          - "Lumpy" scalp syndrome
          - 13-trisomy syndrome
          - 4p-syndrome
          - Ectodermal dysplasia (see Table 7-7)
      - Congenital ectodermal dysplasia of the face
      - Epidermolysis bullosa
      - Epidermal or organoid nevus
        - CHILD syndrome
- II. Onset of hair loss after the first year of life
  - A. Diffuse hair loss
    - 1. Telogen loss
    - 2. Anagen loss
      - Loose anagen syndrome
      - Anagen effluvium
    - 3. Alopecia areata
    - 4. Syndromes with late-onset hereditary hair loss
      - Atrichia with papular lesions
      - Toribio and Quinone's syndrome
      - Bentley-Phillips and Grace's syndrome
      - Petersen's syndrome
      - Monilethrix
    - 5. Ectodermal dysplasias
      - Hidrotic ectodermal dysplasia
      - GAPO syndrome
      - Jorgensen's syndrome
      - Beare's pili torti
    - 6. Dyskeratosis congenita
    - 7. Syndromes associated with premature senility
      - Werner's syndrome
      - Progeria (Hutchinson-Gilford syndrome)
      - Progeroid disorders
        - Fitch-form of bird-headed dwarfism
        - Cockayne's syndrome
        - Rothmund-Thomson syndrome
  - B. Focal hair loss
    - 1. Scarring
      - Conradi-Hünermann chondrodysplasia punctata
      - Incontinentia pigmenti
      - Ankyloblepharon–ectodermal defects–cleft lip/palate syndrome
      - Generalized atrophic benign epidermolysis bullosa
      - Hallermann-Streiff syndrome
      - Neoplasia
      - Primary cutaneous disease, e.g., lichen planus, discoid lupus erythematosus
    - 2. Nonscarring
      - Triangular alopecia
      - Alopecia areata
      - Tinea capitis
      - Traction alopecia
      - Trichotillomania
      - Pityriasis amiantacea

Table 7-2
EVALUATION OF THE CHILD WITH HAIR LOSS

History
- Acquired vs. congenital
- Other family members with similar problem?
- Generalized vs. focal hair loss
- Hair shedding vs. failure of hair growth
- Isolated hair loss vs. association with other symptoms and signs, especially
  - Abnormalities of teeth, nails, sweating?
  - Other cutaneous problems?
  - Failure to thrive?
  - GI, neurological symptoms?

Physical examination and microscopic evaluation of hair
- Generalized or focal hair loss
- Scarring vs. nonscarring process
- Abnormal "growth"
  - Hair window
  - Microscopic examination of shaft
- Abnormal shedding?
  - Hair pull
  - Microscopic examination of hair root
    - Anagen vs. telogen

History

The history should begin with establishing when the abnormal hair growth was first noted and the particulars of the distribution of hair loss. Was the child born with a dense growth of scalp hair which fell out in part or in toto, or did the hair fail to grow in normally? Does the scalp hair seem to have a normal growth rate: i.e., does the hair ever achieve any length or need to be cut? The parents should be questioned about personal knowledge of any hair loss they or other family members experienced as children and whether or not that alopecia persisted into adulthood. A simple genetic tree should be completed if there is any positive family history of hair loss, and parents should be questioned about any of the following symptoms or signs in affected members.

Is this hair loss an isolated problem; i.e., is the child otherwise physically and developmentally normal, or is this one of several other abnormal signs or symptoms the parents or referring physician may have noted? In particular, because hair is one of the four cardinal signs of an ectodermal dysplasia, one should ask whether there is any faulty or delayed tooth development or excess caries, and whether sweating is normal. The latter is often difficult to ascertain, even with special testing, but a history of unexplained pyrexia in an infant or heat intolerance in an older child should create suspicion of a sweat gland problem.

One should inquire about any cutaneous rash, including those attributed to a heat rash or diaper rash. Does the baby or child appear to be eating well, and are the stools normal? Is the infant or child making appropriate gains in height and weight, or is there a failure to thrive? Ask about specific age-appropriate developmental milestones and, if any abnormalities come to light, ask specific questions regarding motor skills. Seizures, including febrile seizures, should be noted.

The alopecia which presents in the toddler or child may be accompanied by increased hair shedding that can be either anagen or telogen in nature. Anagen and telogen hair loss are discussed in further detail in Chapters 9 and 10. The list of causes of telogen effluvium in adults is longer than that in children since drugs and androgen fluctuations or aberrations are not usually causes of telogen effluvium in children.

Physical Examination

The child being evaluated for alopecia should have had a recent physical examination or the clinician should be prepared to do a thorough one. One cannot assume the child is otherwise healthy but must confirm this by physical exam. All abnormalities should be noted, since many syndromes can be diagnosed only by noting a critical recognizable mass of physical findings. In various syndromes that include hair loss, commonly associated anomalies include those of other ectodermal-derived organs, including the teeth, ears, eyes, brain, and mammary glands (Table 7-3). Short stature, abnormal bone development, and cleft lip or palate are also frequently associated with hair loss. Particular attention should be paid to the child's facial features and whether a "distinctive facies" of a syndrome is present.

The focus of the dermatologic examination should be primarily on scalp hair growth. For the purposes of a differential diagnosis, the author has subdivided scalp hair loss into a diffuse process vs. a focal one. *Diffuse hair loss,* as defined here, implies fairly even distribution of hair loss over the scalp and does not address whether the hair loss includes other areas of the

Table 7-3
TISSUES OR STRUCTURES DERIVED FROM ECTODERM

Epidermis
Keratinocytes, melanocytes
Hair
Sebaceous glands
Eccrine glands
Apocrine glands
Nails
Teeth
Lens of eye, conjunctiva
Anterior pituitary gland
Myoepithelium or smooth muscles (sweat, lacrimal, salivary, mammary glands)
Constrictors or dilators (pupils)
Epithelial structures (nose and ears)
Mucosa of mouth, nose, rectum
CNS and peripheral nervous system, including retina and Schwann cells excluding mesolia
Chromaffin tissue (adrenals and sympathetic ganglia)
Part of male ureteral epithelium and all extensions of female external genital organs

Source: Modified from Solomon LM and Keuer EJ[33] and Rosselli D and Gulienetti R[32].

body. *Focal hair loss* is patchy in nature and may be either unifocal or multifocal on the scalp. The hair loss can be either scarring or nonscarring. Scarring hair loss implies attrition of follicles with the clinical finding of smooth, poreless skin, whereas in nonscarring loss, the follicular apparatus is preserved and the follicular pores are generally obvious on clinical inspection. In cases where there is a question about scarring vs. nonscarring, a biopsy of an affected area will lead to the definitive answer. Further differentiation can be made between hair growth abnormalities secondary to (1) failure to initiate hair production, (2) abnormality of maintenance of hair production (increased shedding), and (3) intrinsic breakage.

To determine whether hair is currently growing at a normal rate (approximately 1 cm per month) or at all in a given area of the scalp, a *hair window* can be performed. In this procedure, the hairs in a given area of the scalp are clipped or shaved close to the scalp and the hair growth is then observed a few weeks later. To determine whether abnormal shedding is occurring, a simple *hair pull* can be performed. Finding more than 3 to 5 hairs total after pulling gently on 6 to 8 groups of hair in various areas of the scalp is abnormal.

One also should look for any pigment abnormalities in the patient's skin, eyes, or hair; any cutaneous tumors or nodules (especially of a hamartomatous nature); any perifollicular papules or scale; and any eczema. All of these secondary signs may be part of various hereditary syndromes associated with alopecia.

Microscopic Hair Examination

The proximal hairs obtained by the hair pull should be evaluated microscopically to determine if the hairs are anagen or telogen. The differential diagnosis for anagen or telogen loss can then be pursued.

If the structure of the hair shaft is abnormal, this may lead to frank breakage of the hair close to the scalp or abnormal texture of the affected hair. Any hair growth disturbance in a child should be evaluated by light-microscopic examination of the hair shaft followed by polariscopic examination or scanning electron microscopy if deemed necessary. Polariscopic examination is necessary in cases where trichorrhexis nodosa and trichoschisis are seen on light microscopy, making the diagnosis of trichothiodystrophy a possibility. Scanning electron microscopy should be pursued in cases where the light-microscopic examination is lacking: a surprising number of cases will show anomalies of the cuticle or longitudinal depressions of the hair shaft (the latter especially in cases of unruly hair) under scanning electron microscopy that are not apparent with light microscopy. The etiology of brittle hair can be further pursued by chemical analysis of the hair for sulfur content and/or the presence of individual amino acids.

Together these simple tools—history, physical examination, and microscopic examination of the hair shaft—will help narrow the differential diagnosis of childhood alopecia considerably. The various etiologies of childhood alopecia presented in Table 7-1 will now be discussed in further detail.

HAIR LOSS IN THE FIRST YEAR OF LIFE: DIFFUSE LOSS

Near or Complete Universal Atrichia

Various kindreds have been described with universal alopecia, most of which have had autosomal dominant inheritance.[9] Either the hair loss was obvious at birth or the hair present at birth fell out by the first 1 to 2 years of life without regrowth. An X-linked recessive and autosomal recessive inheritance pattern have also been reported.[9]

SYNDROMES ASSOCIATED WITH MENTAL RETARDATION

There have been other inherited conditions of near or complete universal alopecia presenting in infancy. These include the following four syndromes which are associated with mental retardation:

BARAITSER'S SYNDROME

Universal alopecia from age 1 month plus talipes.[10]

SHOKEIR'S SYNDROME

Near-universal alopecia from birth with pyorrhea and adolescent onset of temporal lobe epilepsy; autosomal dominant inheritance[11] (Fig. 7-2).

Figure 7-2 Young woman with Shokeir's syndrome. (*Reprinted with permission from Shokeir.*[11])

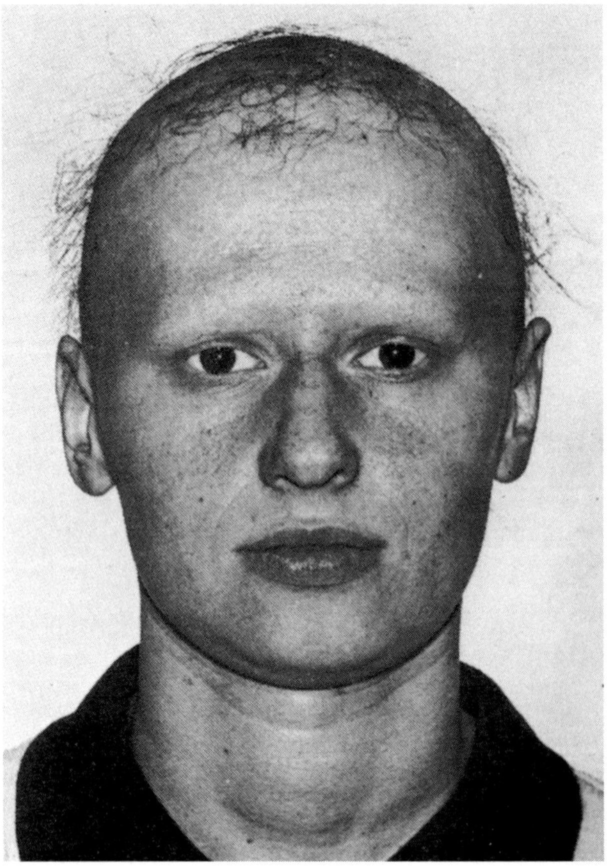

MOYNAHAN'S SYNDROME

Universal alopecia until age 2 to 3; infantile onset of epilepsy; grossly abnormal electroencephalogram.[12]

PERNIOLA'S SYNDROME

Near-universal alopecia with very sparse brittle lanugo hairs; hyperkeratotic follicular papules; seizures plus or minus sensorineural deafness.[13]

MENDES DA COSTA–VAN DER VALK GENODERMATOSIS

The patients described with Mendes da Costa–van der Valk genodermatosis present with complete atrichia either at birth or during the first few months thereafter, accompanied by a reticular brown-red pigmentation on the face and extremities[14] (Fig. 7-3). They develop recurrent intraepidermal blisters without antecedent trauma which disappear by about the third year of life. Some patients have also had associated acrocyanosis, microcephaly with mental retardation, dwarfism, short conic fingers, and nail dystrophy.[15] Inheritance is X-linked recessive. All affected patients have died early due to infections or squamous cell carcinoma.[14]

ATRICHIA WITH PAPULAR LESIONS

Damsté and Prakken described patients born with absent scalp hair, or normal or partial scalp hair which was shed by age 1.[16] Lashes were usu-

Figure 7-3 Mendes da Costa–van der Valk genodermatosis. Note facial poikiloderma and alopecia. (*Reprinted with permission from Carol and Rooij.*[15])

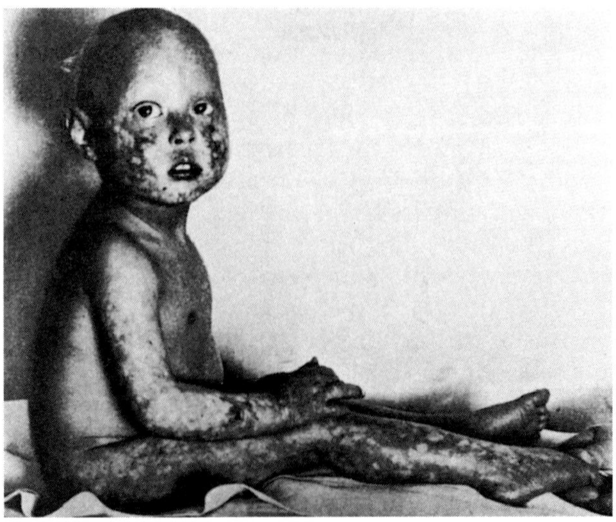

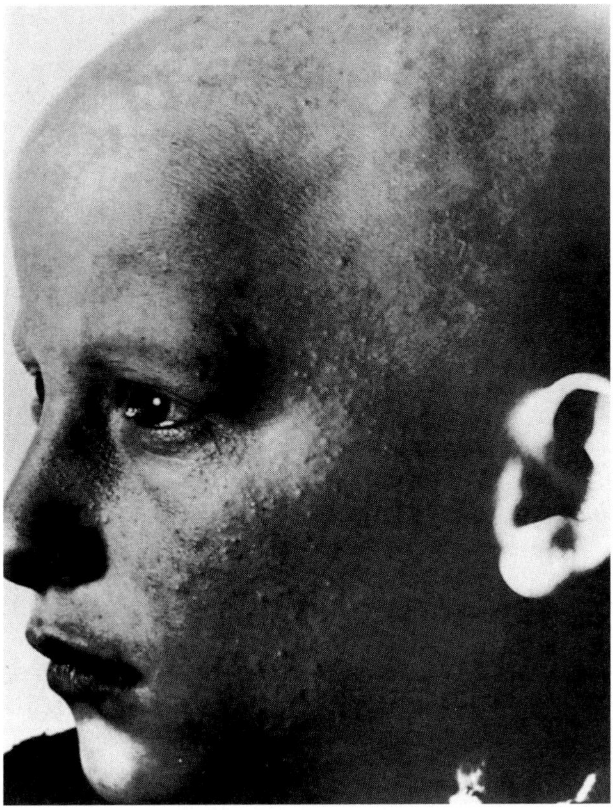

Figure 7-4 Atrichia with papular lesions. (*Reprinted with permission from Loewenthal and Prakken.*[17])

ally sparse but less involved than other hair; brows and body hair were absent. Teeth and nails were normal. These children developed multiple keratin-filled epithelial cysts from age 5 to 18 years (Fig. 7-4). Other similar cases have been reported, some with earlier onset of papular lesions and later onset of alopecia.[17–19] Psychomotor retardation and common variable immunodeficiency have been reported in only a few cases and appear random in nature.[18,19] Inheritance is probably autosomal recessive,[18] but autosomal dominant inheritance has been suggested as well.[19] Other conditions presenting with follicular hyperkeratosis and scalp alopecia are listed in Table 7-4.

ALOPECIA AREATA
Alopecia areata is rare in the first year of life. It has never been documented beyond doubt at birth but has been reported in a 2-month-old.[20] Diffuse hair loss in an infant should thus trigger a search for an explanation other than alopecia areata.

Hypotrichosis

MISCELLANEOUS SYNDROMES
The following syndromes present in infancy with diffuse hypotrichosis but generally not with total alopecia.

HYPOMELIA-HYPOTRICHOSIS-FACIAL HEMANGIOMA SYNDROME (PSEUDOTHALIDOMIDE, SC PHOCOMELIA SYNDROME)
This syndrome is characterized by sparse silver-blond hair, limb reduction abnormalities and flexion positioning of the joints, and distinctive facies, including midfacial hemangioma, hypoplastic nasal alae and septum, anteverted nares, high nasal bridge, and micrognathia. Other common anomalies include talipes; eye abnormalities including blue sclerae and corneal clouding; absent thumbs; and microcephaly.[21] This appears to be an autosomal recessive disorder.

KALLIN'S SYNDROME
These patients present in infancy with a nonscarring blistering eruption primarily on the hands and feet consistent on histology with epidermolysis bullosa, dominant simplex type.[22] The hair has been noted to become sparse and brittle diffusely in infancy or childhood and to either persist or regrow spontaneously (Fig. 7-5). Nails are curved and hypodontia is noted. Inheritance is uncertain.[22]

MARIE UNNA HYPOTRICHOSIS
Marie Unna is credited with the first description of this familial syndrome with sparse or absent scalp hair at birth, very coarse hair regrowth in early childhood and hair loss, especially over the vertex, at puberty (Fig. 7-6).[23–26] Body hair, lashes, and brows are sparse.[23] These patients often have follicular hyperkeratosis with milia-like facial lesions.[23] Hair shaft examination by scanning electron microscopy shows peeling of the cuticle, longitudinal ridging, and pili torti or irregular twisting.[24–26] Inheritance is autosomal dominant.[26]

JEANSELME AND RIME HYPOTRICHOSIS
Jeanselme and Rime presented patients born with abnormal scalp hair (spiral, twisted hair) who then lost all their scalp hair by 8 months of age.[27] These patients also had keratosis pilaris,

Table 7-4
FOLLICULAR HYPERKERATOSIS WITH SCALP ALOPECIA (See Fig. 7-30 on p. 185)

	Inheritance	*Hair*	*Teeth*	*Nails*	*Sweating*	*Skin*	*Other*	*Reference*
Atrichia with papular lesions	? AR, ? AD	Born with normal, partial, or absent scalp coverage but shed by 2 years; lashes ± sparse; usually absent brows; absent body hair	Normal	Normal	± ↓	Keratin-filled epithelial cysts from age 2	Psychomotor retardation; ataxia; hypogonadism; all symptoms may be delayed a few years	16–19,136
Ichthyosis follicularis (Fig. 7-30)	AD or X-linked recessive	Sparse, short, or absent scalp hair; sparse or absent lashes, brows, body hair	Normal	± Dystrophy in childhood (? secondary to infections)	Normal	Extensive follicular hyperkeratosis; chronic skin infections; hyperkeratotic plaques extensor extremities, hands, groin	Marked photophobia ± conjunctivitis, blepharitis, corneal abnormalities; ± hearing loss	137,138
Keratosis follicularis spinulosa decalvans	X-linked recessive or dominant; ? AD	Progressive scarring; loss of scalp hair, lashes, brows, body hair during childhood and adolescence	Normal	Normal	Normal	Generalized follicular hyperkeratosis with marked plugging, especially head and dorsum hands, fingers: these may become atrophic at puberty; palmoplantar hyperkeratosis; may develop telangiectatic pigmentation cheeks and brows late	Atopy; conjunctivitis; photophobia; corneal defects	136,138
Alopecia, keratosis pilaris, cataracts, and psoriasis	AD	Childhood-onset hair loss without preceding inflammation or lesions → scarring alopecia; sparse lashes, brows, body hair	Caries	Small and pitted	Normal	Childhood psoriasis; diffuse follicular hyperkeratosis sparing face and scalp	Keratoconjunctivitis; cataracts	139
Marie Unna hypotrichosis	AD	Scalp hair sparse or absent at birth, coarse hair grows in in early childhood, diffuse loss (especially over vertex) at puberty; hair shaft: cuticle abnormal, longitudinal ridging and irregular twisting; sparse or absent brows, lashes, body hair	Normal	Normal	Normal	Diffuse follicular hyperkeratosis with milia-like facial lesions	± Atopy	23–26
KID syndrome (see Table 7-5)								
Onychotrichodysplasia with neutropenia (Cantú's syndrome) (see Table 7-5)								
Pachyonychia congenita: Jackson-Lawler (see Table 7-5)								
Cystic eyelids, palmoplantar keratosis, hypodontia, and hypotrichosis (Schöpf-Schulz-Passarge syndrome) (see Table 7-5)								

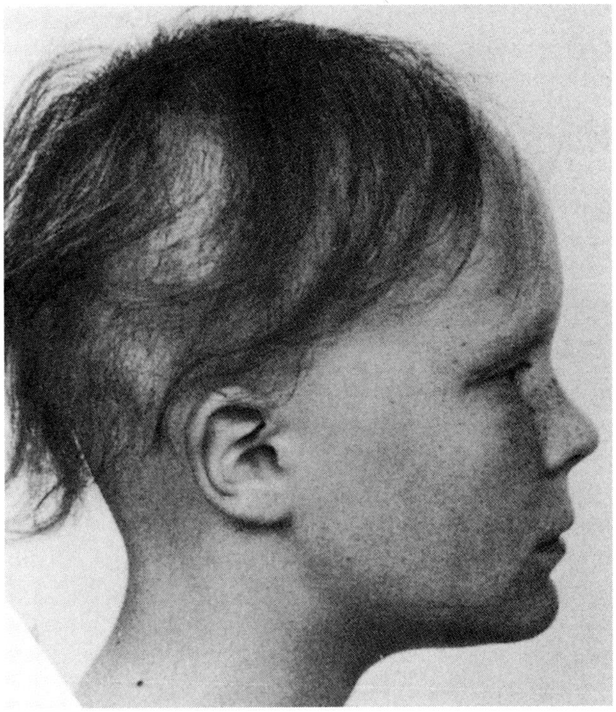

Figure 7-5 Kallin's syndrome. (*Reprinted with permission from Nielson and Sjölund.*[22])

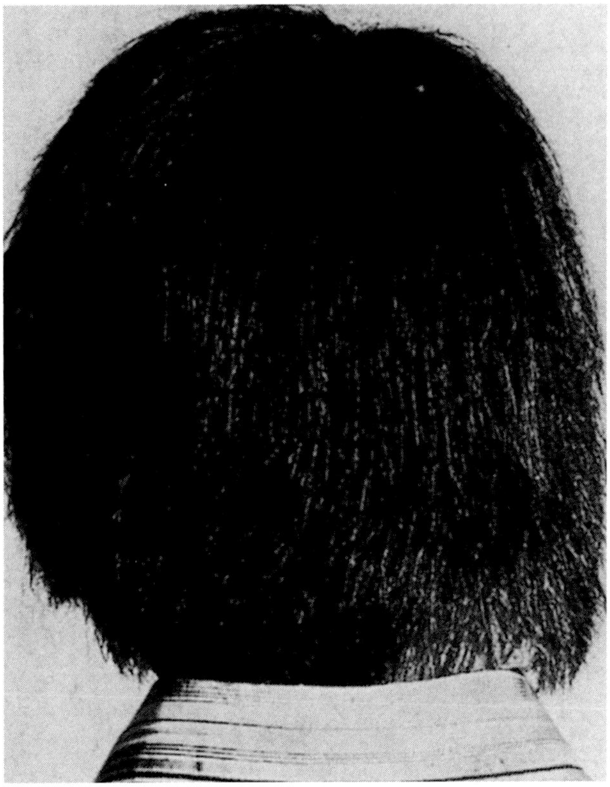

A

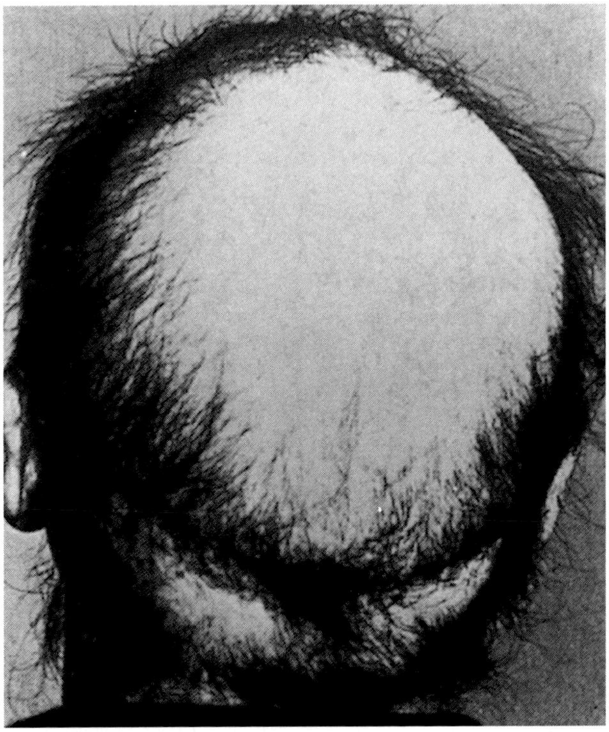

B

Figure 7-6 Patients with Marie Unna hypotrichosis. (*Reprinted with permission from Fortsche Med 97 (44): 2018–2022, 1979.*)

leathery and thickened scalp skin, red blotches on the face, and fragile nails. Inheritance was autosomal dominant.

CARTILAGE-HAIR HYPOPLASIA

This autosomal recessive inherited syndrome includes a distinctive clinical appearance of short-limbed dwarfism and scanty hair. The scalp hair is fine, sparse, and light colored; lashes, brows, and body hair are sparse.[28] Limbs and digits are short secondary to metaphyseal chondrodysplasia. Nails are short but not noted to be dystrophic. These patients have malabsorption abnormalities and an immunodeficiency leading to unusual susceptibility to varicella, vaccinia, and polio viruses.

REGIONAL CHOROIDAL ATROPHY AND ALOPECIA

Two sisters have been reported with fine, sparse, fair scalp hair, sparse lashes and brows, and total choroidal atrophy, the latter developing during childhood. Nails were noted to be "ridged."

Growth and intelligence were normal. Inheritance is uncertain.[29]

Ectodermal Dysplasias

The term *hereditary ectodermal dysplasia* was initially used by Weech in 1929 to describe developmental disorders of ectodermally derived tissue in which hereditary transmission was a constant feature.[30] Freire-Maia has suggested that to qualify as an ectodermal dysplasia, the disorder must demonstrate a *primary* abnormality of two of the following: hair, teeth, nails, or eccrine glands (type A ectodermal dysplasia), or an abnormality of one of these four major anomalies plus one other "ectodermal sign" (type B ectodermal dysplasia).[31] Table 7-3 demonstrates the tissues or structures derived from ectoderm whose aberrations constitute these "ectodermal signs."[32,33] Hereditary ectodermal dysplasias are not exclusively anomalies of ectodermally derived tissues but also include disturbances of tissues or organs originating from other layers.

To facilitate cataloging and understanding these syndromes, particularly the type A ectodermal dysplasias, Freire-Maia has constructed a classification table of ectodermal dysplasia with arbitrary assignment categories, including (1) trichodysplasia (either hypo- or hypertrichosis), (2) odontodysplasia, (3) onychodysplasia, (4) dyshidrosis (either hypo- or hyperhidrosis), and (5) other ectodermal tissues. The existing classification of ectodermal dysplasia is an arbitrary but useful nosologic device to facilitate diagnosis and information retrieval. To that end, this author presents in Table 7-5 those types of ectodermal dysplasias (type A) associated with diminution in hair density or abnormal hair texture. These include patients with either failure to initiate hair growth or fragile, brittle hair. Patients with hypertrichosis who may have a particular ectodermal dysplasia are discussed in Chapter 13.

Clinically, the hair in many of the ectodermal dysplasias is described as coarse, short, and/or brittle or fragile, signaling a potential hair shaft defect, but few reports describe the microscopic charactristics of the abnormal hair. Those ectodermal dysplasias in which the hairs have been studied microscopically have primarily shown, in the cases of brittle hair, either pili torti or trichorrhexis nodosa or, in the cases of unruly hair, longitudinal depressions. Those ectodermal dysplasias with infantile hair loss associated with pili torti are shown in Table 7-6. Affected patients may show more than one hair shaft abnormality.

It is recognized that some syndromes may be merged in the future as more kindred are affected and the full phenotypic expression of a syndrome becomes obvious. It should be noted that hair shaft anomalies inherited as autosomal recessive traits generally constitute but one of many anomalies of a complex syndrome. Expression of these associated defects tends to be relatively constant in autosomal recessive inherited disease as opposed to the variable expression in autosomal dominant inherited disorders.[34] Solomon and Keuer have proposed that hereditary conditions which are progressive in nature (such as Werner's syndrome and Rothmund-Thomson syndrome) are not true ectodermal dysplasias.[33] Cataloguing of these disorders must be continually updated.

Hair Shaft Defects Not Clearly Part of an Ectodermal Dysplasia

The classification system presented here, although inexact, is nonetheless useful in establishing a cause of the hair loss. Many of the hair abnormalities in ectodermal dysplasias are hair shaft abnormalities that are poorly or not at all categorized, and many of the syndromes defined by their hair shaft abnormality have multiple ectodermal defects. A few of the syndromes associated with hair shaft defects that are not clearly type A ectodermal dysplasias, although many could be so classified, are described here. A more detailed discussion of these and other hair shaft anomalies is presented in Chapter 6.

It is worthwhile to point out that many hair shaft abnormalities will require scanning electron microscopy or amino acid analysis (expensive tests) in order to pinpoint the exact diagnosis. Parents of children with hair shaft disorders should be prepared for a thorough evaluation leading to a diagnosis of and prognosis for the child's problem, elucidation of any potentially associated abnormalities now or in the future, and prediction of an inheritance pattern. However, at the present time, treatment options for childhood hair loss are sorely lacking, unless there is a metabolic disturbance that can be aided by dietary manipulation.

HAIR LOSS ASSOCIATED WITH PILI TORTI

Björnstad's dysplasia is an autosomal recessive inherited condition of pili torti and sensorineural deafness[35,36] (Fig. 7-7). Hypogonadotropic hypogonadism and pili torti are found in both *Salti-Salem syndrome*[37] (no other associated findings) and *Crandall's syndrome* (X-linked or autosomal recessive disorder also associated with progressive neurosensory deafness).[38] *Menkes' kinky hair syndrome* is one of the few hereditary syndromes associated with hair loss where a biochemical defect is known (defect in intestinal copper transport).[39] This X-linked recessive disorder is characterized by severe growth and mental retardation, gross neurological disturbances, and dilution of skin and hair pigment.[40] The affected hair shafts show pili torti, trichorrhexis nodosa–like lesions, and monilethrix.

Figure 7-7 Björnstad's dysplasia; 20-year-old patient. (*Reprinted with permission from Voigtländer.*[35])

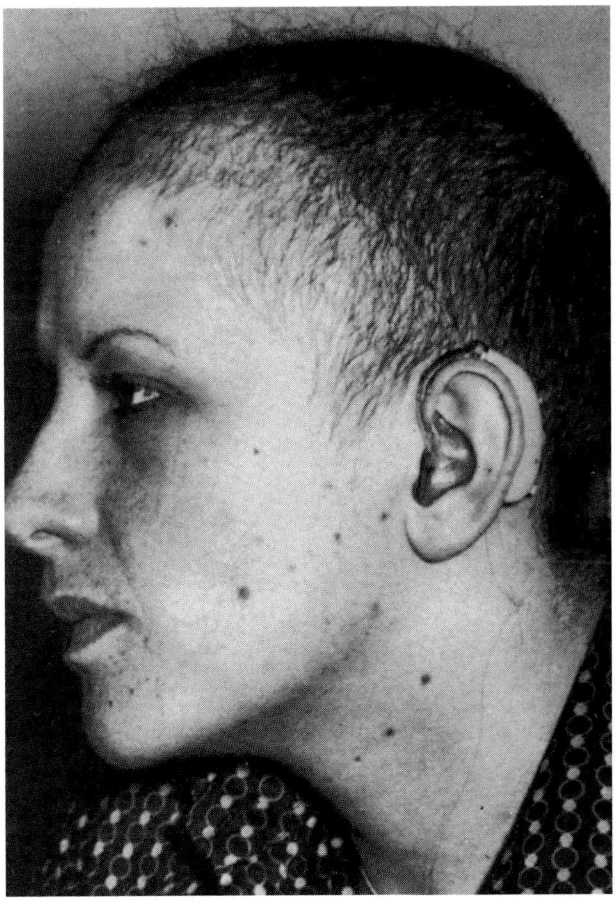

TAY'S SYNDROME

Tay's syndrome is an autosomal recessive disorder characterized by growth retardation, progerialike appearance, mental retardation, short stature, congenital ichthyosiform changes without erythroderma, and palmoplantar keratoderma.[41] Lashes and brows are fine, thin, and fragile. The scalp hair is short and friable from birth, with pili torti and trichoschisis on microscopic examination. Irregularly spaced transverse bands across the shaft with absent birefringence under polarized light indicate a local keratinization defect, and fracture of the shaft occurs through these defective bands. These polariscopic findings are also typical of other autosomal recessive inherited conditions loosely gathered under the nosologic awning of trichothiodystrophy. These include Sabinas syndrome,[42] BIDS,[43,44] IBIDS,[45,46] Pollitt syndrome,[47] PIBIDS,[48] and Marinesco-Sjögren syndrome[49,50] (see Chapter 6, Table 6-2). Trichothiodystrophy is characterized by low hair sulfur content with the variable presence of mental and physical retardation, neurological abnormalities, disturbances of skin and hair keratinization, and other abnormalities.[41,50] Some of these syndromes could be classified as type A ectodermal dysplasias due to the reports of associated brittle nails and/or abnormal teeth.

CONRADI-HÜNERMANN CHONDRODYSPLASIA PUNCTATA

There are two major forms of chondrodysplasia punctata, rhizomelic and nonrhizomelic (also called Conradi-Hünermann syndrome).[51,52] Both types have the characteristic, but not pathognomonic, punctate enchondral ossification termed *chondrodysplasia punctata.*[52] This important radiographic sign disappears by age 3 to 4.

The nonrhizomelic childhood type of chondrodysplasia punctata is characterized by predominantly epiphyseal, frequently asymmetrical calcifications leading to asymmetrical shortening of the extremities.[51] The nonrhizomelic form may be of either autosomal dominant or X-linked dominant inheritance.[51,52] Individuals with nonrhizomelic chondrodysplasia punctata may have a prominent forehead, flat nose, and

(Text continues on p. 166.)

Table 7-5
ECTODERMAL DYSPLASIAS WITH HAIR LOSS PRESENTING IN FIRST YEAR OF LIFE (See Figures 7-31 to 36 on pp. 185–188).

	*I**	*Hair*	*Teeth*	*Nails*
Subgroup 1-2-3-4				
Anhidrotic ectodermal dysplasia (Christ–Siemens–Touraine syndrome) (Fig. 7-31)	Sex-linked recessive; AR type rare	Fine, pale, short, sparse scalp hair ± eyelashes, eyebrows, body hair; may improve after puberty; hair shaft: longitudinal cleft and groove ~ 1 cm distal to bulb	Absent or few; conical canines and incisors; delayed eruption	± Onychodysplasia
Hypohidrotic ectodermal dysplasia: Rapp-Hodgkin with cleft lip/palate syndrome (Fig. 7-32)	AD; can be sporadic	Sparse, light, slow-growing scalp hair like steel wool; scarce body hair, lashes, brows (lateral); hair shaft: ? pili torti, twisting and longitudinal depression on SEM, alternating birefringent bands on polarization	Dental caries; hypodontia; conical teeth; hypoplastic enamel	Narrow and dysplastic
*E*ctrodactyly–*E*ctodermal dysplasia–*C*left lip/palate syndrome (EEC syndrome)	AD	Sparse, light ± wiry scalp hair; scarce body hair, brows, lashes	Partial anodontia; malformed, peg-shaped incisors; early caries; enamel hypoplasia	± Dysplastic, thin, brittle, striated, pitted
Rosselli-Gulienetti syndrome or palate-popliteal pterygia syndrome (? forme fruste EEC syndrome) (Fig. 7-33)	AR	Downy, fair, thin, wooly, short scalp hair; absent eyelashes, eyebrows	Caries; mild dystrophy	Dystrophy with longitudinal and transverse striations; brittle, onychoclasis
*X*eroderma, *T*alipes, *E*namel defect (XTE) syndrome	AD	Sparse, coarse, dry, slow-growing scalp hair; eyelashes absent	Defective enamel	Dystrophic
*A*nkyloblepharon–*E*ctodermal defects–*C*left lip/palate syndrome (AEC syndrome; Hay-Wells syndrome)	AD	Fair, wiry, sparse, or absent scalp and body hair; patchy loss in early childhood during periods of scalp inflammation; sparse lashes and brows; hair shaft: longitudinal depression, trichoclasis, pili torti	Pointed and widely spaced or partial hypodontia; caries; hypoplastic enamel	Onychodystrophy distal > proximal
*K*eratitis–*I*chthyosiform erythroderma–*D*eafness syndrome (KID syndrome) (Fig. 7-34)	AR? AD?	Diffuse fine, sparse, or absent scalp hair which may improve with time; may have patchy scarring alopecia; sparse lashes, brows; hair shaft: trichorrhexis nodosa	± Caries; brittle, malformed, delayed teeth	Leukonychia ± thickened, hypoplastic

Sweating	*MR*[†]	*Distinctive Facies*	*CLP*[‡]	*SS*[§]	*Other*	*Reference*
None or ↓	Un-common	Square forehead; frontal bossing; supraorbital ridge; sunken/flat nasal bridge; hypertelorism; abnormal auricles; short upper lip with thick everted lower lip; radiating wrinkles corners of mouth	No	No	↑ Periorbital pigmentation; atopic dermatitis; absent or supernumerary nipples; ± breast tissue; photophobia; hypoplasia lacrimal duct/gland; hypoplastic mucous glands respiratory tract → recurrent rhinitis and infections	140–143
↓	No	High forehead; narrow nose; hypoplastic maxilla; small mouth; prominent and abnormal auricles	Yes	±	± Ptosis; atretic ear canals; dysplastic eustachian orifices; hypospadias, ± aplasia lacrimal puncta; corneal opacities; photophobia; ± syndactyly	144–148
± ↓	±	Broad nose; small, low-set, and abnormal auricles; pointed chin; malar hypoplasia	Yes	±	± Split hand (ectrodactyly)/split foot deformity; lacrimal gland stenosis; renal abnormalities; photophobia; dacryocystitis → corneal scarring; scaly, hypopigmented skin; ± hypoplastic nipples; syndactyly	50,149–153
± ↓	NED	Epicanthal folds; ± hypoplastic auricles	Yes	No	Syndactyly and ectrodactyly; popliteal and perineal pterygium; renal abnormalities; supernumerary nipples; ± absent thumbs	32,83
↓	No	NED	Yes	No	Blister formation in areas exposed to sunlight; talipes; photophobia; hypoplasia lacrimal puncta; mild oligophrenia	154
± ↓	No	Broad nasal bridge and hypoplastic maxilla; deep-set and dysplastic ears	Yes	No	Papulofollicular erythroderma; ± lacrimal duct stenosis; supernumerary nipples; deformities auricle; episodic scalp dermatitis; ankyloblepharon (congenital eyelid fusion)	132,155,156
± ↓	No	Plaques on face; furrowing about mouth and chin	No	No	Diffuse follicular hyperkeratoses; leathery erythroderma (not scaly) from birth; symmetrical plaques over cheeks, chin, nose, and rim ears in early infancy; verrucous hyperkeratosis over knees; leatherlike changes palms and fingers and keratoderma soles; neurosensory deafness; keratitis	136,157–160

Table 7-5 *Continued*

	*I**	*Hair*	*Teeth*	*Nails*
Pachyonychia congenita: Jadassohn-Lewandowsky type	AD; ? few cases AR	Generalized hypotrichosis; dry hair	Natal teeth; ± caries; malformation	Yellow-brown discoloration; thickened nails (distal ⅔) with pinched margins and upward tilt of distal tips (all cases); paronychial infections
Pachyonychia congenita: Jackson-Lawler type	AD	As above	As above	As above
Focal dermal hypoplasia (Goltz-Gorlin's syndrome) (Fig. 7-35)	X-linked dominant; 10–15% cases are males	± Sparse, brittle scalp hair; small focal areas loss due to aplasia cutis	Dystrophic, spooned, grooved or absent	Anodontia; dysplasia; enamel defects with caries
Zanier-Roubicek syndrome	AD	Scalp hypotrichosis (more striking in men) but normal lashes, brows	Hypodontia; enamel anomalies	Brittle nails
Jorgensen's syndrome	AD	Scalp hypotrichosis; bald by end adolescence; sparse lashes, brows	Caries; hypodontia	Short and thick with longitudinal ridges
Ectodermal dysplasia of Carey	NED	Thin, hypopigmented sparse hair; aplasia cutis congenita scalp	Hypodontia, microdontia, abnormal formation	Dystrophic nails
Ectodermal dysplasia of Tuffli	? AD	Aplasia cutis congenita scalp	Delayed dental eruption and irregular size teeth	± Dysplastic nails
ANOTHER syndrome (*A*lopecia, *N*ail dystrophy, *O*phthalmic complications, *T*hyroid dysfunction, *H*ypohidrosis, *E*phelides and enteropathy, *R*espiratory tract infections)	? AR	Hypotrichosis; ± thin and brittle scalp hair; sparse brows (distal); focal alopecia parietal area; lashes preserved	± Hypodontia; conical teeth	Ridged, shriveled appearance; dystrophic, fragile, brittle

Sweating	*MR*[†]	*Distinctive Facies*	*CLP*[‡]	*SS*[§]	*Other*	*Reference*
↑	No	No	No	No	Palmar-plantar hyperkeratosis; follicular keratosis, esp. knees and elbows; asteatosis; cataracts; hoarseness; painful bullae or ulceration palms and soles; oral leukokeratosis; verrucous lesions extremities; corneal dyskeratosis	161–167
↑	No	No	No	No	As above but no mucous membrane involvement; epidermal cysts	166
± ↓ or ↑	±	Pointed chin; triangular or assymetrical face; protruding ears; notching alae nasi	Uncommon	Yes	Reticular, vermiform or cribiform, frequently linear atrophy skin; hyperkeratotic papules; hyper/hypopigmentation; papillomas, often on mucous membranes; asymmetry of trunk and limbs; syndactyly; longitudinal striations of long bones ± ectrodactyly (lobster-claw hand); scoliosis; anomalies bones, hands/feet; strabismus; nystagmus; colobomas iris, choroid, retina, optic nerve; microphthalmia; lacrimal duct abnormality	95,168–171
↓ Except palms and soles	No	NED	No	No	Decreased tearing; mammary hypoplasia	33,83
↓	↓	Thin nose; long philtrum; thin upper lip	No	No	Unusual dermatoglyphics; hyperextensible joints, posterior fusion labia majora	33,83,106
↓	NL	U-shaped mouth with maxillary hypoplasia, flat nasal bridge	Yes	No	Conductive hearing loss; absent tear ducts; 2-3 syndactyly	83
↓	NL	No	No	No	Nipple and breast hypoplasia; ± adrenal cyst	93
↓	No	No	No	±	Clinodactyly; syndactyly; bilateral epiphora; infantile hypothyroidism; respiratory tract infections; GI problems; dry skin with ephelides; ± absent breast tissue; ± pulmonary stenosis	94,172–174

Table 7-5 ***Continued***

	*I**	*Hair*	*Teeth*	*Nails*
Subgroup 1-2-3				
Coffin-Siris syndrome	? AD ? AR	Sparse scalp hair—may improve with age; bushy brows and lashes; hypertrichosis limbs, back, face	Delayed eruption; microdontia	Absent or hypoplastic, esp. 5th
Hidrotic ectodermal dysplasia (Clouston's syndrome)	AD	Sparse, lusterless, fine, pale, and brittle or absent scalp hair, eyelashes, eyebrows, and body hair; may thicken and darken in adult life	Hypodontia; anodontia; widely spaced; natal teeth; caries	Dystrophic thick and discolored or thin and brittle; unusually small or absent
Odontotrichomelic syndrome (tetramelic syndrome, Freire-Maia's syndrome)	AR ?	Severe hypotrichosis scalp and body	Hypodontia; microdontia; coniform teeth; persistence deciduous teeth	? Hypoplastic
Tricho-dento-osseous syndrome II	AD	Curly, kinky scalp hair and eyelashes that may become straight during childhood	Small and wide-spaced; taurodontia; enamel hypoplasia; discoloration; early caries ± hypodontia; edentulous by 2d–3d decade	Brittle nails; superficial splitting ± white transverse lines
Cranioectodermal syndrome (Sensenbrenner–Dorst–Owen syndrome)	AR	Thin, short, and very fine	Small, gray, and widely spaced; hypodontia; enamel hypoplasia	Broad and short
Incontinentia pigmenti (Bloch-Sulzberger syndrome)	X-linked dominant	Diffuse hypotrichosis; linear and patchy alopecia of scalp (usually of vertex ± scarring) and body	Delayed dentition; pegged teeth; partial anodontia	Uncommon—dystrophic
Fried's tooth and nail syndrome	AR	Sparse scalp hair with some twisting; scanty brows	Hypodontia with peg-shaped "milk" teeth and agenesis permanent teeth	Hypoplastic; small, thin, and concave toenails
Generalized atrophic benign EB	? AR	Thin and lusterless from infancy; atrophic scalp hair loss after adolescence associated with absence pubic, axillary hair; sparse brows, lashes, beard	Caries; enamel abnormality; edentulous by adulthood	Thickened, dystrophic, or absent

Sweating	*MR*[†]	*Distinctive Facies*	*CLP*[‡]	*SS*[§]	*Other*	*Reference*
Normal	+	Thick lips; broad nose; low nasal bridge; anteverted nostrils; microcephaly; coarse facial features	No	Yes	Lax joints; clinodactyly; small or absent patella; absent terminal phalanges, 5th digits and aplasia or hypoplasia mid ± distal phalanges other digits; chronic eczema; ± congenital heart defects; ± perforated ulcers	83,175–178
±	No	No	No	No	Keratoderma; ± patchy hyperpigmentation; strabismus; cataracts; myopia; tufting terminal phalanges; clubbing	103–105,143, 177,179, 180
Normal	No	Protruding lips; enlarged nose; deformed auricles	±	Yes	Hypoplastic or absent areola; tetramelic aplasias; EEG and EKG abnormalities; metabolic abnormalities	83,177
Normal	No	Dolichocephaly; frontal bossing; square jaw	No	No	Sclerosis cortical bone; ± clinodactyly	181–183
Normal	No	Frontal bossing; dolichocephalic; hypotelorism; epicanthal folds, antimongoloid fissures; full cheeks and eversion lower lip; abnormal auricles, broad nasal bridge with anteverted nares	No	Yes	Hypotonia; rhizomelia; disproportionately short fingers and toes; syndactyly, clinodactyly; coronary artery disease; osteoporosis; high arched palate	83,177,184
Normal	±	No	±	±	Successive skin stages: blisters birth or early infancy → clears; successive linear verrucous lesions infancy → clears; whorled hyperpigmentation infancy which fades with age; subungual keratotic tumors adults; ocular abnormalities including strabismus, retinal changes; CNS problems including seizures, motor abnormalities	83,131,185, 186
Normal	No	Prominent lips and chin	Cleft lip one patient	No	Branchial cyst neck	83,177
No	No	No	No	No	Traumatic blisters from birth that heal with atrophy, no milia or syndactyly; junctional EB, non-Herlitz type; ± palmar-plantar hyperkeratosis; ophthalmic abnormalities; dermal nevocytic nevi (shagreen-like plaques)	133

Table 7-5 *Continued*

	*I**	*Hair*	*Teeth*	*Nails*
Hypodontia and nail dysgenesis; tooth and nail syndrome; Witkop's syndrome	AD	Fine and brittle scalp hair—may improve with age; sparse to absent brows	Hypodontia, wide-spaced, cone-shaped; occasional agenesis permanent teeth and supernumerary teeth	Small and spoon-shaped; slow growth in children; longitudinal ridging; toenails most severely affected
Trichorhinophalangeal syndrome, type I (Giedion's syndrome) (Fig. 7-36)	AD or AR	Slow-growing, sparse, fine, hypopigmented, brittle scalp hair; temporal alopecia; ± sparse lashes and lateral eyebrows	± Supernumerary incisors	± Thin, brittle
Trichorhinophalangeal syndrome with exostoses, type II (Giedion-Langer syndrome)	Sporadic	Sparse scalp hair; wide, bushy eyebrows thinned laterally	± Fused lower canines and lateral incisors	Thin
Ellis–van Creveld syndrome or chondroectodermal dysplasia	AR	Thin, brittle, fine, fair, sparse hair (variable degree); scanty brows; may be unremarkable	Oligodontia; neonatal teeth; ± hypoplastic enamel; cone-shaped canines	Small, hypoplastic, or absent; tendency to convexity
Cystic eyelids, palmoplantar keratosis, hypodontia, and hypotrichosis (Schöpf–Schulz–Passarge syndrome)	AR	Marked hypotrichosis, especially scalp; eyebrows and lashes coarse, sparse	Hypodontia; central incisors	Onychodystrophy; longitudinal ridging; splitting; onycholysis
Sălamon's syndrome	AR	Dry, inelastic, wirelike, lusterless, sparse; hair shaft: pili torti, trichorrhexis nodosa	Hypodontia; microdontia	Very dystrophic, brittle; ungues plicatae; toenails most affected
Tricho-oculo-dermo-vertebral syndrome	AR	Dry and rough; hypotrichosis scalp, body, brows (lateral) and lashes	Caries; spaced incisors; gingivitis	Thin and brittle fingernails; wide, short, and dystrophic toenails with paronychia
Oculo-dento-digital syndrome II	NED	Hypotrichosis	Enamel hypoplasia; microdontia; hypodontia; malocclusion; conical incisors	Dysplastic

Sweating	*MR*†	*Distinctive Facies*	*CLP*‡	*SS*§	*Other*	*Reference*
No	No	Premature wrinkles face; everted lips; ± frontal bossing	No	No	NED	83,177,187, 188
Normal	No	Pear-shaped nose and long philtrum with retropositioned alae nasi; thin upper lip and tubercle of skin below lower lip; ± receding chin and midfacial hypoplasia	No	Yes	High-arched palate; brachiophalangeal dystosis with swelling PIP joints secondary to Giedion type 12 cone-shaped epiphyses mid (2d–5th) phalanges	189–193
Normal	Mild to mod-erate	Prominent forehead; bulbous nose with broad nasal bridge; long upper lip with fat accumulation; long philtrum, mandibular retrognathia; large protruding ears	No	Yes	Multiple cartilaginous exostoses (can be delayed until 5th year); hyperextensible joints; redundant skin; winged scapulae; microcephaly	190,194
Normal	±	± Broad nose; prominent frontal bossing	No	Yes	Chondrodysplasia → acromelic dwarfism; ± gingivolabial fusion; bilateral postaxial polydactyly; brachymetacarpy; congenital heart abnormalities	177,195,196
Normal	No	No	No	No	Follicular hyperkeratosis; palmoplantar hyperkeratosis; eyelid apocrine hidrocystomas (develop late)	197
NED	NED	Piriform nose	NED	NED	Chronic blepharoconjunctivitis; punctate keratosis; ocular abnormalities	177
Normal	No	Narrow palpebral fissures; hypoplasia nasal alae; micrognathia; wide nasal bridge	No	Yes	Hyperkeratosis palms and soles; ichthyosiform pigmented macules; nuclear cataracts; entropion; trichiasis; minor skeletal abnormalities (examples: genu valga, enlarged interphalangeal joints); severe kyphoscoliosis; dry skin	83,177,198
NED	No	Hypotelorism; small alae nasi; microstomia with furrowing and overlapping upper lip; micrognathia	No	No	Polydactyly; camptodactyly; syndactyly; hypophalangy; nystagmus; atrophy iris	177,199

Table 7-5 *Continued*

	*I**	*Hair*	*Teeth*	*Nails*
Arthrogryposis and ectodermal dysplasia	NED	Atrichia at birth → hypotrichosis scalp, body, lashes, brows; stretched pili torti on microscopic examination of hair shafts	Enamel hypoplasia	Absent at birth; later tendency to longitudinal breaks
Tricho-odonto-onychial dysplasia of Tsakalakos et al.	AD	Sparse scalp and body hair	Hypodontia; ± conical, widely spaced teeth	Leukonychia punctata; longitudinal ridges; dystrophic nails
GAPO (*G*rowth retardation–*A*lopecia–*P*seudoanodontia–*O*ptic atrophy syndrome)	AR	Generalized loss; progressive since birth (can be delayed to age 2) with atrichia early childhood	Hypodontia, pseudoanodontia (failure to erupt)	Normal or hyperconvexity
Ectodermal dysplasia with syndactyly	AR	Hypotrichosis; brittle scalp hair; sparse brows and lashes; microscopic exam of hair shaft: pili torti	Severe crown hypoplasia; delayed and atypical eruption permanent teeth	Yellow and thickened
Mesomelic dwarfism–skeletal abnormalities–ectodermal dysplasia	NED	Hypotrichosis	Dysmorphic, malpositioned	Hypoplastic toenails
Trichoodontoonychial dysplasia with pili torti	? AD, ? X-linked dominant	Sparse blond scalp hair; hair shaft: pili torti	Hypodontia; widely spaced teeth; peg-shaped incisors; abnormal eruption	Dysplastic; flat with linear grooves
*T*richo*o*dont*o*onycho-*d*ermal syndrome (TOOD syndrome)	NED	Hypotrichosis parieto-occipital region; aplasia cutis congenita scalp; sparse lashes and brows, especially outer ⅔	Enamel hypoplasia; hypodontia; altered size and form; delayed eruption; supernumerary teeth	Severe dystrophy; anychia some fingers
Trichoodontoonychial dysplasia (Pinheiro, Freire-Maia, Roth)	? AR	Generalized hypotrichosis, with remaining scalp hair brittle	Enamel hypoplasia → anodontia	Dystrophic nails, brittle, pigmented
Ectodermal dysplasia with tetramelic disturbances	NED	Scalp hypotrichosis; sparse lashes, brows	Hypodontia; peg-shaped teeth; widely spaced	Platonychia; mildly dysplastic toenails
Odontoonychodys-plasia with alopecia	? AR	Near or total universal alopecia	Enamel hypoplasia; microdontia; abnormal shape; wide spacing; hypodontia	Mild dystrophy; brittle or thick and spoon-shaped

Sweating	*MR*†	*Distinctive Facies*	*CLP*‡	*SS*§	*Other*	*Reference*
Normal	NL to mild	Mongoloid slant	No	Yes	Syndactyly; clinodactyly; talipes equinovarus, arthrogryposis all joints; tendency to excessive bruising and scarring after minor trauma	83,177,200
Normal	No	Focal linear dermal hypoplasia nose and scarlike lesions around mouth	No	No	Dyspigmentation; follicular papules; absent or abnormal breast or nipple development; nerve deafness	201
Normal	No	"Geriatric" appearance; prominent supraorbital ridges; ptosis; lagophthalmos; depressed nasal bridge; protruding lips and micrognathia	No	Yes	Full anterior fontanel at birth; ± abnormal EEG, cerebral angiography; ± hypoplasia breasts; delayed bone age childhood; ± hypogonadism; ± optic atrophy; glaucoma; keratoconus; redundant hyperelastic skin	107,108
Normal	No	No	NED	NED	Dry, hyperkeratotic skin; syndactyly fingers and toes; lordosis; high arched palate; transverse crease of palms	83
Normal	± ↓	Depressed nasal root; micrognathia; hypertelorism; antimongoloid palpebral slant; epicanthal folds; long philtrum; thin lips	No	Yes	Esotropia; short forearms and hands; agenesis proximal radius; broad thumbs and proximal placement; high arched palate; brachycephaly; brachymesophalanges and camptodactyly 5th fingers	83
Normal	No	Mild maxillary hypoplasia; thin lips	No	No	NED	83
Normal	No	Long philtrum; asymmetry face; microstomia; micrognathia; abnormal auricles; hyperpigmentation periorbital area	No	NED	Xerosis and poikiloderma-like spots; abnormal or absent nipple/areola; mild palmar keratosis; abnormal dermatoglyphics; abnormal or absent phalanges; leukoma; hypertrophy frenum linguae; clinodactyly; syndactyly; marked manus cavus	83,177
Normal	No	No	No	Yes	Frontoparietal bone deficiency; ephelides; nevi; xeroderma; mild palmoplantar keratoderma; supernumerary nipples; abnormal dermatoglyphics	83,202
Normal	± Mild	Malformed auricles; protruding lips; wide nasal root; microcephaly	No	Yes	Hypoplastic areola and nipples; esotropia; abnormal clavicle; absence of or duplication of rays; constant tearing, infections conjunctiva	83
Normal	No	No	No	No	Irregular areola; ocular abnormalities; mild palmoplantar keratosis; ± syndactyly	83,203

Table 7-5 *Continued*

	*I**	*Hair*	*Teeth*	*Nails*
Oculotrichodysplasia	AR	Hypotrichosis with sparse scalp, axillary, pubic hair, eyebrows (lateral ⅔) and eyelashes	Hypodontia and caries	Fragile and brittle
Subgroup 1-2-4				
Congenital insensitivity to pain with anhidrosis	AR	± Hypotrichosis areas of scalp	Enamel aplasia	Usually normal; one case dystrophy
Regional ectodermal dysplasia with total bilateral cleft	NED	Near total scalp alopecia; lashes and brows short, thin, fair	Anodontia	Normal
Ectodermal dysplasia with palatal paralysis	NED	Absence frontal hair, brows, lashes	Stunted and peg-shaped; enamel hypoplasia	NED
Subgroup 1-3-4				
Fischer's syndrome	AD	Sparse scalp hair, brows, lashes	Normal	Onychogryposis; onycholysis
Alopecia-onychodysplasia-hypohidrosis-hyperkeratosis-deafness	NED	Severe hypotrichosis scalp and body, brows, lashes	Normal	Normal fingernails; thick, dystrophic toenails
Hayden's syndrome	NED	Almost universal alopecia	Normal	Severe pachyonychia
Alopecia-onychodysplasia-hypohidrosis syndrome	NED	Universal alopecia	Normal	Severely dystrophic
Ectodermal dysplasia with severe mental retardation	NED	Almost universal alopecia	Normal	Almost absent
Dermotrichic syndrome	X-linked recessive	Generalized atrichia from birth	Normal	Dystrophic and hyperconvex fingernails
Subgroup 1-2				
*O*ro*f*acial *d*igital (OFD) syndrome	X-linked dominant; lethal in males	Fine, sparse, and dry	Lower lateral teeth fail to develop; malposition maxillary canines; dental caries	Normal

Sweating	*MR*†	*Distinctive Facies*	*CLP*‡	*SS*§	*Other*	*Reference*
Normal	No	No	No	No	Retinitis pigmentosa; dry skin	204
↓	Yes	No	No	No	Irregular lacrimation; universal sensory loss → sores and fractures; Charcot joints	83,205
↓ On head	No	Bilateral cleft lip; aplasia premaxilla	Yes	Normal	Ectropion; hypoplastic tarsal plates; dermoid cysts scalp; cleft palate	83
↓ On face	No	Frontal bossing; depressed nasal bridge	NED	Normal	Conductive hearing loss; otitis; high arched palate and ↓ sensation, paralysis palate; distorted speech	83
↑ Palms, soles	±	Edema eyelids	NED	NED	Syringomelia; palmoplantar keratosis; clubbing	83
↓	No	Mongoloid slant; prominent nose and bridge of nose; abnormal auricles	No	Yes	Sensorineural deafness; hyperkeratosis palms, soles, knees, elbows; photophobia; hyperopia; estropia	206
↓	NL	Saddle nose; narrow palpebral fissures	No	No	Follicular and plaquelike hyperkeratosis; palmoplantar hyperkeratosis; severe scalp infections; otitis media → deafness; conjunctivitis	83
↓	Yes	Large and prominent ears; protruding lips; saddle nose	No	Yes	Seizures; eczema with thick scaly patches; photophobia; nystagmus; hypospadias	83,206
↓	Yes	Abnormal ears	No	No	Fine, thin, shiny skin; bilateral cataracts; absence nipple/areola	83
↓	Yes	Prominent forehead; large ears; small nose with low nasal bridge; blepharophimosis	No	Yes	Congenital ichthyosis; seizures; psychomotor retardation; arched palate	83
Normal	±	Broad nasal root; dystopia canthorum; micrognathia; alae hypoplasia; hypertelorism; ± facial asymmetry; abnormal auricles	Yes¶	±	Aberrant hyperplastic oral frenula; lobed tongue; tongue nodules; milia at birth; brachydactyly; syndactyly; clinodactyly, polydactyly; ± aplasia alae cartilage; renal abnormalities, basilar skull abnormality	207,208

Table 7-5 *Continued*

	*I**	*Hair*	*Teeth*	*Nails*
Killian's syndrome	NED	Sparse, brittle, and slow-growing scalp hair; exaggerated loss frontal and parietal areas; sparse lashes, brows; hair shaft: partial loss cuticular structure	Delayed and abnormal development	Normal
Oculo-dento-digital syndrome I	AD or AR	Brittle, sparse, dry, slow-growing	General hypoplasia enamel; occasional hypodontia; microdontia; premature loss	Normal
Hallermann-Streiff syndrome	AD or AR	Sparse, light scalp hair; focal areas of alopecia; frontal baldness; absent or sparse brows and lashes; ± sparse body hair; marked cuticle abnormality	Hypodontia; partial anodontia; persistent deciduous teeth; malformation; caries; anomalous implantation	Normal
Mikaelian's syndrome (ectodermal dysplasia with neurosensory deafness)	AR	Sparse, coarse, and brittle scalp hair; may have hair growth late childhood	Carious	Normal
Pili torti and enamel hypoplasia (pili torti hereditaria, Ronchese type)	AR	Thin, dry, fair, brittle; hair shaft: pili torti and monilithrix on microscopic exam; brows sparse, especially lateral ⅔	Enamel hypoplasia; widely spaced teeth; hypodontia; adontia; delayed dentition; irregular in shape	Normal
Trichodental dysplasia	AD	Straight, fine, lusterless hair; cuticle defect; sparse brows, lashes	Hypodontia; peg-shaped teeth; retained deciduous teeth	Normal
Acrorenal-ectodermal dysplasia-lipoatrophic diabetes syndrome	AR	Fine, slow-growing scalp hair; sparse body hair	Enamel dysplasia; anodontia permanent teeth	Normal
Oculoosteocutaneous syndrome (Tuomaala-Haapanen syndrome)	? AR	Scanty, thin, fair scalp hair; thin eyelashes; no axillary, pubic hair	Anodontia	Normal
Walbaum–Dehaene–Schlemmer syndrome	AR	Thin, fair, sparse scalp hair 1st year → alopecia; hypotrichosis body	Hypodontia; supernumerary teeth; microdontia; malposition; delayed eruption	Normal

Sweating	*MR*[†]	*Distinctive Facies*	*CLP*[‡]	*SS*[§]	*Other*	*Reference*
Normal	±	Microencephaly; prominent forehead; hypertelorism; ptosis; exophoria, short nose with anteverted nostrils; long philtrum; thin upper lip with cupid's bow mouth; low-set ears; micrognathia	Bifid uvula	Yes	Short neck; muscle hypotonia and hypermobile joints; ± sensorineural deafness; ± hypopigmented patches; high arched palate	209
Normal	± Mild	Microcephaly; microphthalmia; thin nose; hypoplastic alae and narrow nostrils; orbital hypotelorism	Yes	No	Microcornea; syndactyly and camptodactyly 4th and 5th fingers; aplasia or hypoplasia midphalanges 5th fingers or toes; conductive hearing loss	83,210
Normal	±	Dyscephaly with bird face; brachycephaly; beaked nose; hypoplasia mandible; microstomia	No	Yes	Cataracts; microphthalmia; localized cutaneous atrophy, esp. nose and scalp skin; arched palate; ± cardiac defects	79–83
Normal	Yes	Coarse features	No	No	Hyperkeratotic skin; bilateral sensorineural loss; arachnodactyly	83,211
Normal	No	No	No	No	Generalized keratosis pilaris	83
NED	No	Normal	No	No	NED	83,212
Normal	No	Prominent forehead and bridge of nose; short nasal septum with flat nasal tip; mandibular prognathism; abnormal auricles	No	Yes	Abnormal areola and mammary gland; shortening 4th and 5th metacarpals; tibial abnormalities; lipoatrophic diabetes mellitus	83
Normal	No	Broad nasal base; abnormal auricles; antimongoloid palpebral fissures; prominent mandible; hypoplastic maxilla	No	Yes	Lower micromelia; large big toe and short 2d–5th toes; palmar hyperkeratosis; abnormal nipples/areolae; strabismus, nystagmus; lenticular and corneal opacities; underdeveloped external genitalia	83
Normal	No	Swollen with flat nasal bridge and enlarged tip of nose	No	Yes	Mild gingival hypertrophy	83

Table 7-5 *Continued*

	*I**	*Hair*	*Teeth*	*Nails*
Agammaglobulinemia-thymic dysplasia-ectodermal dysplasia	NED	Alopecia scalp, brows, lashes	Natal; hypoplastic; enamel defects	NED
Alopecia, unusual facies, and preaxial polydactyly (Wilson's syndrome)	NED	Near-universal alopecia	Abnormal enamel; caries	Normal
Alopecia-anosmia-deafness-hypogonadism syndrome	AD	Severe hypotrichosis scalp and body hair, brows, lashes	± Conical teeth; oligodontia; microdontia; abnormal enamel; caries	Normal
Subgroup 1-3				
Palmoplantar hyperkeratosis and alopecia	AD or AR	Sparse to absent scalp, body hair, lashes, and brows	Normal	Short and dystrophic with onycholysis
Congenital atrichia with nail dystrophy, abnormal facies and retarded psychomotor development	? AR	Kinky, sparse hair at birth → lost within weeks; sparse lashes, brows	Normal	Dysplastic, brittle
Onychotrichodysplasia with neutropenia (Cantú's syndrome)	AR	Brittle, lusterless, sparse, short, curly scalp hair; scanty eyebrows, lashes, and body hair; microscopic exam of hair: trichorrhexis nodosa; sparse to absent pubic, axillary hair at puberty	Normal	Dystrophic; koilonychia and onychorrhexis
Trichoonycho-dysplasia with xeroderma	AR	Congenital universal atrichia—regrows later	Normal	Congenital anonychia; convex and dystrophic
Agammaglobulinemia-dwarfism-ectodermal dysplasia	? AR	Hair normal at birth; falls out at a few months with ? no regrowth	NED	Small and dystrophic
Skeletal anomalies–ectodermal dysplasia–growth and mental retardation	NED	Almost complete universal alopecia	Normal	Hypoplastic toenails
Pili torti and onychodysplasia (Beare's type)	AD	Normal in infancy followed in adolescence by hypotrichosis scalp and body hair; hairshaft: pili torti on microscopic exam	Normal	Short, fragile, brittle

Sweating	*MR*[†]	*Distinctive Facies*	*CLP*[‡]	*SS*[§]	*Other*	*Reference*
NED	NED	Normal	No	NED	Infants: bullous lesions face, hands, feet; ichthyosiform erythroderma; agammaglobulinemia with low IgG and IgA	83
Normal	NED	Micrognathia; flat nasal bridge; long upper lip with flat philtrum; malar hypoplasia with down-slanted palpebral fissures	No	No	Preaxial polydactyly feet; notch upper alveolar ridge	213
± ↓	±	Facial asymmetry; mandibular and gingival hypoplasia; periorbital wrinkles; microcephaly; everted lower lip, microtia; epicanthal folds; prominent nose	±	No	Hypogonadotropic hypogonadism; anosmia; conductive hearing loss; hypo- and hyperpigmented spots; anosmia or hyposmia; ± congenital heart defect	214,215
Normal	No	No	No	No	Palmoplantar hyperkeratosis	83,216
Normal	Mild	Depressed nasal bridge; hypertelorism; sunken eyes; broad nose; long philtrum	±	No	NED	20
Normal	Mild to none	Normal	No	No	Chronic neutropenia and recurrent infections; follicular hyperkeratoses; mild hypotonia	83,217,218
Normal	No	No	No	No	Severe xeroderma	83,219
NED	No	NED	NED	Yes	Erythroderma and ichthyosiform lesions; redundant skin; dyschondroplastic dwarfism; lymphopenic agammaglobulinemia with eosinophilia; hypoplastic thymus	83,220
Normal	Yes	Large, prominent nose; upslanting palpebral fissures; short upper lip; abnormal auricles; microbrachycephaly	No	Yes	Dry and hyperkeratotic skin; abnormal hands and feet with short (asymmetrical) digits, gaps between 1st and 2d toes; syndactyly 4th and 5th toes; bone fusions; disproportionate limbs	83,221
Normal	Yes	No	No	No	No	83,109

Table 7-5 *Continued*

	*I**	*Hair*	*Teeth*	*Nails*
Sabinas brittle hair and mental deficiency	AR	Dry, brittle, coarse, and wiry scalp hair; sparse brows and lashes; absent pubic, axillary hair; microscopic exam: ↓ cuticular layer; abnormal amino acid content of hair	Normal	Dystrophic
Cataracts, alopecia, and sclerodactyly	AR	Universal alopecia	Normal	Dystrophic
Subgroup 1-4				
Trichofacio-hypohidrotic syndrome	? X-linked recessive	Sparse, brittle, and fair	Normal	Normal

* I = Inheritance.
† MR = Mental retardation.
‡ CLP = Cleft lip/palate.
§ SS = Short stature.
¶ = Median pseudocleft lip.

small, dysplastic auricles. A congenital ichthyosiform erythroderma with whorls of scale on a diffuse erythematous background (Figure 7-8*A*) commonly disappears by age 3-6 months.[52] Scalp hair may be sparse, coarse, and lusterless with thin brows, especially laterally, and thin lashes (Figure 7-8*B*).[51] Microscopic examination of the hair follicles shows pili torti–like twisting and trichorrhexis nodosa.[51,53] A scarring alopecia can also occur. The nails may be flattened and split in layers and the teeth carious.[51] Cataracts are common, including asymmetrical cataracts. The genetic defect in chondrodysplasia punctata appears to be deficient peroxisomal enzyme activity.[51]

Table 7-6
INFANTILE HAIR LOSS ASSOCIATED WITH PILI TORTI

- Ectodermal dysplasia
  - Rapp-Hodgkin syndrome
  - Sălamon's syndrome
  - Arthrogryposis and ectodermal dysplasia
  - Ectodermal dysplasia with syndactyly
  - Tricho-odonto-onycho-dysplasia with pili torti
  - Pili torti and enamel hypoplasia (Ronchese type)
  - Pili torti and onychodysplasia (Beare's type)
  - Ankyloblepharon-ectodermal defects with cleft lip and palate syndrome
- Björnstad's dysplasia
- Salti-Salem syndrome
- Crandall's syndrome
- Menkes' kinky hair syndrome
- Tay's syndrome and other cases of trichothiodystrophy
- Chondrodysplasia punctata
- Bazex's syndrome
- Citrullinemia

BAZEX'S SYNDROME

Bazex's syndrome is an X-linked dominant or autosomal dominant disorder characterized by various cutaneous abnormalities.[54–57] There is usually short, sparse, and coarse scalp hair, and sparse body hair, lashes, and brows. Microscopic exam of the hair reveals pili torti and trichorrhexis nodosa.[54] Sweating is decreased locally or diffusely. The skin is remarkable for follicular atrophoderma (likened to "ice-pick marks"),[55] primarily on the dorsum of the hands and on the extensor extremities and back (Fig. 7-9). Follicular atrophoderma, though rare, may also be seen with Conradi-Hünermann syndrome, keratosis follicularis, keratosis palmoplantaris dissipata, and hyperhidrosis palmoplantaris.[56] Milia-like cysts are prominent on the face and upper body in Bazex's syndrome (Fig. 7-10), and atopic dermatitis is common. Multiple basal cell carcinomas generally develop in adolescence.

CITRULLINEMIA

Patients with the hereditary deficiency of argininosuccinic acid synthetase may present with fragile hair secondary to pili torti and trichorrhexis nodosa.[49,58]

Sweating	MR†	Distinctive Facies	CLP‡	SS§	Other	Reference
Normal	Yes	Maxillary hypoplasia	No	No	Retinal abnormalities; scalp hyperkeratosis	83
Normal	No	No	No	No	Congenital cataracts; hyperkeratosis palms and soles; poor wound healing; sclerodactyly ± contractures and pseudoainhum	222
↓	No	Wide and deeply depressed base of nose; anteverted nostrils; long philtrum, malar hypoplasia; hypertelorism	No	Yes	Mild upper respiratory problems	83

OTHER HAIR SHAFT ABNORMALITIES ASSOCIATED WITH HAIR LOSS (BREAKAGE)

These are listed in Table 7-1 and discussed further in Chapter 6.

Nutritional Deficiency/Metabolic Disorder

Nutritional deficiency, either of specific elements or a more generalized lack of protein or calories, may lead to diffuse hair loss. The nutritional deficit may be environmental and/or secondary to a hereditary defect in absorption or metabolism.

ZINC DEFICIENCY

Zinc deficiency in childhood may be either secondary to hereditary acrodermatitis enteropathica or acquired secondary to inadequate replacement therapy in the face of malabsorption or short-gut syndrome. *Acrodermatitis enteropathica* is an autosomal recessive disorder thought to be due to impaired intestinal absorption of

Figure 7-8 An infant with X-linked dominant Conradi-Hünermann chondrodysplasia punctata. (*A*) Patterned hyperkeratosis (*B*) Scalp involvement (Photos *courtesy of Dr. Nancy Esterly)*

A

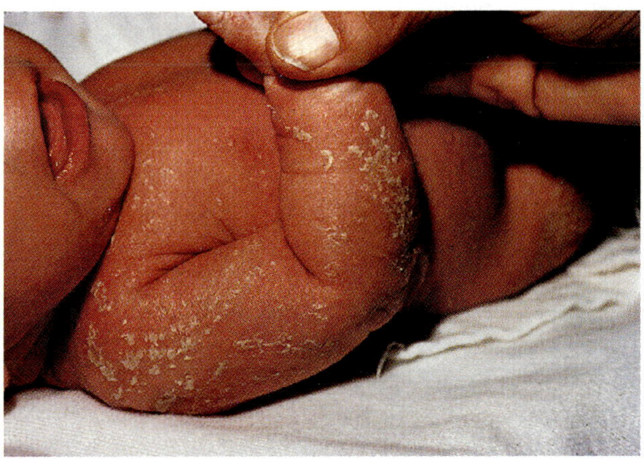

B

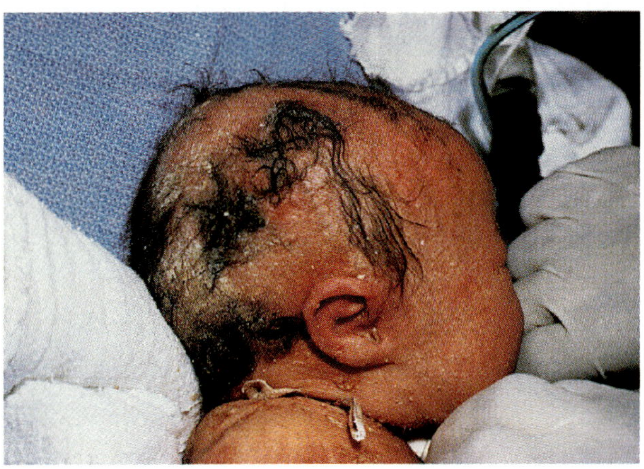

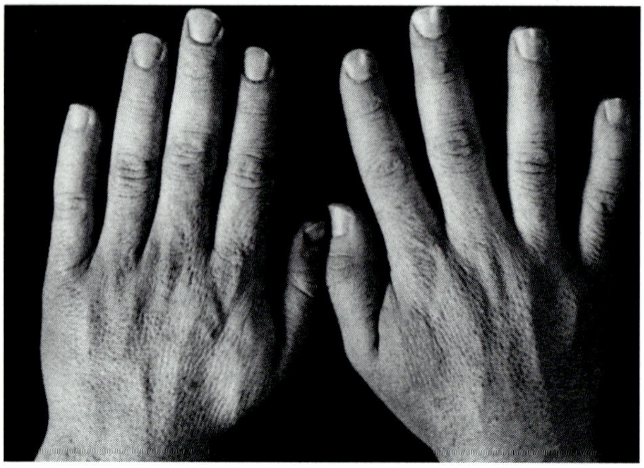

Figure 7-9 Bazex's syndrome. Follicular atrophoderma on hands. (*Reprinted with permission from Viksnins and Berlin.*[55])

Figure 7-10 Bazex's syndrome. Note milia-like cysts, pigmented macules, and marked hypotrichosis. (*Reprinted with permission from Plosila, Kiistala, and Niemi.*[54])

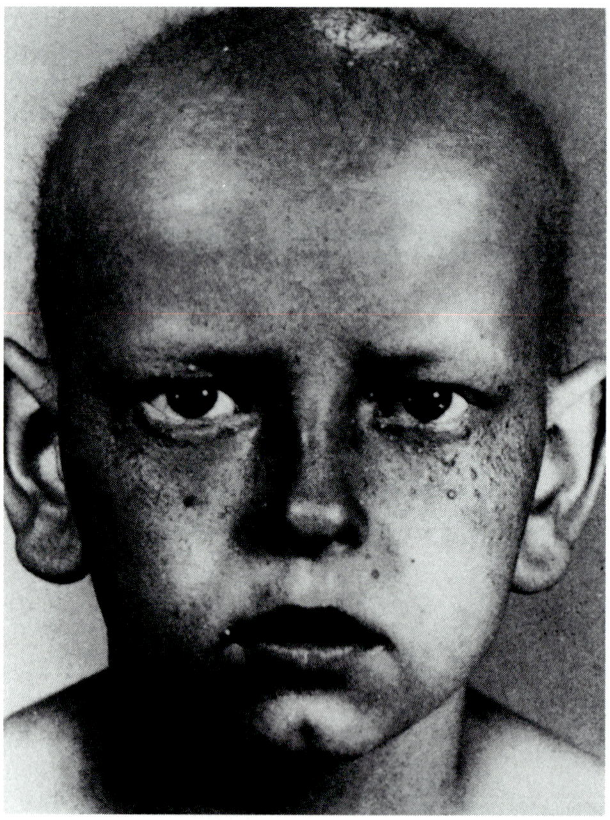

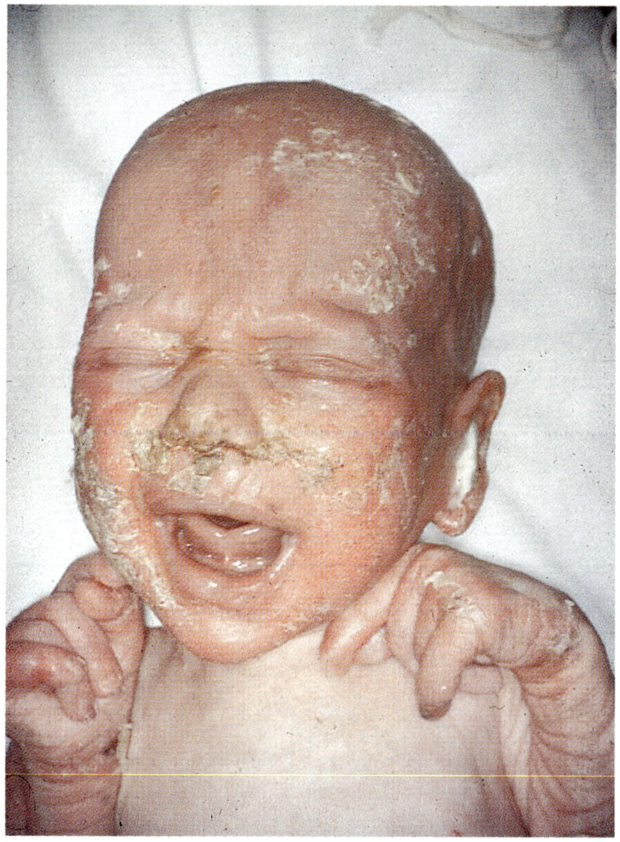

Figure 7-11 Patient with acrodermatitis enteropathica.

zinc.[59] Clinical signs include diarrhea, eczematoid plaques (especially acral and vesiculobullous, and periorificial), glossitis, stomatitis, nail dystrophy, and alopecia[60] (Fig. 7-11). These signs are commonly delayed in appearance in acrodermatitis enteropathica if the infant is breast-fed.[59] The zinc in breast milk is much more biologically available to infants with acrodermatitis enteropathica than the zinc in cows' milk, possibly due to a species-specific zinc binding ligand.[61] Hair growth in acrodermatitis enteropathica is sparse and slow, and pigmentation may be decreased.[59]

The diagnosis of acrodermatitis enteropathica is confirmed by finding low plasma zinc levels. Trace metal contamination is possible from rubber-stoppered vacutainer tubes, and platelet degradation leads to higher serum zinc levels. Because of this, standard venipuncture may need to be modified and plasma levels of zinc are preferred. Normal zinc levels in the face of a positive clinical picture of acrodermatitis enteropathica should not immediately rule out the diagnosis. Zinc levels in hair have been found to correlate with total body zinc, but the slow growth rate of hair in acrodermatitis enteropathica makes interpretation of hair zinc concentration difficult.[59,60] Patients with acrodermatitis enteropathica all respond rapidly to oral zinc with reversal of signs and symptoms.

ESSENTIAL FATTY ACID DEFICIENCY

Essential fatty acid deficiency in children usually occurs after prolonged parenteral alimentation without essential fatty acid supplementation. Clinical findings are a generalized xerotic or eczematous dermatitis, including periorificial dermatitis, poor wound healing, sparse hair growth with lightening of hair color, and thrombocytopenia.[62–64] The ratio of plasma fatty acids of the 20:3 (eicosatrienoic acid) to the 20:4 (eicosatetraenoic acid) type is greater than 0.4.[65] Replacement therapy can be either by the intravenous or percutaneous route (in the latter case, topical linoleic acid may be supplied as safflower oil).[63] The skin generally returns to normal within several weeks, while hair growth and pigmentation are restored within several months of treatment.[63]

BIOTIN DEFICIENCY

Biotin deficiency can be secondary to dietary deficiency or to *hereditary multiple carboxylase deficiency.* The former would occur in situations where malabsorption was known and biotin was not specifically replaced. Two forms of hereditary biotin-responsive multiple carboxylase deficiency exist—neonatal and infantile or juvenile. The neonatal form is generally rapidly fatal.[66,67] In the autosomal recessive infantile form, symptoms and signs generally manifest at 2 to 3 months of age with metabolic acidosis, keratoconjunctivitis, central nervous system dysfunction (seizures, hypotonia, ataxia, hearing loss, and developmental delay), and recurrent infection.[66–69] Diffuse sparse and fine-textured hair loss and a distinctive, sharply marginated dermatitis on the face and groin are present. Superficial erosions with crusting around the mouth are particularly reminiscent of acrodermatitis enteropathica. Diagnosis of both forms of biotin-responsive multiple carboxylase deficiency is by finding ketoacidosis with lactic acidosis, organic aciduria, hyperammonuria, and normal or decreased serum biotin, but acidosis and aciduria can be absent.[67,68] All abnormalities in the infantile form respond rapidly to biotin (5–10 mg per day) unless therapy is instituted late, in which case permanent neurological sequelae may persist[68] (Fig. 7-12).

The neonatal form of hereditary biotin-responsive multiple carboxylase deficiency is due to deficient or abnormal holocarboxylase synthetase activity, whereas the infantile-onset form is secondary to impaired absorption of biotin related to biotinidase deficiency.[66,69] The incidence of biotinidase deficiency (< 5 percent normal activity) is approximately 1 in 50,000 live births per annum.[70] Biotinidase hydrolyzes protein from small biotinyl peptides and biocytin (biotin complexed to lysine) that result from proteolytic degradation of biotin-dependent holocarboxylases.[71] The released biotin can then be reutilized by the body instead of being excreted in the urine.[66] Biotinidase is also important in the processing of biotin from dietary protein–bound sources.[68] Partial biotinidase deficiency (15 to 40 percent normal activity) is about four times as common as severe biotin deficiency. Infants with this condition may be susceptible to developing eczema and alopecia, especially if dietary intake or absorption of biotin is marginal.[70] There is a case report of a patient with Coffin-Siris syndrome and partial biotinidase deficiency in whom the hypotrichosis and dermatitis (ascribed to part of the Coffin-Siris syndrome) disappeared within 1 to 2 weeks of biotin (5 mg per day) supplementation.[70]

The function of as many as three mitochondrial biotin-dependent carboxylases, B-methyl crotonyl CoA carboxylase, propionyl CoA carboxylase, and pyruvate carboxylase, is impaired in biotin-responsive multiple carboxylase deficiency.[67] These enzymes are important in branched-chain amino acid and carbohydrate metabolism. In vitro, the fibroblasts of the neonatal form of multiple carboxylase deficiency have low activities of these carboxylases that respond to high concentrations of biotin added to the culture medium, whereas the fibroblasts of the infantile forms of multiple carboxylase deficiency respond to low levels of biotin.[69] Acetyl CoA carboxylase, a cytosolic enzyme which catalyzes the rate-limiting step for the de novo synthesis of saturated long-chain fatty acids, is a biotin-containing enzyme and is impaired in multiple carboxylase deficiency.[67] Since disturbance in

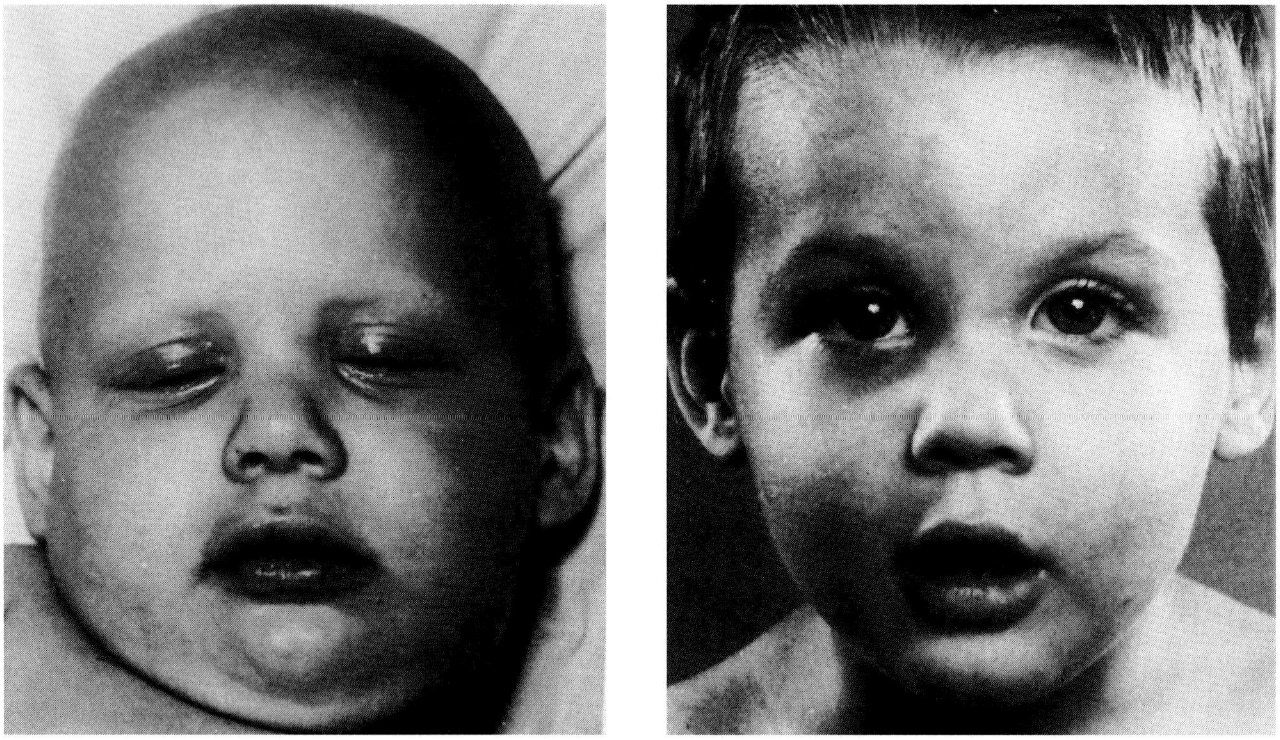

A B

Figure 7-12 Biotin-responsive multiple carboxylase deficiency. (*A*) Patient at 2.75 years before biotin therapy. (*B*) Patient at age 3.1 years, after 4 months of biotin therapy. (*Reprinted with permission from Thoene, Baker, Yoshino, and Sweetman.*[69])

fatty acid metabolism, similar to that seen in essential fatty acid deficiency, also occurs in acrodermatitis enteropathica, a common pathogenic mechanism for the dermatologic changes found in essential fatty acid deficiency, acrodermatitis enteropathica, and biotin-responsive multiple carboxylase deficiency may lie in aberrant lipid biosynthesis.[67] In a case of multiple carboxylase deficiency with alopecia, supplementation with unsaturated fatty acids alone resulted in dramatic improvement in both the dermatologic condition and hair growth.[72]

OTHER AMINOACIDURIAS

Aminoacidurias with hypotrichosis, other than biotin-responsive multiple carboxylase deficiency, include homocystinuria, Hartnup disease, argininosuccinic aciduria, and citrullinemia.[67] The latter two are associated with brittle hair and trichorrhexis nodosa. The cutaneous manifestations of *homocystinuria* include sparse hair, atrophic scars, telangiectases, and elastosis perforans serpiginosa.[67] These patients also have mental retardation, seizures, ectopic lens, marfanoid habitus, and vascular thromboses. The underlying defect of homocystinuria is the enzyme cystathionine synthetase. Treatment is with pyridoxine, methionine restriction, and cysteine supplementation. *Hartnup disease* is caused by faulty renal and intestinal transport of neutral amino acids.[67] Alopecia and premature graying, photosensitivity, nail streaks, and psychiatric disturbances are present. Treatment is with nicotinamide, oral neomycin, and sunscreens.

PROTEIN MALNUTRITION (KWASHIORKOR) OR CALORIC MALNUTRITION (MARASMUS)

Protein malnutrition (kwashiorkor) and caloric malnutrition (marasmus) usually occur concurrently and are still all too common in various parts of the world. The hair in children affected with protein-caloric malnutrition is slow-growing, sparse, and dyspigmented.[73–75] There is anagen bulb atrophy, an increased percentage of telogen hairs, a characteristic diminished hair shaft diameter, and increased hair fragility in affected individuals.[73–78]

HAIR LOSS IN THE FIRST YEAR OF LIFE: FOCAL LOSS

Nonscarring Hair Loss

OCCIPITAL ALOPECIA OF THE NEWBORN

Focal alopecia in the infant can be either of a nonscarring nature, hence potentially transient, or cicatricial. As discussed earlier, the first pelage is slow to be lost in the occipital area of the scalp compared with the remainder of the scalp. Normally, the synchronized shedding in the occipital area occurs 8 to 12 weeks postnatally, accounting for the "occipital alopecia" of the newborn. It is merely a physiological occurrence, and the lost telogen hair is rapidly replaced by anagen hairs with a mosaic pattern of growth and loss.

HALLERMANN-STREIFF SYNDROME (OCULOMANDIBULAR DYSCEPHALY)

The scalp hair loss in Hallermann-Streiff ectodermal dysplasia (Table 7-5) may be diffuse with accentuation over the frontal region, or patchy, particularly over the cranial sutures[79] (Fig. 7-13). Cutaneous atrophy on the scalp, especially in the patches of alopecia, may be evident and appear separate from the aplasia cutis congenita which is also seen in the Hallermann-Streiff syndrome.[79–83] Hair abnormalities seen on scanning electron microscopy include absence or grooving of the cuticle.[79] Eyebrows and eyelashes may be sparse or absent. Patients have a typical "bird facies" due to a sharply curved, thick, pointed nose, and mandibular hypoplasia. Other common associations are brachycephaly and dental and ocular abnormalities. The Hallermann-Streiff syndrome is thought to represent a developmental abnormality (a branchial arch syndrome) occurring at 5 to 7 weeks gestation and to most likely be autosomal recessive in inheritance.[79,81,83]

OTHER CAUSES

Rare causes of patchy nonscarring scalp hair loss at birth and uncommon in infancy include *alopecia areata* and *tinea capitis.*

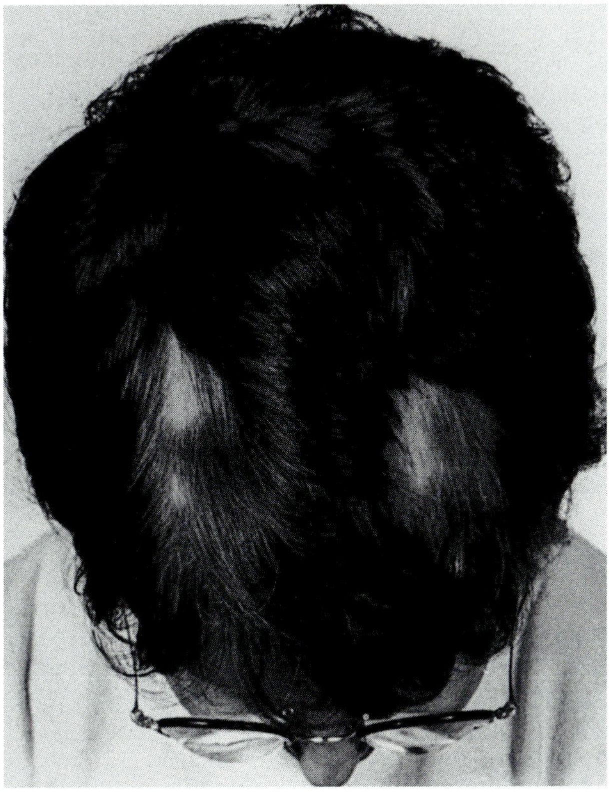

Figure 7-13 Hallermann-Streiff syndrome with patchy hair loss. (*Reprinted with permission from Grattan, Liddle, and Willshaw.*[81])

Scarring Hair Loss

TRAUMA

A number of conditions may be associated with a focal permanent or scarring hair loss during early infancy. Trauma from forceps used at delivery (usually about the ears or sides of the face) or from fetal scalp electrodes can lead to permanent sites of hair loss if prolonged pressure or lacerations occur.

APLASIA CUTIS CONGENITA

Aplasia cutis congenita may also present as ulcerations but can undergo healing in utero, leaving a crust, scar, or sharply demarcated parchmentlike membrane[84] (Fig. 7-14). Aplasia cutis congenita is literally a focal congenital absence of the epidermis and potentially all layers of the dermis and subcutaneous tissue.[85] Biopsy of an area of aplasia cutis congenita with an intact membrane reveals a thin epidermis, decreased or absent elastic fibers, absence or dysplasia of sebaceous and sweat glands, and absence of hair folli-

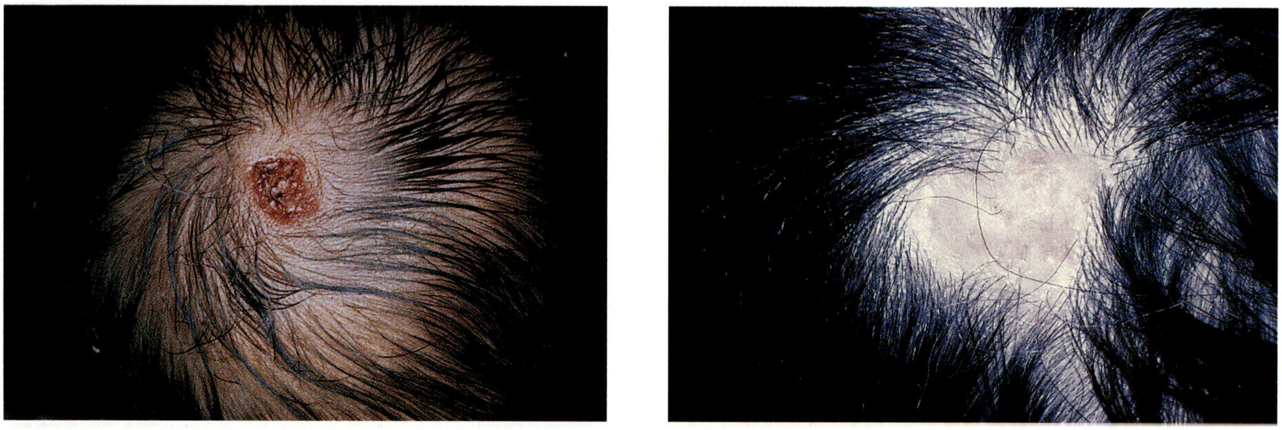

A B

Figure 7-14 Aplasia cutis congenita. (*A*) Superficial ulceration. (*B*) Healed area.

Table 7-7
ECTODERMAL DYSPLASIAS PRESENTING WITH APLASIA CUTIS CONGENITA

	*Inher**	*Hair*	*Teeth*	*Nails*
Johanson-Blizzard syndrome	AR	Aplasia cutis congenita scalp; brittle scalp hair with abnormal frontal upsweep; hypertrichosis elsewhere	Oligodontia; microdontia; aplastic permanent teeth; caries; ± conical incisors	Normal
Ectodermal dysplasia of Carey	?	Thin, hypopigmented sparse hair; aplasia cutis congenita scalp	Hypodontia	Dystrophic nails
Ectodermal dysplasia of Tuffli	? AD	Aplasia cutis congenita scalp	Delayed dental eruption	Dysplastic nails
ANOTHER syndrome See Table 7-5				
Hallerman-Streiff syndrome See Table 7-5				
EEC syndrome See Table 7-5				
Focal dermal hypoplasia See Table 7-5				

* Inheritance.
† Mental Retardation.
‡ Cleft Lip/Palate.
§ Short Structure.

cles.[85] Aplasia cutis congenita is typically located on the vertex of the head near the sagittal suture or over the parietal bone.[84]

Aplasia cutis congenita is generally small and circular except when appearing in one of the cranial suture lines, in which case it is generally elongated and stellate and often quite large.[84] Aplasia cutis congenita can occur anywhere on the body, although about 85 percent of the lesions are on the scalp. Lesions are generally single (70 percent) but can be multiple and are usually in close proximity to the midline and the parietal hair whorl.[84,85] Lesions range in size from 0.5 to 100 cm in diameter, with the larger lesions potentially extending deeper into the dura or meninges.[84,85] As many as 20 to 30 percent of cases of scalp aplasia cutis congenita have absence of the underlying bone, but this usually resolves spontaneously during infancy accompanied by disappearance of radiolucent areas on x-ray.[85,86] The smaller lesions of aplasia cutis congenita will generally cicatrize within several months on their own, but larger lesions, especially those in which the superior sagittal sinus is exposed, should probably be grafted to decrease the incidence of necrosis, infection, and/or hemorrhage.[84–87] Although the area is initially hairless, some hair may grow in the area over time, depending on the depth of the lesion and the degree of abnormal development of the

Sweating	*MR*†	*Distinctive Facies*	*CLP*‡	*SS*§	*Other*	*Reference*
Normal	Yes	Distinctive small beaklike nose due to hypoplasia or aplasia alae nasi; long upper lip with thin vermillion border; small, pointed chin with horizontal groove; maxillary hypoplasia; micrognathia; microcephaly	No	Yes	Exocrine pancreatic insufficiency with failure to thrive; sensorineural deafness; ± imperforate anus; GU anomalies; cardiac abnormalities; lacrimal fistulae; hypotonia; ± nipple/areola abnormality; ± hypothyroidism; ± clinodactyly; ± café-au-lait spots; ± congenital heart defects	91,96, 223,224
↓	?	U-shaped mouth with maxillary hypoplasia	Yes	?	Conductive hearing loss; absent tear ducts; 2-3 syndactyly	83
↓	?	No	No	No	Nipple and breast hypoplasia; adrenal cyst	93

hair follicle.[88] Aplasia cutis congenita as a single defect is usually sporadic or inherited as an autosomal dominant trait.[87]

Aplasia cutis congenita has been reported with other isolated abnormalities such as cleft lip or palate, tracheoesophageal fistula, double cervix and uterus, omphalocele, patent ductus arteriosus, polycystic kidney, mental retardation, and cutis marmorata telangiectasia congenita, each of which is generally of sporadic or autosomal dominant inheritance.[85] Aplasia cutis congenita of the scalp has been associated with limb abnormalities, including limb reduction abnormalities, 2-3 syndactyly, ectrodactyly, and clubfoot; this association is inherited in an autosomal dominant fashion.[85,87] Scalp aplasia cutis congenita has been reported in two phenotypic female siblings with 46 XY genotype and gonadal dysgenesis.[89] Other abnormalities in these patients included unusual facies, cleft lip or palate, overfolded helix, preauricular pits, renal and cardiac abnormalities, and streak gonads. Five generations of one family presented with an autosomal dominant syndrome of aplasia cutis congenita that healed with a "lumpy scalp" and had associated external ear abnormalities, hypoplastic breasts and nipples, hypoplastic uterus, brittle nails, and toe webbing.[90] Aplasia cutis congenita may be seen in the 13-trisomy syndrome and the 4p-syndrome.[91] Aplasia cutis congenita of the scalp and body has been associated with colobomatous orbital cysts and skin tags of the lid margin and nasal septum in the oculocerebro-cutaneous syndrome.[92]

Ectodermal dysplasias associated with aplasia cutis congenita include ectodermal dysplasia of Carey,[83] ectodermal dysplasia of Tuffli,[93] ANOTHER syndrome,[94] and focal dermal hypoplasia[95] (Tables 7-5 and 7-7). Midline scalp defects compatible with aplasia cutis congenita are seen in the Johanson-Blizzard syndrome.[91,96] These patients have very distinctive facies with small beaked nose and absent nasal alae, midfacial hypoplasia, long upper lip with thin vermillion border and downturned corners to the mouth, and a small chin with a horizontal groove (Fig. 7-15). There is an abnormal frontal upsweep to the scalp hair. Deciduous teeth are small and carious, and permanent teeth absent. Sensorineural deafness, pancreatic insufficiency, growth and mental retardation, cutaneous lacrimal duct fistula, hypothyroidism, and anal atresia are other common anomalies. The disorder is transmitted as an autosomal recessive trait.

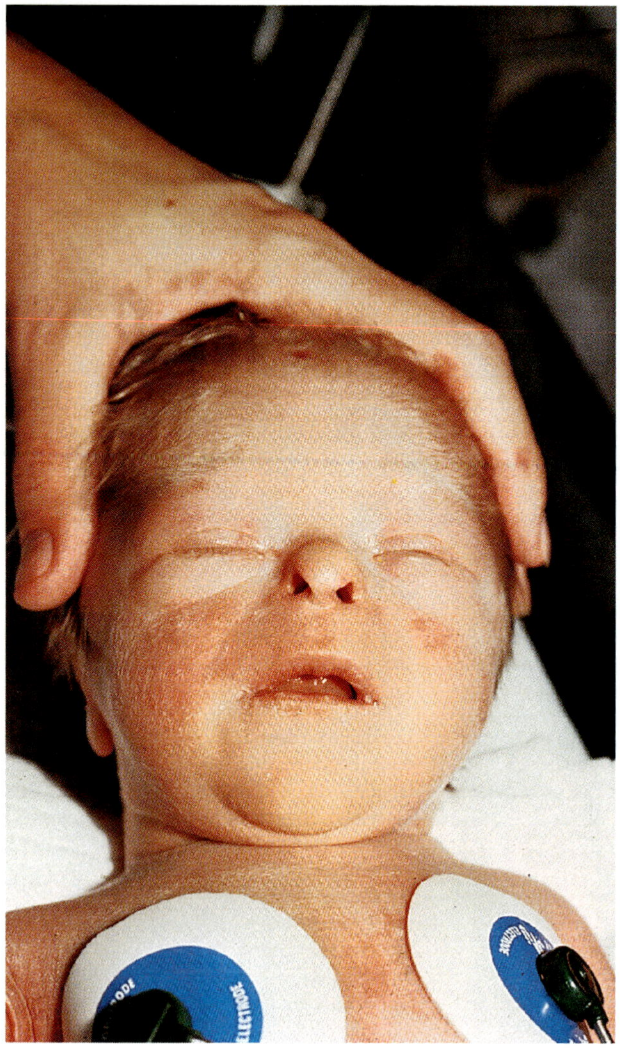

Figure 7-15 Johanson-Blizzard syndrome. (*Courtesy of Dr. Nancy Esterly.*)

CONGENITAL ECTODERMAL DYSPLASIA OF THE FACE

Multiple foci of round to oval atrophic alopecia, variably noted to be hyperpigmented or violaceous and primarily temporal and symmetrical, are present at birth in the autosomal dominant syndrome designated *congenital ectodermal dysplasia of the face*[97] (Fig. 7-16). Biopsy of the scalp reveals absent appendages and markedly decreased dermal elastic tissue. The scalp hair loss is accompanied by linear forehead depressions,

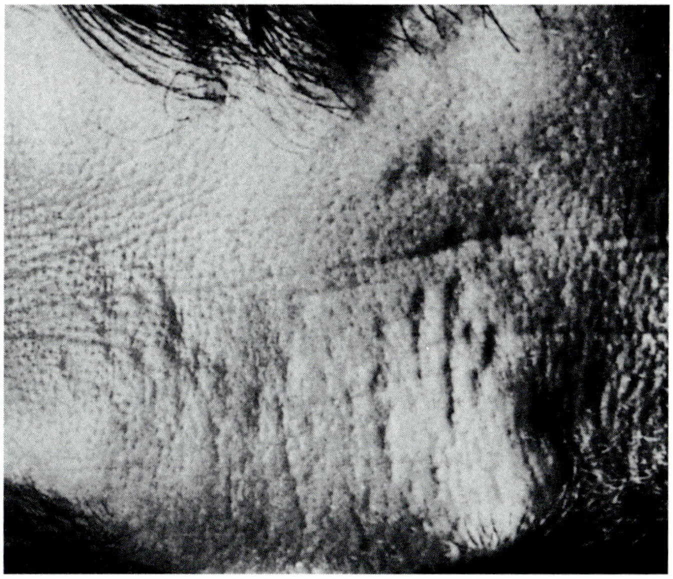

Figure 7-16 Congenital ectodermal dysplasia of the face. Multiple vertical depressions on forehead. (*Reprinted with permission from Jensen.*[97])

sparse lateral two-thirds of the eyebrows, and occasional eyelash abnormalities. Facial deformities, including a flat nasal bridge and soft, flabby nasal tip, are associated with an autosomal recessive variant of this syndrome.

EPIDERMOLYSIS BULLOSA

Congenital focal areas of permanent hair loss have also been seen in epidermolysis bullosa (EB) or EB-like disorders. The hair loss has been related both to EB lesions and to focal absence of skin apparent at birth.[98] The recessive dystrophic forms of EB typically heal with scarring and atrophy, and thus the focal absence of skin at birth may be secondary to in utero blister formation. However, other types of EB-like blisters unassociated with scarring (Bart's syndrome) have been associated with congenital absence of the skin. In these latter cases and perhaps in some cases of dystrophic EB, the local absence of scalp skin at birth is an associated aplasia cutis congenita.

EPIDERMAL OR ORGANOID NEVI

Hair generally does not grow normally in an area affected by an epidermal nevus regardless of the clinical subtype, whether an inflammatory linear epidermal, comedonal, or sebaceous nevus. Epidermal and organoid nevi are usually sporadic events. The nevus sebaceus of Jadassohn generally presents as a congenital focal macular area of hair loss in the scalp that may become verrucoid or elevated at puberty under the influence of androgens (Fig. 7-17). Epidermal or organoid nevi have been reported in close proximity to aplasia cutis congenita and may also be associated with ophthalmologic and neurological abnormalities.[85]

A specific type of ichthyosiform nevus is part of the *CHILD syndrome* (*C*ongenital *H*emidysplasia with *I*chthyosiform *E*rythroderma and *L*imb *D*efects) (Fig. 7-18). In this X-linked dominant inherited disorder, infants at birth or within the first weeks of life develop a unilateral ichthyosiform erythroderma with strict demarcation to the anterior and posterior midline,

Figure 7-17 Nevus sebaceus of Jadassohn. (*Courtesy of Dr. Neil Prose.*)

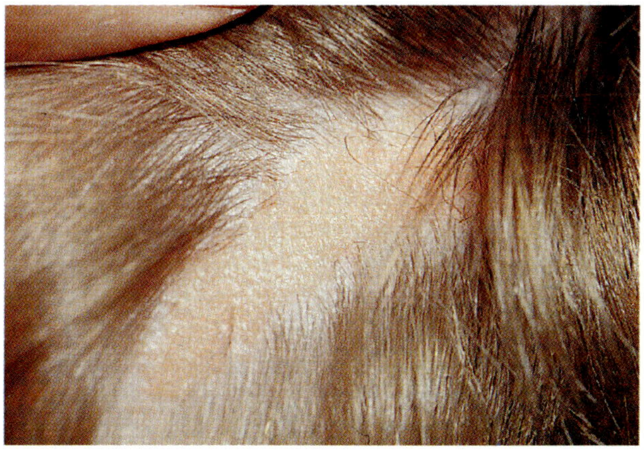

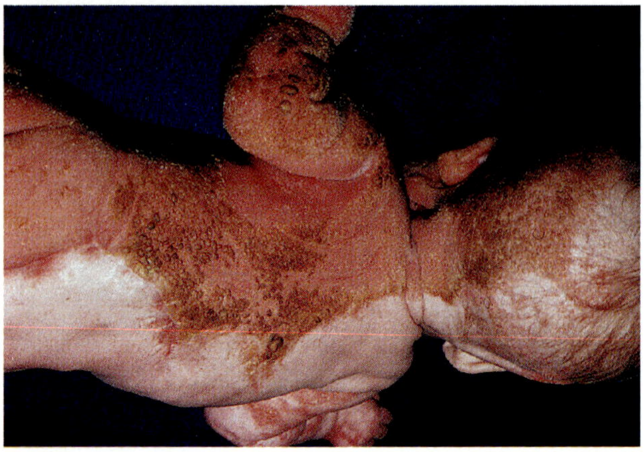

Figure 7-18 CHILD syndrome. (*Courtesy of Dr. Nancy Esterly.*)

sparing the face.[99] This is associated with congenital ipsilateral limb reduction defects and ipsilateral hypoplasia of internal organs, the most serious being cardiovascular defects.[99] The syndrome is secondary to a disorder of peroxisomes with a decrease in peroxisomal content and peroxisomal enzyme activity in the involved skin and, presumably, in the affected embryonic anlage.[100] Peroxisomes are subcellular organelles involved in a variety of metabolic processes, particularly oxidation and lipid metabolism.[100] The Lyon hypothesis of random inactivation of one of the X chromosomes during early fetal development may account for the phenotypic expression of the abnormality. However, unlike incontinentia pigmenti, in which the cutaneous abnormalities follow Blashko's lines, the very distinct anterior-posterior division of the ichthyosis in CHILD syndrome would require any lyonization to have occurred very early in embryological development, perhaps at the first somatic division.[100]

ONSET OF HAIR LOSS AFTER THE FIRST YEAR OF LIFE: DIFFUSE LOSS

TELOGEN AND ANAGEN LOSS

Children are subject to the same causes of telogen and anagen loss as adults and should have a similar evaluation. A "benign" cause of anagen hair loss occurs not uncommonly in children. This *loose anagen syndrome* can be easily distinguished from the more worrisome forms of toxin-related anagen effluvium by microscopic examination of the hair bulbs and lower shafts obtained by a hair pull. An anagen effluvium caused by a toxin in a child potentially signals a more serious problem than that seen in an adult: a child has a lower threshold for toxicity and greater chance for serious central nervous system sequelae or death from the offending agent(s).

ALOPECIA AREATA

Alopecia areata presenting in early childhood more commonly progresses to alopecia totalis and universalis than that presenting in an adult. Alopecia totalis or universalis in children, especially young children under the age of 5, is prone to be persistent and treatment refractory. Since this particular subtype of alopecia areata is frequently associated with nail pitting or dystrophy, the presentation may mimic an ectodermal dysplasia.

SYNDROMES WITH LATE-ONSET HYPOTRICHOSIS

There have been several reports of inherited, diffuse hypotrichosis which first developed after infancy. As noted earlier, affected infants who have the atrichia with papular lesions syndrome (Table 7-4) may have normal hair at birth only to have shedding of scalp hair, brows, and body hair in infancy or early childhood.[19] Toribio and Quinones reported on a large family with the onset of diffuse scalp hair loss at age 5 to 12 years which progressed to near total alopecia by the mid third decade.[101] Brows, lashes, and body hair were preserved. The skin of the scalp was reported as normal-appearing, and no follicular hyperkeratosis or other associated abnormalities were noted. Inheritance was autosomal dominant. Bentley-Phillips and Grace presented another family with an autosomal dominant inherited hair loss in childhood (age 7–13 years) without associated follicular hyperkeratosis or other abnormalities. In this case, the hair loss was generalized, but the scalp skin was noted to be thin and atrophic[27] (Fig. 7-19). Petersen described an autosomal dominant hypotrichosis with hair loss at about age 4 to 5 years and regrowth of short, sparse, fair hair.[101] Patients with monilithrix may have normal-appearing hair at birth only to have the hair shaft abnormality become apparent in early childhood to adolescence.[102]

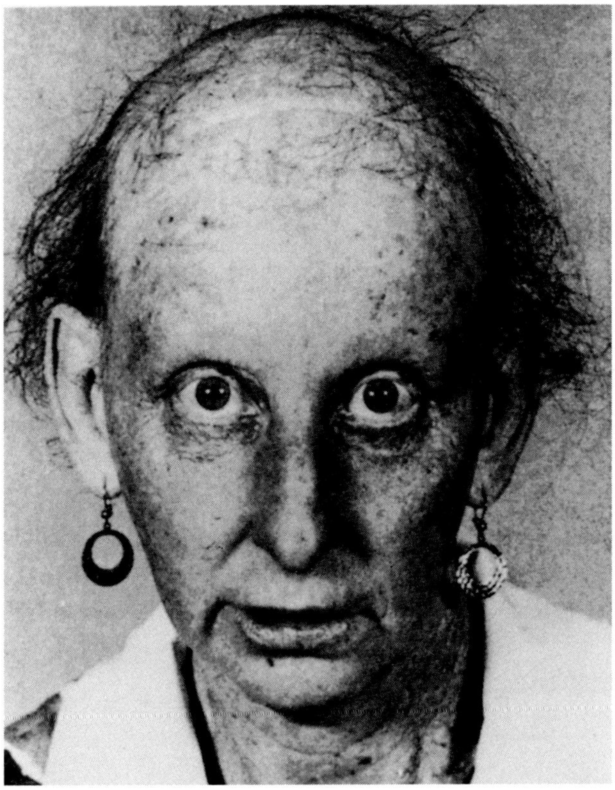

Figure 7-19 Patient with alopecia as described by Bentley-Phillips and Grace. (*Reprinted with permission from Bentley-Phillips and Grace.*[27])

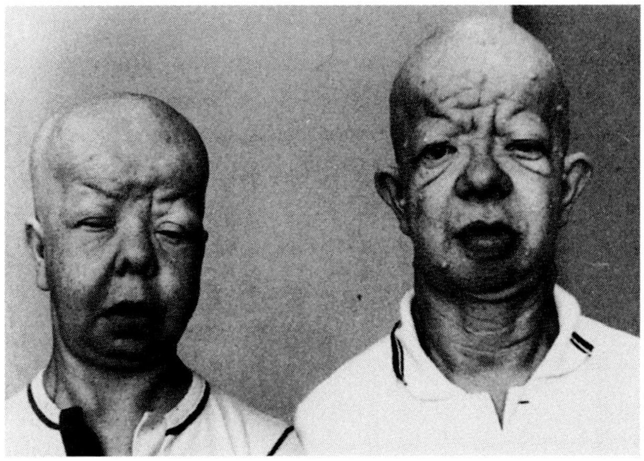

Figure 7-20 Patients with the GAPO syndrome. (*Reprinted with permission from Wajntal et al.*[108])

ECTODERMAL DYSPLASIAS

Certain syndromes classified as ectodermal dysplasias have hair loss that develops only after infancy or the first year of life. The ectodermal dysplasias with late onset of diffuse hair loss (but with other ectodermal anomalies present at birth) include hidrotic ectodermal dysplasia, GAPO syndrome (*G*rowth retardation *A*lopecia, *P*seudoanodontia, and *O*ptic atrophy), Jorgensen's syndrome, and Beare's type of pili torti (Table 7-5). *In hidrotic ectodermal dysplasia,* the hair loss may be apparent at birth or infancy or can be delayed to puberty.[103,104] In full expression, the scalp hair may be sparse or absent and is usually fine and slow-growing. The scalp hair demonstrates decreased tensile strength and is low in disulfide content due to a decrease in the fibrillar or low-sulfur fraction of hair.[105] Androgen-dependent hair is also sparse.[104]

In Jorgensen's syndrome, the scalp hair is generally coarse in infancy and is shed in the second decade.[106] Associated findings are hypohidrosis, dystrophic nails, abnormal teeth, dry skin, and stenotic lacrimal ducts.[83,106] In the *GAPO syndrome* (Fig. 7-20), scalp hair may be present at birth but is generally lost totally within the first few years of life.[107] The primary defect is hypothesized to be one of the enzymes involved in the breakdown of extracellular connective tissue matrix.[108] *In Beare's type of pili torti,* the hair may be normal in infancy, only to become scarce in adolescence.[83,109]

DYSKERATOSIS CONGENITA

Dyskeratosis congenita is usually an X-linked recessive disorder with the abnormal gene assigned to Xq28.[110] However, families have been reported in which autosomal dominant or autosomal recessive inheritance seemed clinically most likely, and this paradox remains unexplained.[110] There are multiple ectodermal defects, primarily of delayed onset, associated with dyskeratosis congenita.[111–115] The cardinal and most constant signs are oral leukoplakia, reticulated hyper- and hypopigmentation with telangiectases and cutaneous atrophy (first on the head and neck, then on the trunk and extremities), and atrophic nails (Fig. 7-21). The nail abnormalities usually appear by early childhood with splitting, peeling, and recurrent paronychia which goes on to atrophy with or without pterygium. The leukoplakia and skin dyspigmentation generally appear in midchildhood to adolescence, although there are sporadic reports of delay of all symptoms until early in the third decade. The hair abnormality generally occurs in early adulthood, with markedly

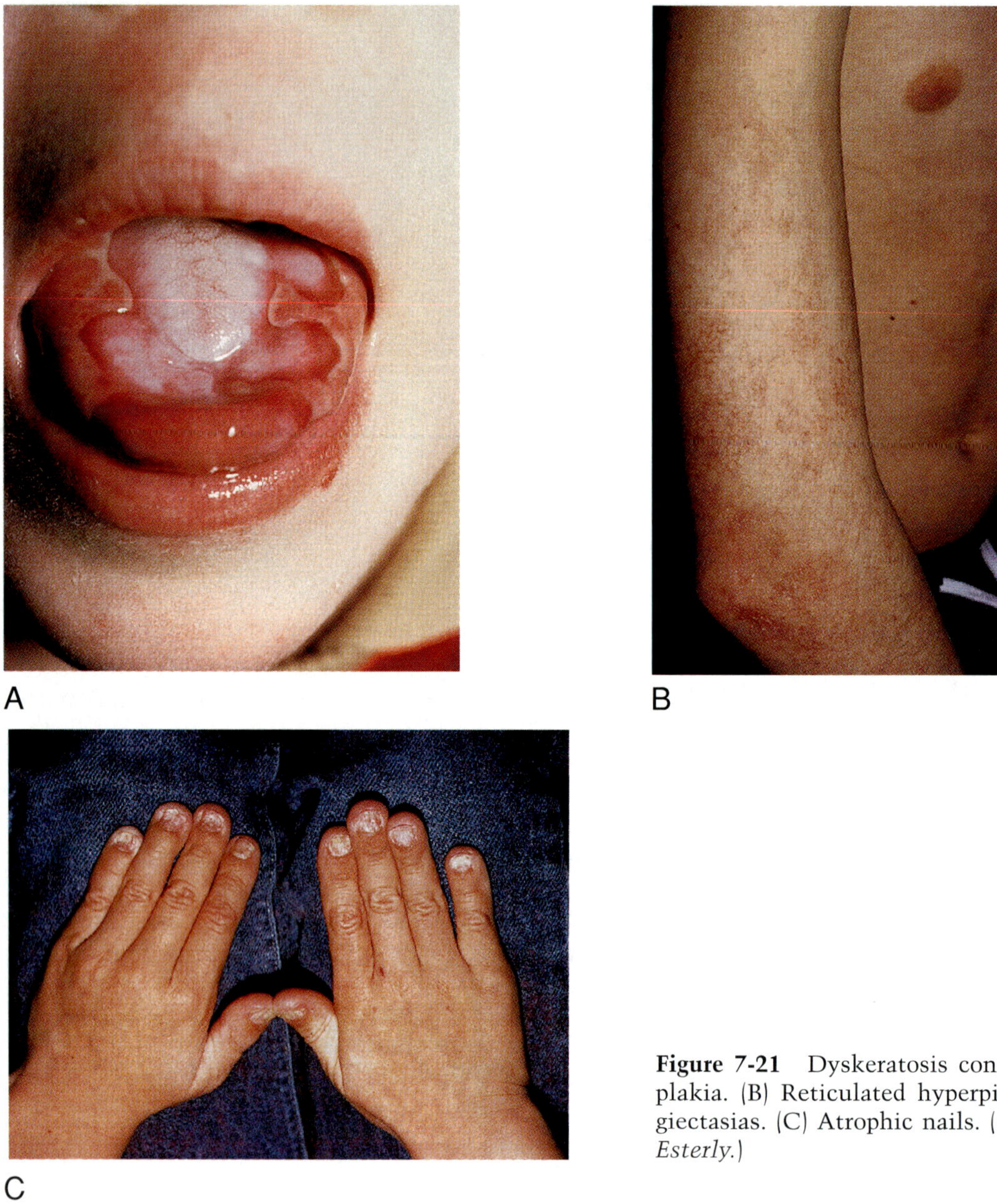

Figure 7-21 Dyskeratosis congenita. (A) Oral leukoplakia. (B) Reticulated hyperpigmentation and telangiectasias. (C) Atrophic nails. (*Courtesy of Dr. Nancy Esterly.*)

thinned, lusterless scalp hair occasionally accompanied by premature graying (Fig. 7-22). Facial hair, brows, and eyelashes are sparse. The teeth may have caries or appear defective. Palms and soles exhibit hyperhidrosis, bullae after trauma, and hyperkeratosis. Pancytopenia and an increased incidence of solid malignancies, especially mucosal (at a mean age of 30), are the most common causes of death. Incomplete syndromes may occur, as shown in one family with pigmentation limited to the neck or intertriginous areas, plus or minus scalp hair thinning and limited nail involvement.[116]

SYNDROMES ASSOCIATED WITH PREMATURE SENILITY

Several syndromes in which diffuse hair loss is a prominent aspect are associated with premature senility (Table 7-8).

WERNER'S SYNDROME

In Werner's syndrome (pangeria), aging begins in late childhood or early adulthood, heralded by premature graying of the scalp hair[115,117–120] (Fig. 7-23). Generalized hair loss develops by age 20 to 25, along with sclerodermatous skin changes,

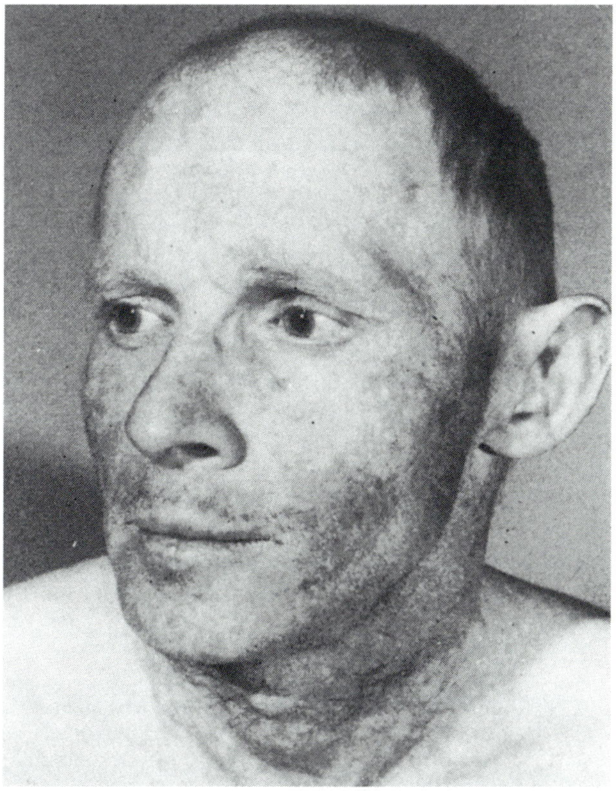

Figure 7-22 Dyskeratosis congenita in an adult. Note alopeica and dyspigmentation. (*Reprinted with permission from Sirinavan and Trowbridge.*[114])

cataracts, degenerative bone and muscle changes, and progressive atherosclerotic disease.

PROGERIA

In contrast, progeria, or Hutchinson-Gilford syndrome, is usually clinically recognizable prior to the second birthday.[117,121] Progressive atrophy of the skin and subcutaneous tissue is accompanied by loss of scalp and body hair, lashes and brows, and by the development of hypoplastic nails (Fig. 7-24). Atherosclerosis is well-developed before age 10, and death generally occurs by the middle of the second decade. The hair loss in this situation is but a minor sign or symptom in these unfortunate children and young adults, and the diagnosis is seldom in question for long.

OTHER "PROGEROID" SYNDROMES

FITCH BIRD-HEADED DWARF

In a case presented by Fitch, male-pattern baldness and graying developed in adolescence along with the distinctive facial features of bird-headed dwarf syndrome, i.e., prominent beaked nose and micrognathia.[122]

COCKAYNE'S SYNDROME

In Cockayne's syndrome, the scalp hair is sparse from infancy with premature graying.[123] These children, like those with Werner's syndrome, are short and have cataracts, hypogonadism, and a loss of subcutaneous fat.[124] However, the early age of onset (generally by age 2) clearly distinguishes patients with Cockayne's from those with Werner's syndrome. Other features such as deafness and ataxia differentiate patients with Cockayne's syndrome from those with early progeria. The patients affected with Cockayne's syndrome carry a mutation in the xeroderma pigmentosa complementation group D (XPD) gene that causes a failure of RNA synthesis to recover to normal levels after ultraviolet exposure, but they maintain normal excision repair of post-ultraviolet DNA damage (in contrast to XP patients).[125,126] These children are photosensitive and develop atrophy, pigmentation, and telangiectasias (poikiloderma) in sun-exposed areas.[127,128]

ROTHMUND-THOMSON SYNDROME

Poikiloderma is also seen with the Rothmund-Thomson syndrome. These children are normal-appearing at birth but at 3 to 6 months of age develop a distinctive inflammation on the cheeks, ears, extensor extremities, and buttocks which is followed by atrophy, telangiectasias, and reticular dyspigmentation[129] (Fig. 7-25). Patients are photosensitive and develop blisters in sun-exposed areas. Cataracts develop by age 4 to 7, and short stature and hypogonadism can also occur. Some of the more distinctive features, such as the warty hyperkeratoses over the joints and palms and soles, may not appear until adolescence. The hair may be sparse on the scalp, body, brows, and lashes at birth, or the loss can be delayed up to about age 3.[115]

Scarring Hair Loss

CONRADI-HÜNERMANN CHONDRODYSPLASIA PUNCTATA

A systematized follicular atrophoderma may develop in childhood in those with Conradi-Hünermann syndrome, usually in the areas of skin previously involved with a whorled ichthyosiform

Table 7-8
SYNDROMES WITH PREMATURE SENILITY AND DIFFUSE HAIR LOSS OCCURRING AFTER INFANCY

Disorder	*Inher**	*Onset Symptoms*	*Hair*	*Stature and Bone Changes*	*Ocular Changes*
Werner's syndrome (Pangeria)	AR	Adolescence	Premature graying by age 20; general hair loss age 20–25	Short stature; osteoporosis; osteoarthritis peripheral joints	Cataracts 20–25 years; keratopathy; glaucoma
Progeria (Hutchinson-Gilford syndrome)	AR	2–12 months	Loss of scalp and body hair, brows, lashes first 2 years	Dwarfism; fibrosis joints; skeletal dysplasia and hypoplasia	None
Fitch bird-headed dwarfism	NED‡	Birth	Early male-pattern baldness and graying; sparse facial, axillary, and pubic hair at puberty	Short stature; osteoporosis	None
Cockayne's syndrome	AR	By age 2	± Sparse scalp hair; premature graying	Short stature; dorsal kyphosis; disproportionately long extremities	Retinal pigment degeneration; optic atrophy; cataracts; inadequate response mydriatics
Rothmund-Thomson syndrome	AR	Usually by 6 months	± Sparse scalp and body hair, brows, and lashes (0–3 years)	Short stature; ± asymmetrical limbs; short digits	Cataracts (3–7 years)

* Inher = inheritance.
† Cancer = increased risk malignancy.
‡ NED = not enough data.

hyperkeratosis.[52] Histologically, the follicular atrophoderma is a retention hyperkeratosis with calcium in keratotic plugs, focal hyperpigmentation of the basal keratinocytes, and selective atrophy of the hair follicles.[130] Coarse, lusterless hair and cicatricial alopecia are commonly present. (Fig. 7-26).

INCONTINENTIA PIGMENTI

Incontinentia pigmenti is another X-linked dominant condition in which patients may develop cicatricial alopecia secondary to whorled hyperkeratotic lesions. In incontinentia pigmenti, vesicular lesions at birth or early infancy are followed by linear verrucous lesions which clear and are replaced by whorled hyperpigmentation (Fig. 7-27). A permanent linear or patchy scalp alopecia may result, in addition to the reported more diffuse background scalp hypotrichosis (Fig. 7-28).[131]

ANKYLOBLEPHARON, ECTODERMAL DEFECT, CLEFT LIP OR PALATE (AEC) SYNDROME

In AEC syndrome (Table 7-5), the hair may be fine or wiry and sparse or absent since birth. The hair loss may become patchy in childhood coincidental with the development of recur-

Cutaneous Changes	*Hypogonadism*	*Cancer*†	*Other*	*Reference*
Atrophy skin and subQ; acral sclerosis; ischemic and neurotropic ulcerations; mottled pigmentation and telegiectasias; normal or dystrophic nails; hyperkeratoses over bony prominences	Yes	Yes	Calcification peripheral and cardiac arteries and soft tissue; gross foot abnormalities; voice changes; muscle atrophy; diabetes; atherosclerotic vascular disease; peripheral vascular disease; ± typical facies with beaked nose	115,117–120
Atrophic with loss subcutaneous tissue; hypoplastic nails; midface cyanosis; mottled hyperpigmentation	Absence sexual maturation	No	Birdlike facies; death mid-2d decade; anomalous dentition; severe atherosclerosis by age 10; hypercholesterolemia	117,120
Facial eczema age 1; deficiency subQ tissue with skin redundancy	Cryptorchid testes	No	Carious teeth with malocclusion; hyperhidrosis; high-arched palate; ptosis; nystagmus; palmar creases; low-set ears with abnormal auricles; gradual onset bird-headed appearance with prominent beaked nose and micrognathia in adolescence; recurrent infections	122
Lack of subcutaneous tissue; photosensitivity; poikilodermatous changes in sun-exposed skin	± Cryptorchidism	No	Partial deafness; flexion contractures; mental retardation; ataxia; cerebral calcifications; microcephaly	123,124, 128,129, 225
Photosensitivity ± blisters; distinctive erythema → poikilodermatous changes cheeks, ears, extensors, buttocks first at 3–6 months; warty hyperkeratosis; nails normal or small and dystrophic	Yes	Yes	Frontal bossing; broad depressed nasal bridge; microcephaly but mental retardation uncommon; teeth abnormalities uncommon but occasional microdontia, delayed eruption, supernumerary teeth, hypodontia	115,123, 124,128, 129,226

rent episodes of scalp inflammation and/or infection.[132]

GENERALIZED ATROPHIC BENIGN EPIDERMOLYSIS BULLOSA (EB)

Generalized atrophic benign EB, as well as any other forms of dystrophic EB, may lead to focal scarring alopecia. In generalized atrophic benign EB, the scalp hair loss distribution is primarily over the vertex and is associated with an atrophic appearance to the underlying skin. Biopsy of atrophic areas shows fibrosis and an absence of skin appendages. Beard, lashes, brows, and pubic and axillary hair are also sparse or absent but without associated skin atrophy. Alopecia generally does not occur until adolescence,[133] although the blistering process is present from birth. Whether the scalp alopecia is related to the blistering process is unclear, but hair loss certainly occurs in areas without blisters and without cutaneous atrophy.

HALLERMANN-STREIFF SYNDROME

As noted earlier, Hallermann-Streiff syndrome may be associated with diffuse scalp hair thinning, frontal baldness, and patchy nonscarring hair loss, as well as patchy scarring alopecia.[81]

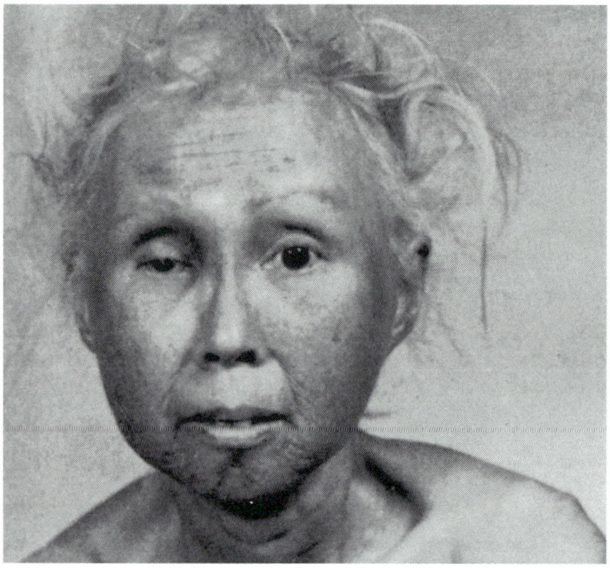

Figure 7-23 A 48-year-old woman with Werner's syndrome. (*Reprinted with permission from Epstein, Martin, Schultz, and Motulsky.*[119])

Figure 7-24 Patient age $6^{1}/_{2}$ years with progeria. Note alopecia, craniofacial dysproportion, prominent eyes, prominent scalp veins, sculptured nose with grooved tip, and spotty skin pigmentation. (*Reprinted with permission from DeBusk.*[121])

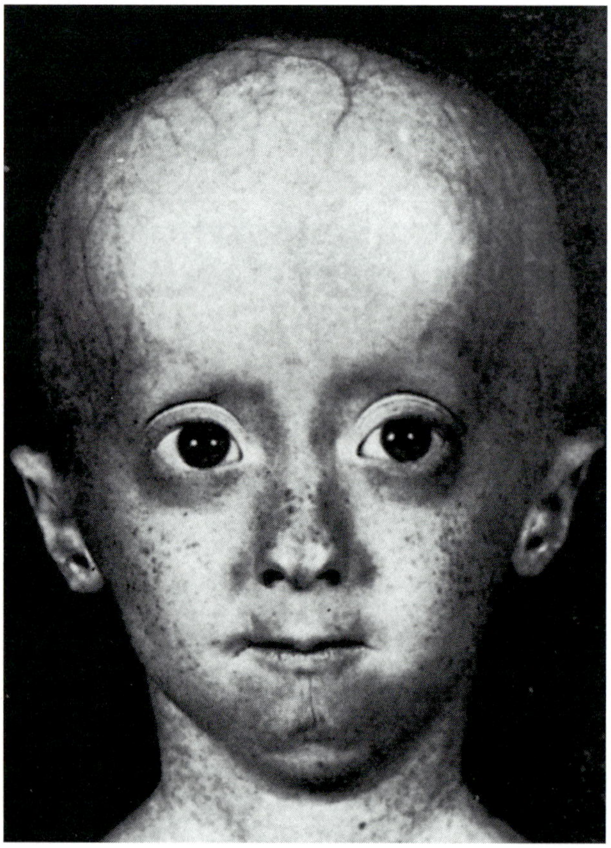

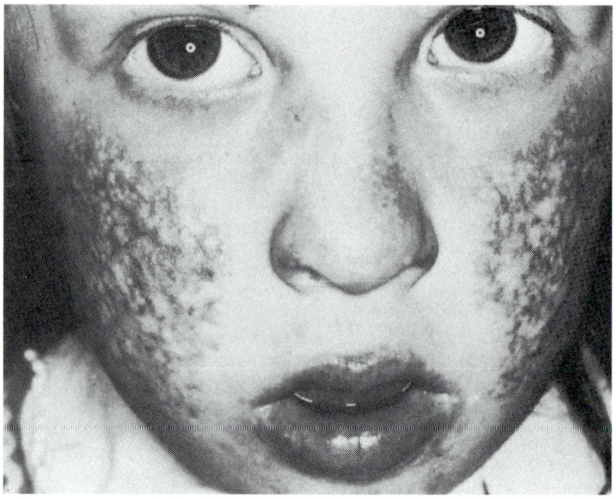

Figure 7-25 Facial poikiloderma seen in Rothmund-Thomson syndrome. (*Reprinted with permission from Gorlin, Pindborg, and Cohen.*[129])

Figure 7-26 Hair loss in a patient with Conradi-Hünermann chondrodysplasia punctata. (*Courtesy of Dr. Nancy Esterly.*)

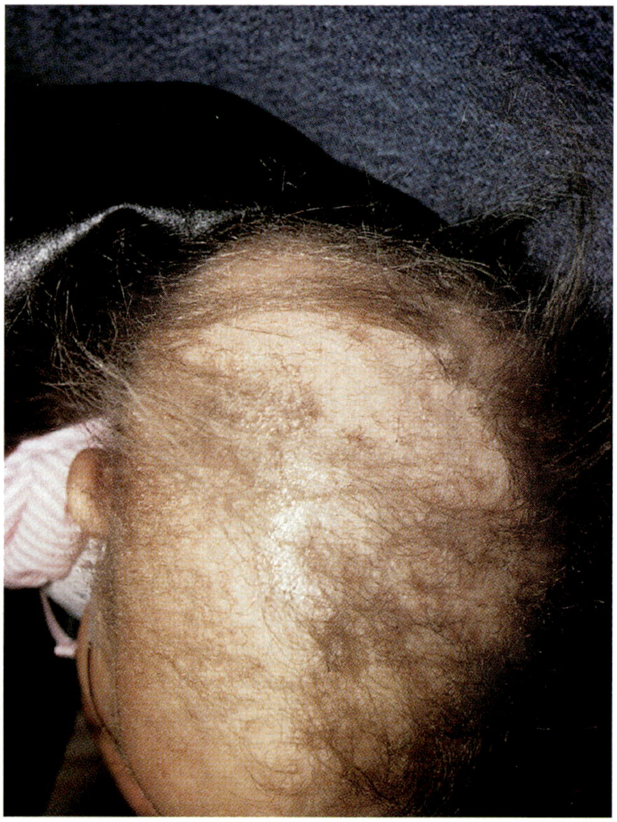

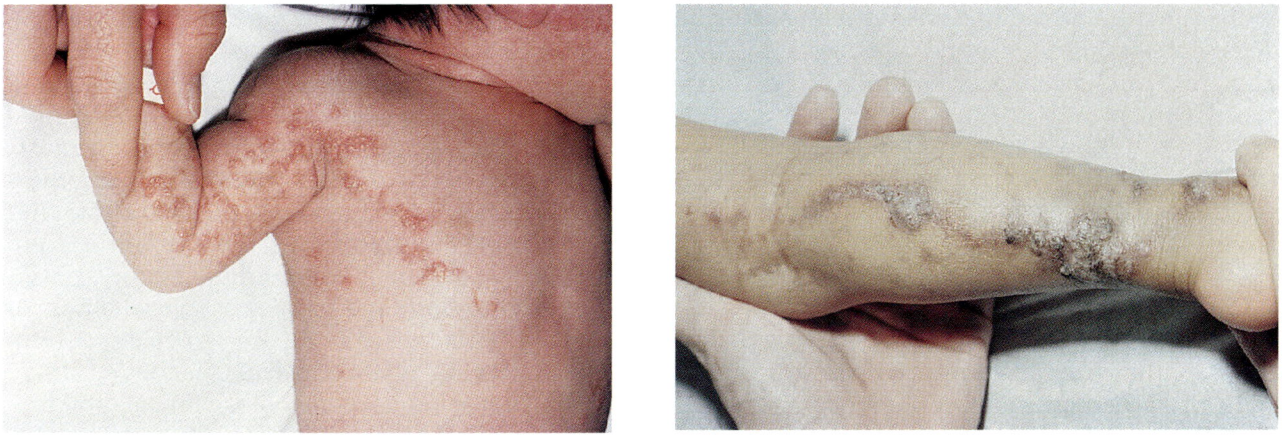

A B

Figure 7-27 Incontinentia pigmenti. (A) Vesicular lesions on the trunk. (B) Verrucous hyperpigmented lesions on the leg. (*Courtesy of Dr. Nancy Esterly.*)

CUTANEOUS TUMOR OR PRIMARY CUTANEOUS DISEASE

Neoplasia, benign or malignant, can lead to focal hair loss in childhood. Primary cutaneous diseases such as lichen planus and discoid lupus erythematosus, although uncommon in children, can lead to a focal scarring or permanent alopecia.

Figure 7-28 Incontinentia pigmenti: scalp involvement in an infant. (*Courtesy of Dr. Nancy Esterly.*)

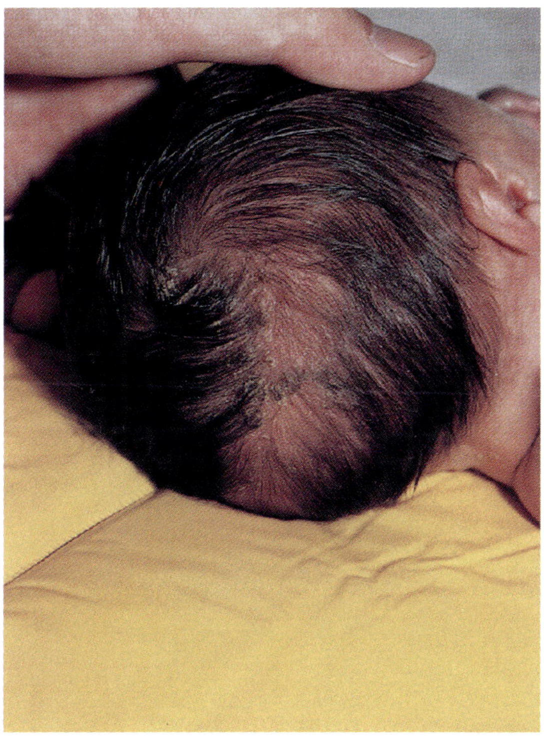

Nonscarring Hair Loss

TRIANGULAR ALOPECIA

Triangular alopecia generally appears at age 2 to 5 but may be present at birth.[134] There is a triangular area of nonscarring hair loss with the base

Figure 7-29 Congenital triangular alopecia. (*Courtesy of Dr. Nancy Esterly.*)

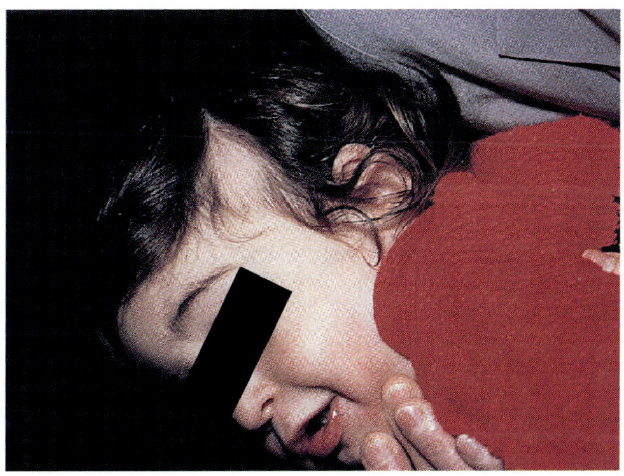

at the junction of the frontal and temporal hairlines and sparing the frontal hairline (Fig. 7-29). The areas of alopecia may be unilateral or bilateral. Histologically, there is a transformation of hairs from terminal to vellus but no signs of destruction of hair follicles. The areas of hair loss are generally persistent.[135] The condition is not inherited.

OTHER CAUSES

Other causes of focal nonscarring alopecia in a child include the relatively common *alopecia areata, tinea capitis, traction alopecia* (which can become scarring), *and trichotillomania. Pityriasis amiantacea* is uncommon and can lead to nonscarring or scarring hair loss. These conditions are all discussed in detail elsewhere in this book (see Chapters 5 and 8).

CONCLUDING REMARKS

The admittedly arbitrary system of classification of hair loss in infancy and childhood presented here should facilitate recognition and diagnosis of the myriad uncommon syndromes or disorders in which hair loss is but a single sign. Dermatologists are in a unique situation as pertains to children with hair loss; by simple history, physical examination, and microscopic evaluation of affected hairs, we may be able to make an elusive or previously unconsidered diagnosis.

Additional microscopic, biochemical, and molecular analyses of affected hairs in these numerous syndromes need to be done: understanding of the mechanism of hair derangement may shed light on the primary abnormality in these disorders and into control of hair growth in general.

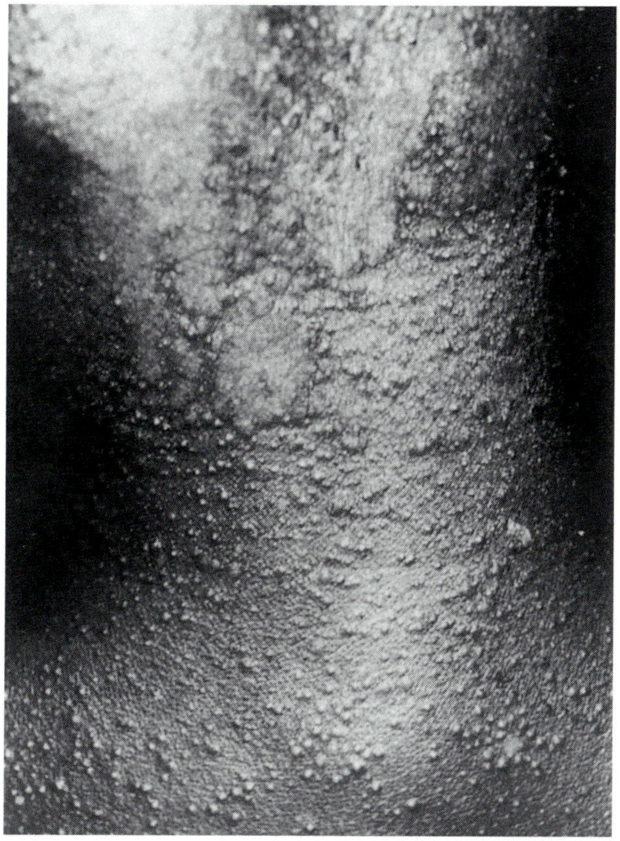

Figure 7-30 Ichthyosis follicularis. Close-up of nape of neck showing follicular spinous papules (See Table 7-4). (*Reprinted with permission from Rothe et al.*[137])

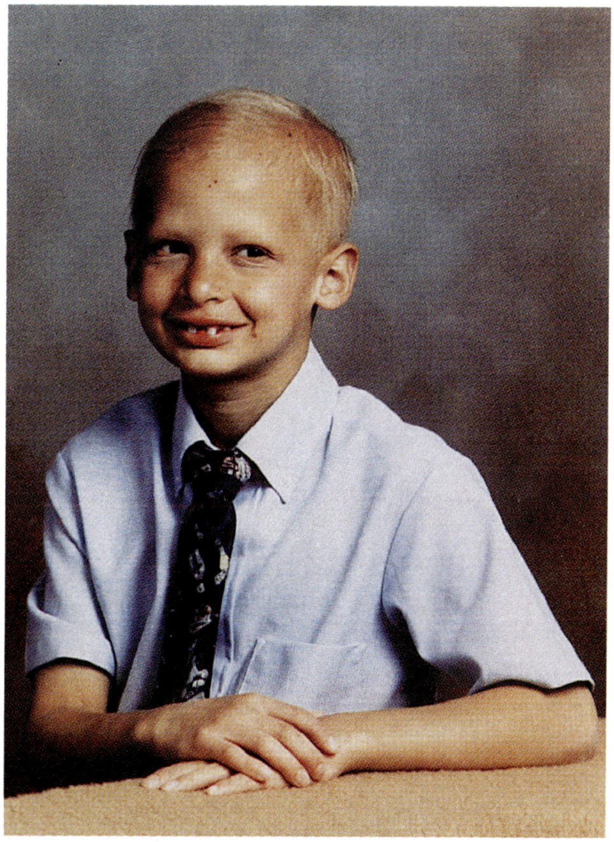

Figure 7-32 Patient with hypohidrotic ectodermal dysplasia (See Table 7-5). (*Courtesy of Dr. Daniel B. Jones.*)

Figure 7-31 Anhidrotic ectodermal dysplasia (See Table 7-5). Patient at age 3 years (left) and 14 years (right). Note characteristic facies and periorbital pigmentation. (*Reprinted with permission from Reed, Lopez, and Landing.*[140])

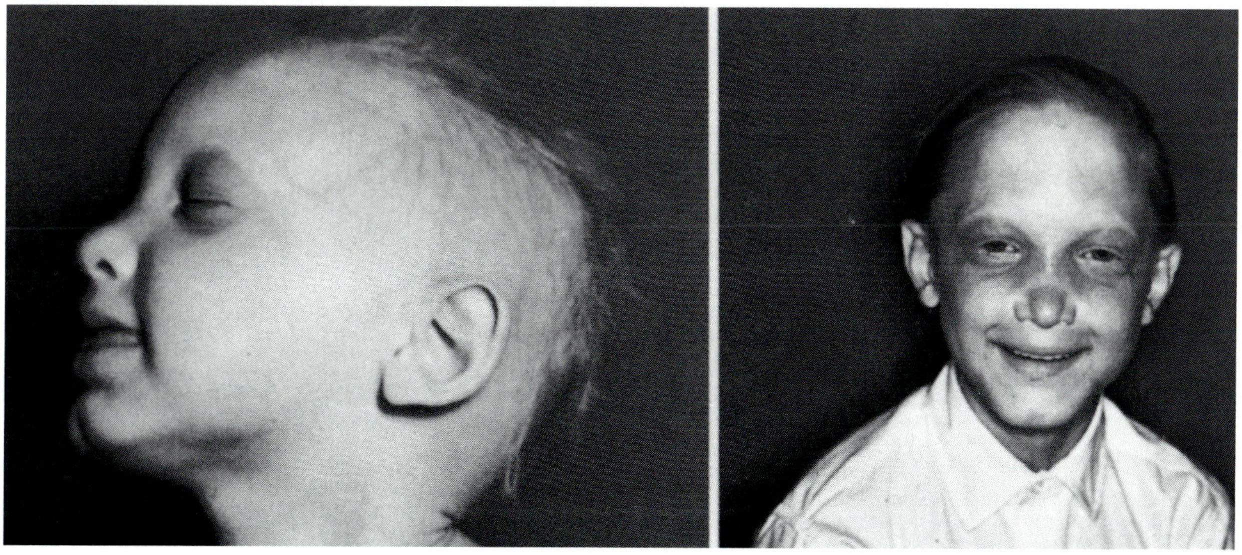

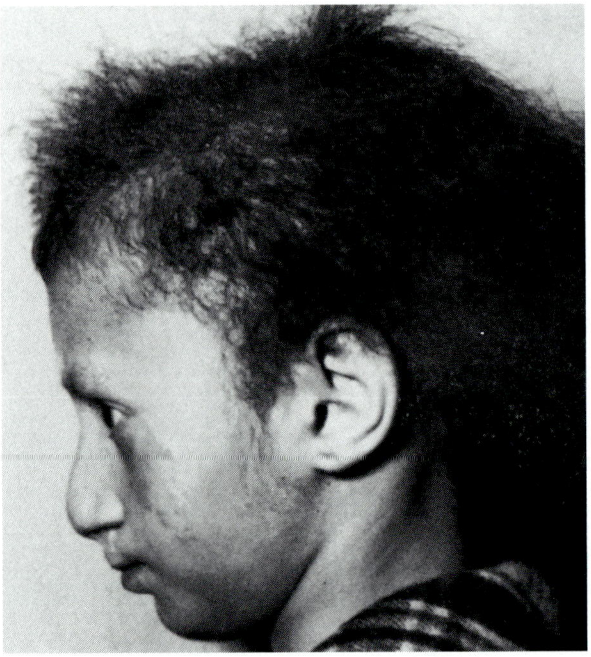

Figure 7-33 Ectodermal dysplasia of Rosselli and Gulienetti (See Table 7-5). (*Reprinted with permission from Rosselli and Gulienetti.*[32])

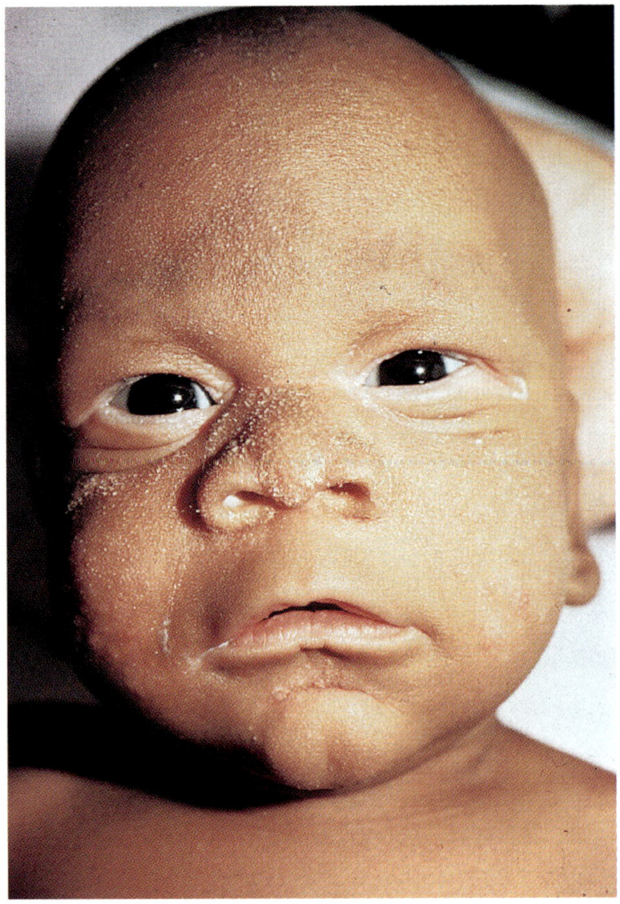

B

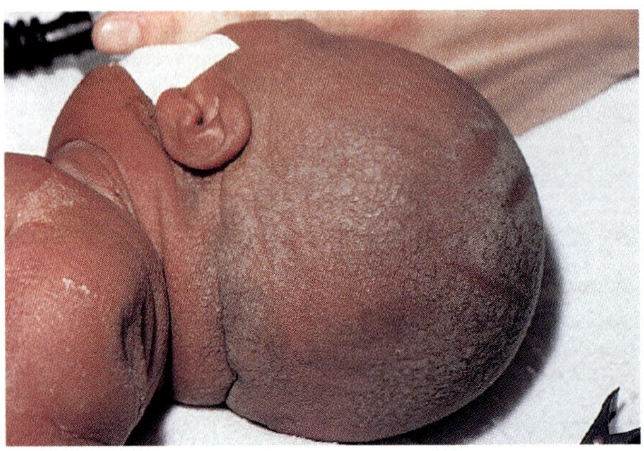

A

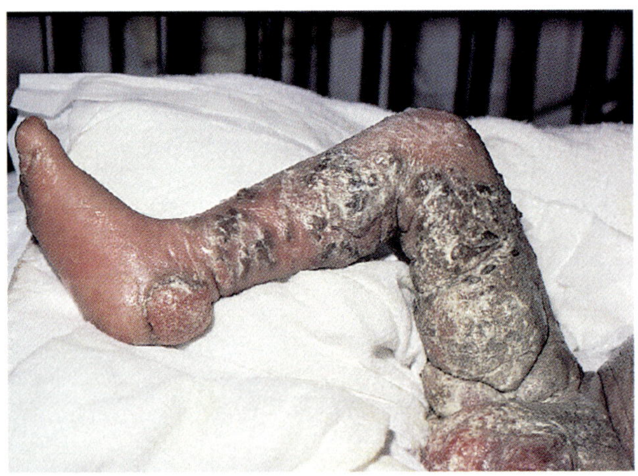

C

Figure 7-34 KID syndrome (See Table 7-5). (*A*) Scalp involvement in an infant. (*B*) Symmetrical facial scaling and plaques. (*C*) Verrucoid hyperkeratosis. (*Courtesy of Nancy Esterly.*)

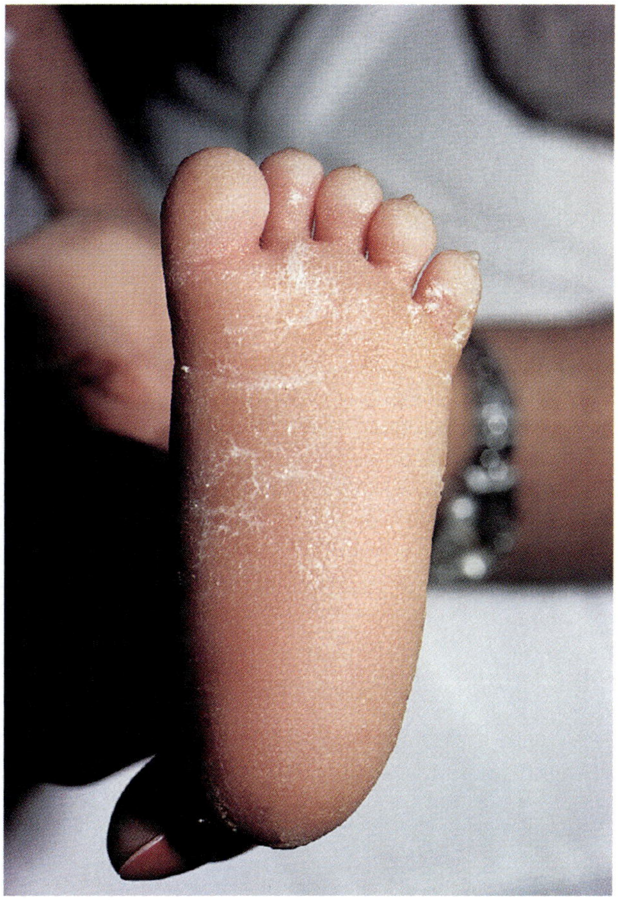

D

Figure 7-34 (*Continued*) (*D*) Leathery Keratoderma soles of feet. (*Courtesy of Dr. Nancy Esterly.*)

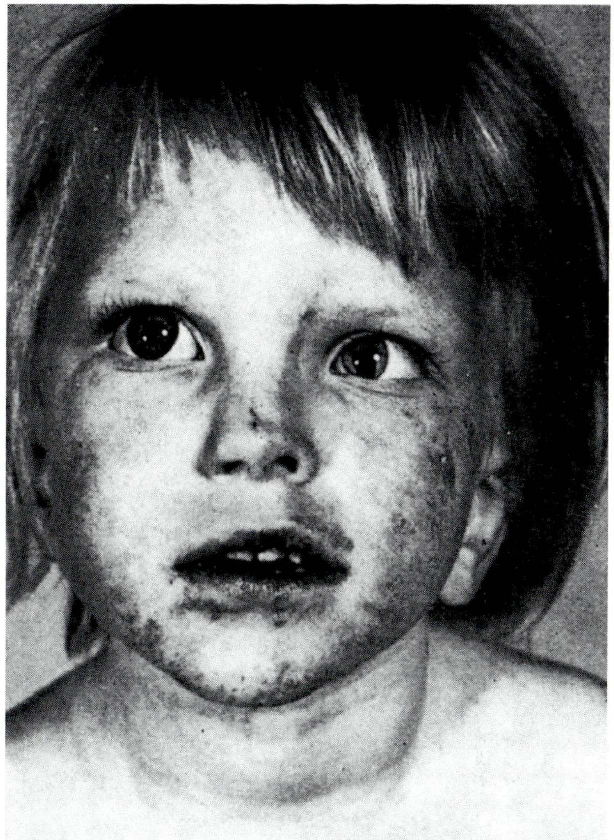

A

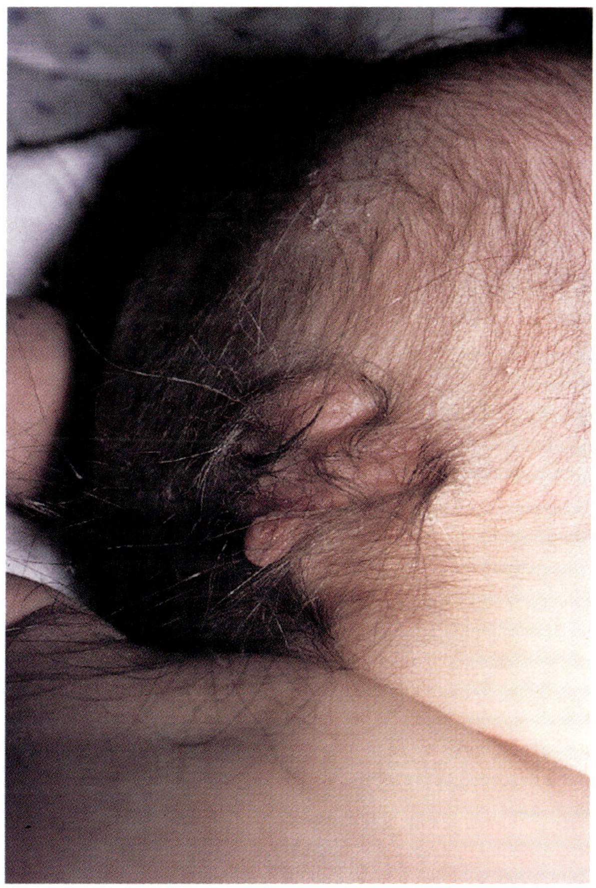

B

Figure 7-35 Focal dermal hypoplasia syndrome (See Table 7-5). (*A*) Underdevelopment left side of face, coloboma left iris, reticular hypoplasia of skin of the nose, cheeks, and chin, papillomas of the lip. (B) papillomas on the scalp. (*Courtesy of Dr. Nancy Esterly.*)

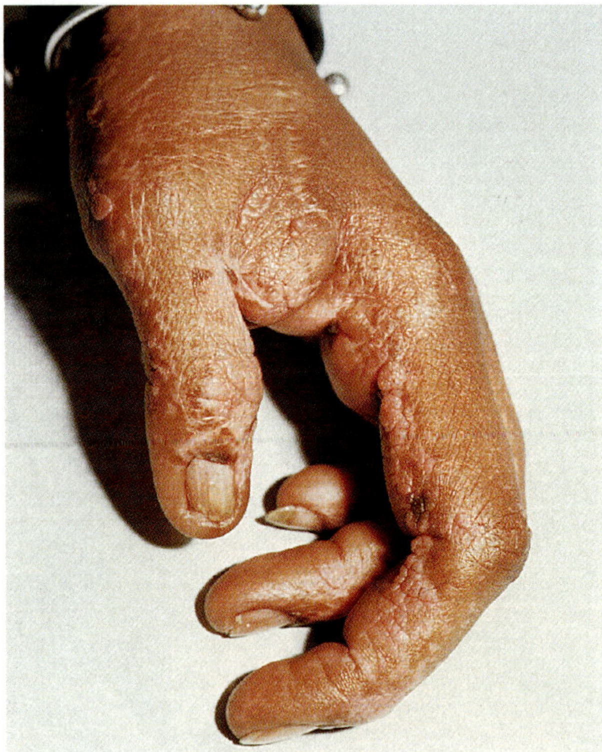

C

Figure 7-35 (*Continued*). (C) Reticular (*Courtesy of Dr. Nancy Esterly.*) (*Reprinted with permission from Goltz, Henderson, Hitch, and Ott.*[95])

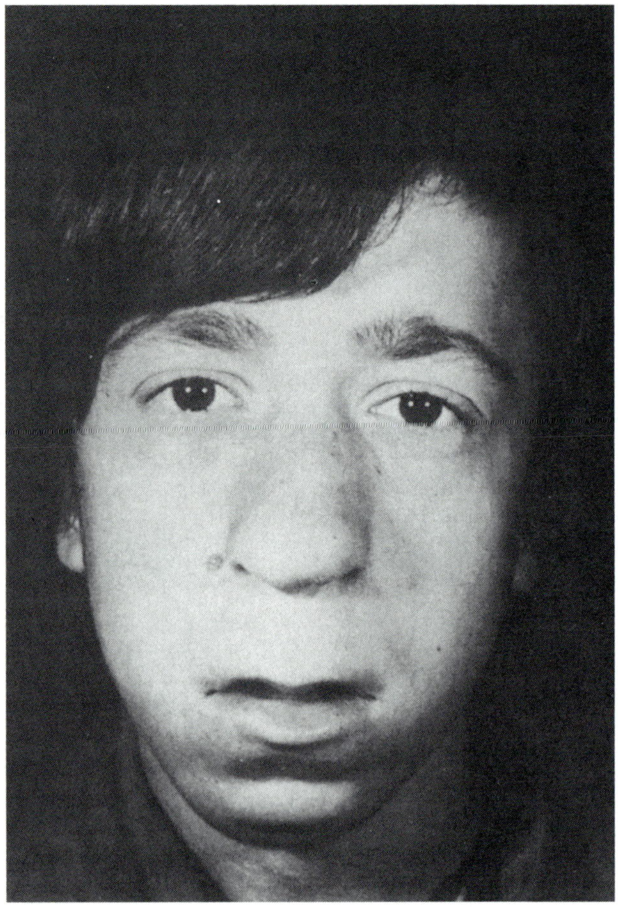

Figure 7-36 Trichorhinophalangeal syndrome. Note pear-shaped nose and long philtrum. (*Reprinted with permission from Kuna, Collipp, and Balsam.*[192])

REFERENCES

1. Barth JH: Normal hair growth in children. Pediatr Dermatol 4:173–184, 1987.
2. Barman JM, Pecoraro V, Astore I, Ferrer J: The first stage in the natural history of the human scalp hair cycle. J Invest Dermatol 48:138–142, 1967.
3. Giacometti L: The anatomy of the human scalp. In *Advances in Biology of Skin,* vol. 6. Oxford, Pergamon Press, 1965, pp 97–120.
4. Oxfords Pergamon Press Duggins OH, Trotter M: Age changes in head hair from birth to maturity: II. Medullation in hair of children. Am J Phys Anthropol 8:399–415, 1950.
5. Trotter M, Duggins OH: Age changes in head hair from birth to maturity: I. Index and size of hair of children. Am J Phys Anthropol 6:489–506, 1948.
6. Danforth CH: Studies on hair, with special reference to hypertrichosis. 12:76–94, 1925.
7. Duggins OH, Trotter M: Changes in morphology of hair during childhood. Ann NY Acad Sci 53:569–575, 1951.
8. Bogaty H: Differences between adult and children's hair. J Soc Cosmetic Chem 20:159–171, 1969.
9. Lundbäck H: Total congenital hereditary alopecia. Acta Derm Venereol 25:189–206, 1945.
10. Baraitser M, Carter CO, Brett EM: A new alopecia/mental retardation syndrome. J Med Genet 20:64–75, 1983.
11. Shokeir MHK: Universal permanent alopecia, psychomotor epilepsy, pyorrhea and mental subnormality. Clin Genet 11:13–17, 1977.
12. Moynahan EJ: Familial congenital alopecia, epilepsy, mental retardation with unusual electroencephalograms. Proc R Soc Med 55:411–412, 1962.
13. Perniola T, Krajewska G, Carnevali F, Lospalluti M: Arch Dermatol Syphilol 12:76–94, 1925 Congenital alopecia, psychomotor retardation, convulsions in two sibs of a consanguineous marriage. J Inher Metab Dis 3:49–53, 1980.
14. Hassing JH, Doeglas HMG: Dystrophia bullosa hereditaria, typus maculatus (Mendes da Costa–van der Valk): A rare genodermatosis. Br J Dermatol 102:474–476, 1980.
15. Carol WLL, Rooij R: Typus Maculatus der Bullosen Hereditaren Dystrophie. Acta Derm Venereol 18:265–283, 1937.
16. Damsté TJ, Prakken JR: Atrichia with papular lesions, a variant of congenital ectodermal dysplasia. Dermatologica 108:114–121, 1954.
17. Loewenthal LJA, Prakken JR: Atrichia with papular lesions. Dermatologica 122:85–89, 1961.
18. del Castillo V, Ruiz-Maldonado R, Carnevale A: Atrichia with papular lesions and mental retardation in two sisters. Int J Dermatol 13:261–265, 1974.
19. Kanzler MH, Rasmussen JE: Atrichia with papular lesions. Arch Dermatol 122:565–567, 1986.
20. Vogt BR, Traupe H, Hamm H: Congenital atrichia with nail dystrophy, abnormal facies, and retarded psychomotor development in two siblings: A new autosomal recessive syndrome? Pediatr Dermatol 5:236–242, 1988.
21. Hall BD, Greenberg MH: Hypomelia-hypotrichosis-facial hemangioma syndrome. Am J Dis Child 123: 602–604, 1972.
22. Nielsen PG, Sjölund E: Epidermolysis bullosa simplex localisata associated with anodontia, hair and nail disorders: A new syndrome. Acta Derm Venereol (Stockh) 65:526–530, 1985.
23. Stevanovic DV: Hereditary hypotrichosis congenita: Marie Unna type. Br J Dermatol 83:331–337, 1970.
24. Wirth G, Bindewald I, Küster W, Goerz G: Hypotrichosis congenita hereditaria Marie Unna. Hautarzt 36:577–580, 1985.
25. Mende B, Kreysel HW: Hypotrichosis Congenita Hereditaria Marie Unna mit Ehlers-Danlos-Syndrom und Atopie. Hautarzt 38:532–535, 1987.
26. Solomon LM, Esterly NB, Medenica M: Hereditary trichodysplasia: Marie Unna's hypotrichosis. J Invest Dermatol 57:389–400, 1971.
27. Bentley-Phillips B, Grace HJ: Hereditary hypotrichosis: A previously undescribed syndrome. Br J Dermatol 101:331–339, 1979.
28. Blackston RD, Brown AC: Cartilage-hair hypoplasia. In Brown AC, Crounse RG (eds): *Hair, Trace Elements and Human Illness.* New York, Praeger, 1980, pp 257– 272.
29. Moloney J: Regional choroidal atrophy and alopecia: A new syndrome. Bull Soc Belge Ophtalmol 224:39–41, 1987.
30. Weech AA: Hereditary ectodermal dysplasia (congenital ectodermal defect). Am J Dis Child 37:766–790, 1929.
31. Freire-Maia N: Ectodermal dysplasias. Hum Hered 21:309–312, 1971.
32. Rosselli D, Gulienetti R: Ectodermal dysplasia. Br J Plast Surg 14:190–204, 1961.
33. Solomon LM, Keuer EJ: The ectodermal dysplasias: Problems of classification and some newer syndromes. Arch Dermatol 116:1295–1299, 1980.
34. Happle R: Genetic diseases of the hair. In Baden HP (ed): *Symposium on Alopecia.* New York, HP Publishing Co., 1987, pp 3–11.
35. Voigtländer V: Pili torti with deafness (Björnstad syndrome): Report of a family. Dermatologica 159:50–54, 1979.
36. Robinson GC, Johnston MM: Pili torti and sensory neural hearing loss. J Pediatr 70:621–623, 1967.
37. Salti IS, Salem Z: Familial hypogonadotropic hypogonadism with alopecia. Can Med Assoc J 121:428–434, 1979.
38. Crandall BF, Samec L, Sparkes RS, Wright SW: A familial syndrome of deafness, alopecia, and hypogonadism. J Pediatr 82:461–465, 1973.
39. Danks DM et al.: Menkes' kinky-hair syndrome. Lancet 1:1100–1102, 1972.
40. Menkes JH et al.: A sex-linked recessive disorder with retardation of growth, peculiar hair, and focal cerebral and cerebellar degeneration. Pediatrics 29:764–779, 1962.
41. Tay CH: Ichthyosiform erythroderma, hair shaft abnormalities, and mental and growth retardation: A new recessive disorder. Arch Dermatol 104:4–13, 1971.
42. Arbisser AI et al.: A syndrome manifested by brittle hair with morphologic and biochemical abnormalities, developmental delay and normal stature. Birth Defects 12:219–228, 1976.
43. Baden HP et al.: The physicochemical properties of hair in the BIDS syndrome. Am J Hum Genet 28:514–521, 1976.

44. Jackson CE, Weiss L, Watson JHL: "Brittle" hair with short stature, intellectual impairment and decreased fertility: An autosomal recessive syndrome in an Amish kindred. Pediatrics 54:201–207, 1974.
45. Jorizzo JL, Crounse RG, Wheeler CE Jr: Lamellar ichthyosis, dwarfism, mental retardation and hair shaft abnormalities: A link between the ichthyosis-associated and BIDS syndromes. J Am Acad Dermatol 2:309–317, 1980.
46. Jorizzo JL, Atherton DJ, Crounse RG, Wells RS: Ichthyosis, brittle hair, impaired intelligence, decreased fertility and short stature (IBIDS syndrome). Br J Dermatol 106:705–710, 1982.
47. Pollitt RJ, Jenner FA, Davies M: Sibs with mental and physical retardation and trichorrhexis nodosa with abnormal amino acid composition of the hair. Arch Dis Child 43:211–216, 1968.
48. Crovato F, Borrone C, Rebora A: Trichothiodystrophy—BIDS, IBIDS and PIBIDS? Br J Dermatol 108:247–251, 1983.
49. Porter PS: The genetics of human hair growth. In Bergsma D (ed): *Birth Defects,* 7(8): 69–85, 1971.
50. Birnbaum PS, Baden HP: Heritable disorders of hair. Dermatol Clin 5:137–153, 1987.
51. Manzke H, Christophers E, Wiedemann H-R: Dominant sex-linked inherited chondrodysplasia punctata: A distinct type of chondrodysplasia punctata. Clin Genet 17:97–107, 1980.
52. Edidin DV, Esterly NB, Bamzai AK, Fretzin DF: Chondrodysplasia punctata: Conradi-Hünermann syndrome. Arch Dermatol 113:1431–1434, 1977.
53. Happle R: X-linked dominant chondrodysplasia punctata: Review of literature and report of a case. Hum Genet 53:65–73, 1979.
54. Plosila M, Kiistala R, Niemi K-M: The Bazex syndrome: follicular atrophoderma with multiple basal cell carcinomas, hypotrichosis and hypohidrosis. Clin Exp Dermatol 6:31–41, 1981.
55. Viksnins P, Berlin A: Follicular atrophoderma and basal cell carcinomas: The Bazex syndrome. Arch Dermatol 113:948–951, 1977.
56. Curth HO: The genetics of follicular atrophoderma. Arch Dermatol 114:1479–1483, 1978.
57. France D: Follicular atrophoderma and hypotrichosis: ? Bazex's syndrome. Br J Dermatol (suppl) 17:32–33, 1979.
58. Patel HP, Unis ME: Pili torti in association with citrullinemia. J Am Acad Dermatol 12:203–206, 1985.
59. Neldner KH, Hambidge KM, Walravens PA: Acrodermatitis enteropathica. Int J Dermatol 17:380–387, 1978.
60. Tucker SB, Schroeter AL, Brown PW, McCall JT: Acquired zinc deficiency: Cutaneous manifestations typical of acrodermatitis enteropathica. JAMA 235:2399–2402, 1976.
61. Eckhert CD, Sloan MV, Duncan JR, Hurley LS: Zinc binding: A difference between human and bovine milk. Science 195:789–790, 1977.
62. Caldwell MD, Jonsson HT, Othersen HB Jr: Essential fatty acid deficiency in an infant receiving prolonged parenteral alimentation. J Pediatr 81:894–898, 1972.
63. Skolnik P, Eaglstein WH, Ziboh VA: Human essential fatty acid deficiency: Treatment by topical application of linoleic acid. Arch Dermatol 113:939–941, 1977.
64. Hansen AE et al.: Role of linoleic acid in infant nutrition. Pediatrics 31(2):171–192, 1963.
65. Holman RT: The ratio of trienoic:tetraenoic acids in tissue lipids as a measure of essential fatty acid requirement. J Nutr 70:405–410, 1960.
66. Burlina AB et al.: Neonatal screening for biotinidase deficiency in north eastern Italy. Eur J Pediatr 147:317–318, 1988.
67. Williams ML, Packman S, Cowan MJ: Alopecia and periorificial dermatitis in biotin-responsive multiple carboxylase deficiency. J Am Acad Dermatol 9:97–103, 1983.
68. Wolf B et al.: Neonatal screening for biotinidase deficiency: An update. J Inher Metab Dis 9(suppl 2):303–306, 1986.
69. Thoene J, Baker H, Yoshino M, Sweetman L: Biotin-responsive carboxylase deficiency associated with subnormal plasma and urinary biotin. N Engl J Med 304:817–820, 1981.
70. Burlina AB, Sherwood WG, Zacchello F: Partial biotinidase deficiency associated with Coffin-Siris syndrome. Eur J Pediatr 149:628–629, 1990.
71. Oizumi J et al.: Partial deficiency of biotinidase activity. J Pediatr 110:818–819, 1987.
72. Munnich A et al.: Fatty-acid-responsive alopecia in multiple carboxylase deficiency. Lancet 1(2):1080–1081, 1980.
73. Johnson AA, Latham MC, Roe DA: An evaluation of the use of changes in hair root morphology in the assessment of protein-calorie malnutrition. Am J Clin Nutr 29:502–511, 1976.
74. Sims RT: Hair growth in kwashiorkor. Arch Dis Child 42:397–400, 1967.
75. Bradfield RB, Jelliffe EFP: Early assessment of malnutrition. Nature 225:283–284, 1970.
76. Bradfield RB, Bailey MA, Cordano A: Hair-root changes in Andean Indian children during marasmic kwashiorkor. Lancet 2(2):1169–1170, 1968.
77. Bradfield RB, Cordano A, Graham GG: Hair-root adaptation to marasmus in Andean Indian children. Lancet 2(2):1395–1397, 1969.
78. Bradfield RB, Bailey MA, Margen S: Morphological changes in human scalp hair roots during deprivation of protein. Science 157:438–439, 1967.
79. Golomb RS, Porter PS: A distinct hair shaft abnormality in the Hallermann-Streiff syndrome. Cutis 16:122–128, 1975.
80. Falls HF, Schull WJ: Hallermann-Streiff syndrome: A dyscephaly with congenital cataracts and hypotrichosis. Arch Ophthalmol 63:409–420, 1960.
81. Grattan CEH, Liddle BJ, Willshaw HE: Atrophic alopecia in the Hallermann-Streiff syndrome. Clin Exp Dermatol 14:250–252, 1989.
82. Francois J: A new syndrome: Dyscephalia with bird face and dental anomalies, nanism, hypotrichosis, cutaneous atrophy, microphthalmia, and congenital cataract. Arch Ophthalmol 60:842–862, 1958.
83. Freire-Maia N, Pinheiro M: *Ectodermal Dysplasias: A Clinical and Genetic Study.* New York, Alan R. Liss, 1984.
84. Peer LA, van Duyn J: Congenital defect of the scalp: Report of a case with fatal termination. Plast Reconstr Surg 3:722–726, 1948.

85. Frieden IJ: Aplasia cutis congenita: A clinical review and proposal for classification. J Am Acad Dermatol 14:646–660, 1986.
86. Ruiz-Maldonado R, Tamayo L: Aplasia cutis congenita, spastic paralysis, and mental retardation. Am J Dis Child 128:699–701, 1974.
87. Sybert VP: Congenital scalp defects with distal limb anomalies (Adams-Oliver syndrome—McKusick 10030): Further suggestion of autosomal recessive inheritance (letter). Am J Med Genet 32:266–267, 1989.
88. Anderson NP, Novy FG Jr: Congenital defect of the scalp. Arch Dermatol 46:257–263, 1942.
89. Brosnan PG et al.: A new familial syndrome of 46,XY gonadal dysgenesis with anomalies of ectodermal and mesodermal structures. J Pediatr 97:586–590, 1980.
90. Finlay AY, Marks R: An hereditary syndrome of lumpy scalp, odd ears and rudimentary nipples. Br J Dermatol 99:423–430, 1978.
91. Mardini MK, Ghandour M, Sakati NA, Nyhan WL: Johanson-Blizzard syndrome in a large inbred kindred with three involved members. Clin Genet 14:247–250, 1978.
92. Baruchin AM, Nahieli O, Golan Y: Oculo-cerebro-cutaneous syndrome: First description in an adult. J Cranio-Maxillo-Facial Surg 20(2):70–72, 1992.
93. Tuffli GA, Laxova R: Brief clinical report: New, autosomal dominant form of ectodermal dysplasia. Am J Med Genet 14:381–384, 1983.
94. Pinheiro M, Penna FJ, Freire-Maia N: Two other cases of ANOTHER syndrome: Family report and update. Clin Genet 35:237–242, 1989.
95. Goltz RW, Henderson RR, Hitch JM, Ott JE: Focal dermal hypoplasia syndrome: A review of the literature and report of two cases. Arch Dermatol 101:1–11, 1970.
96. Gershoni-Baruch R et al.: Johanson-Blizzard syndrome: Clinical spectrum and further delineation of the syndrome. Am J Med Genet 35:546–551, 1990.
97. Jensen NE: Congenital ectodermal dysplasia of the face. Br J Dermatol 84:410–416, 1971.
98. Bart BJ: Epidermolysis bullosa and congenital localized absence of skin. Arch Dermatol 101:78–81, 1970.
99. Happle R, Koch H, Lenz W: The CHILD syndrome: Congenital hemidysplasia with ichthyosiform erythroderma and limb defects. Eur J Pediatr 134:27–33, 1980.
100. Emami S et al.: Peroxisomal abnormality in fibroblasts from involved skin of CHILD syndrome. Arch Dermatol 128:1213–1222, 1992.
101. Toribio J, Quiñones PA: Hereditary hypotrichosis simplex of the scalp. Br J Dermatol 91:687–696, 1974.
102. Gilchrist TC: A case of monilethrix with an unusual distribution. J Cutan Dis 16:157, 1898.
103. Wilkinson RD: Hidrotic ectodermal dysplasia of Clouston: Clinical and histopathological features. In Brown AC (ed): *The First Human Hair Symposium.* New York, Medcom Press, 1973, pp 61–71.
104. Rajagopalan K, Tay CH: Hidrotic ectodermal dysplasia: Study of a large Chinese pedigree. Arch Dermatol 113:481–485, 1977.
105. Gold RJM, Scriver CR: Properties of hair keratin in an autosomal dominant form of ectodermal dysplasia. Am J Hum Genet 24:549–561, 1972.
106. Jorgenson RJ: C47—Ectodermal dysplasia with hypotrichosis, hypohidrosis, defective teeth, and unusual dermatoglyphics (Basan syndrome?). Birth Defects 10:323–325, 1974.
107. Tipton RE, Gorlin RJ: Growth retardation, alopecia, pseudo-anodontia, and optic atrophy—The GAPO syndrome: Report of a patient and review of the literature. Am J Med Genet 19:209–216, 1984.
108. Wajntal A et al.: GAPO syndrome (McKusick 23074)—A connective tissue disorder: Report on two affected sibs and on the pathologic findings in the older. Am J Med Genet 37:213–223, 1990.
109. Beare JM: Congenital pilar defect showing features of pili torti. Br J Dermatol 64:366–372, 1952.
110. Connor JM et al.: Assignment of the gene for dyskeratosis congenita to Xq28. Hum Genet 72:348–351, 1986.
111. Drachtman RA, Alter BP: Dyskeratosis congenita: Clinical and genetic heterogeneity. Am J Pediatr Hematol/Oncol 14(4):297–304, 1992.
112. Connor JM, Teague RH: Dyskeratosis congenita: Report of a large kindred. Br J Dermatol 105:321–325, 1981.
113. Dodd HJ, Devereux S, Sarkany I: Dyskeratosis congenita with pancytopenia. Clin Exp Dermatol 10:73–78, 1985.
114. Sirinavin C, Trowbridge AA: Dyskeratosis congenita: Clinical features and genetic aspects: Report of a family and review of the literature. J Med Genet 12:339–354, 1975.
115. Rook A, Davis R, Stevanovic D: Poikiloderma Congenitale Rothmund-Thomson Syndrome. Acta Derm Venereol 39:392–420, 1959.
116. Tchou P-K, Kohn T: Dyskeratosis congenita: An autosomal dominant disorder. J Am Acad Dermatol 6:1034–1039, 1982.
117. Ruvalcaba RHA et al.: Children who age rapidly—Progeroid syndromes. Clin Pediatr 16:248–252, 1977.
118. Zalla JA: Werner's syndrome. Cutis 25:275–278, 1980.
119. Epstein CJ, Martin GM, Schultz AL, Motulsky AG: Werner's syndrome: A review of its symptomatology, natural history, pathologic features, genetics and relationship to the natural aging process. Medicine 45:177–221, 1966.
120. Gilkes JJH, Sharvill DE, Wells RS: The premature ageing syndromes: Report of eight cases and description of a new entity named metageria. Br J Dermatol 91:243–262, 1974.
121. DeBusk FL: The Hutchinson-Gilford progeria syndrome: Report of 4 cases and review of the literature. J Pediatr 80:697–724, 1972.
122. Fitch N, Pinsky L, Lachance RC: A form of bird-headed dwarfism with features of premature senility. Am J Dis Child 120:260–264, 1970.
123. Landing BH, Sugarman G, Dixon LG: Eccrine sweat gland anatomy in Cockayne syndrome: A possible diagnostic aid. Pediatr Pathol 1:349–353, 1983.
124. Moyer DB, Marquis P, Shertzer ME, Burton BK: Brief clinical report: Cockayne syndrome with early onset of manifestations. Am J Med Genet 13:225–230, 1982.
125. Johnson RT, Squires S: The XPD complementation group: Insights into xeroderma pigmentosum, Cockayne's syndrome and trichothiodystrophy. Mutat Res, DNA Repair 273:97–118, 1992.
126. Greenhaw GA et al.: Xeroderma pigmentosum and Cockayne syndrome: Overlapping clinical and biochemical phenotypes. Am J Hum Genet 50:677–689, 1992.

127. Macdonald WB, Fitch KD, Lewis IC: Cockayne's syndrome: An heredo-familial disorder of growth and development. Pediatrics 25:997–1007, 1960.
128. Lasser AE: Cockayne's syndrome. Cutis 10:143–148, 1972.
129. Gorlin RJ, Pindborg JJ, Cohen MM Jr: Rothmund-Thomson syndrome. In *Syndromes of the Head and Neck,* 2d ed. New York, McGraw-Hill, 1976, pp 652–656.
130. Kolde G, Happle R: Histologic and ultrastructural features of the ichthyotic skin in X-linked dominant chondrodysplasia punctata. Acta Derm Venereol (Stockh) 64:389–394, 1984.
131. Carney RG Jr: Incontinentia pigmenti: A world statistical analysis. Arch Dermatol 112:535–542, 1976.
132. Hay RJ, Wells RS: The syndrome of ankyloblepharon, ectodermal defects and cleft lip and palate: An autosomal dominant condition. Br J Dermatol 94:277–289, 1976.
133. Hintner H, Wolff K: Generalized atrophic benign epidermolysis bullosa. Arch Dermatol 118:375–384, 1982.
134. Kubba R, Rook A: Congenital triangular alopecia. Br J Dermatol 95:657–659, 1976.
135. Minars N: Congenital temporal alopecia. Arch Dermatol 109:395–396, 1974.
136. Eramo LR et al.: Ichthyosis follicularis with alopecia and photophobia. Arch Dermatol 121:1167–1174, 1985.
137. Rothe MJ et al.: Ichthyosis follicularis in two girls: An autosomal dominant disorder. Pediatr Dermatol 7:287–292, 1990.
138. Rand R, Baden HP: Keratosis follicularis spinulosa decalvans: Report of two cases and literature review. Arch Dermatol 119:22–26, 1983.
139. Appell ML, Sherertz EF: A kindred with alopecia, keratosis pilaris, cataracts, and psoriasis. J Am Acad Dermatol 16:89–95, 1987.
140. Reed WB, Lopez DA, Landing B: Clinical spectrum of anhidrotic ectodermal dysplasia. Arch Dermatol 102:134–143, 1970.
141. Passarge E, Nuzum CT, Schubert WK: Anhidrotic ectodermal dysplasia as autosomal recessive trait in an inbred kindred. Humangenetik 3:181–185, 1966.
142. Clarke A, Phillips DIM, Brown R, Harper PS: Clinical aspects of X-linked hypohidrotic ectodermal dysplasia. Arch Dis Child 62:989–996, 1987.
143. Clouston HR: The major forms of hereditary ectodermal dysplasia. Can Med Assoc J 40:1–7, 1939.
144. Rapp RS, Hodgkin WE: Anhidrotic ectodermal dysplasia: Autosomal dominant inheritance with palate and lip anomalies. J Med Genet 5:269–272, 1968.
145. Wannarachue N, Hall BD, Smith DW: Ectodermal dysplasia and multiple defects (Rapp-Hodgkins type) (letter). J Pediatr 81(2):1217–1218, 1972.
146. Bocian M, Rimoin DL: A new autosomal dominant syndrome of hypohidrotic ectodermal dysplasia and unusual facies. Birth Defects 15(5B):239–251, 1979.
147. Summitt RL, Hiatt RL: Hypohidrotic ectodermal dysplasia with multiple associated anomalies. Birth Defects. 7(8):121–124, 1971.
148. Salinas CF, Montes-G GM: Rapp-Hodgkin syndrome: Observations on ten cases and characteristic hair changes (pili canaliculi). Birth Defects 24:149–168, 1988.
149. Brill CB, Hsu LYF, Hirschhorn K: The syndrome of ectrodactyly, ectodermal dysplasia and cleft lip and palate: Report of a family demonstrating a dominant inheritance pattern. Clin Genet 3:295–302, 1972.
150. Penchaszadeh VB, de Negrotti TC: Ectrodactyly-ectodermal dysplasia-clefting (EEC) syndrome: Dominant inheritance and variable expression. J Med Genet 13:281–284, 1976.
151. Preus M, Fraser FC: The lobster claw defect with ectodermal defects, cleft lip-palate, tear duct anomaly and renal anomalies. Clin Genet 4:369–375, 1973.
152. Küster W, Majewski F, Meinecke P: EEC syndrome without ectrodactyly? Report of 8 cases. Clin Genet 28:130–135, 1985.
153. Rüdiger RA, Haase W, Passarge E: Association of ectrodactyly, ectodermal dysplasia, and cleft lip-palate. Am J Dis Child 120:160–163, 1970.
154. Moynahan EJ: XTE syndrome (xeroderma, talipes and enamel defect): A new heredo-familial syndrome. Two cases: Homozygous inheritance of a dominant gene. Proc R Soc Med 63:447–448, 1970.
155. Spiegel J, Colton A: AEC syndrome: Ankyloblepharon, ectodermal defects, and cleft lip and palate. J Am Acad Dermatol 12:810–815, 1985.
156. Greene SL, Michels VV, Doyle JA: Variable expression in ankyloblepharon-ectodermal defects-cleft lip and palate syndrome. Am J Med Genet 27:207–212, 1987.
157. McGrae JD Jr: Keratitis, ichthyosis, and deafness (KID) syndrome. Int J Dermatol 29:89–92, 1990.
158. Cram DL, Resneck JS, Jackson WB: A congenital ichthyosiform syndrome with deafness and keratitis. Arch Dermatol 115:467–471, 1979.
159. Senter TP, Jones KL, Sakati N, Nyhan WL: Atypical ichthyosiform erythroderma and congenital neurosensory deafness—A distinct syndrome. J Pediatr 92:68–72, 1978.
160. Rycroft RJG, Moynahan EJ, Wells RS: Atypical ichthyosiform erythroderma, deafness and keratitis. Br J Dermatol 94:211–217, 1976.
161. Soderquist NA, Reed WB: Pachyonychia congenita with epidermal cysts and other congenital dyskeratoses. Arch Dermatol 97:31–33, 1968.
162. Su WPD, Chun SI, Hammond DE, Gordon H: Pachyonychia congenita: A clinical study of 12 cases and review of the literature. Pediatr Dermatol 7:33–38, 1990.
163. Tidman MJ, Wells RS, MacDonald DM: Pachyonychia congenita with cutaneous amyloidosis and hyperpigmentation—A distinct variant. J Am Acad Dermatol 16:935–940, 1987.
164. Feinstein A, Friedman J, Schewach-Millet M: Pachyonychia congenita. J Am Acad Dermatol 19:705–711, 1988.
165. Stieglitz JB, Centerwall WR: Pachyonychia congenita (Jadassohn-Lewandowsky syndrome): A seventeen-member, four-generation pedigree with unusual respiratory and dental involvement. Am J Med Genet 14:21–28, 1983.
166. Clementi M et al.: Pachyonychia congenita Jackson-Lawler type: A distinct malformation syndrome. Br J Dermatol 114:367–370, 1986.
167. Haber RM, Rose TH: Autosomal recessive pachyonychia congenita. Arch Dermatol 122:919–923, 1986.
168. Ruiz-Maldonado R, Carnevale A, Tamayo L, de Montiel EM: Focal dermal hypoplasia. Clin Genet 6:36–45, 1974.

169. Hall EH, Terezhalmy GT: Focal dermal hypoplasia syndrome: Case report and literature review. J Am Acad Dermatol 9:443–451, 1983.
170. Goltz RW: Focal dermal hypoplasia syndrome: An update. Arch Dermatol 128:1108–1111, 1992.
171. Gorlin RJ, Chaudhry AP, Moss ML: Craniofacial dysostosis, patent ductus arteriosus, hypertrichosis, hypoplasia of labia majora, dental and eye anomalies: A new syndrome? J Pediatr 56:778–785, 1960.
172. Pabst HF, Groth O, McCoy EE: Hypohidrotic ectodermal dysplasia with hypothyroidism. J Pediatr 98:223–227, 1981.
173. Pike MG, Baraitser M, Dinwiddie R, Atherton DJ: A distinctive type of hypohidrotic ectodermal dysplasia featuring hypothyroidism. J Pediatr 108:109–111, 1986.
174. Morris CA, Carey JC, Demsey SA: Another case of another syndrome (hypohydrotic ectodermal dysplasia with hypothyroidism). Proc Greenwood Genet Center 6:145–146, 1987.
175. Coffin GS, Siris E: Mental retardation with absent fifth fingernail and terminal phalanx. Am J Dis Child 119:433–439, 1970.
176. Meinecke P, Engelbrecht R, Schaefer E: Coffin-Siris Syndrom bei einem 5jährigen Mädchen. Monatsschr Kinderheilkd 134:692–695, 1986.
177. Pinheiro M, Pereira LC, Freire-Maia N: A previously undescribed condition: Tricho-odonto-onycho-dermal syndrome. A review of the tricho-odonto-onychial subgroup of ectodermal dysplasias. Br J Dermatol 105:371–382, 1981.
178. Carey JC, Hall BD: The Coffin-Siris syndrome. Am J Dis Child 132:667–671, 1978.
179. Wilsch L, Haneke E, Schaidt G: Structural hair abnormalities in hidrotic ectodermal dysplasia (HED). Arch Dermatol Res 259:101–103, 1977.
180. Fulk CS: Hidrotic ectodermal dysplasia: Report of a case with reticulated acropigmentation. J Am Acad Dermatol 6:476–480, 1982.
181. Quattromani F et al.: Clinical heterogeneity in the tricho-dento-osseous syndrome. Hum Genet 64:117–121, 1983.
182. Crawford PJM, Aldred MJ: Amelogenesis imperfecta with taurodontism and the tricho-dento-osseous syndrome: Separate conditions or a spectrum of disease? Clin Genet 38:44–50, 1990.
183. Lichtenstein J et al.: The tricho-dento-osseous (TDO) syndrome. Am J Hum Genet 24:569–582, 1972.
184. Sensenbrenner JA, Dorst JP, Owens RP: R–New syndrome of skeletal, dental and hair anomalies. Birth Defects 11(2):372–379, 1975.
185. Happle R: Lyonization and the lines of Blaschko. Hum Genet 70:200–206, 1985.
186. El-Benhawi MO, George WM: Incontinentia pigmenti: A review. Cutis 41:259–262, 1988.
187. Ellis J, Dawber RPR: Ectodermal dysplasia syndrome: A family study. Clin Exp Dermatol 5:295–304, 1980.
188. Witkop CJ Jr, Brearley LJ, Gentry WC Jr: Hypoplastic enamel, onycholysis, and hypohidrosis inherited as an autosomal dominant trait. Oral Surg 39:71–86, 1975.
189. Giedion A et al.: Autosomal-dominant transmission of the tricho-rhino-phalangeal syndrome: Report of 4 unrelated families, review of 60 cases. Helv Paediatr Acta 28:249–259, 1973.
190. Langer LO Jr et al.: The tricho-rhino-phalangeal syndrome with exostoses (or Langer-Giedion syndrome): Four additional patients without mental retardation and review of the literature. Am J Med Genet 19:81–111, 1984.
191. Gorlin RJ, Cohen MM Jr, Wolfson J: Tricho-rhino-phalangeal syndrome. Am J Dis Child 118:595–599, 1969.
192. Kuna GB, Collipp PJ, Balsam D: Trichorhinophalangeal dysplasia (Giedion syndrome). Clin Pediatr 17:96–98, 1978.
193. Pashayan HM, Solomon LM, Chan G: The tricho-rhino-phalangeal syndrome. Am J Dis Child 127:257–261, 1974.
194. Hall JG: Tricho-rhino-phalangeal syndrome, type II. In Bergsma D (ed): *Birth Defects Compendium,* 2d ed. New York, Alan R. Liss, 1979, p 1043.
195. Gorlin RJ, Pindborg JJ, Cohen MM Jr: Chondroectodermal dysplasia (Ellis-van Creveld syndrome). In *Syndromes of the Head and Neck,* 2d ed. New York, McGraw-Hill, 1976, pp 80–85.
196. Ellis RWB, van Creveld S: A syndrome characterized by ectodermal dysplasia, polydactyly, chondro-dysplasia and congenital morbus cordis. Arch Dis Child 15:65–84, 1940.
197. Burket JM, Burket BJ, Burket DA: Eyelid cysts, hypodontia, and hypotrichosis. J Am Acad Dermatol 10:922–925, 1984.
198. Alves AFP, dos Santos PAB, Castelo-Branco-Neto E, Freire-Maia N: Brief clinical report: An autosomal recessive ectodermal dysplasia syndrome of hypotrichosis, onychodysplasia, hyperkeratosis, kyphoscoliosis, cataract, and other manifestations. Am J Med Genet 10:213–218, 1981.
199. O'Rourk TR Jr, Bravos A: H—An oculo-dento-digital dysplasia. Birth Defects 5(2):226–227, 1969.
200. Coté GB, Adamopoulos D, Pantelakis S: Arthrogryposis and ectodermal dysplasia. Hum Hered 32:71–72, 1982.
201. Tsakalakos N, Jordaan FH, Taljaard JJF, Hough SF: A previously undescribed ectodermal dysplasia of the tricho-odonto-onychial subgroup in a family. Arch Dermatol 122:1047–1053, 1986.
202. Pinheiro M, Freire-Maia N, Roth AJ: Trichoodonto-onychial dysplasia—A new meso-ectodermal dysplasia. Am J Med Genet 15:67–70, 1983.
203. Pinheiro M, Freire-Maia N, Gollop TR: Odonto-onychodysplasia with alopecia: A new pure ectodermal dysplasia with probable autosomal recessive inheritance. Am J Med Genet 20:197–202, 1985.
204. Cecatto-de-Lima L, Pinheiro M, Freire-Maia N: Oculotrichodysplasia (OTD): A new probably autosomal recessive condition. J Med Genet 25:430–432, 1988.
205. Swanson AG: Congenital insensitivity to pain with anhydrosis. Arch Neurol 8:299–306, 1963.
206. Freire-Maia N, Cat I, Rapone-Gaidzinski R: An ectodermal dysplasia syndrome of alopecia, onychodysplasia, hypohidrosis, hyperkeratosis, deafness and other manifestations. Hum Hered 27:127–133, 1977.
207. Gorlin RJ, Psaume J: Orodigitofacial dysostosis—A new syndrome. J Pediatr 61:520–530, 1962.
208. Whelan DR, Feldman W, Dost I: The oro-facial-digital syndrome. Clin Genet 8:205–212, 1975.
209. Killian W, Zonana J, Schroer RJ: Abnormal hair, cranio-

facial dysmorphism, and severe mental retardation—A new syndrome? J Clin Dysmorphol 1(3):6–13, 1983.
210. Martinez B, Monasterio L, Pinheiro M, Freire-Maia N: Cleft lip/palate-oligodontia-syndactyly-hair alterations, a new syndrome: Review of the conditions combining ectodermal dysplasia and cleft lip/palate. Am J Med Genet 27:23–31, 1987.
211. Mikaelian DO, der Kaloustian VM, Shahin NA, Barsoumian VM: Congenital ectodermal dysplasia with hearing loss. Arch Otolaryngol 92:85–89, 1970.
212. Salinas CF, Spector M: Tricho-dental syndrome: A new syndrome with autosomal dominant inheritance? (abstract). J Dent Res 58:268, 1979
213. Wilson WG et al.: "New" ectodermal dysplasia syndrome with distinctive facial appearance and preaxial polydactyly of feet. Am J Med Genet 34:227–229, 1989.
214. Johnston K et al.: Alopecia-anosmia-deafness-hypogonadism syndrome revisited: Report of a new case. Am J Med Genet 26:925–927, 1987.
215. Johnson VP, McMillin JM, Aceto T Jr, Bruins G: A Newly Recognized Neuroectodermal Syndrome of Familial Alopecia, Anosmia, Deafness, and Hypogonadism. Am J Med Genet 15:497–506, 1983.
216. Stevanovic DV: Alopecia congenita. Acta Genet 9:127–132, 1959.
217. Hernández A, Olivares F, Cantú J-M: Autosomal recessive onychotrichodysplasia, chronic neutropenia and mild mental retardation. Clin Genet 15:147–152, 1979.
218. Verhage J et al.: A patient with onychotrichodysplasia, neutropenia and normal intelligence. Clin Genet 31:374–380, 1987.
219. Freire-Maia N, Pinheiro M, Fernandes-dos-Santos A: Xerodermia como sinal mais grave num quandro de displasia ectodérmica pura com etiologia genética. Cienc Cult Suppl 34:764, 1982.
220. Gatti RA et al.: Hereditary lymphopenic agammaglobulinemia associated with a distinctive form of short-limbed dwarfism and ectodermal dysplasia. J Pediatr 75:675–684, 1969.
221. Schinzel A: A case of multiple skeletal anomalies, ectodermal dysplasia, and severe growth and mental retardation. Helv Paediatr Acta 35:243–251, 1980.
222. Wallis C, Ip FSL, Beighton P: Cataracts, alopecia, and sclerodactyly: A previously apparently undescribed ectodermal dysplasia syndrome on the island of Rodrigues. Am J Med Genet 32:500–503, 1989.
223. Zerres K, Holtgrave E-A: The Johanson-Blizzard syndrome: Report of a new case with special reference to the dentition and review of the literature. Clin Genet 30:177–183, 1986.
224. Daentl DL, Frias JL, Gilbert EF, Opitz JM: The Johanson-Blizzard syndrome: Base report and autopsy findings. Am J Med Genet 3:129–135, 1979.
225. Greenhaw GA et al.: Xeroderma pigmentosum and Cockayne syndrome: Overlapping clinical and biochemical phenotypes. Am J Hum Genet 50:677–689, 1992.
226. Taylor WB: Rothmund's syndrome—Thomson's syndrome. Arch Dermatol 75:236–244, 1957.

Chapter

8

ALOPECIA AREATA

Maria K. Hordinsky

CLINICAL FEATURES

Hair

Alopecia areata is a nonscarring, recurrent, sometimes treatment-refractory hair disease which can potentially cause hair loss in any hair-bearing area. Alopecia areata commonly presents as round or oval patches of hair loss, loss of all scalp hair (alopecia totalis), loss of all body hair (alopecia universalis), or an ophiasis (bandlike) pattern of hair loss. Examples of these forms are shown in Figure 8-1. Patients with the reticular variant of patchy alopecia areata experience loss of hair in one site concurrent with spontaneous hair regrowth in another area of hair loss. This type of activity may go on for months to years. Less common presentations include diffuse scalp alopecia areata and perinevoid alopecia areata. Individuals with the diffuse variant of alopecia areata are unable to grow long anagen hairs in involved areas and may appear as if they have androgenetic alopecia or trichotillomania when the disease process is restricted to the top of the head (Fig. 8-2). Perinevoid alopecia areata is quite rare and is characterized by alopecia areata developing around pigmented nevi.[1]

In early, active alopecia areata, the hair cycle is disrupted and the expected ratio of anagen, catagen, and telogen for that site is abnormal, with most hair follicles entering the telogen or late catagen stage.[2] To the patient, the hairs which fall out have "roots" and, when examined under the microscope, these are telogen hairs. Fractured hairs (which appear as black dots) can also be seen at the active margins of alopecia areata. These hairs are commonly described by the clinician as "exclamation-mark" hairs because the distal segment is broader than the proximal end (Fig. 8-3). Such hairs are telogen hairs and, as such, are easily extracted from the scalp.[3] Damage involving both the cortex and the medulla in these exclamation-point hairs may result in distal fractures. The cuticular architec-

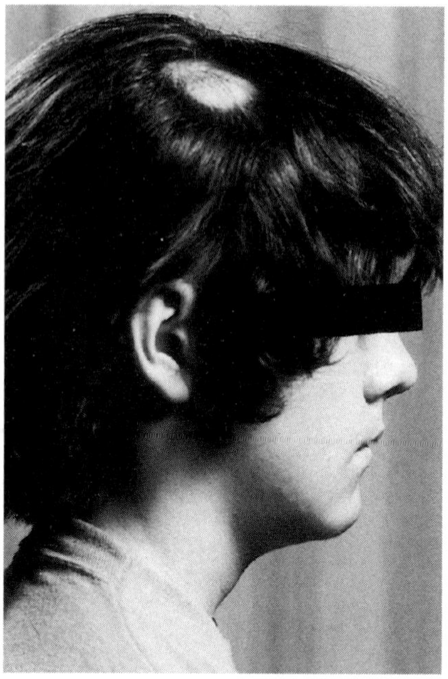

A

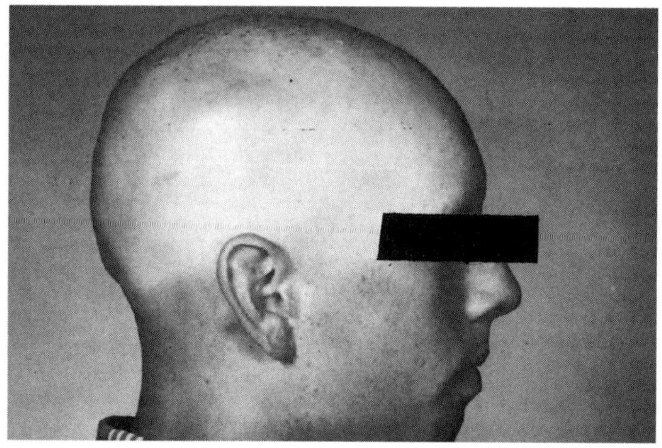

B

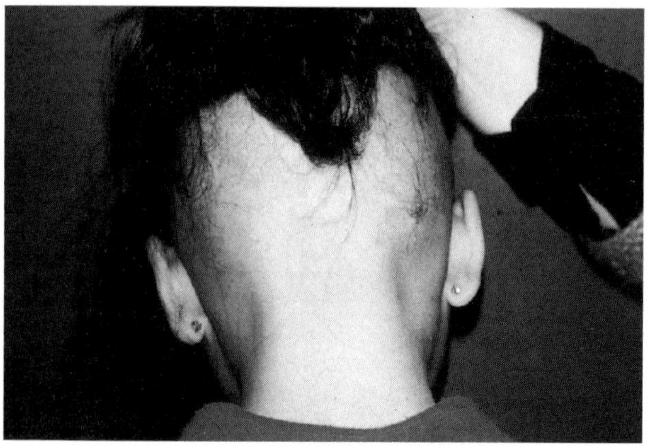

C

Figure 8-1 (*A*) Classic presentation of patchy alopecia areata. (*B*) Extensive scalp hair loss as seen in patients with alopecia totalis or alopecia universalis. (*C*) Alopecia areata in the ophiasis region.

ture is generally preserved to the distal fracture, but a longitudinal fissure may be present.[3]

Hair pigment is often affected in alopecia areata. Frequently, alopecia areata will affect only pigmented hairs and spare unpigmented or white hairs. The initial regrowth in alopecia areata is often white.

Patients who do not recover completely from their episode of active alopecia areata may experience persistent, chronic loss of hair characterized by the affected hair follicles arresting in either late telogen or early anagen. Other patients may experience partial telogen-to-anagen conversion and show short, white, "fuzzy" hairs on the surface of affected areas.[4]

Nails

The frequency of nail changes in patients with alopecia areata ranges from 10 to 66 percent.[5] Nail pitting is the most commonly seen abnormality, but other reported nail plate changes include longitudinal ridging, koilonychia, brittle nails, spotting of the lunula, onycholysis, and onychomadesis (Fig. 8-4). Anonychia and scarring are not seen. These changes have been ob-

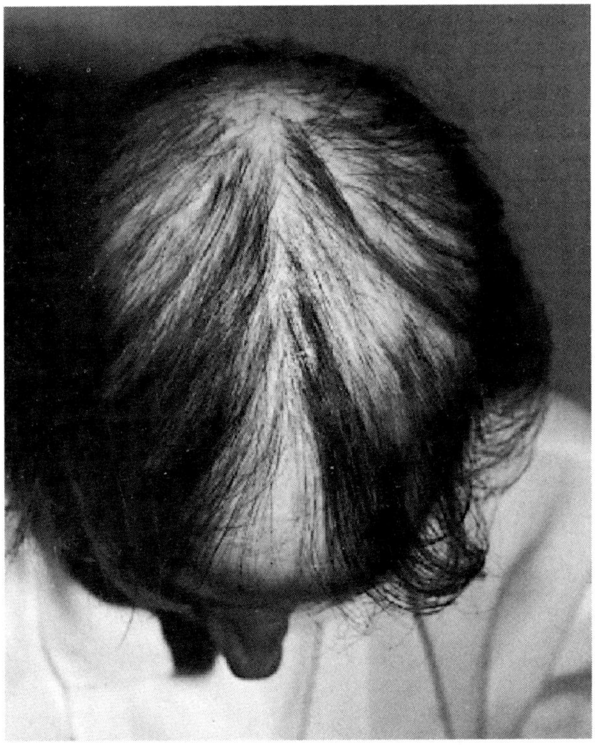

Figure 8-2 Diffuse variant of alopecia areata mimicking androgenetic alopecia. (*Courtesy of Dr. Elise A. Olsen.*)

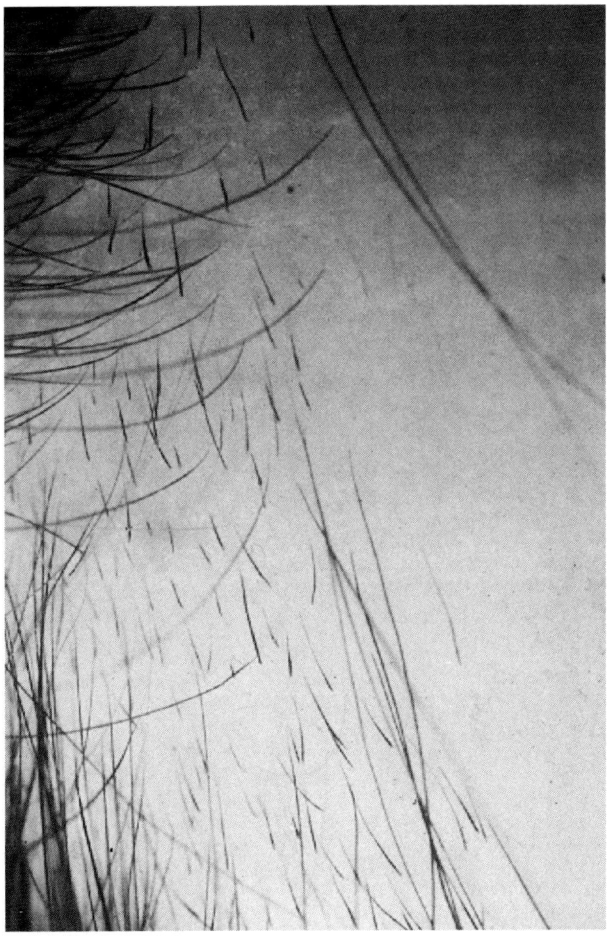

Figure 8-3 Example of the exclamation-mark hairs commonly seen in alopecia areata. (*Courtesy of Dr. David A. Fenton.*)

served to precede, follow, or occur concurrently with hair loss activity.[6,7]

Other Epidermal Appendages

A decrease in sebaceous gland volume, epidermal thickness, and the number of hair matrix and hair papilla cells labeling with ^{3}H-TdR has been documented in scalp affected by alopecia areata as compared with normal scalp. No differences in the density of labeled cells in the reticular dermis between normal scalp and alopecia areata scalp have been observed.[8] More recently, Elieff, Sundby, Kennedy, and Hordinsky examined sweat gland number and function in 20 patients with alopecia areata compared with age- and sex-matched controls. As a group, patients with alopecia areata had significantly decreased activated sweat gland number and function as measured by pilocarpine stimulation and analysis of sweat droplets in Silastic mounts (Fig. 8-5). The degree of sweat gland dysfunction was not related to the extent of hair loss, therapy, or concurrent diseases.[9]

Disease Associations

Common disease associations with alopecia areata include allergic rhinitis, asthma, and atopic dermatitis. Atopic features can be found in more than 40 percent of alopecia areata patients, while the prevalence of atopic diseases in the general population is estimated to be 20 percent.[10–13]

Diseases of the thyroid gland are also frequently seen in association with alopecia areata. Muller and Winkelmann found that 59 of 736 patients with alopecia areata had a clinical thyroid abnormality. These 59 patients represented

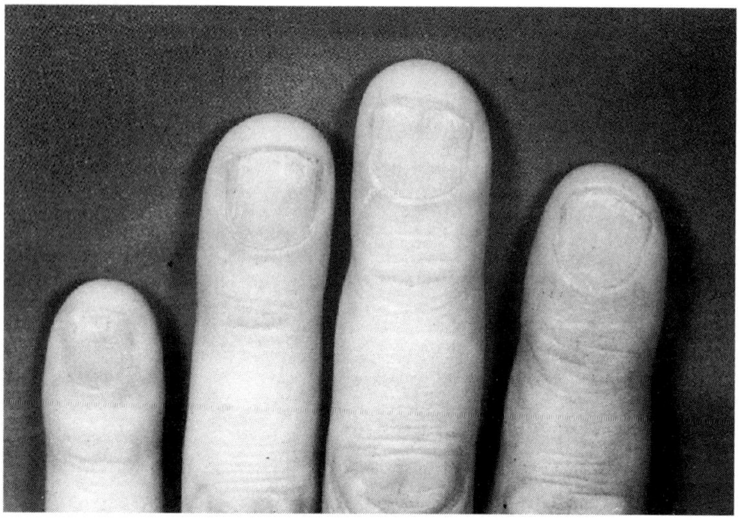

A

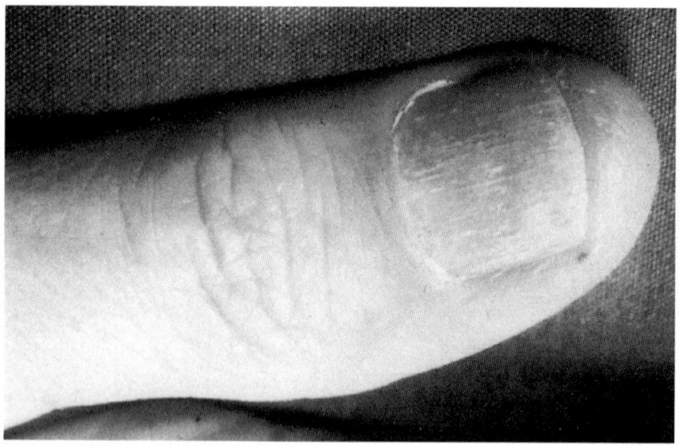

B

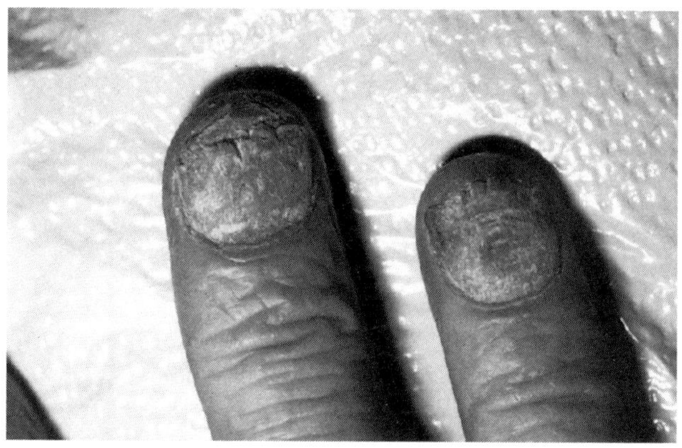

C

Figure 8-4 Nail abnormalities seen in patients with extensive alopecia areata. (*A*) Brittle nails with longitudinal ridging and distal onycholysis. (*B*) Close-up of affected thumbnail. (*C*) Severely affected nails.

14 cases of exophthalmic goiter, 27 cases of simple goiter, 7 cases of myxedema, 6 cases of Hashimoto's thyroiditis, and 5 cases of previous thyroidectomy.[10] Cunliffe, Hall, Stevenson, and Weightman found the incidence of these same diseases to be increased in patients with alopecia areata.[14] Others, however, have not been able to confirm these findings.[15]

Alopecia areata has also been associated with other diseases, most of which are autoimmune in nature.[16–18] Some of these diseases include vitiligo, lupus erythematosus, discoid lupus erythematosus, rheumatoid arthritis, pernicious anemia, scleroderma, ulcerative colitis, myasthenia gravis, and lichen planus. Alopecia areata has been associated with diabetes mellitus[19] and has also been described in patients seropositive for the human immunodeficiency virus.[20,21] Alope-

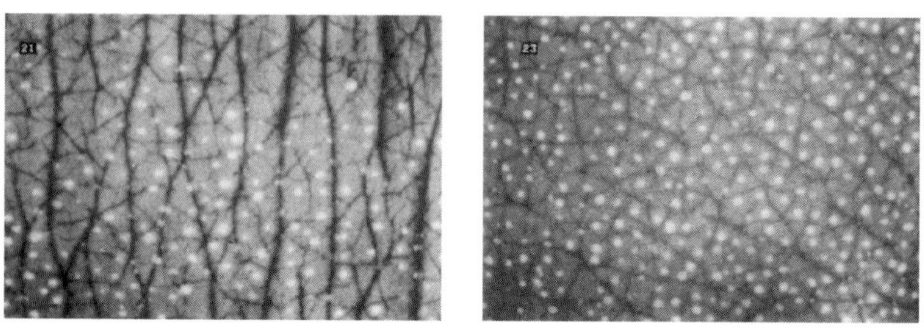

Figure 8-5 Sweat gland droplets as determined with the Silastic mold method. The panel on the left is a mold taken from a patient with alopecia areata; the panel on the right is a mold taken from a control matched for age, sex, weight, and height. There is a decrease in sweat gland number, as well as abnormal-appearing sweat droplets, in the patient with alopecia areata.

cia areata may be seen in association with two chromosome disorders—Down's syndrome and Turner's syndrome.[22–24] In one study, alopecia areata was found in 60 of 1000 Down's syndrome patients compared with 1 of 1000 control subjects with mental retardation related to other causes.[24] Unusual associations with alopecia areata include testicular atrophy or dysfunction, and ophthalmologic changes such as iris color change, pigment hyperplasia of the choroid and retinal epithelium, and depressed Arden's ratio (ratio of light peak to dark trough as measured by electrooculography) in some patients.[25,26]

HISTOLOGY

Hair

Lymphocytic infiltrates and granulomatous inflammation have been observed around late anagen hairs as well as within the hair follicle in the acute progressive stage of alopecia areata[4] (Fig. 8-6). Inflammatory cells, primarily CD4+ lymphocytes and Langerhans' cells, are present in the peribulbar and perivascular areas and in the external root sheath of the follicular epithelia.[27] Three different patterns of hair follicle cellular degeneration have been observed in acute alopecia areata, including necrosis, apoptosis, and dark cell transformation.[28] Apoptosis, or cell death, has not been limited to the outer root sheath keratinocytes, as in normal catagen, but has also been found in matrix keratinocytes, melanocytes, Langerhans' cells, and dermal dendritic cells. Another type of follicular degeneration described in alopecia areata is a circumscribed cystic change in the suprabulbar region above the dermal papillae (Fig. 8-7).

Early anagen and telogen hair follicles are reportedly affected only in advanced stages of the disease[29,30] (Fig. 8-8). In long-standing alopecia areata, melanin incontinence, trichomalacia, and foreign body tissue reaction have been found. The following may also be seen in long-standing alopecia areata: epithelial buds and small ball-shaped protrusions from the outer root sheath, enlarged sebaceous glands, reduced numbers of anagen hair follicles, undifferentiated dermal nerves, and perifollicular mononuclear cell infiltrates.[30–33] Infiltration of hair follicles by mononuclear cells is, therefore, independent of the duration of the disease.

The expression of autologous class I major histocompatibility (MHC) antigens is necessary for interaction between target cells and specific cytotoxic T lymphocytes, whereas class II MHC antigens are involved in the afferent limb of the immune response.[34] Normal anagen hair bulb keratinocytes normally lack expression of MHC class I and class II antigens.[35] However, in alopecia areata, human leukocyte antigen (HLA)-A, HLA-B, HLA-C, and HLA-DR antigens are all expressed on anagen hair bulbs.[34,36] HLA-DR expression has also been found on telogen hair bulbs of alopecia areata but to a much lower extent. Focal, partial, or complete staining of anagen hairs in alopecia areata with HLA-DQ has been described.[37]

The expression of HLA-A, HLA-B, and HLA-C antigens in alopecia areata would permit the interaction of cytotoxic T lymphocytes with hair matrix cells.[34] The expression of HLA-DR by hair follicle keratinocytes is not believed to be a primary event in alopecia areata but rather a secondary event induced by cytokines such as gamma interferon released from cells in the perifollicular inflammatory infiltrate.[38] The functional role of HLA-DQ antigens in alopecia areata is not understood.[37]

Homing of T lymphocytes to lesions of alopecia areata may be regulated by adhesion molecules. Cell adhesion molecules, which mediate cell-cell and cell-matrix interaction, are expressed in alopecia areata. Endothelial cells lining postcapillary venules normally release cell adhesion molecules in response to certain soluble inflammatory mediators such as tumor necrosis factor-alpha and gamma interferon. E-selectin (ELAM), vascular cell adhesion molecule-1 (VCAM-1), and intracellular adhesion molecule-1 (ICAM-1) have all been described on endothelial cells in alopecia areata.[39] ICAM-1 has also been found to be expressed on the follicular epithelium in areas of alopecia areata and is known to regulate interactions between leukocytes and keratinocytes.[39,40] However, none of these observations explain how T cells migrate to hair follicles and penetrate the outer root sheath basement membranes to interact with ICAM-1 positive cells.

Alterations in connective tissue composition are not believed to play a prominent role in the pathogenesis of alopecia areata. Gollnick, Imcke, and Orfanos studied the expression of basement membrane proteins in hair follicles from alopecia areata patients. Using antibodies directed toward laminin, the lamina lucida, and type IV collagen, they found that the expression of laminin around hair follicles in alopecia areata was weak and sometimes totally lacking. They concluded that any changes seen were related to the severity of injury to the hair follicle and, most likely, represented secondary events.[41] Van Baar et al. also found the expression of laminin in alopecia areata hair follicles to be weak and sometimes totally lacking. They also examined the patterns of tenascin, fibronectin, and heparan sulfate proteoglycan expression and found no major differences between the scalp skin samples from normal controls and those from alopecia areata patients.[42]

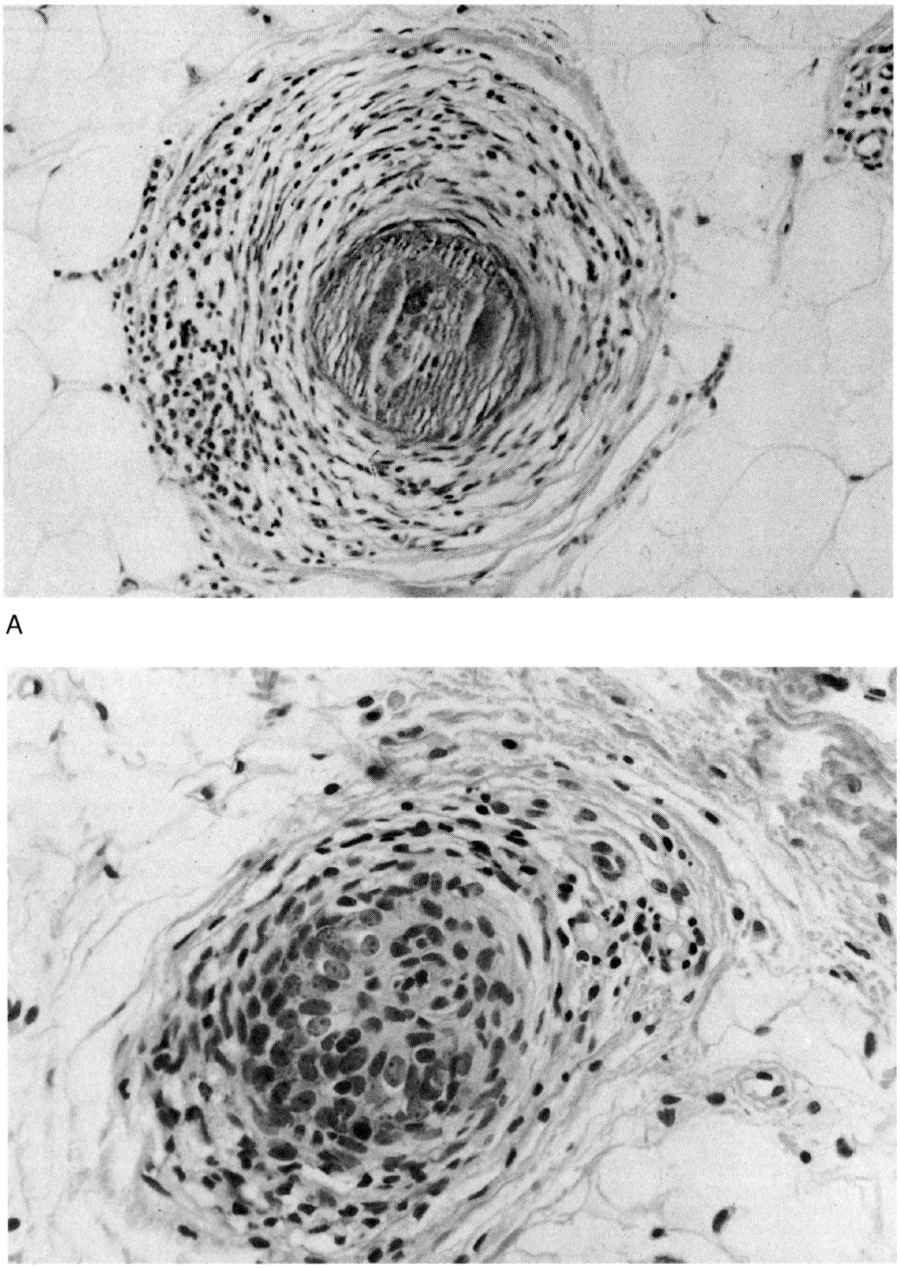

A

B

Figure 8-6 Histology of alopecia areata. (*A,B*) Mild to moderate inflammation involving the external root sheath of the hair follicle in acute alopecia areata. (× 100) (*continued*)

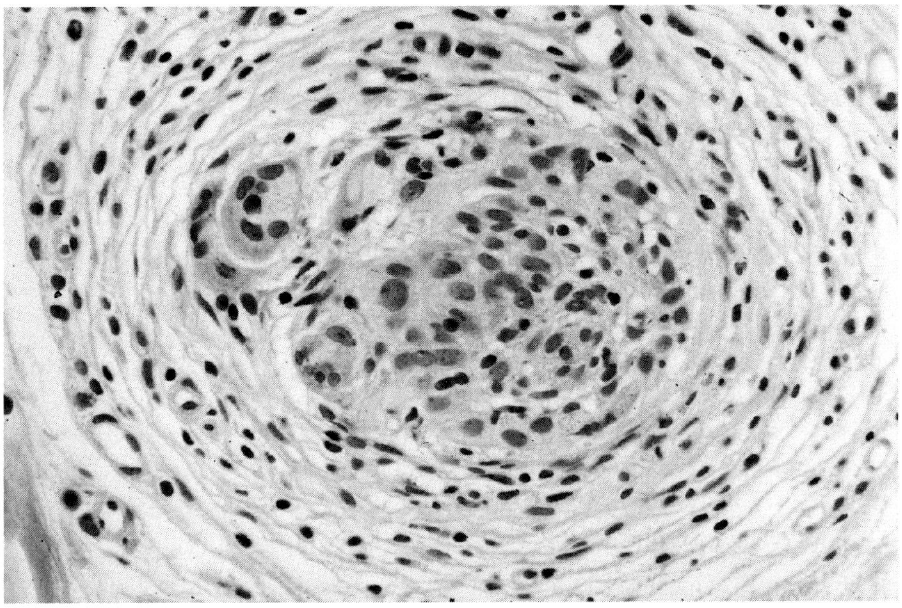
C

Figure 8-6c (*C*) Granulomatous inflammation in a patient with acute onset of hair loss. (× 100)

Nails

Using both light- and electron-microscopic techniques, most of the nail changes seen in alopecia areata have been found to be related to changes within the proximal matrix.[43] However, examination of nail biopsies taken from 12 patients with trachyonychia (from the Greek word *trakos,* meaning rough) showed a mild to moderately dense lymphocytic infiltrate, exocytosis, and spongiosis in the proximal nail fold, nail matrix, nail bed, and/or hyponychium in 11 of 12 specimens. The twelfth specimen showed classic changes of lichen planus. Six months after the biopsy was taken, this latter patient developed (clinical) cutaneous lichen planus. The authors

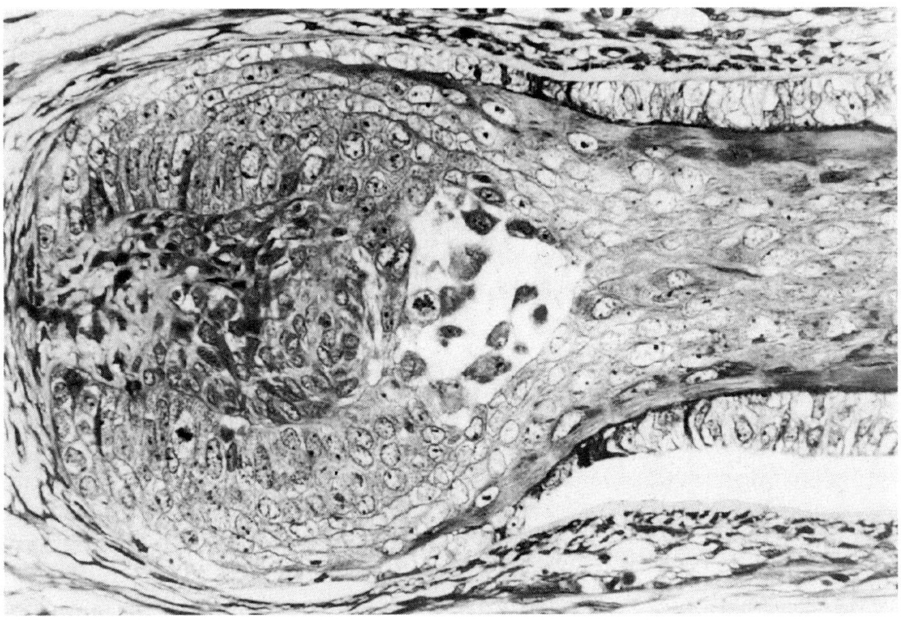

Figure 8-7 Follicular degeneration in alopecia areata characterized by a circumscribed cystic change in the suprabulbar region above the dermal papilla (× 250). (*Courtesy of Dr. Hideo Uno* with permission of *Scope Publications, The Upjohn Company.* In Current Concepts [monograph], *p 38.*)

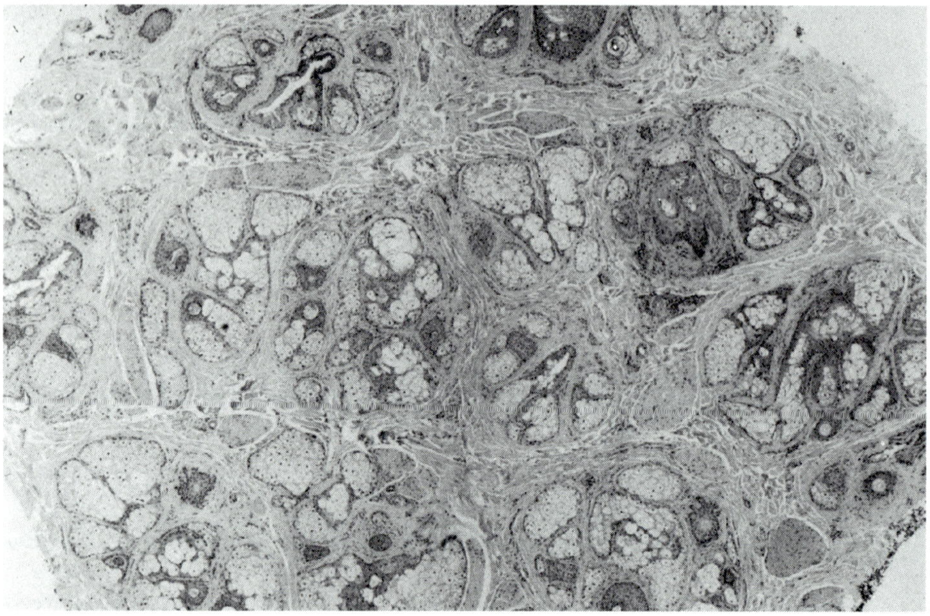

Figure 8-8 Transverse section at the level of the sebaceous gland in a patient with alopecia areata showing an average of 10 follicular units with approximately two hairs per unit. Seventy percent of the hairs are in telogen or catagen. A modest perifollicular inflammatory infiltrate is found around several follicles. (× 40)

concluded that the clinical association of trachyonychia with alopecia areata does not preclude that the nail abnormalities could be due to lichen planus or other disorders.[44]

EPIDEMIOLOGY

Alopecia areata can occur at any age, but approximately 50 percent of cases appear before age 20.[45] The prevalence of alopecia areata in the United States, as determined from the First National Health and Nutrition Examination Survey conducted from 1971 through 1974, was 158 per 100,000 persons, or roughly 0.1 to 0.2 percent of the population.[46] Conflicting reports have shown a higher incidence of alopecia areata in females or males.[47,48]

Ikeda reviewed the case histories of 1989 patients with alopecia areata at Kyoto University in Japan and assigned them to one of four types.[49] Other investigators subsequently confirmed many of her conclusions.[50,51] Under the Ikeda classification system, type I alopecia areata was the most common form (83 percent) and was characterized as the "round" or patchy type. Individuals with type I alopecia areata had no family history of alopecia areata and carried a good prognosis (no history of hypertension, atopy, or endocrinologic disorders). Type II alopecia areata was described as being clinically round or reticular, with a frequency of 10 percent of cases in this study. Patients with type II alopecia areata had a history of asthma, allergic rhinitis, or dermatitis. The hair loss in these patients lasted longer than those with type I alopecia areata and was associated with seasonal recurrences. Over 75 percent of these patients went on to develop alopecia totalis. Patients with type III alopecia areata had chronic disease activity and a reticular pattern of hair loss. The frequency of this type of alopecia areata was 4 percent, and alopecia totalis developed in 39 percent of these individuals. Interestingly, the incidence of parental hypertension in this group was 95 percent, as compared with 10 percent in the common type, 11 percent in the atopic group, and 21 percent in a control population. Patients with type IV alopecia were usually over 40 years of age, had some type of endocrinologic disease, and experienced round-, reticular-, or ophiasis-pattern alopecia areata for a prolonged time period. The frequency of this type of alopecia areata was 3 percent, and alopecia totalis developed in 10 percent of this group.

Muller and Winkelmann conducted a historical review of 736 patients with alopecia areata seen at the Mayo Clinic between 1945 and 1954. They reported that 30 percent of patients developed alopecia totalis (54 percent of the children, 24 percent of the adults) and that the proportion of patients presenting with alopecia totalis declined with each decade of life.[10] Walker and Rothman studied 230 patients with alopecia areata who were seen in the University of Chicago Clinics during the period from 1928 to 1948.[52] They reported that the duration of the initial alopecia areata episode until complete hair regrowth was less than 6 months in 33 percent of the patients and less than 1 year in 50 percent, but that 33 percent never recovered from the initial episode. The overall incidence of relapse or of experiencing another episode of alopecia areata was 86 percent, although it reached 100 percent if patients were followed for 20 years. Of those patients who developed alopecia areata before puberty, 50 percent eventually developed alopecia totalis and none fully recovered from the episode. In contrast, only 23 percent of those who developed patchy alopecia areata after puberty became totally bald, and only 5 percent of these patients fully recovered.[52] Those patients with alopecia totalis tended to remain persistently bald.

ETIOLOGY

The etiology of alopecia areata is unknown. A number of potential etiologies have been postulated over the past century, the most popular one being that alopecia areata is an autoimmune disease. Other theories to explain the etiology of this disease include exposure to chemicals or infectious agents, inheritance, or mediation by the nervous system. Recently, it has been suggested that alopecia areata is directly related to intrinsically abnormal keratinocytes or melanocytes.[53] Stress and anxiety are frequently blamed by patients as the cause of their hair loss.

Genetics

Genetic factors have been implicated in alopecia areata. The familial incidence has been reported to range between 10 and 27 percent.[10,11,54] The mode of inheritance has been proposed to be autosomal dominant with variable penetrance.[55] Alopecia areata has been reported to occur concurrently or sequentially in both monozygotic and fraternal twins.[56–58]

Other autoimmune diseases such as insulin-dependent diabetes mellitus, rheumatoid arthritis, and pemphigus vulgaris have been associated with an increase in certain HLA-region genes or haplotypes.[59] Moreover, since the predisposition to autoimmunity has been associated with HLA-D alleles and alopecia areata is hypothesized to be a T-cell–mediated autoimmune hair loss disorder, many investigators have looked for a significant association between HLA and alopecia areata. Investigators have attempted to correlate their results with disease susceptibility, resistance, and extent.

An increased prevalence of the following markers has been found in alopecia areata patients: HLA-A9, HLA-B7, and HLA-B8;[60] HLA-B12;[61] HLA-B18;[62] HLA-DR4 and HLA-DR5, with HLA-DR5 being linked to the early-onset form of alopecia areata and more extensive hair loss;[63–65] HLA-Cw1, HLA-Cw3, HLA-B13, HLA-B27, and HLA-DR7;[66] and HLA-DPw4 and HLA-DR4.[67] HLA-DRa4 and HLA-DRw11, with their associated DQw7(w3) and DQw8(w3) specificities, may be associated with susceptibility to alopecia areata, while the presence of DRw523a may confer resistance.[59] Clark, Welsh, Reveille, and Duvic oligotyped for HLA-DPB1 alleles in 84 Caucasian alopecia areata patients and 62 controls to subdivide the DPw4 specificities. DPB1 allele frequencies were neither increased nor decreased significantly in the patients vs. controls, suggesting the HLA-DPB1 alleles are not associated with alopecia areata.[68] In families with multiple affected members, common haplotypes have been reported for those affected members.[69] The variability of these results could be due to ethnic factors or to the methods involved in performing the HLA analyses. Immunoglobulin G heavy-chain determinants (Gm), which are present on chromosome 14, have been studied in alopecia areata and found to be significantly associated with an increased frequency of Gm 1,2,3,17;5,13,21 and a decreased frequency of Gm 1,3,17;5,13,21.[70] These results suggest that Gm 1,2,3,17;5,13,21 is associated with disease susceptibility and Gm 1,3,17;5,13,21 with resistance toward developing alopecia areata.

Immune Hypothesis

Alopecia areata has been proposed to be an autoimmune disorder involving T-cell interaction with aberrant HLA-DR antigens expressed by hair follicle keratinocytes.[34,38] There are no specific studies that have determined the role of T cells in the pathogenesis of alopecia areata, but indirect evidence exists suggesting the importance of T cells in this disease. Increased, decreased, and normal peripheral blood T and B lymphocyte number and function have been reported in alopecia areata patients.[71–74] In five of seven alopecia areata patients, autoreactive T cells, defined as cells which proliferate to irradiated autologous peripheral blood mononuclear cells in the absence of exogenous antigen, were found to be enriched in lesional scalp skin as compared to blood.[75] Other indirect evidence suggesting the importance of T cells in this disease comes from a study reported by Gilhar and Krueger.[76] They showed that 2-mm sections of scalp skin from patients with patchy or extensive alopecia areata would grow hair when engrafted onto congenitally athymic nu/nu mice. These findings suggest that alopecia areata is mediated by immune cells not present in athymic mice (i.e., T cells) or by dermal components which can affect the hair bulb. The strongest evidence for a primary role of T cells in the pathogenesis of alopecia areata in vivo comes from clinical data involving the successful use of immunosuppressive agents, such as glucocorticoids or cyclosporine, in treating this disease.[77,78]

The DEBR rat, which displays a T-lymphocytic perifollicular and intrabulbar infiltration of hair follicles arrested in a state of dystrophic anagen, has been suggested as an animal model for alopecia areata.[79] Interestingly, when this animal is treated with cyclosporine, virtually complete hair regrowth occurs. This is in marked contrast to the lack of regrowth when FK 506, another drug which selectively inhibits T-cell activation and proliferation, is administered to these animals.[80] Another proposed animal model for alopecia areata is the aging C3H/HEJ mouse. These mice develop a nonscarring alopecia on their ventral abdomen which histologically shows anagen follicles infiltrated and surrounded by T lymphocytes.[81]

The Keratinocyte

From the data presented at the 1990 research workshop on alopecia areata held at the National Institutes of Health, Goldsmith postulated that there is an intrinsic, genetic abnormality in the follicular keratinocyte of those with alopecia areata.[53] Under the influence of a variety of stimuli (external or internal), keratinocytes produce proinflammatory cytokines, including interleukin-1 beta, interleukin-8, and tumor necrosis factor-alpha, plus other T-cell chemotactic factors.[53] T cells attracted to the follicular keratinocyte may interact with the follicular keratinocyte and possibly release additional cytokines as well as cellular components, some of which could be potential antigens. Examples would include melanocytic antigens or newly exposed antigens on the keratinocyte.

The Pigment Cell

It is not well understood why pigmented hairs are frequently affected preferentially and white hairs spared in alopecia areata, or why regrowing hair is often initially white (Fig. 8-9). Messenger and Bleehen examined (with light and electron microscopy) biopsies of regrowing white hairs from seven patients with alopecia areata.[82] They described decreased numbers of melanocytes and melanosomes, decreased melanization, and poorly developed dendritic processes. Melanosomes were rarely found within keratinocytes,

Figure 8-9 White terminal hair regrowth in alopecia areata.

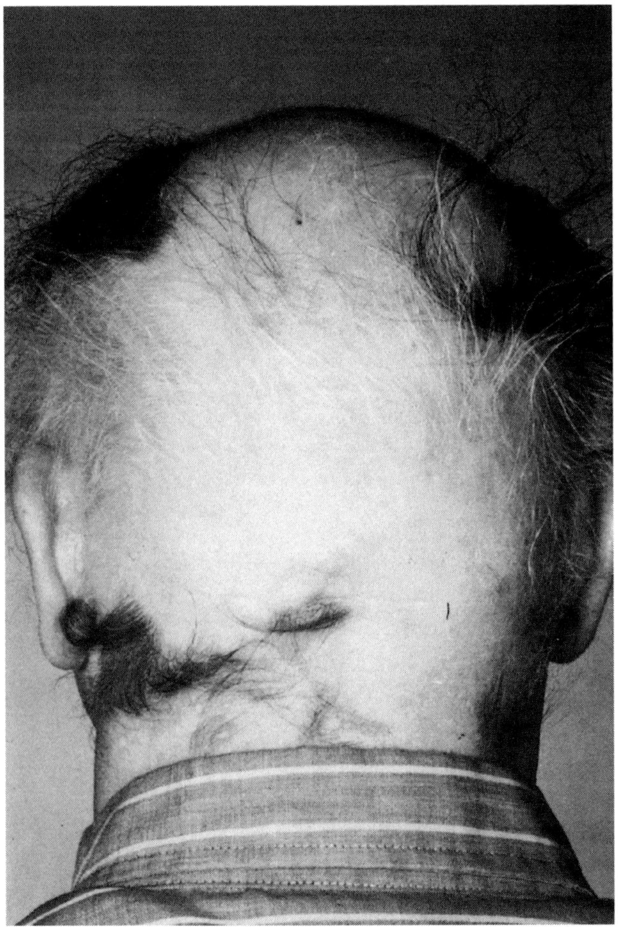

and autophagocytosis of melanosomes within melanocytes was seen. Very prominent upper cortical keratinocyte degeneration was noted in 7 of the 15 hair bulbs examined, suggesting that the primary target cells in alopecia areata are the upper bulb precortical keratinocytes. However, the normal anagen-to-catagen transformation seen in alopecia areata could account for some of these changes.

Tobin, Fenton, and Kendall studied scalp biopsy specimens from untreated areas of alopecia in 10 adults and from the scalps of 3 unaffected adults.[83] They found increased numbers of bizarre melanosomes in affected melanocytes in the follicles from the alopecia areata patients as compared with the normal controls. These melanosomes showed incomplete or "aborted" melanization and appeared disrupted, enlarged, and rounded, with loss of their normal ellipsoid shape. An unusual outer root sheath distribution of hair bulb melanocytes was also seen. Though these findings are interesting, it is unclear what role, if any, these abnormal morphological findings play in the pathogenesis of alopecia areata.

Neural Hypothesis

The idea of a generalized neuronal defect in alopecia areata is supported by reports of abnormal electroencephalographic (EEG) examinations in patients with alopecia areata and the fact that many patients experience occasional itching, tingling, formication, or slight local pain during combing, touching, or tension on the hair.[84–86] A lack of differentiation of dermal nerves has also been reported in areas of alopecia areata. However, similar changes have also been reported around other appendages, larger blood vessels, and the dermoepidermal region when no inflammatory processes are present.[30,33]

Using iontophoresis of pilocarpine, Elieff, Sundby, Kennedy, and Hordinsky recently found activated sweat gland number and function to be decreased in alopecia areata patients.[9] Iontophoresis of the cholinergic agonist pilocarpine is believed to stimulate eccrine glands directly, thereby testing the postganglionic innervation in conjunction with the function of the sweat gland itself. It is presently not clear whether the sweating deficiency described in patients with alopecia areata is a reflection of subclinical dysfunction of autonomic nerves or reflects a problem with the sweat gland itself.

Emotional Stress

Stressful life events and psychiatric disorders have been studied as they relate to both the onset and the progression of alopecia areata. The results of these studies are conflicting. Anderson found that 23 percent of 114 patients with alopecia areata had "acute anxiety" or "mental shock" before their first episode of hair loss.[87] Mehlman and Griesemer evaluated 20 children with alopecia areata and found that a stressful event had frequently occurred in the 2-week period prior to the development of hair loss.[88] Perini et al. found that 48 patients with alopecia areata, compared with 30 with common baldness and 30 with tinea capitis, had a significantly higher number of stressful life events in the 6 months preceding hair loss.[89] A Belgian study of 164 adult alopecia areata patients concluded that stressful events in the 1 to 6 months just prior to hair loss were double the number of stressful events in the preceding 6 to 12 months.[90] Using a mailed questionnaire, Koo and colleagues recently studied 294 patients with alopecia areata and found that the onset of alopecia areata was not usually associated with a preceding stressful life event (Koo J, Shellow WVR, Edwards JE, Yager J, Fairbanks L: Psychiatric, immunologic and atopic aspects of alopecia areata: An epidemiological study of 321 patients. Abstract, International Symposium on Dermatology and Psychiatry, Vienna, Austria, 1987).

It has been suggested that psychiatric diagnoses are more prevalent in patients with alopecia areata. Anderson held that 26 of his 114 patients with alopecia areata had some form of mental disturbance.[87] Muller and Winkelmann in their review of 736 patients with alopecia areata found that 22 percent of the children and 17 percent of the adults exhibited psychoneuroses, personality disorders, or neurotic behavior.[10] More recently, an attempt has been made to systematically diagnose psychiatric disorders in adults with alopecia areata. Colon et al. studied 31 patients using a structured psychiatric interview.[91] High lifetime prevalence rates of major depression (39 percent) and generalized anxiety disorders (39 percent) were found. In addition, patients reported an increased incidence of psychiatric disorders in first-degree relatives. These included anxiety disorders (58 percent), affective disorders (35 percent), and substance abuse (35 percent). Patients with patchy alopecia areata were more likely to have a lifetime diagnosis of generalized anxiety disorder.

TREATMENT

There is no one "best" treatment for alopecia areata, and there is no strong evidence to suggest that drug-induced remissions or therapies alter the course of alopecia areata. It is believed that the available treatments at best only suppress the underlying process.[92] Most of the published studies on the treatment of alopecia areata have focused on determining the efficacy of regrowth (defined very variably) and correlating the clinical results of therapy with disease extent, disease duration, and historical factors such as previous treatment or history of atopy. Very few studies have been done examining the effect of treatment on hair follicle differentiation or the inflammatory perifollicular-peribulbar infiltrate. No studies have been done examining the effect of treatment on activated sweat gland number and function or epidermal and sebaceous gland size.

There are many treatments available which may help stimulate regrowth in patients with alopecia areata. The efficacy, risks, and benefits of each treatment have to be considered when choosing a treatment plan.

Immunomodulating Agents

STEROIDS

TOPICAL

Topical steroids are frequently used to treat patchy alopecia areata and, in some cases, extensive alopecia areata.[93,94] Pascher, Kurtin, and Andrade conducted a placebo-controlled trial using 0.2% fluocinolone acetonide in a cream base (Synalar-HP), applied twice daily with occlusion each night for 6 months to paired comparison sites.[93] A satisfactory to excellent (total to near-total) therapeutic response was obtained to active drug in 17 of the 28 evaluable patients. Disease extent did not affect the outcome, but age and disease duration were factors. Every child between the ages of 3 and 10 years showed 100 percent regrowth, whereas only approximately 50 percent of older children and 33 percent of adults responded. Outcome was good when the alopecia areata process was present less than 1 year and poor, particularly in adults, if the disease had been present for longer periods of time. Children who had the disease for up to 7 years still did well.

Montes examined the use of 0.1% halcinonide cream applied daily with or without occlusion, but not more than 60 g per month, to seven patients with patchy hair loss and three patients with extensive hair loss.[94] All patients attained full hair regrowth, with the duration of treatment ranging from 6 to 18 months. In four patients in whom biopsies were performed, the inflammatory infiltrate seen before treatment was not markedly reduced after treatment, despite clinical hair regrowth.

Fiedler reported the successful use of 0.05% betamethasone dipropionate cream in a nonoptimized vehicle (Diprosone 0.05%), applied twice daily without occlusion, in children and some adults.[92] Similar to Pascher, she found that at least 3 months of uninterrupted treatment was necessary before evaluating hair regrowth. She further suggested that this treatment may be helpful to individuals experiencing actively flaring alopecia areata.

The minimum effective strength or class of topical steroid in alopecia areata has not been determined, although it would appear that 1% hydrocortisone is too weak. The maximum effective strength remains to be determined. Side effects of topical steroid therapy include folliculitis, hypertrichosis, acneiform eruption, and the potential for developing local atrophy and telangiectasias. In children with extensive alopecia areata applying more than 45 g per month of class I or II topical steroids, there may be associated significant systemic absorption and the attendant systemic side effects.

INTRALESIONAL

Intralesional steroids are used frequently to treat alopecia areata,[95–97] particularly localized patches of alopecia areata. Once disease extent exceeds 50 percent of the scalp, intralesional steroid use is hampered by the total amount of drug required to cover the affected area. Typically, the steroid is delivered using a 1-ml tuberculin syringe and a 30-gauge $^1/_2$-inch or 1-inch needle, depending on the operator's preference. Delivery with a jet injector has also been reported.[96] The steroid should be injected just below the epidermis and not into the fat. The hair follicles are so small that if one injects the steroid into the middermis, one could be injecting below the follicles.

Studies have been done comparing the use of different steroid preparations.[95,97] Commonly used preparations for intralesional use are triamcinolone acetonide or triamcinolone hexacetonide. Ten mg/ml is typically administered to scalp lesions and 3 to 5 mg/ml to eyebrow areas. Intralesional steroids have also been used to initiate eyelash hair regrowth. The average time from injection of steroid to the emergence of hair at the injected site of alopecia is 2 to 6 weeks.[95,96]

Abell and Munro treated 84 patients with varied degrees of alopecia areata using a "Porto Jet" needleless injector. They administered injections of 0.1 ml of 5 mg/ml of triamcinolone acetonide every 1 to 2 weeks × 3.[96] At 6 weeks, satisfactory regrowth (predominantly pigmented terminal hair regrowth) was present in 92 percent of patients with patchy disease and in 61 percent of those with alopecia totalis. A substantial proportion of both groups lost this regrowth by 12 weeks (regrowth maintained in 71 percent of patients with alopecia areata and 28 percent of those with alopecia totalis). Patients with rapidly progressive alopecia areata, those with extensive alopecia areata, and those in whom the duration of alopecia areata was ≥ 2 years responded poorly to this form of therapy.

The complications of intralesional steroid therapy include pain with drug delivery and transient atrophy. Large depot injections should be avoided, as this can lead to tissue loss and severe depression of the skin.[97] If injections are given too frequently and if atrophied areas are reinjected, this atrophy may become permanent and interfere with hair regrowth. Blood vessel occlusion and uniocular amaurosis have been reported with the administration of intralesional hydrocortisone suspension and methylprednisolone acetate suspension to the frontal and/or temporoparietal region.[98] Now, however, this complication is rarely seen because of the availability of solutions containing microsize steroid particles. If injections are done on a regular basis in the periocular area, a baseline eye exam and regular follow-up examination at least every 12 months are recommended to check for glaucoma and/or cataracts.

INTRAMUSCULAR

The use of intramuscular triamcinolone acetonide 40 to 80 mg q 1 to 6 weeks for $4^1/_2$ to 18 months was evaluated in nine patients with alopecia totalis and two with alopecia universalis.[99] The average total dose given was 919 mg. Eight patients attained cosmetically acceptable hair regrowth, but relapse occurred 4 to 9 weeks off therapy. Side effects of intramuscular steroids are the same as those with prolonged use of oral steroids and are discussed below.

ORAL

Dillaha and Rothman were the first to report on the use of orally administered cortisone for the treatment of alopecia areata.[100] They treated 22 patients (4 with alopecia totalis, 11 with alopecia universalis, 7 with patchy hair loss) with cortisone acetate tablets: initially 100 or 150 mg daily in three or four divided doses and then a decreased dose after 4 weeks if hair growth was well under way. Sixteen of the 22 patients regrew hair, with the onset of regrowth within 3 to 6 weeks. Regrowth was patchy in 10, diffuse in 6, and complete in none. Cessation of therapy or a decrease in the dose below 50 to 75 mg q.d. was associated with a relapse. A longer duration of the last episode of alopecia areata (average 11.7 years in the nonresponders vs. 4.7 years in the responders) and having a history of active disease during adolescence were associated with failure to respond to oral cortisone acetate.

Kern, Hoffman, Hambrick, and Blizzard treated 27 patients, 13 with patchy alopecia areata and 14 with alopecia universalis or totalis with prednisone.[101] The starting doses were 40 to 60 mg per day in adults and 20 to 30 mg per day in children. After 1 month, either the daily dose was tapered (e.g., from 60 to 40 mg) or the patient was switched directly to an alternate-day treatment schedule. Prednisone was eventually tapered during therapy to the lowest alternate-day dosage consistent with cosmetically acceptable hair regrowth. A relapse was treated with an increase in prednisone.

Results were encouraging in that all patients showed significant hair regrowth which usually began 3 to 6 weeks after initiation of prednisone therapy. Of the 18 patients who received steroids for longer than 6 months, all but 2 patients (with alopecia universalis) regrew their hair completely or to the degree that the patient could discontinue use of a hair prosthesis. A follow-up report, by Winter, Kern, and Blizzard, on these same patients after a mean of 15 months after discontinuation of the drug[102] showed that 5 of the 18 prednisone-treated patients showed lasting improvement off drug, but the rest experienced worsening (usually rapid hair loss) with discontinuation of prednisone. The authors concluded that the effect of oral corticosteroids on alopecia areata fit the described natural course of the disease, i.e., that one-third of affected individuals with alopecia areata spontaneously improve, one-third show no change, and the remaining one-third worsen.[102]

In contrast, Unger and Schemmer described the advantageous use of combination therapy with topical, intralesional, and oral corticosteroids in 15 patients with alopecia totalis or alopecia universalis.[103] Thirty to 40 mg of prednisone daily was prescribed in combination with 0.025% fluocinolone acetonide cream under occlusion for 12 hours per day. Resistant areas were also treated with intralesional triamcinolone acetonide, 3.3 mg/ml. Seven of the 15 patients who were able to regrow virtually all of their scalp hair were able to discontinue oral corticosteroids without recurrence of their disease for an average follow-up of 32 months (2 months to $7^1/_2$ years).

Olsen, Carson, and Turney treated 32 patients (16 patchy alopecia areata, 16 totalis or universalis) with a 6-week tapering dose of oral prednisone beginning at 40 mg q.d. in adults, tapering by 5 mg q.d. weekly over 4 weeks, then by 5 mg q.d. every 3 days.[77] Children < 40 kg were given 0.75 mg/kg q.d. × 1 week and had their daily dose decreased by one-eighth each week over 4 weeks, then by one-eighth every 3 days over 2 weeks. At the end of 6 weeks of prednisone therapy, 15 out of 32 patients (47 percent) had at least 25 percent regrowth, including 8 out of 32 patients (25 percent) with near-complete (> 75 percent) regrowth. The authors felt that the critical threshold for hair growth with systemic steroids was less than 0.8 mg/kg daily, or well under the 100 mg noted earlier by Dillaha and Rothman to be necessary to initiate hair growth in the average adult. Olsen and colleagues questioned the duration of the hair regrowth off prednisone and further randomized patients to topical minoxidil or vehicle for 14 weeks. They found that only 17 percent of vehicle-treated patients were able to maintain or expand on the prednisone-induced hair growth at 12 weeks and none at 20 weeks.

Burton and Shuster tested the hypothesis that if a single intradermal injection of corticosteroid into a patch of alopecia areata can produce prolonged hair regrowth, then the use of a pulse high-dose systemic glucocorticoid might produce a prolonged response in patients with severe (totalis) alopecia areata.[104] They used either prednisolone as a single 2-g dose intravenously (22 patients) or 500 mg of oral prednisolone daily for 5 days (13 patients). Four of the latter patients also applied 0.4% fluocinolone acetonide in 80% dimethyl sulfoxide topically to the bald areas twice daily. Of the patients given oral prednisolone, 5 had no response to treatment, 7 had only a poor response, and 1 had a good response. The use of topical fluocinolone did not influence the response. Of the 22 patients who had intravenous prednisolone, 14 had no response to treatment, 5 had a poor response, and 3 had a good response (generalized regrowth sufficient to be cosmetically acceptable).

Side effects were seen with systemic steroids in all of the preceding studies. Dillaha and Rothman reported weight gain, hypokalemia, acneiform eruptions, and menstrual disturbances.[100] Kern, Hoffman, Hambrick, and Blizzard described finding subcapsular opacities in three patients.[101] Unfortunately, these patients were not routinely examined prior to therapy. Winter, Kern, and Blizzard reported acne and obesity.[102] In addition, these investigators described hypertension in three patients and small, posterior subcapsular cataracts in three of eight patients examined. In contrast, Unger and Schemmer reported side effects mainly limited to weight gain.[103] One of their patients had a small, asymptomatic subcapsular lens opacity which was discovered $1^1/_2$ years after prednisone therapy was discontinued, and a small cataract developed within 2 months of starting prednisone therapy in one patient.[103] Hypertension did not develop in any of the patients. One patient had moderately severe gastrointestinal pain when prednisone was started. Olsen, Carson, and Turney reported weight gain as the most common side effect of oral prednisone use.[77] Mood changes and emotional lability, acne and/or seborrhea, and headaches were reported in more than 10 percent of their patients.

CYCLOSPORINE

Both oral and topical cyclosporine have been used in the treatment of alopecia areata.[105–108] DeProst and colleagues evaluated a topical cyclosporine preparation (100 mg/ml in an oil base) in 43 patients with severe alopecia areata (20 with alopecia universalis, 7 with alopecia totalis, and 16 with alopecia areata).[105] The mean disease duration was 11 years.[107] Twenty-two patients applied topical cyclosporine and 21 applied the vehicle alone to one-half of the scalp daily. Diffuse vellus hair growth was observed on the treated side in 5 patients treated with cyclosporine and in 3 controls. In 7 patients treated with active cyclosporine, small (0.5–2 cm in diameter) tufts of terminal hairs were observed to appear between the second and sixth months in the treated area. Gilhar, Pillar, and Etzioni used a similar 10% topical cyclosporine preparation twice daily in an open-label study of 10 patients with severe alopecia areata.[106] No beneficial effect was seen after 12 months of therapy. Coulson and Holden treated 6 patients with alopecia totalis with 10% (w/w) cyclosporine in an alcoholic gel in an open-label 3-month trial in which patients applied the drug to half of the scalp and the gel vehicle to the other half of the scalp. No hair regrowth was seen.[107] McCarley and Olsen (unpublished data) used a 2% wt/wt cyclosporine in petrolatum preparation applied to one-half of the scalp in a blinded fashion to treat 10 patients with alopecia areata for 6-plus months. No patient had any significant hair regrowth.

No systemic cyclosporine blood levels were detected in the three preceding published studies.[105–107] In contrast, Parodi and Rebora described a patient with a 3-year duration of alopecia universalis who applied cyclosporine, 250 mg in 80 ml of an alcohol–propylene glycol–water vehicle, to his entire scalp once daily.[108] At 16 months after beginning therapy and with hair growth, he was noted to have a blood cyclosporine level of 101 ng/ml (usual serum level 500–1500 ng/ml in organ transplant patients). This patient was also observed to experience a steady but slow rise in his white blood cell and absolute lymphocyte counts while on topical cyclosporine.

Coulson and Holden examined cyclosporine levels in scalp punch biopsies of patients with alopecia areata performed after cyclosporine therapy. These patients had had no response to therapy. No cyclosporine was detected in biopsies 6 hours after the first application, but in three of six biopsies performed at 1 month, the mean cyclosporine concentration was 16 mg/kg.[107]

Side effects of topical cyclosporine were uncommon. Transient folliculitis and irritation may have been secondary to the oily vehicle.[105]

Gupta et al. treated six patients with oral cyclosporine, three patients with alopecia universalis, one with alopecia totalis, and two with patchy alopecia areata.[78] Treatment was 6 mg/kg of oral cyclosporine per day for 12 weeks. Cosmetically acceptable hair regrowth occurred in the one patient with alopecia totalis and the two patients with patchy alopecia areata. However, 3 months after therapy was discontinued, significant hair loss occurred. The degree of terminal hair regrowth correlated significantly with decreases in follicular epithelial human lymphocyte antigen-DR and intercellular adhesion molecule expression, T cells, helper-inducer (CD4) T cells, suppressor-cytotoxic (CD8) T cells, and Langerhans' cells ($CD1^+DR^+$) from the hair follicles during cyclosporine therapy.[78]

Several side effects typical of oral cyclosporine use were seen in these patients. One patient each developed a headache, dysesthesia, fatigue, or diarrhea. Gingival hyperplasia, flushing, and myalgias developed in two patients each. One patient developed multiple cutaneous papules and nodules consistent histologically with a benign lymphocytic infiltrate. Elevated serum blood urea nitrogen and creatinine levels were also observed. All of these abnormalities disappeared after therapy was discontinued.

ISOPRINOSINE

Isoprinosine (Inosiplex) potentiates T-lymphocyte and phagocyte function.[109–111] Lowy, Ledoux-Corbusier, Achten, and Wybran treated 10 patients with alopecia universalis and 4 patients with patchy alopecia areata with isoprinosine, 50 mg/kg per day three times a day, for 6 months.[109] Nine of the 14 patients showed a positive clinical response, including 5 with total hair regrowth. Interestingly, only 1 of the 5 nonresponders vs. 7 of the 9 responders had various autoantibodies (including nuclear, smooth muscle, thyroid, striated muscle, skin, and/or gastric parietal cells) prior to treatment. These disappeared after therapy. After treatment, both groups showed an increase in T-cell rosette formation with human transformed B lymphocytes, also known as *interactive rosetting.* The authors suggested that alopecia areata may be a heterogeneous disease which can be subclassified by the presence or absence of autoantibodies.

Galbraith, Thiers, and Fudenberg used inosiplex to treat nine patients with alopecia totalis who had known associated T-cell function defects, such as diminished production of leukocyte migration inhibition factor in response to mitogen stimulation and reduced T-cell rosette formation.[110] Inosiplex was administered at an initial dose of 50 mg/kg per day (with the maximum dose being 3 g per day) × 3 weeks and then the dose was reduced on day 14 to 50 mg/kg per day for 3 days a week. Subsequent dosage adjustment was made according to clinical and laboratory responses. All nine patients developed enhanced T-cell function, and seven attained clinically obvious hair regrowth. When therapy was discontinued after 6 months, acute hair loss associated with immune defects occurred within 2 weeks of inosiplex discontinuation. Stabilization and continued hair growth followed reinstitution of therapy.

Twenty-five patients with alopecia totalis and cell-mediated immune defects completed 40 weeks of a double-blind, placebo-controlled crossover trial of inosiplex therapy.[111] One group of patients received inosiplex for a total of 20 weeks at a dose of 50 mg/kg per day, up to a maximum of 5 g per day with temporary dose reduction of 50 mg/kg three times a week at weeks 3 to 8. Group 2 received placebo. After 20 weeks, the two groups crossed over therapy. Eleven patients on inosiplex were clinically identified as "responders," i.e., had some terminal hair regrowth either on the scalp (9 patients) or elsewhere (2 patients); 5 patients had spontaneous regrowth. Evaluation of scalp skin biopsies showed reduced inflammation in 8 patients on inosiplex and 2 patients on placebo, although comparison between the two treatment groups did not reveal any significant enhancement of immune function related to inosiplex therapy. The 11 patients on inosiplex who had hair regrowth had a significant increase in interactive T-cell rosetting 20 weeks after therapy compared with nonresponders.

The major side effect of inosiplex seen in this study was a minor increase in serum uric acid levels. Mild, transient symptoms reported by patients occurred with approximately equal frequency in both the drug and placebo phases of the study and included nausea, headache, drowsiness, and dry skin.

THYMOPENTIN

Thymopentin is a synthetic pentapeptide which represents the active site of thymopoietin and has been shown experimentally to induce T-cell differentiation and modulate the function of mature lymphocytes.[112,113] Tosti, Manuzzi, and Gasponi treated 20 patients with extensive (> 50 percent scalp hair loss) alopecia areata, using thymopentin 50 mg/ml diluted in physiological saline intravenously three times a week for 3 weeks.[112] Ten of the patients had progressive alopecia areata. Regrowth began an average of 3 months (1–5 months) after start of therapy. At a 6-month follow-up, 7 of the 20 patients (35 percent) experienced complete scalp hair regrowth. Orecchia treated 37 patients with alopecia areata affecting more than 50 percent of the scalp with thymopoietin, either 25 mg injected intradermally in the left scalp 10 times weekly (14 patients) or 50 mg intravenously three times a week for 4 weeks.[113] At the 6-month evaluation, 2 patients had complete hair regrowth and 4 others showed partial regrowth at the injection site. All 6 of these patients had had patchy alopecia areata. At 6 months, 8 of the 23 patients treated with thymopentin intravenously had a partial response, including 5 with alopecia areata and 3 with alopecia universalis. Three of 23 patients, all with alopecia areata, had complete regrowth. No complications of thymopentin therapy were reported in these studies.

NITROGEN MUSTARD

Eleven patients (five with 25 to 99 percent scalp hair loss and six with alopecia totalis) between the ages of 16 and 65 were treated with topical nitrogen mustard.[114] Patients applied an aqueous solution containing 0.2 mg/ml of mechlorethamine hydrochloride over the entire scalp daily until terminal hair growth was noted. At that time, the frequency of applications was decreased to three times a week, and once good hair regrowth was obtained, topical therapy was maintained at a frequency of once a week for 2 additional months. Of the six patients with alopecia totalis, two attained complete regrowth, one had 60 percent regrowth, one had 20 percent regrowth, and two were failures. In the latter case, therapy was suspended due to drug allergy. Of the five patients with localized alopecia areata, three had 100 percent regrowth and two had 10 percent regrowth. Side effects were mild hyperpigmentation and two cases of contact sensitization.

AZATHIOPRINE

Although the use of azathioprine has never been examined in controlled studies for the treatment of alopecia areata, there is an interesting report in the literature of a patient with Crohn's disease who developed alopecia totalis while on a daily dose of 7.5 mg prednisolone.[115] Even though his Crohn's disease was quiescent, azathioprine 50 mg twice daily was added to assess its potential effect on the hair loss. Hair started to regrow after 4 months and was normal-appearing by 8 months. After 4 months off azathioprine, the patient lost all of his hair again. Following reinstitution of therapy, he regrew all of his hair. Throughout this period, his prednisolone dose was maintained at 7.5 mg per day.

PHOTOTHERAPY WITH ULTRAVIOLET B LIGHT

The use of phototherapy with ultraviolet B light has been reported to be useful in some patients with alopecia areata.[116] Thirty-two patients between the ages of 6 and 70 years with extensive alopecia areata were treated with a Kromayer's ultraviolet lamp. The 5-cm-diameter quartz glass of the lamp, which emits biologically active wavelengths of less than 3000 Å, was applied directly to each of the bald patches with moderate pressure. The time of exposure varied between 3 and 60 seconds, with each patient receiving enough light to cause an erythematous reaction. Treatments were repeated weekly or every other week. Interestingly, 25 of the 32 patients observed hair growth within the first 3 months of treatment. Full hair and beard regrowth occurred in 14 of 25 patients with alopecia areata, and "almost full regrowth" was noted in 4 patients with alopecia areata and 1 patient with alopecia totalis. Neither of the other 2 patients with alopecia totalis and none of the patients with alopecia universalis made further progress after the initiation of insignificant regrowth in the first 3 months of therapy. Several of the patients experienced hair loss after treatment was discontinued.

PSORALEN + ULTRAVIOLET A LIGHT (PUVA)

Both topical and oral psoralens combined with exposure to ultraviolet A (UVA) light have been used to treat alopecia areata.[117–120] Weissmann et al. treated one patient with alopecia universalis and two with alopecia areata using topical photochemotherapy with 8-methoxypsoralen (8-MOP) and application of UVA light.[117] A 0.15% 8-MOP solution was applied 1 hour prior to UVA irradiation to a 4.5-cm-diameter area and treated five times weekly. The initial UVA dose was 1 J/cm^2, which was increased to about 7 J/cm^2. Controls included painted but unirradiated and irradiated but unpainted sites in alopecia areata lesions. Following 27 to 32 treatments, two patients developed prominent hair regrowth in the actively treated sites. The other patient dropped out in the initial stage of the study. Subsequently, these investigators treated additional patients with extensive scalp disease using a standard stand-up PUVA box and found induction of hair growth after 19 to 32 treatments.[117]

Claudy and Gagnaire reported on their 5-year experience with PUVA treatment for 23 patients with alopecia areata.[118] Seven patients had patchy alopecia areata, 13 had alopecia totalis, and 3 had alopecia universalis. The UVA source was a hexagonal stand-up box of fluorescent tubes emitting 320 to 400 nm irradiation. Seventeen patients received methoxsalen orally 2 hours prior to total body exposure, and 3 had only scalp UVA therapy. The dosages of psoralen ranged from 10 mg for < 25 kg of body weight up to 60 mg for weights > 90 kg. Three patients with alopecia totalis applied a 0.1% solution of methoxsalen to the scalp 2 hours prior to irradiation of the scalp only. Patients received UVA irradiation three times a week, and the UVA dosage was increased by 1 J/cm^2 on each odd-numbered exposure, with the average intensity for any session between 8 and 8.5 J/cm^2 at 50 cm. The mean energy required was 505 J/cm^2, and the mean follow-up period was 18.6 months.

Vellus hair regrowth appeared at around the 30th session and complete hair regrowth between the 50th and 80th sessions. Eleven of 17 patients treated with oral methoxsalen and total body irradiation had ≥ 90 percent regrowth. Four of the 7 patients with patchy alopecia areata, 5 of 7 patients with alopecia totalis, and 2 of 7 patients with alopecia universalis had complete hair regrowth. The 3 patients who used topical methoxsalen and UVA to the scalp were treatment failures, and the 3 who received oral methoxsalen and UVA to the scalp only were only partially responsive. The side effects seen in this study were minor. The most significant side effect was nausea in about 30 percent of patients taking oral methoxsalen.

Van der Schaar and Smitt treated 30 patients with alopecia areata—5 with alopecia totalis and the remainder with patchy alopecia areata[119]—with 8-MOP orally combined with whole-body UVA. A dose of 10 mg for those weighing 30 kg or less and up to 60 mg for those weighing greater than 90 kg was prescribed. Medication was taken 2 hours before light exposure in a stand-up light box with 62 fluorescent tubes emitting 310 to 380 nm irradiation. Patients were given total-body irradiation three times a week, with the initial dose being 1 J/cm^2. Treatment duration was 7 to 9.4 months. One patient had an excellent result, 8 had good results (including 3 of the 5 with alopecia totalis), 7 patients had poor results, 10 patients were treatment failures, and 4 patients stopped treatment for personal reasons. All the patients who had good results had recurrences within a mean time of 7.7 months after discontinuation of therapy.

In contrast, Lassus, Kianto, Johansson, and Juvakoski treated 41 patients, 15 with patchy alopecia areata, 8 with ophiasis-pattern alopecia areata, and 18 with either alopecia totalis or alopecia universalis.[120] 8-MOP was administered either orally (0.6 mg/kg) 2 hours before light application or topically with 1% 8-MOP ointment applied on the treated area 1 hour prior to UVA exposure. The initial UVA dose was approximately 1 J/cm^2, which was gradually increased to about 9 J/cm^2. The treatment was given as either local 8-MOP application plus local irradiation, oral 8-MOP plus local irradiation, or oral 8-MOP plus whole-body irradiation. The type of treatment given was selected according to the type of alopecia or for technical reasons, i.e., tall patients had local irradiation, and patients with a considerable amount of scalp hair were never treated with the ointment. Treatments were given twice a week, and the treatment results were evaluated after every 10 treatments. If no regrowth was seen after 20 treatments or a regrowth of less than 30 percent of the involved area was seen after 40 treatments, the treatment was interrupted.

Fifteen patients had < 30 percent regrowth, including 11 with either alopecia totalis or alopecia universalis. Six patients had 30 to 60 percent regrowth, and 20 had > 60 percent regrowth, including 12 with complete regrowth. Of these 20 patients, 5 had alopecia totalis or alopecia universalis. These 20 patients were followed 6 to 12 months off treatment and only 2 had recurrences. Two of 3 patients with an episode of alopecia areata of less than 5 years duration had an excellent response, compared with no or poor response in over 50 percent of patients with an episode of alopecia areata of greater than 5 years duration. There appeared to be no significant difference in response between the different treatment groups.

Hair Follicle Stimulant

MINOXIDIL

Minoxidil has a well-recognized effect on the prolongation of keratinocyte growth in vitro[121] and on increasing the proportion of hairs in anagen in monkeys and humans with androgenetic alopecia.[122,123] Weiss et al. treated 48 patients with alopecia areata, 24 with alopecia areata and 24 with alopecia totalis or universalis, with a 1% topical minoxidil solution.[124] These were all patients who were treatment failures to at least one other modality, if not several, used to treat alopecia areata. Patients applied the drug twice a day with a glass rod applicator only to the right side of the scalp and used a thin layer of petrolatum for occlusion at night. Duration of treatment ranged from 2 to 15 months. Cosmetically acceptable regrowth was defined as the patient no longer needing a wig or cap to conceal the hair loss on the treated side. Hair growth was noted approximately 2 months after the initiation of treatment but was not well-maintained after therapy was discontinued. A total of 25 patients had terminal hair regrowth, and 11 of the 25 had cosmetically acceptable hair regrowth. Six patients showed vellus hair regrowth, and 17 patients showed no regrowth. No positive correlation was seen between the response to minoxidil therapy and either disease severity, gender, duration of disease, or current episode of hair loss. There was also no correlation with the presence of personal or family history of autoimmune disease or atopy. Except for 1 patient developing an allergic contact dermatitis reaction to the minoxidil solution, no systemic side effects were seen.

Fiedler-Weiss, West, Buys, and Runsfield subsequently went on to study the use of 5% topical minoxidil in 47 patients with severe alopecia areata (only 9 patients had < 50 percent scalp hair loss), including 26 patients previously treated with 1% topical minoxidil.[125] The study duration was 60 weeks. For the first 12 weeks, therapy was double-blind and thereafter it was open-label. The solution was applied every 12 hours with a mesh applicator (Dab-O-Matic bottle). Thirty minutes after the evening application, a thin layer of petrolatum was used for occlusion. Forty of the 47 patients had terminal hair regrowth after 48 to 60 weeks of treatment. However, cosmetically acceptable hair regrowth (as defined earlier) was seen in 4 of 37 patients with 25 to 74 percent scalp hair loss and 2 of 6 patients with 75 to 100 percent hair loss. When compared with the data from the previous study on the use of topical 1% minoxidil solution, both the percentage of responders and the quality of hair regrowth were significantly greater with the 5% topical minoxidil compared with the 1% topical minoxidil solution.

In a corollary to the preceding study, Fiedler-Weiss further compared the efficacy of topical 1% and 5% minoxidil used in two similar but separate studies in the treatment of patients with alopecia areata.[126] Patients in both studies applied topical minoxidil every 12 hours to the areas of scalp hair loss, with petrolatum occlusion at night. Those on 5% topical minoxidil were treated in a double-blind fashion for 12 weeks and then open-label for the remainder of 60 weeks. Those on 1% minoxidil were treated with such from baseline. Of patients with extensive (75 percent or greater) scalp hair loss, 38 percent had terminal hair growth with 1% topical minoxidil vs. 81 percent of patients using 5% topical minoxidil. In patients with < 75 percent baseline hair loss, response was seen in 67 percent of those on 1% minoxidil vs. 100 percent of those on 5% minoxidil. Nonresponders in both studies were more likely to have severe alopecia areata. Cosmetically acceptable hair growth was also much more likely to be found and maintained in patients with patchy disease. The mean time to response in both studies was 2 to 3 months, and maximum achievable response generally occurred by 1 year.

In two studies, Price examined the use of 3% topical minoxidil applied twice daily for the treatment of alopecia areata.[127] In the double-blind, placebo-controlled, year-long trial, topical minoxidil–treated patients responded better than placebo-treated patients. In a second study, 30 patients were treated for 3 years with 3% topical minoxidil. No patient with 100 percent hair loss had a cosmetically acceptable response. In those patients with less than full scalp involvement (25–99 percent hair loss) who showed cosmetically acceptable hair growth (9 of 20 at 1 year), the response was apparent after 1 to 2 years of therapy. The third year of treatment did not produce additional cosmetically acceptable regrowth in any patient.

The use of topical minoxidil to treat alopecia areata is associated with few side effects. These include minor scalp irritation and mild facial hypertrichosis. Rare cases of allergic contact dermatitis and photoallergic contact dermatitis have been reported with topical minoxidil use.[125–128]

Fiedler-Weiss et al. have also examined the safety and efficacy of oral minoxidil in the treatment of alopecia areata. They evaluated 65 patients with severe treatment-resistant alopecia areata, including 34 patients previously treated with 5% topical minoxidil.[129] Forty-four patients had 75 to 100 percent scalp hair loss, 19 had 25 to 74 percent loss, and 2 had zero to 24 percent loss. Mean duration of alopecia areata was 6 years, and ages were 13 to 55 years. Patients took minoxidil 5 mg every 12 hours for a mean of 53 weeks (20–115 weeks). All patients were also asked to strictly follow a 2-g sodium diet. Hair regrowth progressed more rapidly and was more extensive with oral minoxidil than with 5% topical minoxidil. A cosmetically acceptable response was seen in 18 percent of patients. The mean time to response was 9.3 weeks, and mean time to cosmetic response was 34.8 weeks. Side effects included fluid retention (when the patient did not adhere to the 2-g sodium diet); occasional episodes of headaches, depression, or lethargy in women; occasional episodes of palpitations or tachycardia after ingestion of caffeine, alcohol, or decongestants; and facial hypertrichosis. Thirty-three patients, including 19 with a lack of response, discontinued oral minoxidil. Seven of the 14 who discontinued the drug for personal reasons experienced hair loss within 2 to 8 weeks after discontinuing therapy.

Topical Sensitizers

Three major chemical sensitizers have been used to treat alopecia areata. These are dinitrochlorobenzene (DNCB), squaric acid dibutyl ester (SADBE), and diphencyprone. None of these have been subjected to rigorous testing for stability, purity, absorption, metabolism, excretion, toxic effects, or carcinogenicity. Naldi et al. recently summarized the data published in English, French, and Italian, between January 1977 and January 1988, on sensitization therapy for alopecia areata.[130] Of the 26 studies, 19 were judged to present positive results, 4 negative results, and 3 equivocal results.

The mechanism of action of chemical sensitizers in alopecia areata is unclear but has been hypothesized to be antigen competition. Support for this hypothesis comes from studies demonstrating a relative increase in OKT8+ cells in the peribulbar infiltrate of patients treated with contact allergans.[131,132] Patients with active alopecia areata have perifollicular lymphocytic infiltrates with ratios of helper-inducer to suppressor-cytotoxic lymphocytes of 4:1, whereas patients with stable alopecia areata have ratios of 2:1. However, Johansson et al. reported no specific alterations in lymphocyte subsets of patients treated with topical SADBE[133] but did notice that during SADBE treatment the relative number of infiltrating helper-inducer cells increased. Bröcker, John, Steinhausen, and Hamm have shown no correlation of the in vivo change in delayed hypersensitivity with contact sensitizers to the clinical hair growth response.[134] The mechanism of action remains unknown.

The treatment of alopecia areata with repeated topical applications of DNCB was introduced by Rosenberg.[135] However, DNCB is mutagenic in the Ames test and, therefore, is now rarely used to treat alopecia areata.[136,137] SADBE, although negative in the Ames test, is reported to be unstable in acetone solution and is also now uncommonly used.[138,139] Diphencyprone is currently the most commonly used topical sensitizer[139–143] and is nonmutagenic[144] in the Ames assay. However, it is very photolabile, and the potential photomutagenic property of diphencyprone as well as the mutagenic properties of a synthetic precursor of diphencyprone, α,α'-dibromodibenzylketone, have been demonstrated.[144,145]

To initiate sensitization therapy, the following procedure is typically used. Since diphencyprone is readily degraded by ultraviolet light, it is usually made up with acetone, ethanol, or cyclohexane stored in dark glass bottles at room temperature.[145] The patient is normally sensitized to a 2% solution. After sensitization is complete, typically at 14 days, weekly applications of a concentration sufficient to elicit a mild allergic contact dermatitis are used.[146,147] Weekly concentrations may range from 1.0, 0.5, 0.1, 0.05, 0.01, 0.001, to 0.0001%. Diphencyprone concentrations needed to maintain a mild allergic contact dermatitis, i.e., mild eczema without blistering or oozing, may vary during treatment. In some studies, the weekly applications have been made by the patient; in others, by a physician or nurse. Studies on the stability of diphencyprone in solution with acetone have shown that appreciable evaporation of the acetone occurs by the third month, suggesting that the shelf life of diphencyprone in acetone is 3 months.[146]

The first trial of diphencyprone in the treatment of alopecia areata was reported in 1983 by Happle, Hausen, and Wiesner-Menzel.[140] Twenty-seven patients, 5 with ≥ 25 percent scalp hair loss and 22 with alopecia totalis, were treated with topical diphencyprone. Sensitization was obtained with a 2% solution applied once to one-half of the scalp: the other side of the scalp served as the control. At the weekly applications, dose adjustments were made according to the patient's reactivity against the allergen. The duration of treatment ranged from 4 to 17 months. Unilateral induction of hair growth was observed in 23 of 27 patients.

Subsequent to this trial, numerous investigators reported the successful use of diphencyprone in the therapy of alopecia areata.[139,141–143,147] However, the response rates varied greatly among these studies. Recently, the use of diphencyprone for the treatment of childhood alopecia areata has been described.[148] In this pediatric study, 12 children with extensive alopecia areata or alopecia totalis were treated with diphencyprone for 5 to 12 months. Eight of the 12 patients regrew hair, including 4 patients with complete hair regrowth. Six months after treatment was discontinued, 3 of the 4 children with complete hair regrowth had maintained their hair and 1 lost all of the regrowth.

Van der Steen et al. ascertained prognostic factors in 139 patients with extensive alopecia areata treated with topical diphencyprone.[149] The following three factors were found to be of negative prognostic significance: type of alopecia areata as documented before treatment, duration of the disease before therapy, and presence of nail changes. Factors which did not significantly influence the response to topical immunotherapy were the following: age of onset, sex, presence of atopic features, extent of variation in the range of diphencyprone concentrations during treatment, or sleep disturbances caused by pruritus.

MacDonald-Hull and Cunliffe reported that if the alopecia areata process becomes active, diphencyprone is unable to reverse this process.[146] During phases of disease activity, not only is the newly regrown hair lost but there is a simultaneous reduction in sensitivity to diphencyprone.

Side effects associated with the contact dermatitis induced by the use of topical sensitizers include pruritus, a mild to severe dermatitis, and regional lymphadenopathy. Sleep disturbances have also been reported. Less common side effects include contact urticaria, erythema multiforme–like reactions, vitiligo, arthralgias, and fever.[139–143,147–148]

Irritants

Anthralin is an irritant that can induce hair regrowth in alopecia areata. The mechanism is unknown, but hair growth does not occur with topical application of other potential irritants (croton oil, sodium lauryl sulfate, topical tretinoin).[150–152] Schmoeckel, Weissmann, Plewig, and Braun-Falco were the first to try inducing hair growth in patients with alopecia areata by producing a noninflammatory nonallergic dermatitis.[153] They treated 32 patients, 8 with alopecia totalis and 24 with moderate hair loss, including 6 with the ophiasis-pattern alopecia areata. Anthralin in 0.2% to 0.8% concentrations in an ointment base was applied once daily. A visible dermatitis was usually induced. Treatment was interrupted for several days if severe itching, blistering, or regional lymph node swelling developed. Treatment was continued for several weeks after regrowth of hair had become visible. Hair regrowth was first visible after 5 to 8 weeks and first presented as thin, white hairs which later became repigmented. Of the 24 patients with patchy alopecia areata, 18 had cosmetically good results, 3 grew hair only transiently, and 3 showed no response. Of the 8 patients with alopecia totalis, 2 had cosmetically good results, 1 grew hair only for a short period, 2 grew only vellus hairs, and 3 had no response.

Subsequently, Fiedler-Weiss and Buys examined the efficacy of anthralin cream in the treatment of 66 patients with severe alopecia areata.[154] The patients ranged in age from 4 to 68 years. A 0.5% anthralin cream (Drithocreme) was applied at bedtime on alternate days for the first 2 weeks and daily thereafter for a mean duration of 28 weeks. Eight hours after application, patients shampooed with zinc pyrithione (Head and Shoulders). If no regrowth was seen after 6 months or no additional growth was seen in the preceding 3 months, the concentration of anthralin was increased to 0.75%. If there was no regrowth after another 6 months or no additional improvement in the preceding 3 months, the anthralin concentration was increased to 1%. Exposure time to 1% anthralin was initially 30 minutes, and the time then increased to tolerance. Examinations were every 3 months.

A response was seen during the first 3 months of treatment with 0.5% anthralin in 15 of 29 patients with 75 to 100 percent scalp hair loss, in 16 of 33 patients with 25 to 74 percent scalp hair loss, and in all 4 patients with 0 to 24 percent scalp hair loss. Response was eventually achieved in 44 of the 66 patients (67 percent), with the mean time to response being 11 weeks. A cosmetic response, defined as sufficient terminal hair regrowth such that a wig or cap was not necessary to conceal hair loss, occurred in 13 of 66 patients treated with 0.5% anthralin and in 17 of the 68 patients treated with 0.5% to 1.0% anthralin. The mean time of therapy to attain a cosmetic response was 23 weeks. Expected side effects were pruritus, erythema, and scaling. Local pyoderma (if the patient did not shampoo with zinc pyrithione) and regional lymphadenopathy were occasionally seen.

Combination Therapy

Many combination therapies have been tried in alopecia areata. Some of those involving the combination of topical, intralesional, and/or systemic steroids were reviewed earlier. Other combinations which have been tried include the following.

Prednisolone 5 mg/kg was administered for 2 months followed by oral administration of 2.5 mg/kg of cyclosporine in six patients with treatment-refractory alopecia universalis.[155] Cyclosporine was used for 5 months, and prednisolone therapy was continued during the cyclosporine therapy and gradually decreased after the cyclosporine therapy was discontinued. One month after the addition of cyclosporine, hair began to grow in all six cases and continued for more than 6 months after the cessation of cyclosporine.

Olsen, Carson, and Turney examined the effect of 2% topical minoxidil on prednisone-induced hair growth.[77] At the completion of 6 weeks of a tapering dose (as noted previously in the section on steroids) of prednisone, patients were randomly prescribed either 2% topical minoxidil or vehicle. For 14 weeks after completion of the steroid taper, up to 1 ml of topical minoxidil was applied three times a day by patients who weighed 40 kg or more and up to 0.5 ml three times a day by patients who weighed less than 40 kg. The results of this study were compared with an open trial of 48 patients with alopecia areata treated with a similar taper of prednisone with concomitant 2% topical minoxidil applied twice a day. Sixteen of 32 patients in the controlled trial vs. 13 of 43 in the open trial had alopecia totalis or universalis. At the end of 6 weeks of prednisone therapy, 15 of 32 (47 percent) patients had an objective response (≥ 25 percent regrowth). At 3 months after discontinuing prednisone, 6 of 7 2% topical minoxidil–treated patients vs. 1 of 6 vehicle-treated patients who had an objective response to prednisone maintained or improved their hair growth. At 20 weeks, these numbers were 3 of 7 and 0 of 4 patients, respectively. In the open trial, an objective response to the combination of prednisone and 2% topical minoxidil was seen in 13 of 43 (30 percent) at the end of 6 to 8 weeks, and this growth persisted in more than 50 percent of patients at 6 months with the continued use of 2% topical minoxidil. The authors concluded that 2% topical minoxidil appears to limit or slow poststeroid hair loss in patients with alopecia areata.

In a controlled, double-blind study in patients with severe, chronically treatment-resistant alopecia areata, twice-daily application of 5% topical minoxidil followed 30 minutes later by the application of 0.05% betamethasone dipropionate cream (Diprosone, nonoptimized vehicle) vs. either therapy alone, or placebo, was evaluated (J. J. Ferry and V. C. Fiedler, AAD poster presentation, 1991). Thirteen percent treated with placebo, 22 percent treated with steroid alone, 27 percent treated with minoxidil alone, and 56 percent treated with the combination therapy showed a fair to good regrowth of hair after 16 weeks of therapy. This synergism may include different mechanisms of action. The authors postulated that the concomitant use of topical steroid increases the local tissue concentration of minoxidil, probably through vasoconstriction and a secondary reduced clearance of drug.[156]

The use of topical 5% minoxidil plus 0.5% anthralin (Drithocreme) was evaluated in an open-label study of severe treatment-resistant alopecia areata.[157] One milliliter of 5% topical minoxidil was applied twice a day and the anthralin applied 2 hours after the evening minoxidil dose and left on overnight. Terminal hair regrowth was seen in 39 of 50 patients at week 12. Cosmetically acceptable response (patient no longer needing to wear a wig to conceal hair loss) was achieved in 5 of 45 patients by week 24, and 4 of these 5 patients maintained good regrowth with continued treatment up to 84 weeks. Side effects were mild to moderate scaling and pruritus. Although minoxidil blood levels increased over topical minoxidil alone, there was no clinical evidence of systemic minoxidil effects.

The combination of diphencyprone and inosiplex therapy was evaluated for the treatment of alopecia totalis.[158] Three groups matched for age and sex were studied. One group received inosiplex 50 mg/kg per day, another group was treated with diphencyprone topically, and the third group received both treatments. The duration of therapy was 6 months. In contradistinction to the earlier reported studies with inosiplex,[109–111] none of the 22 patients treated with inosiplex responded and only 2 of 22 patients responded to diphencyprone alone.

Shapiro, Tan, and Tron sensitized 15 patients with alopecia areata to diphencyprone and then weekly treated one-half of the scalp of each patient.[159] Therapy with either 5% topical minoxidil or placebo twice daily to the diphencyprone-treated half of the scalp was randomly assigned. After 24 weeks, 5 of the 15 patients showed significant unilateral regrowth, including 3 of 5 on diphencyprone and vehicle and 2 of 5 on diphencyprone and topical minoxidil 5%. The use of topical minoxidil did not appear to add to the success rate of diphencyprone alone.

Zinc

Oral zinc has been reported to be helpful in treating alopecia areata. Wolowa and Jablonska reported successful treatment of two patients with alopecia areata with 600 mg of zinc sulfate daily.[160] Both patients regrew their hair after treatment for weeks to a few months. Serum zinc levels were normal in both patients before treatment. Ead subsequently designed a double-blind trial to investigate the effect of zinc therapy for alopecia areata.[161] Forty-two patients with alopecia areata participated in this study. One-half were given 220 mg of zinc sulfate twice daily for 3 months, and the other half received an identical placebo capsule. There was no improvement in disease extent or activity with zinc treatment.

Cryotherapy

An interesting therapy for alopecia areata is the use of liquid nitrogen. Huang, Huans, and Wei first reported treating 123 patients with liquid nitrogen spray, with a "cure rate" of 71.5 percent.[162] Lei et al. subsequently used liquid nitrogen to treat 72 patients between the ages of 3 and 59 years who had patchy alopecia areata.[163] A cotton swab application of liquid nitrogen was applied to the involved area until it became slightly frozen. After the area thawed, a second treatment of comparable duration was administered. Treatments were repeated every week for 4 weeks. A comparable control group of 40 patients with patchy alopecia areata was treated with 2% glacial acetic acid lotion t.i.d. for 4 weeks. New hair growth occurred in over 60 percent of the areas treated with liquid nitrogen in 70 of 72 (97 percent) patients. Hair growth with liquid nitrogen was usually seen after just one or two treatments. Fourteen of 40 (35 percent) patients in the control group had new hair growth over more than 60 percent of the scalp, and 22 of 40 (55 percent) control group patients had no improvement. Side effects of liquid nitrogen therapy were transient swelling, hyperesthesia, and itching.

Treatments With No Benefit or Proven Efficacy

Fiedler, in her excellent review of the therapy of alopecia areata, also reviewed the treatments used for alopecia areata which have shown no benefit or proven efficacy.[92] Those treatments which have been studied and shown to be of no benefit include the vitamin D analogue calcipotriol,[164] intralesional interferon alpha-2,[165] and the irritants croton oil[150] and sodium lauryl sulfate.[151] Other treatments which have been studied and shown no proven efficacy in the management of alopecia areata include the use of staphylococcus-streptococcus vaccine, griseofulvin, relaxation, topical tretinoin, or the irritants benzyl benzoate and phenol.[92,152,166–168]

No Treatment

Tosti, Bardazzi, and Guerra posed the question of whether treating patients with alopecia areata who are nonresponders to sensitizing therapies is useful.[169] Twenty-six patients with alopecia totalis or universalis who did not respond to 1 year of sensitizing therapies were randomly assigned to receive either topical 10% cyclosporine in an oily solution (8 patients), PUVA (8 patients), or intravenous thymopentin (10 patients). After 6 months of therapy, none of the patients had any cosmetically acceptable improvements. The authors concluded that patients with 100 percent scalp hair loss who had failed previous treatments should not be placed in clinical trials evaluating new therapeutic agents, as the inclusion of such patients may lead to misleading results.

Tosti, De Padova, Minghetti, and Veronesi also examined whether patchy alopecia areata treated with various topical therapies produced different results from the use of placebo.[170] One hundred nineteen patients between 5 and 74 years of age with patchy alopecia areata affecting less than 40 percent of the scalp were studied. Forty-four patients were treated with topical squaric acid dibutylester, 35 with topical diphencyprone, 20 with 1% topical minoxidil, and 20 with placebo. In all cases, treatment was carried out for at least 6 months. No significant differences were seen comparing the different therapies and the placebo-treated group, suggesting that these treatments do not actually affect the natural course of hair regrowth in mild forms of alopecia areata.

Cosmetic Management

HAIR REPLACEMENT OPTIONS

The use of turbans and scarves, hairpieces, or custom prostheses is an exceptionally important part of therapy for patients with extensive alopecia areata. Turbans and scarves are relatively inexpensive and can be purchased at hair replacement centers, better wig shops, department stores, and beauty product outlets. Machine-made hairpieces, commonly referred to as *wigs*, averaging $60.00 to $300.00 can also be purchased at hair replacement centers, department stores, and wig shops. Custom hairpieces (cranial prostheses) are made by hand, not machine, and can be purchased in better wig shops or hair replacement centers. These cost in the range of

$350.00 to $700.00. Full-custom hairpieces (full cranial prostheses) are made by taking a mold of the head and the hairpiece is then constructed by hand. Such full-custom hairpieces cost from $900.00 to $2000.00 and can usually be purchased only through a hair replacement center.

TATTOOS

Tattooing has been used to mask the loss of eyebrows and eyelashes. The main drawbacks to this procedure are its cost and its permanence. In an alopecia areata patient who has no eyebrows, the technician has no visible guidelines for placement of the eyebrow tattoo. Patients should be forewarned that their natural eyebrows may grow back eventually in a different location than the tattoo and may then necessitate plucking or electrolysis to remove hairs outside the tattoo.

CONCLUDING REMARKS

The clinical features, histology, and epidemiology of alopecia areata were reviewed in this chapter. The postulated etiologies of alopecia areata were presented, including the immune and neural hypotheses, and the theory that alopecia areata is related to intrinsically abnormal keratinocytes or melanocytes. The chapter concluded with a summary of the many treatments that have been utilized to treat both patchy and extensive alopecia areata.

REFERENCES

1. Yesudian P, Thambiah AS: Perinevoid alopecia. Arch Dermatol 112:1432–1434, 1976.
2. Messenger AG, Slatter DN, Bleehen SS: Alopecia areata: Alterations in the hair growth cycle and correlation with the follicular pathology. Br J Dermatol 114:337–347, 1986.
3. Peereboom-Wynia JDR, Koerten HK, Van Joost TH, Stolz E: Scanning electron microscopy comparing exclamation mark hairs in alopecia areata with normal hair fibres, mechanically broken by traction. Clin Exp Dermatol 14:47–50, 1989.
4. Headington JT: The histopathology of alopecia areata (abstract). J Invest Dermatol 96:69S, 1991.
5. Orecchia G, Douville H, Marelli MA: Nail changes and alopecia areata. Ital Gen Rev Dermatol 25:179–184, 1988.
6. Klingmuller G, Rech E: Nagelgrubchen und deren Familiare Haufungen bei der Alopecia Areata. Arch Klin Exp Dermatol 201:574–584, 1955.
7. Baden HP: Nail abnormalities associated with cutaneous diseases. In Baden HP (ed): *Diseases of the Hair and Nails.* Chicago, Year Book Medical Publishers, 1987, pp 134–143.
8. Pierard-Franchimont C, Pierard GE: Corroborative evidence that alopecia areata involves the epidermis and the sebaceous glands. Am J Dermatopathol 9:111–113, 1987.
9. Elieff D, Sundby S, Kennedy W, Hordinsky M: Decreased sweat-gland number and function in patients with alopecia areata. Br J Dermatol 125:130–135, 1991.
10. Muller SA, Winkelmann RK: Alopecia areata. Arch Dermatol 88:290–297, 1963.
11. DeWeert K, Temmerman L, Kint A: Alopecia areata: A clinical study. Dermatologica 168:224–229, 1984.
12. Young E, Bruns HM, Berrens L: Alopecia areata and atopy. Dermatologica 156:306–308, 1978.
13. Blumenthal MN: Family, twin, and population studies of allergic responsiveness. In Marsh DJ, Lochart A, Holgate ST (eds): *The Genetics of Asthma.* Oxford, Blackwell Scientific Publications, 1993, pp 133–142.
14. Cunliffe WJ, Hall R, Stevenson CJ, Weightman D: Alopecia areata, thyroid disease, and autoimmunity. Br J Dermatol 81:877–881, 1969.
15. Main RA et al.: Smooth muscle antibodies and alopecia areata. Br J Dermatol 92:389–393, 1975.
16. Mitchell AJ, Krull EA: Alopecia areata: Pathogenesis and treatment. J Am Acad Dermatol 11:763–775, 1984.
17. Hordinsky MA: Alopecia areata. In Jordan RE (ed): *Immunologic Diseases of the Skin.* East Norwalk, CT, Appleton and Lange, 1991, pp 427–434.
18. Nelson DA, Spielvogel RL: Alopecia areata (review). Int J Dermatol 24:26–34, 1985.
19. Aw TC, Cheah JS: Diabetes mellitus presenting with alopecia areata totalis (letter). Lancet 1(2):268, 1978.
20. Schonwetter RS, Nelson EB: Alopecia areata and the acquired-immunodeficiency-syndrome-related-complex. Ann Intern Med 104:287, 1986.
21. Ostlere LS, Langry JAA, Staughton RCD, Samrasinghe PL: Alopecia universalis in a patient seropositive for the human immunodeficiency virus. J Am Acad Dermatol 27:630–631, 1992.
22. Carter DM, Jegasothy BV: Alopecia areata and Down syndrome. Arch Dermatol 112:1397–1399, 1976.
23. Du Vivier A, Munro DD: Alopecia areata, autoimmunity and Down's syndrome. Br Med J 1:191–192, 1975.
24. Casteels Van Daele M, Proesmans W, Van den Berghe H, Verresen H: Down's anomaly (21 trisomy) and Turner's syndrome (46, XXqi) in the same sibship. Helv Paediatr Acta 25:412–420, 1970.
25. Brown AC, Pollard ZF, Jarrett WH: Ocular and testicular abnormalities in alopecia areata. Arch Dermatol 118:546–554, 1982.
26. Tosti A et al.: Retinal pigment epithelium function in alopecia areata. J Invest Dermatol 86:553–555, 1986.
27. MacDonald-Hull SP et al.: Immunohistologic and ultrastructural comparison of the dermal papilla and hair follicle bulb from "active" and "normal" areas of alopecia areata. J Invest Dermatol 96:673–681, 1991.
28. Tobin DJ, Fenton DA, Kendall MD: Cell degeneration in alopecia areata. Am J Dermatopathol 13:248–256, 1991.
29. Goos M: Zur Histopathologie der Alopecia Areata: Mit Besonderer Berucksichtigung ihrer Beziehung zur Dauer, Lokalisation und Progression des Haarausfalls. Arch Dermatol Forsch 240:160–172, 1971.
30. Thies W: Vergleighende Histologische Untersuchungen bei Alopecia Areata und Narbig-Atrophisierenden Alopecian. Arch Klin Exp Dermatol 227:541–549, 1966.
31. Van Scott EJ: Evaluation of disturbed hair growth in alopecia areata and other alopecias. Ann NY Acad Sci 83:480–490, 1959.
32. Klingmuller G: Alopecia Areata: Mit be sonderer Berücksichtigung der Therapie. Hautarzt 9:97–108, 1958.

33. Prieto JG, Gonzalez GG, Uria-Rico MA: Inervación del folíaculo piloso en las alopecias universales. Actas Dermosifiliogr 65(9–10):477–484, 1974.
34. Bröcker E-B, Echternacht-Happle K, Hamm H, Happle R: Abnormal expression of class I and class II major histocompatibility antigens in alopecia areata: Modulation by topical immunotherapy. J Invest Dermatol 88:564–568, 1987.
35. Harrist TJ, Ruiter DJ, Mihm MC Jr, Bhan AK: Distribution of major histocompatibility antigens in normal skin. Br J Dermatol 109:623–633, 1983.
36. Messenger AG, Bleehen SS: Expression of HLA-DR by anagen hair follicles in alopecia areata. J Invest Dermatol 85:569–572, 1985.
37. Hamm H et al.: HLA-DR and HLA-DQ antigen expression of anagen and telogen hair bulbs in long-standing alopecia areata. Arch Dermatol Res 280:179–181, 1988.
38. Khoury EL, Price VH, Greenspan JS: HLA-DR expression by hair follicle keratinocytes in alopecia areata: Evidence that it is secondary to the lymphoid infiltration. J Invest Dermatol 90:193–200, 1988.
39. Nickoloff BJ, Griffiths CEM: Aberrant intercellular adhesion molecule-1 (ICAM-1) expression by hair follicle epithelial cells and endothelial leukocyte adhesion molecule-1 (ELAM-1) by vascular cells are important adhesion-molecule alterations in alopecia areata. J Invest Dermatol 96:91S–92S, 1991.
40. Dustin LM, Singer KH, Tuck DT, Springer TA: Adhesion of T lymphoblasts to epidermal keratinocytes is regulated by interferon gamma and is mediated by intercellular adhesion molecule (ICAM-1). J Exp Med 167:1323–1340, 1988.
41. Gollnick H, Imcke E, Orfanos CE: Immunohistochemical study of the expression of cytokeratins, filaggrin, and basement membrane proteins in hair follicles of alopecia areata patients (abstract). Arch Dermatol Res 281:145, 1989.
42. Van Baar HMJ et al.: Expression of tenascin in perifollicular connective tissue: Comparison of normal scalp and alopecia areata. Arch Dermatol Res 283:86–90, 1991.
43. Laporte M, Stouffs-Vanhoof JA, Achten G: Nail changes in alopecia areata: Light and electron microscopy. Arch Dermatol Res 280:S85, 1988.
44. Tosti A, Fanti PA, Morelli R, Bardazzi F: Trachyonychia associated with alopecia areata: A clinical and pathologic study. J Am Acad Dermatol 25:266–270, 1991.
45. Brown WH: The etiology of alopecia areata and its relationship to vitiligo and possibly scleroderma. Br J Dermatol Syph 41:299–323, 1929.
46. Safavi K: Prevalence of alopecia areata in the First National Health and Nutrition Examination Survey (letter). Arch Dermatol 128:702, 1992.
47. Gollnick H, Organos CE: Alopecia areata: Pathogenesis and clinical picture. In Orfanos CE, Happle R (eds): *Hair and Hair Diseases.* Berlin, Springer-Verlag, 1990, pp 529–569.
48. Runne U: Alopecia areata. In Orfanos CE (ed): *Haar und Haarkrankheiten.* Stuttgart, Fischer, 1979, pp 505–544.
49. Ikeda T: A new classification of alopecia areata. Dermatologica 131:421–445, 1965.
50. Penders AJ: Alopecia areata and atopy. Dermatologica 136:395–399, 1968.
51. Mali JWH: Alopecia areata. Br J Dermatol 93:605–606, 1975.
52. Walker SA, Rothman S: Alopecia areata: A statistical study and consideration of endocrine influences. J Invest Dermatol 14:403–413, 1950.
53. Goldsmith LA: Summary of alopecia areata research workshop and future research directions. J Invest Dermatol 96:98S–100S, 1991.
54. De Waard Van der Spek FB, Orange AP, De-Raeymaecker DM, Peereboom-Wynia JDR: Juvenile versus maturity-onset alopecia areata: A comparative retrospective clinical study. Clin Exp Dermatol 14:429–433, 1989.
55. Sauder DN: Alopecia areata: An inherited autoimmune disease. In Brown AC, Crounse RG (eds): *Hair, Trace Elements and Human Illness.* New York, Praeger, 1980, pp 343–347.
56. Hendren OS: Identical alopecia areata in identical twins. Arch Dermatol 60:793–795, 1949.
57. Cole GW, Herzlinger D: Alopecia universalis in identical twins. Int J Dermatol 23:283, 1984.
58. Scerri L, Pace JL: Identical twins with identical alopecia areata. J Am Acad Dermatol 27:766–767, 1992.
59. Duvic M, Hordinsky MK, Fiedler VC, O'Brien WR: HLA-D locus associations in alopecia areata. Arch Dermatol 127:64, 1991.
60. Kuntz BM, Selzle D, Braun-Falco O: HLA antigens in alopecia areata. Arch Dermatol 113:1717, 1977.
61. Kianto U et al.: HLA-B12 in alopecia areata. Arch Dermatol 113:1716, 1977.
62. Hacham-Zaden S, Brautbar C, Cohen CA, Cohen T: HLA and alopecia areata in Jerusalem. Tissue Antigens 18:71–74, 1981.
63. Orecchia G et al.: Human leukocyte antigen region involvement in the genetic predisposition to alopecia areata. Dermatologica 175:10–14, 1987.
64. Frentz G, Thomsen K, Jakobsen BK, Svejgaard A: HLA-DR4 in alopecia areata. J Am Acad Dermatol 14:129, 1982.
65. Mikesell JF, Bergfeld WF, Braun WE: HLA-DR antigens in alopecia areata. Cleve Clin Q 53:189–191, 1986.
66. Averbakh EV, Pospelo LE: HLA antigens in patients with alopecia areata. Vestn Dermatol Venerol 1:24–26, 1986.
67. Odum N et al.: HLA-DP antigens in patients with alopecia areata. Tissue Antigens 35:114–117, 1990.
68. Clark HH, Welsh E, Reveille JD, Duvic M: Alopecia areata is not associated with HLA-DPB1 (abstract). Clin Res 40:497A, 1992.
69. Hordinsky MK, Hallgren H, Nelson D, Filipovich AH: Familial alopecia areata. Arch Dermatol 120:464–468, 1984.
70. Galbraith GMP, Thiers BH, Pandey JP: Gm allotype associated resistance and susceptibility to alopecia areata. Clin Exp Immunol 56:149–152, 1984.
71. Valsecchi R, Bontempelli M, Vicari O: Peripheral T-cell subsets in patients with alopecia areata in different clinical phases. Dermatologica 171:170–174, 1985.
72. Bystryn JC, Tamesis J: Immunological aspects of hair loss. J Invest Dermatol 96:88S, 1991.
73. Galbraith GMP et al.: Increased ratio of helper to suppressor T cells in alopecia areata. Br J Dermatol 110:171–175, 1984.
74. Majewski BBJ et al.: Increased ratio of helper to suppressor T cells in alopecia areata. Br J Dermatol 110:171–175, 1984.
75. Kalish RS, Johansson KL, Hordinsky MK: Autoreactive T-cells are variably enriched relative to peripheral blood in the scalp lesions of alopecia areata. Arch Dermatol 128:1072–1077, 1992.
76. Gilhar A, Krueger GG: Hair growth in scalp grafts from patients with alopecia areata and alopecia universalis grafted onto nude mice. Arch Dermatol 123:44–50, 1987.
77. Olsen EA, Carson SL, Turney EA: Systemic steroids with or without 2% topical minoxidil in the treatment of alopecia areata. Arch Dermatol 128:1467–1473, 1992.
78. Gupta AK et al.: Oral cyclosporine for the treatment of

alopecia areata: A clinical and immunohistochemical analysis. J Am Acad Dermatol 22:242–250, 1990.
79. Oliver RF et al.: The DEBR rat model for alopecia areata. J Invest Dermatol 96:97S, 1991.
80. Sainsbury TSL et al.: Differential effects of FK 506 and cyclosporine on hair regrowth in the DEBR model of alopecia areata. Transplant Proc 23:3332–3334, 1991.
81. Sundberg JP, King LE: An alopecia areata-like disease in aging C3M/MEJ mice (abstract). Clin Res 40:781A, 1992.
82. Messenger AG, Bleehen SS: Alopecia areata: Light and electron microscopic pathology of the regrowing white hair. Br J Dermatol 110:155–162, 1984.
83. Tobin DJ, Fenton DA, Kendall MD: Ultrastructural observations on the hair bulb melanocytes and melanosomes in acute alopecia areata. J Invest Dermatol 94:803–807, 1990.
84. Nonemann VW, Hofer W: Bestehen Beziehungen Zwischen der Lokalisation der Alopecia-Areata-Herde und der Nervalen Versorgung des Kopfes? Dermatol Monatsschr 156:683–689, 1970.
85. Watanabe Y et al.: A special trial in the treatment of alopecia areata by occipital nerve blockage with electron microscopical studies. In Kobori T, Montagna W (eds): *Biology and Disease of the Hair.* Tokyo, University of Tokyo Press, 1976, pp 529–542.
86. Ishizaki F, Sasaki K, Shimoda Y, Shimao S: EEG findings, rapid ACTH test and autonomic nervous symptoms in patients with alopecia areata. J Neural Transm 39:71, 1976.
87. Anderson I: Alopecia areata: A clinical study. Br Med J 1250–1252, 1950.
88. Mehlman RD, Griesemer RD: Alopecia areata in the very young. Am J Psychiatry 125:605–614, 1968.
89. Perini GI et al.: Life events and alopecia areata. Psychother Psychosom 41:48–52, 1984.
90. Van Moffaert M: Psychosomatics of alopecia. Dermatologica 171:501, 1985.
91. Colon EA et al.: Lifetime prevalence of psychiatric disorders in patients with alopecia areata. Compr Psychiatry 32:245–251, 1991.
92. Fiedler VC: Alopecia areata: A review of therapy, efficacy, safety, and mechanism. Arch Dermatol 128:1519–1529, 1992.
93. Pascher F, Kurtin S, Andrade R: Assay of 0.2% fluocinolone acetonide cream for alopecia areata and totalis. Dermatologica 141:193–202, 1970.
94. Montes LF: Topical halcinonide in alopecia areata and in alopecia totalis. J Cutan Pathol 4:47–50, 1977.
95. Porter D, Burton JL: A comparison of intralesional triamcinolone hexacetonide and triamcinolone acetonide in alopecia areata. Br J Dermatol 85:272–273, 1971.
96. Abell E, Munro DD: Intralesional treatment of alopecia areata with triamcinolone acetonide by jet injector. Br J Dermatol 88:55–59, 1973.
97. Orentreich N, Sturm HM, Weidman AI, Pelzig A: Local injection of steroids and hair regrowth in alopecias. Arch Dermatol 82:894–902, 1960.
98. Selmanowitz VJ, Orentreich N: Cutaneous corticosteroid injection and amaurosis. Arch Dermatol 110:729–734, 1974.
99. Michalowski R, Kuczynska L: Long-term intramuscular triamcinolon-acetonide therapy in alopecia areata totalis and universalis. Arch Dermatol Res 261:73–76, 1978.
100. Dillaha CJ, Rothman S: Therapeutic experiments in alopecia areata with orally administered cortisone. JAMA 150:546–550, 1952.
101. Kern F, Hoffman WH, Hambrick GW, Blizzard RM: Alopecia areata: Immunologic studies and treatment with prednisone. Arch Dermatol 107:407–412, 1973.
102. Winter RJ, Kern F, Blizzard RM: Prednisone therapy for alopecia areata. Arch Dermatol 112:1549–1552, 1976.
103. Unger WP, Schemmer RJ: Corticosteroids in the treatment of alopecia totalis: Systemic effects. Arch Dermatol 114:1486–1490, 1978.
104. Burton JL, Shuster S: Large doses of glucocorticoid in the treatment of alopecia areata. Acta Derm Venereol (Stockh) 55:493–496, 1975.
105. DeProst Y et al.: Placebo-controlled trial of topical cyclosporine in severe alopecia areata (letter). Lancet 2(2):803–804, 1986.
106. Gilhar A, Pillar T, Etzioni A: Topical cyclosporin A in alopecia areata. Acta Derm Venereol (Stockh) 69:252–253, 1989.
107. Coulson IH, Holden CA: Topical cyclosporine A in alopecia totalis: Failure of therapeutic effect due to lack of penetration. Br J Dermatol 121(suppl 34):53–54, 1989.
108. Parodi A, Rebora A: Topical cyclosporine in alopecia areata (letter). Arch Dermatol 123:165–166, 1987.
109. Lowy M, Ledoux-Corbusier M, Achten G, Wybran J: Clinical and immunologic response to isoprinosine in alopecia areata and alopecia universalis: Association with autoantibodies. J Am Acad Dermatol 12:78–84, 1985.
110. Galbraith GMP, Thiers BH, Fudenberg HH: An open-label trial of immunomodulation therapy with Inosiplex (isoprinosine) in patients with alopecia totalis and cell-mediated immunodeficiency. J Am Acad Dermatol 11:224–230, 1984.
111. Galbraith GMP, Thiers BH, Jensen J, Hoehler F: A randomized double-blind study of Inosiplex (isoprinosine) therapy in patients with alopecia totalis. J Am Acad Dermatol 16:977–983, 1987.
112. Tosti A, Manuzzi P, Gasponi A: Thymopentin in the treatment of severe alopecia areata. Dermatologica 177:170–174, 1988.
113. Orecchia G: Thymopentin in the treatment of alopecia areata (letter). Dermatologica 178:231–232, 1989.
114. Arrazola JM, Sendagorta E, Harto A, Ledo A: Treatment of alopecia areata with topical nitrogen mustard. Int J Dermatol 24:608–610, 1985.
115. Goddard CJR, August PJ, Whorwell PJ: Alopecia totalis in a patient with Crohn's disease and its treatment with azathioprine. Postgrad Med J 65:188–189, 1989.
116. Krook G: Treatment of alopecia areata with Kromayer's ultraviolet lamp. Acta Derm Venereol (Stockh) 41:178–181, 1961.
117. Weissmann I et al.: PUVA-therapy for alopecia areata. Arch Dermatol Res 262:333–336, 1978.
118. Claudy AL, Gagnaire D: PUVA treatment of alopecia areata. Arch Dermatol 119:975–978, 1983.
119. van der Schaar WW, Smitt JHS: An evaluation of PUVA-therapy for alopecia areata. Dermatologica 168:250–252, 1984.
120. Lassus A, Kianto U, Johansson E, Juvakoski T: PUVA treatment for alopecia areata. Dermatologica 161:298–304, 1980.
121. Baden HP, Kubilus J: Effect of minoxidil on cultured keratinocytes. J Invest Dermatol 81:558–560, 1983.
122. Uno H, Cappas A, Brigham P: Action of topical minoxidil in the bald stump-tail macaque. J Am Acad Dermatol 16:657–668, 1987.
123. Headington JT, Novak E: Clinical and histological studies of male pattern baldness treated with topical minoxidil. Curr Ther Res 36:1098–1106, 1984.
124. Weiss VC et al.: Alopecia areata treated with topical minoxidil. Arch Dermatol 120:457–463, 1984.
125. Fiedler-Weiss VC, West DP, Buys CM, Runsfield JA:

Topical minoxidil dose-response effect in alopecia areata. Arch Dermatol 122:180–182, 1986.
126. Feidler-Weiss VC: Topical minoxidil solution (1% and 5%) in the treatment of alopecia areata. J Am Acad Dermatol 16:745–748, 1987.
127. Price VH: Topical minoxidil in extensive alopecia areata, including 3-year follow-up. Dermatologica 175(suppl 2):36–41, 1987.
128. Tosti A et al.: Contact dermatitis to minoxidil. Contact Derm 13:275–276, 1985.
129. Fiedler-Weiss VC et al.: Evaluation of oral minoxidil in the treatment of alopecia areata. Arch Dermatol 123:1488–1490, 1987.
130. Naldi L et al.: Role of topical immunotherapy in the treatment of alopecia areata: Quality analysis of articles published between January 1977 and January 1988 about three treatments. J Am Acad Dermatol 22:654–656, 1990.
131. Happle R, Perret C, Wiesner-Menzel L: Treatment of alopecia areata with diphencyprone induces hair regrowth and affects the composition of peribulbar infiltrates. In MacDonald DM (ed): *Immunodermatology.* London, Butterworths, 1984, pp 279–286.
132. Happle R, Klein M, Macher E: Topical immunotherapy changes the composition of the peribulbar infiltrate in alopecia areata treated with squaric acid dibutylester (SADBE). Arch Dermatol Res 278:214–218, 1986.
133. Johansson E et al.: Immunohistological evaluation of alopecia areata treated with squaric acid dibutylester (SADBE). Acta Derm Venereol (Stockh) 66:485–490, 1986.
134. Bröcker E-B, John SM, Steinhausen D, Hamm H: Topical immunotherapy with contact allergens in alopecia areata: Evidence for non-specific systemic suppression of cellular immune reactions. Arch Dermatol Res 283:133–134, 1991.
135. Rosenberg WE (ed): Society transactions. Arch Dermatol 112:255–256, 1976.
136. Summer KH, Goggelmann W: 1-Chlor-2, 4-dinitrobenzene depletes glutathione in rat skin and is mutagenic in *Salmonella typhimurium.* Mutat Res 77:91–93, 1980.
137. Kratka J, Goerz G, Vizethum W, Strobel R: Dinitrochlorbenzene influence on the cytochrome P-450 system and mutagenic effects. Arch Dermatol Res 266:315–318, 1979.
138. Strobel R, Röhrborn G: Mutagenic and cell transforming activities of 1-chlor-2, 4-dinitrobenzene (DNCB) and squaric acid-dibutylester (SADBE). Arch Toxicol 45:307–314, 1980.
139. Monk B: Induction of hair growth in alopecia totalis with diphencyprone sensitization. Clin Exp Dermatol 14:154–157, 1989.
140. Happle R, Hausen BM, Wiesner-Menzel L: Diphencyprone in the treatment of alopecia areata. Acta Derm Venereol (Stockh) 63:49–52, 1983.
141. Van der Steen PHM, Van Baar HMJ, Perret CM, Happle R: Treatment of alopecia areata with diphenylcyclopropenone. J Am Acad Dermatol 24:253–257, 1991.
142. Hoting E, Boehm A: Therapy of alopecia areata with diphencyprone. Br J Dermatol 127:625–629, 1992.
143. MacDonald-Hull SP, Cunliffe WJ: Successful treatment of alopecia areata using the contact allergen diphencyprone. Br J Dermatol 124:212–213, 1991.
144. Wilkerson MG et al.: Assessment of diphenylcyclopropenone for photochemically induced mutagenicity in the Ames assay. J Am Acad Dermatol 17:606–611, 1987.
145. Wilkerson MG, Henkin J, Wilkin JK: Diphenylcyclopropenone: Examination for potential contaminants, mechanisms of sensitization, and photochemical stability. J Am Acad Dermatol 11:802–807, 1984.
146. MacDonald-Hull SP, Cunliffe WJ: Treatment of alopecia areata with diphenylcyclopropenone (letter). J Am Acad Dermatol 26:276–277, 1992.
147. MacDonald-Hull SP, Norris JFB: A new contact sensitizer, diphencyprone, in the treatment of alopecia areata. Br J Dermatol 117(suppl 32):22, 1987.
148. MacDonald-Hull SP, Pepall L, Cunliffe WJ: Alopecia areata in children: Response to treatment with diphencyprone. Br J Dermatol 125:164–168, 1991.
149. Van der Steen PHM et al.: Prognostic factors in the treatment of alopecia areata with diphenylcyclopropenone. J Am Acad Dermatol 24:227–230, 1991.
150. Swanson NA et al.: Topical treatment of alopecia areata: Contact allergen vs primary irritant therapy. Arch Dermatol 117:384–387, 1981.
151. Büchner U, Echternacht-Happle K, Happle R: Irritant versus allergic contact dermatitis for the treatment of alopecia areata (abstract). Arch Dermatol Res 264:123–124, 1979.
152. Ashworth J, Tuyp E, Macke RM: Allergic and irritant contact dermatitis compared in the treatment of alopecia totalis and universalis: A comparison of the value of topical diphencyprone and tretinoin gel. Br J Dermatol 120:397–401, 1989.
153. Schmoeckel C, Weissmann I, Plewig G, Braun-Falco O: Treatment of alopecia areata by anthralin-induced dermatitis. Arch Dermatol 115:1254–1255, 1979.
154. Fiedler-Weiss VC, Buys CM: Evaluation of anthralin in the treatment of alopecia areata. Arch Dermatol 123:1491–1493, 1987.
155. Teshima H et al.: Alopecia universalis treated with oral cyclosporine A and prednisolone: Immunologic studies. Int J Dermatol 31:513, 1992.
156. Ferry JJ, Fielder VC: Pilot study to evaluate the effect of topical betamethasone dipropionate on the percutaneous absorption of minoxidil from 5% topical solution (abstract). J Invest Dermatol 94:524, 1990.
157. Fiedler VC et al.: Treatment-resistant alopecia areata: Response to combination therapy with minoxidil plus anthralin. Arch Dermatol 126:756–759, 1990.
158. Berth-Jones J, Hutchinson PE: Treatment of alopecia totalis with a combination of inosine pranobex and diphencyprone compared to each treatment alone. Clin Exp Dermatol 16:172–175, 1991.
159. Shapiro J, Tan J, Tron V: Diphencyprone and minoxidil in alopecia areata: A clinical and immunopathologic evaluation (abstract). J Invest Dermatol 98:562, 1992.
160. Wolowa F, Jablonska S: Zinc in the treatment of alopecia areata. In Kobori T, Montagna W (eds): *Biology and Disease of the Hair.* Baltimore, University Park Press, 1976, pp 305–308.
161. Ead RD: Oral zinc sulphate in alopecia areata—A double blind trial. Br J Dermatol 104:483–484, 1981.
162. Huang P, Huans S, Wei G: One hundred twenty-three cases of alopecia areata treated with liquid nitrogen cryotherapy. J Clin Dermatol 15:269, 1986.
163. Lei Y et al.: Effect of superficial hypothermic cryotherapy with liquid nitrogen on alopecia areata (letter). Arch Dermatol 127:1851–1852, 1991.
164. Berth-Jones J, Hutchinson PE: Alopecia totalis does not respond to vitamin D analogue calcipotriol. J Dermatol Treat 1:293–294, 1991.
165. Magee KL, Hsu SM, Tucker SB: Trial of intralesional interferon alfa in the treatment of alopecia areata. Arch Dermatol 126:760–762, 1990.
166. Baird KA: Alopecia areata. Arch Dermatol 104:562–563, 1971.
167. Franz E: Zur Histodynamik der Alopecia Areata in Ab-

hangigkeit von der Griseofulvin: Induzierten Epithelian Proliferation. Arch Dermatol Res 263:297–306, 1978.
168. Much T: Behandlung von Alopecia Areata mit Vitamin A Saure. A Hautkr 51:993, 1976.
169. Tosti A, Bardazzi F, Guerra L: Alopecia totalis: Is treating nonresponder patients useful? J Am Acad Dermatol 24:455–456, 1991.
170. Tosti A, De Padova MP, Minghetti G, Veronesi S: Therapies versus placebo in the treatment of patchy alopecia areata. J Am Acad Dermatol 15:209–210, 1986.

Chapter

9

ANAGEN HAIR LOSS

Karyn L. Grossman and Joseph C. Kvedar

INTRODUCTION

Few dermatologic complaints carry as much psychosocial anxiety as hair loss. The obvious altered appearance and the various common associations between aging and hair loss are some of the reasons for this anxiety. In addition to its obvious psychosocial importance, hair loss may be a symptom of systemic disease. This chapter addresses causes of hair loss that result in the shedding of large numbers of hairs in the anagen phase of growth. The common thread which binds most of these etiologies together is a direct toxic insult to the rapidly dividing keratinocytes in the hair germ. The cessation of metabolic activity in the growing hair shaft results in the weakening of the partially keratinized, proximal portion of the structure and subsequent breakage of the hair. The morphological consequence of this abrupt interruption of hair growth is the dystrophic hair, which is best visualized via a microscopic analysis of plucked hairs.

In anagen effluvium (Fig. 9-1*A* and *B*), copious hair loss occurs since up to 90 percent of scalp hair may be in anagen at a given time. This may be difficult to distinguish clinically from the more common telogen effluvium, but the history of exposure to a toxin and/or finding a majority of dystrophic anagen hairs on a hair pull or pluck can help the clinician in making this diagnosis. Because the hair loss is not dependent on the transition from anagen to telogen and subsequent release of telogen hairs, the time course for typical anagen effluvium contrasts sharply with that for telogen effluvium. In classic anagen effluvium, ingestion or exposure to a toxin is followed in days to a few weeks by breakage of the weakened shafts and resultant hair loss. If the insult is removed, regrowth should be prompt since normal anagen growth has been only temporarily interrupted. In telogen effluvium, the period of time from stimulus (because a transition from anagen through telogen is required) to noticeable hair loss is 3 to 4 months, and re-

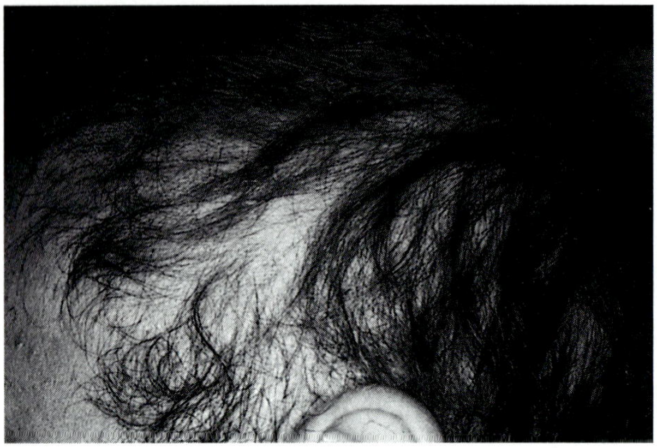

A

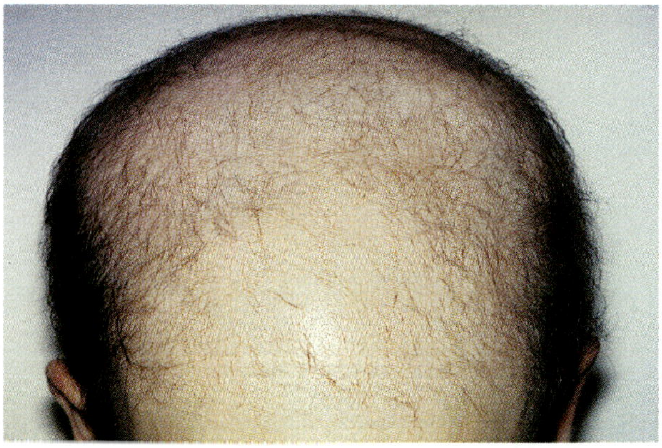

B

Figure 9-1 Typical patterns of hair loss seen with acute anagen effluvium. Patient *A* is day 30 after taking oral VP-16. (*Courtesy of Dr. Elise A. Olsen.*) Patient *B* had multiagent chemotherapy for a brain tumor. (*Courtesy of Dr. Howard P. Baden.*)

growth is also much slower. Between these extremes there exists a group of patients who have a stimulus and initial pattern of hair loss consistent with anagen effluvium but in whom the hair loss is prolonged and regrowth is slow. At least in terms of radiation, this effect appears to be dose-related. The literature is unclear on the mechanism, but it seems possible that "mixed" syndromes can occur in which a toxic insult is sufficient to provoke not only the standard anagen effluvium but some component of telogen effluvium and, in some cases, even permanent scarring alopecia.

In evaluating patients with generalized hair loss, the first hairs chosen for microscopic analysis should be those obtained by gentle pulling of hair from several representative areas of the scalp. In patients with acute anagen or telogen effluvium, such hairs will be easy to obtain, whereas normally no anagen and few telogen hairs may be obtained in this fashion. The common dystrophic hairs prominent in anagen effluvium break easily with even gentle pulling: examination of the proximal shaft obtained by this method usually shows a tapered tip where the weakened damaged shaft has broken (Fig. 9-2*A*). This contrasts with the club-shaped, unpigmented proximal end and cornified root sheath of telogen hairs seen in telogen effluvium (Fig. 9-2*B*).

When the gentle pulling of hair does not yield helpful information, a more forceful hair pluck with a hemostat should be undertaken. In performing this type of pluck, the hairs should be removed with a sharp tug in the direction of hair growth with a tightly closing rubber-shod hemostat placed as close to the skin as possible.[1] The hair may be trimmed to 1 to 2 cm above the

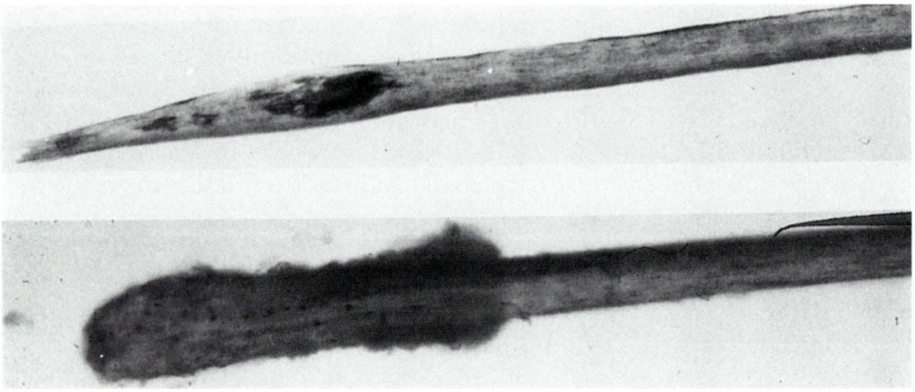

Figure 9-2 Light-microscopic analysis of hairs obtained from gentle pulling. (*Top*) A dystrophic anagen hair shaft. (×100) Note the tapered proximal end and lack of root sheaths. (*Bottom*) A telogen or club hair. (×100) Note the absence of pigment, the clubbed end, and the cornification of the root sheaths.

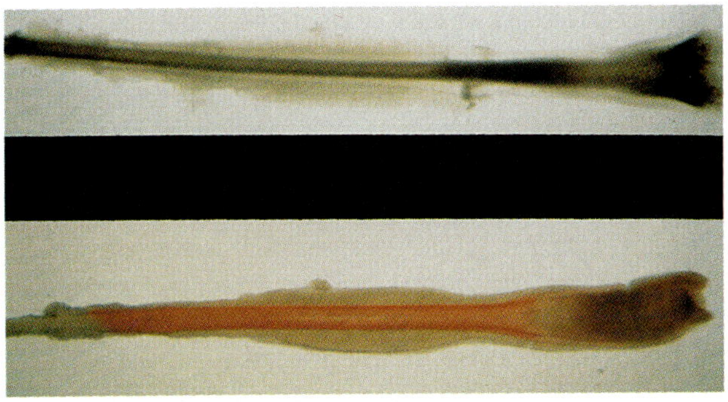

Figure 9-3 (*A*) Normal anagen hair. (×40) Note the broom-shaped bulb and the presence of inner as well as outer root sheaths. (*B*) Same hair as *A* but stained with 4-dimethylaminocinnamaldehyde. (×40) Note the red staining of the inner root sheath which completely encircles the cortex through most of the photograph. Also, note the lack of staining of the bulb, external root sheath, and cortex.

scalp prior to the procedure to facilitate the pluck. Only about 20 hairs should be extracted at a time, and several contiguous areas should be sampled to reach a total of approximately 50 hairs. The hairs should be mounted on a glass slide under a coverslip with water, glycerin, or cyanoacrylic glue. If the insult is still occurring, the roots of anagen hairs will be dystrophic compared with those seen normally. Analysis of dystrophic hairs from this type of sample is difficult because forceful pulling of the hair can result in broken hairs which have identical morphology to dystrophic hairs but are artifactual in their origin. Telogen (club) hairs are also seen in this type of analysis since 10 to 20 percent of all scalp hair is in telogen normally, and the percentage may artifactually increase as anagen hairs break off. One percent 4-dimethylaminocinnamaldehyde (DACA), which stains the inner root sheath of anagen hairs, may be added to the slide to help differentiate anagen from telogen hairs[2] (Fig. 9-3*A* and *B*).

The following is a detailed discussion of some of the important causes of anagen effluvium.

RADIATION

Within months of the discovery of radiation by Röntgen, reports about the effects of radiation on hair and skin began to appear.[3] Years later, single doses of low-voltage radiation of 300 to 1,000 rad (or cGy) administered to mice were found to induce anagen effluvium.[4,5] At relatively low doses (200–300 rad), most anagen follicles recovered quickly and completely. High doses of 3000 rad resulted in marked inhibition of matrix cell proliferation with little recovery of proliferative capacity,[5] perhaps secondary to the effect on the more radioresistant dermal papillae.[6] Telogen hairs were noted to be more resistant than anagen hairs in rodents exposed to x-irradiation, and recovery of hair growth was superior when the animal's hair was in the telogen vs. anagen phase.[6,7] Telogen effluvium could be produced in addition to an anagen effluvium with higher doses of irradiation.[6,7] Thus, more than one physiological response may occur after exposure to ionizing radiation; i.e., it may vary from temporary anagen and/or telogen effluvium to permanent hair loss.

In man, both a temporary and a permanent epilation has been reported following irradiation. The doses required to cause epilation vary between individuals and in different areas of the body. Scalp hair is the most sensitive to radiation effects, with axillary hair, beard hair, pubic hair, and eyelashes showing a progressive increase in radioresistance:[3] this may be explained by the variable percentages of hair in anagen and duration of anagen in different body areas. The dose of radiation necessary to cause temporary alopecia will also depend on the quantum energy of the respective type of radiation and the size of the radiation field.[3] X-rays generated at 100 keV under 0.5 mm Al filtration produce temporary epilation in man at 350 rad/air, while at 200 keV under 2 mm Cu filter, as much as 650 to 700 rad/air may be required for this effect. In general, temporary epilation begins 8 to 10 days after a single dose of irradiation and continues for 2 to 3 weeks, with full hair regrowth by 8 to 12 weeks.[3] From 1910 to 1959 (the time of introduction of griseofulvin), x-ray was a widely accepted therapy for tinea capitis. The standardized Adamson-Kienbock procedure was used which involved five fields of exposure to 100 keV unfiltered x-ray of 300 to 400 rad each: a total of 450 to 850 rad was delivered to any particular area on the scalp.[8] Epilation of the infected hairs was followed by resolution of the process and hair regrowth.

Ellinger noted that the single dose for permanent epilation is remarkably uniform for different animal species, varying between 2000 and

3000 rad/air.[3] Permanent epilation in humans has been reported with deep x-ray doses of > 300 rad (180–200 keV, 0.5–0.1 mm Cu filter) or 5000 to 6000 cGy of soft x-rays (50 keV, 1 mm Al filter).[9] In clinical practice for the treatment of malignancy, dose fractionation is employed and epilation is dependent here on both the daily dose and the time interval between doses. Increasing the time over which the radiation is given allows larger total doses to be given without the sequela of permanent alopecia.

The explosion of the atomic bomb in Japan gave further clinical information on the effects of gamma radiation on human hair. Individuals within 1500 yards of the hypocenter of the explosion developed a sudden epilation approximately 2 weeks after the event. The histological changes were similar to those observed in the normal cycle of loss except for a relative increase in membrane thickening and pigment dispersion.[10] For those who survived a prolonged period, the hair began to regrow in 6 to 8 weeks.

Morphologically, there is a "tailing," or progressive narrowing, of the proximal hair after x-ray exposure. The length of the "tail" is proportional to the intensity of x-ray exposure and duration.[11] Work on mice or rat vibrissae has elucidated the ultrastructural changes in hair secondary to x-irradiation. The most striking feature is the development of autophagic vacuoles in the cytoplasm of both matrix and root sheath cells within an hour of moderate-dose (1000–1500 rad) x-ray that continues for up to several weeks afterward.[12,13] A "smudging" of the cytoplasm develops early.

The use of ^{3}H-thymidine has allowed more complete investigations into the cell kinetics of the matrix after irradiation. Cattaneo, Quastler, and Sherman found that a single dose of 800 rad to mouse skin, in which all hairs were in anagen, resulted in complete cessation of matrix cell mitosis within 1 hour.[5] DNA synthesis was reduced to 50 percent at 30 minutes and had ceased completely by 6 hours. Overall after therapy, the matrix population was reduced by about 50 percent. No change in effect was noted over a range of 800 to 3000 rad. However, following a lower dose of 200 rad, the effect on thymidine incorporation and matrix cell mitosis was markedly reduced but was highly variable from follicle to follicle.[5] Recovery was, as expected, inversely proportional to the dose of irradiation, with cells exposed to ≤ 200 rad completely recovering.[5] DNA synthesis resumed within 12 hours after exposure to 3000 rad, but abnormal morphology and growth rate persisted for some time afterward.[5]

Protein synthesis in matrix cells has been examined by looking at the uptake of isotopically labeled amino acids. For single doses of x-ray, mouse hairs irradiated during anagen revealed a dose-dependent decrease in uptake of ^{3}H-serine and ^{35}S-methionine. If the preceding telogen generation of hair was treated, the uptake of these amino acids in the succeeding anagen generation was decreased in a dose-dependent fashion.[14] However, to achieve comparable results to those irradiated during anagen growth, it was necessary to expose the telogen hairs to 2 to 2 1/2 times the radiation dose of the anagen hairs.[14] These differences are probably secondary to the fact that telogen matrix cells are principally G_1 cells which are more resistant to radiation damage than the rapidly proliferating anagen matrix cells.[14] Radiosensitivity is greatest in M and G_2, followed by G_1, early S, and late S phases of mitosis.[15] The nondividing matrix cells of telogen follicles may sustain and store radiation damage secondary to decreased cellular metabolism and the inability to eliminate damaged matrix cells.[16] The radiation damage may be expressed later following an appropriate mitotic stimulus.[16]

Today, pre- and postoperative radiation to the skull for the treatment of cancer characteristically ranges from 2000 to 5000 rad in divided doses[17] depending upon the individual protocol. These patients predictably develop alopecia, which should be temporary. Occasionally, the hair will not regrow completely or will grow back a different color or texture from that seen before treatment.[3,18] It should be noted that pigment loss in mouse hairs is greatest in those follicles x-rayed in catagen or telogen.[19]

DRUGS

Any drug which disrupts either cell cycling or the production of a specific component of hair may cause an interruption in the development of the hair shaft or an alteration in the hair follicle with resultant alopecia. Many substances, including medications, chemotherapy, and environmental hazards, may contribute to the development of hair loss.

Chemotherapy

The efficacy of antineoplastic agents is based on their ability to target and kill cells undergoing mitosis. Since most somatic cells have a slow turnover and most cancer cells are rapidly dividing, the drugs are relatively specific for cancer cells. Certain tissues which have naturally rapid turnover, such as bone marrow, gastrointestinal epithelia, and hair matrix, will also be affected and manifest the major toxicities of these drugs. In the case of hair, this manifestation is in the form of anagen alopecia (Table 9-1). Because it is generally transient and not life-threatening, this phenomenon is not of great concern to most oncologists. Patients, on the other hand, tend to fear hair loss as among the most dreaded side effects of cancer chemotherapy.[20]

The hair loss characteristically begins 1 to 2 weeks after the initial chemotherapeutic dose and is most apparent at 1 to 2 months after the initiation of therapy. The process is usually reversible. In some cases, regrowth has been noted during continuation of the chemotherapeutic drugs;[20] an explanation for this "escape" phenomenon may help elucidate development of tumor resistance to chemotherapy agents. The new hair may be of different color, shape, or texture, and these changes may persist for several years.[21]

Anagen effluvium as a manifestation of cancer chemotherapy is a result of a direct toxic insult to the rapidly dividing cells of the hair matrix. The root sheaths may become necrotic or, in less severe cases, form a weak, constricted hair shaft which then breaks upon reaching the follicular orifice. The scalp is the most common location for hair loss, but other terminal hairs may be variably affected depending on the percentage of hairs in anagen.[22] The beard, eyebrows, eyelashes, and axillary and pubic hairs may become involved with multiple exposures over a long time period. The incidence and severity of the loss are variable but are frequently dose-dependent. Table 9-1 lists the chemotherapeutic agents associated with hair loss.

Microscopic studies of epilated hairs have been conducted after in vivo exposure to individual chemotherapeutic agents.[23] With methotrexate as a prototype,[23] a decrease in the diameter of the hair bulb and keratogenous zone can be noted 4 to 6 days after a single dose (dose unspecified). As the hair recovers, growth of the matrix resumes and the shaft produced within the next 2 to 5 days is noted to contain a small constricted section. The constriction moves distally with growth; with repeated doses, successive constrictions of the shaft are noted. These have been termed *Pohl-Pinkus marks* and are analogous to Beau's lines of the nails.[24] Total scalp hair loss can occur with high doses or even low doses (5 mg qd × 3 of methotrexate) in the face of impaired renal function.[23] Methotrexate has also been noted to produce a unique change in blond hair called the "flag sign": with multiple doses, dark bands alternating with the normal blond color have been seen in the scalp hair, eyebrows, and cilia. Its likely mechanism is a direct effect on the epidermal melanocytes stimulating melanin production.[25,26]

Intraarterial perfusion of nitrogen mustard has been reported to cause an unusual localized alopecia in the areas of distribution of the injected vessel.[27] Cutaneous edema and erythema plus or minus ulceration were followed by epila-

Table 9-1
CHEMOTHERAPEUTIC AGENTS ASSOCIATED WITH ANAGEN ALOPECIA

Amsacrine[25]
Bleomycin[20]
Chlorambucil (rare)[97]
Colcemid[23]
Cyclophosphamide (Cytoxan)[20]
Cytarabine (Ara-C)[25]
Dacarbazine (DTIC)[96]
Dactinomycin (Actinomycin D)[20]
Daunorubicin (Daunomycin; Cerubidine)[20]
Dichloromethotrexate[23]
Doxorubicin (Adriamycin)[25]
Endoxan[21]
Etoposide[25,98]
Fluorouracil (5-FU)[25]
Fludarabine[96]
Floxuridine (FUDR)[98]
Hexamethylmelamine[98]
Hydroxyurea[22]
Idarubicin[96]
Ifosfamide[96]
Lomustine (CCNU)[96]
Mechlorethamine (nitrogen mustard)[27]
Melphalen (Alkeran)[96]
Methotrexate[20]
Mitomycin (Mutamycin)[22]
Mitoxantrone[96]
Nitrosureas[25]
Procarbazine[96]
Triethylenethiophosphoramide (Thiotepa)[23]
Vinblastine (Velban)[22]
Vincristine (Oncovin)[22]

tion in the involved area by approximately day 12. Histological evaluation at that time showed follicular edema, a perifollicular homogenous eosinophilic zone, and the absence of sebaceous glands and hair shafts. Hair shafts appeared to recover by 3 months after infusion.[27]

Multiple efforts have been made to reduce the alopecia produced upon the administration of chemotherapeutic agents. It should be noted that patients with neoplasms in which the scalp may serve as a reservoir for malignant cells or in which scalp metastasis has occurred should not receive any measures to prevent alopecia. These include patients with brain tumors, lymphomas, leukemias, or other hematologic malignancies. Also, while some of the efforts have been shown to delay or decrease the chemotherapy-related alopecia, none of the modalities clearly prevent it.

Many of these efforts to reduce alopecia following chemotherapy have been aimed at reducing the amount of blood flow and thus probable delivery of drug to the scalp by means of hypothermia[28–33] alone or with a tourniquet application. Various devices such as cryopacks and cooling caps have been utilized. The cooling cap is capable of reducing the mean epidermal temperature to 14.2°C and decreasing scalp blood flow to 35 percent of baseline. It is employed just prior to, during, and for approximately 1 hour after infusion. However, because of questions involving (1) the effectiveness in preventing hair loss, (2) the potential increased risk of metastasis to the scalp, and (3) the potential effect on circulation to the skull and brain, as of 1990 the Food and Drug Administration rescinded marketing approval for these scalp-cooling devices until proof of efficacy and safety is obtained.[34]

Alternative methods to prevent chemotherapy-related hair loss have been preliminarily explored in animal models using various agents. These studies not only demonstrate some potential methods of preventing chemotherapy-related hair loss but also highlight the differential mechanisms by which hair loss is caused by these drugs.[35–37] ImuVert is a biologic response modifier derived from *Serratia marcescens* which is being studied as a chemotherapeutic agent. In rats treated with cytosine arabinoside (ara-C) and doxorubicin (both cell cycle–specific agents) plus or minus ImuVert prior to injection of chloroleukemic cells, ImuVert protected against alopecia as well as increased the survival rate of the animals.[35] ImuVert did not, however, protect against alopecia induced by cyclophosphamide (a cell cycle–non-specific agent). In a separate but related experiment, interleukin I protected against alopecia induced by ara-C but not that produced by cyclophosphamide.[36] Whether interleukin I is the cytokine through which ImuVert offers this protection from follicular toxicity is still uncertain. Supplementation of the diet with alphatocopherol in Angora rabbits and humans has been reported to prevent doxorubicin-dependent inhibition of hair growth,[37] but its effectiveness in humans has been disputed.[38,39]

The combination of irradiation and chemotherapy may have variable effects on the expected alopecia from either agent alone. Administration of phase- or cycle-specific chemotherapy agents may induce partially synchronous cell populations which, dependent on the position in the cell cycle, can either enhance or decrease the toxicity of a subsequent administration of radiation.[40]

Colchicine

Colchicine is an antimitotic agent derived from the plant *Colchicum autumnale* which has long been used to treat arthritic pain and gout.[41] Another alkaloid isolated from the same plant, deacetyl-N-methyl-colchicine, or demecolcine, has also been shown to possess antimitotic capabilities similar to colchicine and has been used for the treatment of gout and other diseases such as mycosis fungoides, Hodgkin's disease, leukemia, and lymphosarcoma. Toxicity of the two agents is similar.

Multiple cases of alopecia following the administration of colchicine or demecolcine have been reported.[42–44] Diffuse hair loss has been reported in psoriasis patients within 2 to 3 weeks of taking colchicine in doses of 2 to 3 mg daily.[44] The scalp is most commonly affected, but the beard area may become involved in men. Hair loss is only rarely seen on the extremities and, if so, it is usually mild. The severity ranges from mild hair loss to an almost complete effluvium.[44] Typically, there are increased numbers of telogen hairs, although morphological abnormalities in anagen hairs can rarely be seen: these include matrix atrophy and constriction of the hair shaft. Hair loss generally persists for several weeks to about 3 months and is reversible, in some cases even when the patient continues to take the medication.

The amount and timing of hair loss vary with

the dose, the timing of administration, and the percentage of individual follicles in anagen. Most frequently, hair loss occurs after a relatively large dose of colchicine or demecolcine (36–150 mg).[44] However, hair loss occurred in one patient only after receiving continuous administration of demecolcine (450 mg) over 4 1/2 months. Alternatively, hair loss has been reported with a single dose of 10 mg of demecolcine or 21 g of colchicine spread over five injections.[44]

The mechanism involved in colchicine-induced alopecia is presumed to be secondary to its antimitotic activity. In animal studies, one sees an increased number of mitotic figures secondary to an arrest of nuclear division in metaphase. In high concentrations, evidence of further damage, including nuclear pyknosis, disintegration of the nuclear membrane, and complete nuclear disintegration, may be seen.[45]

PLANTS

Few cases of diffuse alopecia following the ingestion of plants or plant parts, in particular the seeds, have been reported. The two offending species are the "coco de mono," or *Lecythis ollaria,* and the *Leucaena glauca.*

Coco de mono is the name used in Venezuela for various species of trees belonging to the genus *Lecythis,* a member of the same family, Lecythidaceae, as the common Brazil nut. The trees are located throughout a vast zone which extends from Costa Rica to Brazil, with an abundance in the flatlands of Venezuela. The plant derives its name, monkeypod, from the configuration of its fruit[46] (Fig. 9-4). There are popular beliefs among the native people that the oil of the nut has hemostatic properties and that eating the almonds will cause a diffuse hair loss.[47]

There are only a few reports in the medical literature describing the effects of this plant.[47–50] Ingestion of the seeds results in rapid signs of toxicity, often within 30 minutes. Patients typically experience anxiety, nervousness, and vertigo followed by gastrointestinal upset. Patients may have severe nausea, vomiting, and diarrhea followed by persistent anorexia and vague complaints of abdominal pain. All of the reported cases described some form of alopecia occurring with the other signs of toxicity. There is also one report of a patient eating eight seeds without the development of any ill effects.[47]

Kerdel-Vegas examined the effect of coco de mono nut ingestion in mice. He found that the nuts inhibited the anagen phase of hair growth, an effect which was reversible if the almond extract was discontinued.[47] Subsequently, a cytotoxic component from concentrated coco de mono nuts was isolated and purified by two separate groups simultaneously.[51] This compound was identified as selenocystathionine, the selenium-containing analogue of the sulfur amino acid cystathionine. The cytotoxic effects of both the crude extract of the nut as well as the purified selenocystathionine could be reversed by *l*-cystine, and to a lesser extent by *d,l*+ allocystathionine and *l*-cystathionine. Selenocystathionine has also been isolated from *Astragalus pectinatus*[52] and *Stanleya pinnata.*[53] While human intoxication with seleniferous plants has not been extensively described, there have been isolated reports from parts of Colombia. In the United States, selenium poisoning has been associated with hair loss in certain Indians.[51]

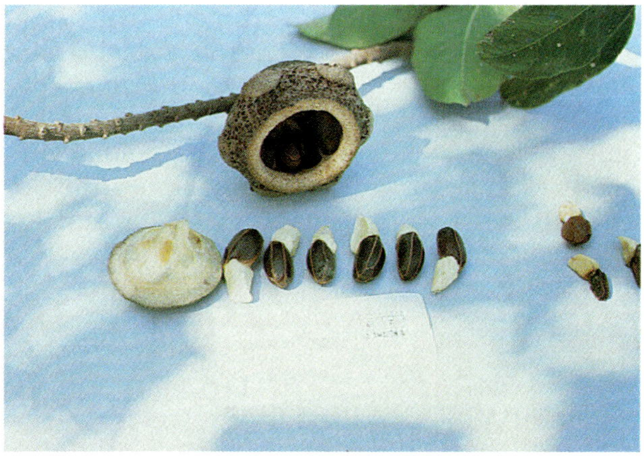

Figure 9-4 *Lecythis ollaria,* or coco de mono, plant and nut. (*Courtesy of Professor Ghillean T. Prance.*)

Hair loss has also been described after the consumption of leaves and seeds from the *Leucaena glauca* plant. The sudden loss of hair of native women has been ascribed to the consumption of the seeds,[54] and several investigators have documented hair loss in rodents secondary to ingestion of the seeds and leaves.[54,55] The toxin in the plant appears to be the amino acid leucenol or leucenine. This substance has been given the alternative name of mimosine.

Several theories regarding the mechanism of damage with mimosine have evolved. Some suggest that leucenol may interfere with keratinization by displacing alanine via competitive inhibition.[56] Others have shown that leucenol can act as a tyrosine analogue and postulate that it may inhibit tyrosine decarboxylase or tyrosinase or even be substituted into proteins instead of tyrosine.[54] Another theory is that leucenol inhibits mitosis, specifically in the matrix, similar to those effects seen with x-irradiation or cytotoxic chemicals.[55] Further studies need to be done to elucidate the mechanism of action involved in hair loss from mimosine.

ENVIRONMENTAL AND OCCUPATIONAL EXPOSURE

Occupational exposure to hazardous chemicals has decreased over the years due to more stringent government regulations; however, significant exposure to agents which may have alopecia as a sign of toxicity can still occur in industrial settings. Furthermore, several chemicals still available in household products or encountered in the home have alopecia as a sign of toxicity. While most adults generally avoid ingestion and contact with these agents, children may inadvertently become exposed to chronic low levels or acute large doses of these toxins. Rapid recognition of the agents may be essential to decrease the mortality and morbidity from these potential poisonings.

Boric Acid

Alopecia may be the most obvious sign of chronic boric acid poisoning. Boric acid is a colorless, odorless compound which is available in multiple forms including a white powder, crystals, and granules. While the medicinal uses of boric acid have gradually dropped within the United States, it is still widely used in multiple industries including laundering, fireproofing wood and fabric, manufacturing leather, and producing pottery glazes and enamel.[57,58] It is also sold commercially as a household pesticide.

The symptoms of acute boron intoxication are primarily those of the gastrointestinal tract, central nervous system, and kidneys, as well as a hemorrhagic diathesis.[57,59] Skin signs include erythroderma, exfoliation, and/or bullae: this may be confused with staphylococcal scalded skin syndrome in infants.[57,59,60] Total scalp alopecia has been reported following acute intoxication of ingested boric acid powder.[58] Characteristically, chronic exposure can lead to symptoms much like those of the acutely intoxicated but are generally milder in nature. Several incidents of hair loss related to chronic exposure to boric acid compounds have been reported since the late 1800s. The scalp hair becomes dry and falls out. The hair loss may extend to the eyebrows and pubic and axillary hair. The nails may grow white and crumbly.[57]

Absorption of boric acid may be through the skin or gastrointestinal tract. Boric acid in "medicated" talcum powder can be absorbed in sufficient degree to give toxic symptoms[57] through intact as well as irritated skin.[57,58] Occupational exposure in one patient to powdered borax (washing powder) for 6 years resulted in a diffuse alopecia involving the scalp and beard area, which resolved after removal from exposure to the offending product.[57] Diffuse alopecia has been reported secondary to chronic ingestion of boric acid–containing mouthwash.[59]

The diagnosis can be made by measuring blood boric acid levels: normal values are up to 0.3 mg/100 ml blood as boron.[59] The acute lethal dose of boric acid varies for children and adults. The minimal lethal dose appears to be 18 to 20 g in adults and 5 to 6 g in children.[58] There is no antidote for acute boric acid poisoning. Various investigators have tried plasma exchange and/or hemodialysis or peritoneal dialysis[58,61,62] with mixed success. In general, supportive care is needed, with close attention to fluid balance. Despite these measures, mortality remains high, particularly in children. In more chronic cases, dramatic regrowth of scalp, eyebrows, and pubic and axillary hair has been seen following strict avoidance of borate-containing compounds.[59]

Heavy Metals

Many heavy metals are capable of disrupting the formation of the hair shaft. They are able to form covalent bonds with the numerous sulfhydryl groups in keratin, leading to abnormal development and potential fragmentation of the hair shaft. The hair is also a unique analytic tool for studying exposure to heavy metals. The metals can only bind to that portion of the hair which is undergoing terminal differentiation and thus become a component of the hair shaft. The hair, then, provides a lasting record of the long-term exposure to these toxins. While many metals may be capable of causing alopecia, several are well known because of the more frequent exposure to them.

THALLIUM

Prior to the ban of its use commercially in 1972, thallium sulfate was a common and inexpensive pesticide and rodenticide and a frequent cause of toxin-induced alopecia.[63,64] It is also used as a catalyst in fireworks, in optical lenses, in industry as an alloy, and in cardiac perfusion imagery.[65] Prior to 1940, thallium was used to treat tinea capitis secondary to its ability to epilate hair.[66] It is a cumulative poison which is absorbed through the skin, pulmonary tree, or gastrointestinal tract. Excretion is by both renal and gastrointestinal routes and occurs very slowly.[67] Thallium binds to sulfhydryl groups in mitochondrial membranes at intracellular sites.[65]

Neurological signs, especially ataxia, tremor, paresthesias, somnolence, and weakness, and gastrointestinal symptoms (often vague) are the most prominent presentations within hours to days of acute thallium poisoning.[66,67] Alopecia, however, is the most common symptom[68] and usually begins 10 days after ingestion as a diffuse shedding of abnormal anagen hairs.[69] Doses of 7 to 8 mg/kg will lead to epilation, although adolescents appear to have a lower threshold for toxicity than do younger children.[67] Complete epilation generally occurs within 1 month.[66] With lower doses of thallium, the onset of hair loss may be delayed up to 3 weeks after the initial ingestion, with a gradual shedding of club hairs occurring over 3 to 4 months.[69] Hair loss may be the only symptom in mild poisoning.[63]

Trichogram analysis reveals an irregularity of the dark keratogenous zone and air bubbles within the hair shaft near the tapered tips, giving a distinctive appearance.[69] The pattern of alopecia is not consistent but is most marked on the crown.[63] There is sparing of the axilla and facial hair, including the inner half of the eyebrow.[66] After discontinuance of exposure, the hair will usually regrow completely within 6 months.[69] The length of time to regrow suggests a component of telogen effluvium as well, but this has not been documented.

Other dermatologic manifestations include xerosis and thick, pruritic, white scale on the scalp, which may lead to the incorrect diagnosis of seborrheic dermatitis.[63] Nail dystrophy may develop as evidenced by white transverse bands (Mees' lines) 3 to 4 weeks after exposure. A bluish line may develop in the gums at the same time.[66]

Several studies have implicated alterations in keratin formation as the mechanism for thallium-induced alopecia.[69] In mice, experimental alopecia from thallium can be reduced with the addition of 1% to 2% cystine.[70] These supplemented animals also demonstrated better growth and survival rates. As keratin contains a significant portion of the sulfur found in hair, an interruption or alteration in the formation of this protein or proteins may lead to hair loss.

The diagnosis of poisoning is best made by demonstrating the presence of the metal in the urine, as any amount greater than zero is considered abnormal.[63,67] However, excretion may be sudden and massive, and daily excretion rates are irregular. Thus, a negative thallium test may not rule out thallium toxicity,[63] and repeat testing should be performed as traces of urinary thallium can be detected for months after ingestion.[63,67] Idiometric analysis is the method of choice as it is more sensitive than photometric analysis.[63] Thallium is radiopaque and evident on an x-ray of the abdomen.[65]

Treatment recommendations for thallium poisoning are based on attempts to increase excretion or bind thallium. The major problem with both of these approaches is that by the time the diagnosis of toxicity is made, thallium is widely distributed in the intracellular compartment of most body organ systems and is slowly removed; hence, thallium is relatively inaccessible to treatment.[66] Whether treatment affects the course of thallium toxicity is unclear, but the following recommendations are valid:

1. Remove any recently ingested thallium by gastric lavage or ipecac-induced vomiting. Prussian blue absorbs thallium in the gastrointestinal tract and is given as a single dose of 250 mg/kg.[65]
2. Increase urinary excretion of thallium by increasing the intake of fluids and administering potassium chloride 3 to 5 mg per day for 5 to 10 days. Potassium chloride also frees intracellular stores of thallium, and thus treatment is limited by the amount of thallium that can be released into the blood without worsening symptoms.[68]
3. Use a laxative to enhance gastrointestinal removal.
4. Symptomatic and supportive care should be undertaken for severe neuralgiform pain, tremors, and convulsions.[66]
5. Peritoneal dialysis or hemodialysis should be used as indicated.

6. The use of diethyldithiocarbonate (dithocarb) is no longer recommended in cases of thallium intoxication due to the potential of dithocarb-thallium complexes to diffuse into the brain with subsequent clinical and electroencephalographic worsening.[65]

Thallium poisoning is a serious event. Death has occurred following a dose of 15 mg/kg.[65] Twenty-six out of 48 patients who presented with neurological symptoms associated with thallium intoxication continued to have neurological defects when followed for an average of 4 years.[66] This entity should be considered in any person presenting with acute central nervous system and gastrointestinal signs of toxin exposure and alopecia, as well as in those with chronic unexplained hair loss, particularly in the setting of psychiatric or neurological symptoms.[63]

MERCURY

Mercury is another elemental metal which may cause intoxication and dermatologic symptoms, including diffuse alopecia.[71,72] Mercury exists in a variety of inorganic and organic forms which exhibit variable absorption, excretion, and toxicity. The organic mercuric forms (alkyl mercurials) are much more dangerous than the elemental or inorganic forms due to better absorption and slower elimination.[73] Methylmercury is the most common organic form and is readily absorbed through skin or mucous membranes, ingestion, or vaporization, although the direct threat to humans from methylmercury exposure comes from dietary consumption of fish and other seafoods.[74] Methylmercury is extremely lipid-soluble, is resistant to biotransformation, and has a long half-life (~ 70+ days).[71,73,74] The alkyl mercurials readily cross the placenta and blood-brain barrier and, as the fetal brain is much more sensitive to methylmercury than the adult brain, in utero exposure to toxic levels can lead to brain damage.[73,74] Bacteria found widely in soil and water sources (bottom sediments) can biosynthesize methylmercury from other forms of mercury. Both organic and inorganic mercury compounds inhibit sulfhydryl enzymes by binding to cysteinyl groups.[73,74]

During the early twentieth century, mercury intoxication was common from medicinal compounds used to treat syphilis, ointments used to treat various dermatologic conditions, teething powder (Calomel), purgatives (Calomel), or from exposure to mercury-containing antiseptics. Today, the exposure to mercury in medications is limited to an organomercury diuretic and various phenylmercuric derivatives used as bacteriostatic agents such as thimerosal, merbromin in Mercurochrome, phenylmercuric acetate in a contraceptive jelly, and phenylmercuric nitrate in a hemorrhoid preparation.[71] Intoxication is primarily through chronic industrial exposure (such as mercury thermometer factory workers),[75] industrial pollution of water sources and consumption of affected seafood, or inadvertent exposure to mercury used as fungicides or antiseptics. The bioaccumulation of methylmercury in tissues of higher organisms, including fish, is diffusion-controlled and rapid. Freshwater fish from contaminated waters or large, carnivorous ocean fish at the end of the food chain, such as tuna and swordfish, are the most dangerous sources of mercury toxicity.[74] Ingestion of bread made from grain seeds treated with a methylmercury fungicide has been responsible for numerous epi-demic outbreaks of mercury poisoning, including those in Iraq,[76,77] Pakistan,[78] Guatemala,[79] and Ghana.[80] Methylmercury in paint has led to toxicity not only from direct ingestion or cutaneous exposure but through inhalation of the vapor for weeks after application of the paint.[81] Intoxication has also been reported from the inadvertent exposure to mercury in hair bleach.[82] Inorganic mercury is also widely used today in dental amalgams.

The lowest observable "safe" level of blood mercury is unknown, but symptoms generally do not occur until blood mercury levels are >340 ng/ml.[74] The Food and Agriculture Organization/World Health Organization has set the provisional tolerable (not acceptable) weekly intake for humans at 5 μg/kg body weight of mercury and 3.3 μg/kg body weight of methylmercury.[74] The U.S. National Occupational Standards of Health sets threshold limit values for occupational exposure to mercury, but the cumulative effects of occupational and environmental exposure to mercury are unclear.

The symptoms of acute mercury poisoning, which can first appear weeks to months after exposure,[74] are primarily neurological and include sensory impairment, constriction of visual fields, hearing impairment, ataxia, and speech disturbances (Hunter-Russell syndrome).[73] Paresthesia is the earliest and most persistent symptom.

Gastrointestinal symptoms are rare with methylmercury poisoning but common with ethyl mercury and mercuric chloride intoxication.[73] Hair loss has been reported even without other symptoms.[72] In children, chronic exposure to inorganic mercury compounds leads to a distinctive clinical picture of dermatologic, cardiovascular, and neurobehavioral abnormalities termed *acrodynia,* or *pink disease.*[73] Manifestations may include pain in the abdomen, extremities, and joints; desquamation or pink color of the palms and soles; headache; irritability; photophobia; hyperhidrosis; and diffuse hair loss.[81]

Diagnosis is made through measuring urine, blood, or hair levels of mercury. Blood levels > 35 ng/ml and urine mercury > 150 ng/liter are abnormal.[65] The concentration of mercury in hair is proportional to blood, with 100,000 ng/g mercury in hair equaling approximately 400 ng/ml in blood.[74]

Emesis or gastric lavage should be done if the source is ingested mercury. Activated charcoal is not helpful as this does not bind metals. Treatment is aimed at providing excess sulfhydryl groups to bind the mercury. Dimercaprol (BAL: British anti-Lewisite) is most effective for preventing renal damage with acute inorganic mercury poisoning but is of little value in methylmercury poisoning.[73] Sulfhydryl agents such as D-penicillamine, N-acetylpenicillamine, cysteine, and N-acetylcysteine are capable of reversing the protein binding of methylmercury and can be used in the treatment of both acute and chronic inorganic mercury or organic mercury poisoning.[73] Other treatments include polythiols, selenium, vitamin E, hemodialysis, and exchange transfusion.[73] Concomitant selenium occurring naturally in contaminated waters raises the threshold for mercury toxicity.[74]

ARSENIC

Inorganic arsenic compounds are found in insecticides, rodenticides, fungicides, wood preservatives, and herbicides, and in glass manufacturing.[65] Organic arsenic compounds have been used in the past to treat syphilis, epilepsy, psoriasis, and amebiasis. Arsine (arsenous hydride) is used in the smelting and refining of metals, in galvanizing and etching, in lead plating, and in the silicon microchip industry. Acute toxicity today follows either accidental ingestion or exposure (e.g., working with chromium-copper-arsenic–treated wood in closed spaces or burning of the same),[83] industrial accidents, or suicidal or homicidal intoxications. Chronic toxicity follows low-level exposure in industry or chronic consumption of contaminated food, water, or medications. Arsenic is absorbed through the skin, lungs, and gastrointestinal tract, the inorganic form more readily than the organic form. Excretion is 90 percent renal, and arsenic can be detected in the urine for 7 to 10 days after a single dose. Arsenic is concentrated in the hair and detectable for much longer time periods (months) after intoxication than in urine or blood.

Acute arsenic intoxication generally presents with gastrointestinal symptomatology (nausea, vomiting, diarrhea, difficult swallowing, abdominal pain, and a garlic odor on the breath), along with hypotension, cyanosis, shortness of breath, delirium, seizures, coma, acute tubular necrosis, and hemolysis. One to 3 weeks after ingestion, polyneuritis may be evident. One to 6 weeks later, diffuse brawny desquamation with hyperpigmentation and mucous membrane irritation may occur.[84] Approximately 6 weeks following ingestion, one may see Mees' lines in nails[84] (Fig. 9-5). Mees originally described these transverse white nail lines in three patients surviving acute arsenic intoxication and ascribed them to actual deposition of arsenic in the nails.[85] Others have ascribed the white lines to a sudden growth arrest of the nail plate at the level of the lunula.[86] Other nail findings in arsenic intoxication include onychomadesis, longitudinal brown bands, and diffuse brown nails.[87] Diffuse hair loss has

Figure 9-5 Mees' lines. (*Courtesy of Dr. Elise A. Olsen.*)

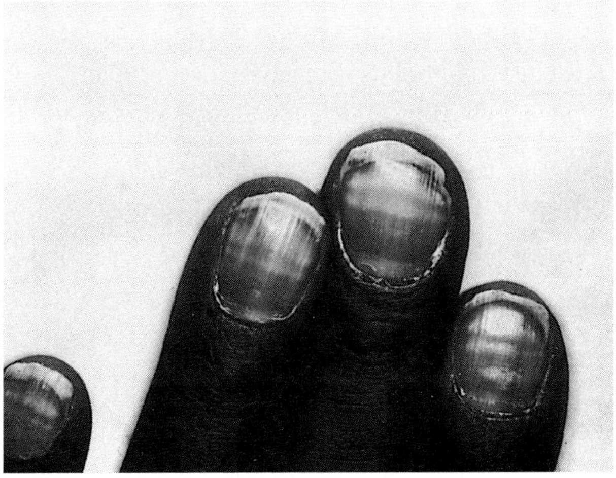

been reported approximately 1 to 2 months after exposure but is not prominent and certainly does not lead to epilation as seen in thallium poisoning.[88] Toxicity is produced by binding to tissue sulfhydryl groups.

Diagnosis of arsenic poisoning can be proved by several methods. Arsenic is radiopaque and can be seen on x-ray of the abdomen. Normal arsenic levels in blood should not exceed 3 μg/dl or 100 μg/liter in urine. Hair clippings can be useful if enough time has elapsed from exposure (> 1 month) to allow the affected hair to reach the skin surface, or hair plucks can be useful within days of intoxication.[84] Scalp hair is the best place to sample due to the high proportion of anagen hairs. A half-gram bundle of hairs should be cut at the roots and the orientation maintained so that the proximal hair is noted. The hairs may be sent for arsenic analysis to National Medical Services (2300 Strait Ave, PO Box 433A, Willow Grove, PA 19090). Analysis of hair for arsenic is particularly useful in cases where the patient is seen sometime after the acute stage, when arsenic has ceased to be eliminated in the urine and feces in diagnostic quantities.[88] Normal arsenic levels in hair are < 0.65 parts per million (ppm).[83] Nails can also be used to document arsenic intoxication (normal level < 1.8 ppm).[83]

Treatment of acute arsenic poisoning should include induction of vomiting or gastric lavage, Dimercaprol (ineffective for arsine poisoning), D-penicillamine, and/or hemodialysis if acute renal failure occurs.

OTHER HEAVY METALS

Copper intoxication has been found to be associated with an acute diffuse alopecia.[89] The exposure to copper was most likely due to ingestion of tap water containing a high concentration of copper salts, presumably from either low pH, the presence of chelating agents, or connection of electric ground wires to copper water pipes which caused the current to ionize the metal.

Alopecia has been reported with cadmium and bismuth intoxication.[89,90] A line of grayish pigmentation on the gingiva has been seen in the latter situation.[69]

LOOSE ANAGEN SYNDROME

Loose anagen syndrome is a recently described entity in which loose anagen hairs can easily be pulled from the scalp. The syndrome was initially reported by Zaun[91] in 1984 at the First Congress of the European Society for Pediatric Dermatology and then further elaborated on by Nodl, Zaun, and Zinn.[92] Since that time, there have been increasing reports of this entity. Nodl, Zaun, and Zinn[92] described a new disease in which all children affected had hair which could easily be pulled out in bundles without pain, and left large areas of alopecia. The hair regrew promptly. The trichogram almost exclusively revealed thinned anagen hairs. In the case report of a 6 year old female with fair hair, the authors noted that there was no alopecia or scalp changes but that the hair could be pulled out easily. The trichogram revealed 12 percent anagen hairs with intact root sheaths and 78 percent anagen hairs without root sheaths. The hair shafts were not round in cross section but of an irregular oval or droplike shape. On histological exam, a cleft was noted between the internal and outer root sheaths, and the internal root sheaths appeared homogenized. The authors concluded that while the clinical and histological pictures were in concordance, no conclusions regarding pathogenesis could be made.

Subsequently, several other reports of this disorder have appeared.[93–95] Loose anagen syndrome is currently defined as a disorder characterized by easily pluckable hairs, which on trichogram analysis are revealed to be in anagen. It occurs predominantly in children aged 1 to 9, although there have been cases in which adults have had similar findings.[94,95] The parents of affected children complain that their child's hair grows very slowly and only rarely needs to be cut. The condition appears to be more prevalent in females and in children with fair hair.[95] The clinical picture varies only slightly (Fig. 9-6). All patients demonstrate easily pluckable hair with a preponderance (> 97 percent) of anagen hairs on trichogram. Some have a diffuse involvement with generally sparse hair with uneven distal ends, while others appear to have more focal areas of hair loss with the development of several ill-defined areas of balding. Most of the hair is dry and lusterless. The children are otherwise healthy and have no history of infection or toxin exposure. They have normal central nervous system development, as well as normal nails and skin.

Trichogram analysis can be obtained by gently plucking hairs and is remarkable for the pres-

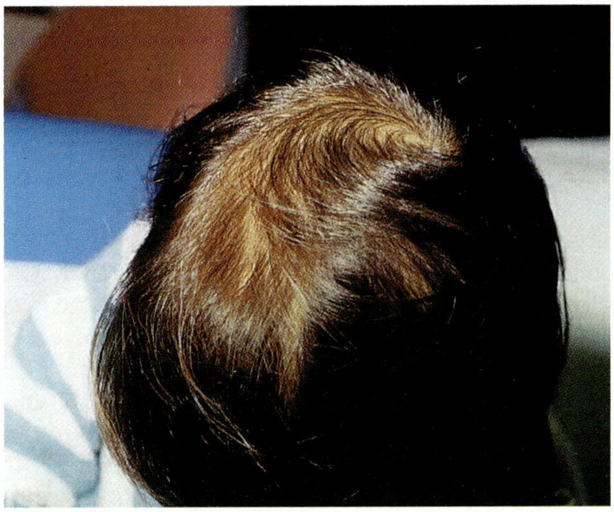

Figure 9-6 Loose anagen syndrome. Note the mild diffuse thinning as evidenced by the visibility of the scalp.

ence of 98 to 100 percent of anagen hairs. Some atrophic anagen[79] and telogen[95] hairs have been noted. Frequently the hair bulb is distorted, some being at acute angles to the hair shaft and others with either twisted or long and tapered bulbs.[94] Pronounced cuticle ruffling just distal to the bulb and a short segment of twisted hair shaft between the bulb and the roughened cuticle are characteristic[94] (Fig. 9-7).

Figure 9-7 A typical loose anagen hair as seen by light microscopy. (×160) The arrow points to the fraying of the cuticle which is characteristic of this disease. (*Reprinted from Baden, Kvedar, and Magro.*[95])

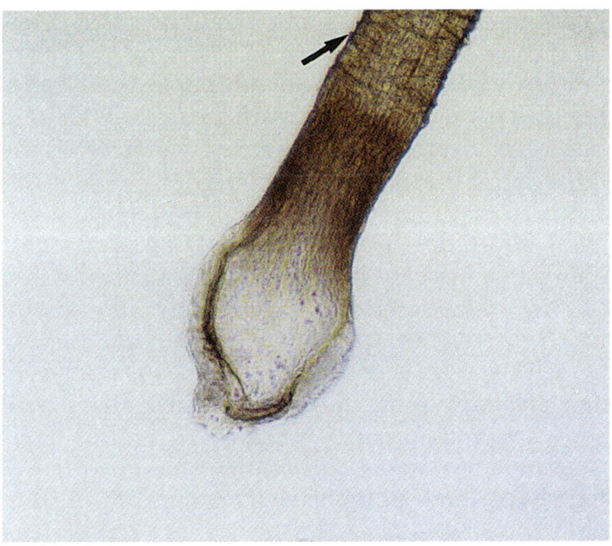

The hair shafts are typically not round in cross section.[92–95] Using shrink-tube analysis,[93] about 20 percent of the plucked hairs were noted to have abnormal shapes, including triangular, quadrangular, trapezoid, kidney-shaped, heart-shaped, and droplike configurations. Electron microscopy has confirmed this as well as noting the presence of longitudinal grooves and a slight twisting of the hair on its axis, similar to that seen in pili trianguli et canaliculi.[93] Polarized light has revealed anisotropic patches in the shaft[92] as well as an irregularly "freckled" pattern of small dark and light patches in small intervening lengths of otherwise normal hair.[93] These may be the cause of the occasional unevenness in color noted.

Histological studies of scalp biopsies have revealed changes both in the hair shaft and in the root sheaths of the follicle. Notably, there have been no reports of any inflammatory infiltrates or evidence of scarring. Nodl, Zaun, and Zinn reported abnormal clefting between the internal and outer root sheaths,[92] and Hamm and Traupe noted marked clefting between the internal root sheath and the hair shaft.[93] The internal root sheath also revealed homogenization with a crumbling degeneration.[93] Price and Gummer reported evidence of premature keratinization of Henle's and Huxley's layers, noting large amounts of trichohyalin granules in Huxley's layer at the level of the lower hair bulb.[94] The cross section of the hair revealed grossly abnormal fibers. Baden, Kvedar, and Magro have confirmed these previous findings as well as further elucidating some of the histological changes regarding epithelial cell adhesion in this disorder. They noted that while there are consistently reproducible abnormalities, not all hair follicles are involved. The internal root sheath reflects premature keratinization with trichohyalin granules in the inferior portion of the bulb. Distal to this region there are varying degrees of cuticle separation, with splits between the hair cuticle and cortex and between the hair cuticle and internal root sheath cuticle. Furthermore, hair bulbs demonstrated markedly contorted morphology proximally, with disadhesive outer root sheaths without attachment to the vitreous layer.[95]

Electron-microscopic studies of hair obtained by gentle pulling[94,95] reveal a distorted bulb end with absence of both root sheaths and of the cuticle just distal to the bulb. Just distally, the cuticle scales are present but are rolled backward, creating a rippled appearance, then gradually become normal. There are also notable ridges and grooves in the hair shaft. The outer root sheath displays the most prominent abnormalities. In the lower portion of the follicle, from the bulb through the keratogenous zone, the epithelium displays poor intercellular cohesion as manifested by prominent cytoplasmic processes and decreased numbers of desmosomes. The internal root sheath cuticle and the hair cuticle cells demonstrate cytoplasmic vacuolization with nuclear degeneration and disruption of the plasmalemma. There is no exocuticle on the hair shaft. After the level of complete keratinization of the internal root sheath, these structures appear normal.[95]

Several theories have developed as to the interrelationships between the various clinical and histological findings. Many have focused on the insufficient adherence between the hair shaft and the root sheath.[92–94] The internal root sheath is of paramount importance in the anchoring of the shaft to the follicle. It is possible that the premature and abnormal keratinization of the internal root sheath could interfere with the interdigitation of the two cuticle cell layers.[94] Also, as the internal sheath is critical in the formation of the shaft, alterations in it could result in misshapen hairs.[93] Hair folliculograms[94] reveal that many of the follicles are generally smaller in size. Twenty-seven percent of the scalp hairs in one study were in telogen, while 73% were in anagen, suggesting that the cyclic interval of anagen is shorter than normal. Also, the apparent resolution of the loose anagen syndrome with age may be a function of the normal growth of hair follicles at the latter part of the first decade or first part of the second which then results in thicker individual hairs, masking the previous sparseness.

Baden, Kvedar, and Magro put forth several ideas as to the possible mechanisms involved.[95] They note that all epithelial components of the follicle appear to be disturbed. Since it is likely that the differentiation of the various layers is coordinated and mediated by intercellular signals, a possible defect in an early signaling pathway could result in multiple abnormalities. An alternative hypothesis involves altered cell adhesion. Cells appear separated in many layers, and the separation of the cuticle from the cortex occurs low in the follicle before significant differentiation has occurred.

While loose anagen syndrome is described as a new entity, it is possible that affected children may have carried other diagnoses in the past. In fact, several reported cases had been given the original diagnosis of alopecia areata. In alopecia areata, however, the lesions are typically well-demarcated with few remaining terminal hairs. Exclamation-point hairs can be found, and the trichogram reveals an increase in dystrophic anagen hairs and telogen hairs. Also, biopsies of involved areas of alopecia areata reveal peribulbar inflammatory changes. Loose anagen syndrome may be confused with a telogen effluvium if the proximal end of shed hairs is not evaluated. Telogen effluvium, however, rarely occurs in children, while loose anagen syndrome rarely first presents in adulthood. The acute active stage of certain cicatricial alopecias may also initially present with easily extractable anagen hairs. Some of these include lichen planopilaris, pseudopelade, and discoid lupus erythematosus. In these conditions, however, the hair shafts are normal, and scarring is either present or will develop. Uncombable hair syndrome has similar alterations in hair shaft shape and longitudinal grooving, but there are rare complaints of hair loss.

CONCLUDING REMARKS

Anagen effluvium manifests as an acute loss of hair, usually days to weeks following a stimulus which interrupts the mitotic activity of rapidly dividing cells in the hair bulb. The most common causes of this type of hair loss in the United States today are cancer chemotherapy and ionizing radiation. Poisoning with heavy metals and other toxic substances must be considered in the differential diagnosis. The condition is often difficult to distinguish from the more common telogen effluvium because, in both cases, copious quantities of scalp hair are lost in a short period of time. Characteristics which may help distinguish the two are the acuity of onset and history of exposure to a potentially toxic substance. In anagen effluvium, loosely plucked hairs will show a predominance of tapered broken ends whereas in telogen effluvium, the majority of hairs will show a clubbed appearance of the proximal ends. In the case of anagen effluvium, withdrawal of the toxic substance, which is the only treatment, should result in prompt reversal of the shedding and hair breakage. Most cases of anagen effluvium should resolve without scarring. However, some patients, especially those exposed to multiple chemotherapeutic regimens and ionizing radiation, do not regrow their hair completely, suggesting that some scarring has occurred. In some cases, it appears that an overlap between telogen effluvium and anagen effluvium exists.

Most cases of this entity will not prompt consultation with a dermatologist. However, when the dermatologist is asked to see a patient with the clinical features of anagen effluvium, careful attention to detail in searching for an offending toxic agent may save the patient a great deal of morbidity and, in some cases, it may possibly save the patient's life.

REFERENCES

1. Caserio RJ: Diagnostic techniques for hair disorders: III. Clinical hair manipulations and clinical findings. Cutis 40:442–448, 1987.
2. Baden HP, Kubilus J, Baden L: A stain for plucked anagen hairs. J Am Acad Dermatol 1:121–122, 1979.
3. Ellinger F: Effects of ionizing radiation on growth and replacement of hair. Ann NY Acad Sci 53:682–687, 1951.
4. Chase HB, Montagna W: Relation of hair proliferation to damage induced in the mouse skin. Proc Soc Exp Biol Med 76:35–37, 1951.
5. Cattaneo SM, Quastler H, Sherman FG: DNA synthesis in irradiated hair follicles of the mouse. Radiat Res 12:587–593, 1960.
6. Geary JR Jr: Effect of roentgen rays during various phases of the hair cycle of the albino rat. Am J Anatomy 91:51–96, 1952.
7. Argyris TS: The relationship between the hair growth cycle and the response of mouse skin to x-irradiation. Am J Anatomy 94:439–463, 1954.
8. Shore RE, Albert RE, Pasternack BS: Follow-up study of patients treated by x-ray epilation for tinea capitis: Resurvey of post-treatment illness and mortality experience. Arch Environ Health 31:21–28, 1976.
9. Goerz G, Kind R, Lehmann P: Cicatricial alopecias. In Orfanos CE, Happle R (eds): *Hair and Hair Diseases.* Berlin, Springer-Verlag, 1990, pp 611–639.
10. Liebow AA: Effects produced on hair by atomic bombs. Ann NY Acad Sci 53:688–689, 1951.
11. Williams AW: A note on certain appearances of x-rayed hairs. Br J Dermatol 18:63–65, 1906.
12. Pearson RW, Malkinson FD: Ultrastructural changes in rat vibrissae following irradiation. J Invest Dermatol 53:95–106, 1969.
13. Pearson RW, Malkinson RD, Marianovic R: The ultrastructural effects of x-irradiation or hydroxyurea on vibrissae matrix cells. Radiat Res 76:565, 1976.
14. Malkinson FD, Griem ML: Radiation injury and recovery in anagen and telogen rodent hairs. Radiat Res 33:554–562, 1968.
15. Sinclair WK, Morton RA: X-ray sensitivity during the cell generation cycle of cultured chinese hamster cells. Radiat Res 29:450–474, 1966.
16. Malkinson FD, Griem ML, Marianovic R: Persistent impairment of hair growth after single large doses of x-rays. Radiat Res 43:83–91, 1970.
17. Perez CA, Marks J, Powers WE: Preoperative irradiation in head and neck cancer. Semin Oncol 4(4):387–397, 1977.
18. Gauci L, Serrou B: Changes in hair pigmentation associated with cancer chemotherapy (letter). Cancer Treat Rep 64:193, 1980.
19. Chase HB: Growth of the hair. Physiol Rev 34:113–126, 1954.
20. Bronner AK, Hood AF: Cutaneous complications of chemotherapeutic agents. J Am Acad Dermatol 9:645–663, 1983.
21. Falkson G, Schulz EJ: Changes in hair pigmentation associated with cancer chemotherapy. Cancer Treat Rep 65:529, 1981.
22. Hood AF: Cutaneous side effects of cancer chemotherapy. Med Clin North Am 70:187–209, 1986.
23. Crounse RG, Van Scott EJ: Changes in scalp hair roots as a measure of toxicity from cancer chemotherapeutic drugs. J Invest Dermatol 35:83–90, 1960.
24. Sims RT: "Beau's lines" in hair: Reduction of hair shaft diameter associated with illness. Br J Dermatol 79:43–49, 1967.
25. Kerker BJ, Hood AF: Chemotherapy-induced cutaneous reactions. Semin Dermatol 8:173–181, 1989.
26. Wheeland RG, Burgdorf WHC, Humphrey GB: The flag sign of chemotherapy. Cancer 51:1356–1358, 1963.
27. Sullivan RD, Mescon H, Jones R: The effect of intra-arterial nitrogen-mustard therapy on human skin. Cancer 6:288–293, 1953.
28. Hillen HFP, Breed WPM, Botman CJ: Scalp cooling by cold air for the prevention of chemotherapy-induced alopecia. Neth J Med 37:231–235, 1990.
29. Satterwhite B, Zimm S: The use of scalp hypothermia in the prevention of doxorubicin-induced hair loss. Cancer 54:34–37, 1984.
30. Luce JK et al.: Prevention of alopecia by scalp cooling of patients receiving adriamycin. Cancer Chemother Rep 57:108–109, 1973.
31. Edelstyn GA et al.: Doxorubicin-induced hair loss and possible modification by scalp cooling. Lancet 2:253–254, 1977.
32. Dean JC et al.: Prevention of doxorubicin-induced hair loss with scalp hypothermia. N Engl J Med 301: 1427–1429, 1979.
33. Aderson J, Hunt J, Smith K: Prevention of doxorubicin-induced alopecia by scalp cooling in patients with advanced breast cancer. Br Med J 282:423–424, 1981.
34. Perlin E, Amin D: Protection from chemotherapy-induced alopecia. Med Pediatr Oncol 19:129–130, 1991.
35. Hussein AM et al.: Protection from chemotherapy-induced alopecia in a rat model. Science 249:1564–1565, 1990.
36. Hussein AM: Interleukin 1 protects against 1-ß-D-arabinofuranosylcytosine-induced alopecia in the newborn rat animal model. Cancer Res 51:3329–3330, 1991.
37. Powis G, Kooistra KL: Doxorubicin-induced hair loss in the angora rabbit: A study of treatments to protect against the hair loss. Cancer Chemother Pharmacol 20:291, 1987.
38. Wood LA: Possible prevention of adriamycin-induced alopecia by tocopherol. N Engl J Med 312:1060, 1985.
39. Perez JE et al.: High-dose alpha-tocopherol as a preven-

tive of doxorubicin-induced alopecia. Cancer Treat Rep 70(10):1213–1214, 1986.
40. Malkinson FD, Keane JT: Hair matrix cell kinetics: A selective review. Int J Dermatol 17:536–551, 1978.
41. Malkinson FD, Lynfield YL: Colchicine alopecia. J Invest Dermatol 33:371–384, 1959.
42. Rook A: Some chemical influences on hair growth and pigmentation. Br J Dermatol 77:115–129, 1965.
43. Flesch P: Inhibition of keratinizing structures by systemic drugs. Pharmacol Rev 15:653–671, 1963.
44. Malkinson FD, Lynfield YL: Colchicine alopecia. J Invest Dermatol 33:371, 1959.
45. Levine M: The action of colchicine on cell division in human cancer, animal, and plant tissues. Ann NY Acad Sci 51:1365–1408, 1951.
46. Menninger EA: *Flowering Trees of the World.* New York, Hearthside Press, 1962.
47. Kerdel-Vegas F: Generalized hair loss due to the ingestion of "coco de mono" (*Lecythis ollaria*). J Invest Dermatol 42:91–94, 1964.
48. Vegas M: Acción depilatoria del coco de mono. Rev Pol Caracas 27:1843–1845, 1936.
49. Vélez-Boza F: Cuatro observaciones clínicas de los efectos producidos por la ingestión de las semillas del coco de mono. Mem Soc Cien Nat La Salle 8:28, 1943.
50. Dao L: Experiencias sobre enfermedades tropicales en zonas rurales de Venezuela. Corporación Universaro, 1958.
51. Aronow L, Kerdel-Vegas F: Seleno-cystathionine, a pharmacologically active factor in the seeds of *Lecythis ollaria.* Nature 205:1185–1187, 1965.
52. Horn MJ, Jones DB: Isolation from *Astragalus pectinatus* of a crystalline amino acid complex containing selenium and sulfur. J Biol Chem 139:649–660, 1941.
53. Virupaksha TK, Shrift A: Biosynthesis of a selenocystathionine from selenate in *Stanleya pinnata.* Biochem Biophys Acta 74:791–793, 1963.
54. Crounse RG, Maxwell JD, Blank H: Inhibition of growth of hair by mimosine. Nature 194:694–695, 1962.
55. Montagna W, Yun JS: The effects of the seeds of the *Leucaena glauca* on the hair follicles of the mouse. J Invest Dermatol 40:325–332, 1963.
56. Rothman S: *Physiology and Biochemistry of the Skin.* Chicago, University of Chicago Press, 1955.
57. Tan TG: Occupational toxic alopecia due to borax. Acta Derm Venereol 50:55–58, 1970.
58. Schillinger BM, Berstein M, Goldberg LA, Shalita AR: Boric acid poisoning. J Am Acad Dermatol 7:667–673, 1982.
59. Stein KM et al.: Toxic alopecia from ingestion of boric acid. Arch Dermatol 108:95–97, 1973.
60. Rubenstein AD, Musher DM: Epidemic boric acid poisoning simulating staphylococcal toxic epidermal necrolysis of the newborn infant: Ritters disease. J Pediatr 77:884–887, 1970.
61. Boggs RF Jr, Anrode HG: Boric acid poisoning treated by exchange transfusion. Pediatrics 16:109–114, 1955.
62. Baliah T, MacLeish H, Drummond KN: Acute boric acid poisoning. Can Med Assoc J 101:166–168, 1969.
63. Hubler WR: Hair loss as a symptom of chronic thallotoxicosis. South Med J 59:436–442, 1966.
64. Desendos JA, Wilder MH, Coppenger GW: Thallium poisoning: An outbreak in Florida. South Med J 85:1203–1206, 1988.
65. Graef JW, Lovejoy FJ Jr: Heavy metal poisoning. In Braunwald E et al. (eds): *Harrison's Principles of Internal Medicine,* 11th ed. New York, McGraw-Hill, 1987, pp 850–855.
66. Reed D et al.: Thallotoxicosis: Acute manifestations and sequelae. JAMA 183:516–522, 1963.
67. Chamberlain PH et al.: Thallium poisoning. Pediatrics 22:1170–1182, 1958.
68. Bank WJ et al.: Thallium poisoning. Arch Neurol 26:456–464, 1972.
69. Dawber RPR, Ebling FJG, Wojnarowska FT: Disorders of hair. In Champion RH, Burton JL, Ebling FJG (eds): *Textbook of Dermatology,* 5th ed. Oxford, Blackwell Scientific Publications, 1992, pp 2582–2584.
70. Gross P, Runne E, Wilson JW: Studies on the effect of thallium poisoning of the rat: The Influence of cystine and methionine on alopecia and survival periods. J Invest Dermatol 10:119–134, 1948.
71. Ciaccio EI: Mercury: Therapeutic and toxic aspects. Semin Drug Treat 1:177–194, 1971.
72. Pierard GE: Toxic effects of metals from the environment on hair growth and structure. J Cutan Pathol 6:237–242, 1979.
73. Elhassani SB: The many faces of methylmercury poisoning. J Toxicol 19:875–906, 1982.
74. An Assessment of Mercury in the Environment. A Report prepared by the Panel on Mercury of the Coordinating Committee for Scientific and Technical Assessments of Environmental Pollutants, National Research Council. Washington, National Academy of Sciences, 1978.
75. Richter ED, Peled N, Luria M: Mercury exposure and effects at a thermometer factory. Scan J Work Environ Health 8(suppl 1):161–166, 1982.
76. Jalili MA, Abbasi AH: Poisoning by ethylmercury toluene sulphonamide. Br J Ind Med 18:303–308, 1961.
77. Bakir F et al.: Methylmercury poisoning in Iraq, an interuniversity report. Science 181:230–241, 1973.
78. Haq IU: Agrosan poisoning in man. Br Med J 1:1579–1582, 1963.
79. Ordonez JV et al.: Estudio epidemiologico de una enfermedad considerada como encefalititis en la region de Los Altos de Guatemala. Bull Pan Am Sanit Bur 60:510–519, 1966.
80. Derlan LKA: Outbreak of food poisoning due to alkylmercury fungicide on southern Ghana state farm. Arch Environ Health 28:49–52, 1974.
81. Hirschman SZ, Feingold M, Boylen G: Mercury in house paint as a cause of acrodynia: Effect of therapy with N-acetyl-D, L-penicillamine. N Engl J Med 65:889–893, 1963.
82. Wustner H et al.: Nail changes and loss of hair: Cardinal signs of mercury poisoning from hair bleaches (author's transl) (Ger). Dtsch Med Wochenschr 100(34):1694–1697, 1975. H. Wüstner, C.E. Orfanos Nagelverfärbung und Haarausfall: Leitsymptome eíner Quecksilbervergiftung durch kosmetische bleichmittel. Dtsch Med Wochenschr 100(34): 1694–1697, 1975.)
83. Peters HA et al.: Hematological, dermal and neuropsychological disease from burning and power sawing chromium-copper-arsenic (CCA)-treated wood. Acta Pharmacol Toxicol 59(6–7):39–43, 1986.
84. Heyman A, Pfeiffer JB Jr, Willett RW, Taylor HM: Peripheral neuropathy caused by arsenical intoxication. N Engl J Med 254(9):401–409, 1956.
85. Mees RA: The nails with arsenical polyneuritis. JAMA 72:1337, 1919.
86. De Nicola P, Morsiani M, Zavagli G: *Nail Diseases in Internal Medicine.* Springfield, Illinois, Charles C Thomas, 1974.
87. Daniel CR, Scher RK: Nail changes secondary to systemic drugs or ingestants. J Am Acad Dermatol 10:250–258, 1984.
88. Althausen TL, Gunther L: Acute arsenic poisoning: A report of seven cases and a study of arsenic excretion with especial reference to the hair. JAMA 92:2002, 1929.

89. Pierard GE: Toxic effects of metals from the environment on hair growth and structure. J Cutan Pathol 6:237–242, 1979.
90. Goltner VE: Versenatbehandlung einer Alopezie nach Wismuttherapie. Z Haut u-Geschl Kr 31:164, 1961.
91. Zaun H: Differential diagnosis of alopecia in children. In Happle R, Grosshans E (eds): *Pediatric Dermatology.* Berlin, Springer, 1987, pp 157–166.
92. Nodl F, Zaun H, Zinn HK: Gesteigerte Epilierbarkeit von Anagenhaaren bei Kindernals Folge eines Reifungsdefekts der Follikel mit Gestorter Verhaftung von Haarschaft und Wurzelscheiden: Das Phanomen der Leicht Ausziehbaren Haare. Aktüel Dermatol 12:55–57, 1986.
93. Hamm H, Traupe H: Loose anagen hair of childhood: The phenomenon of easily pluckable hair. J Am Acad Dermatol 20:242–248, 1989.
94. Price VH, Gummer CL: Loose anagen syndrome. J Am Acad Dermatol 20:249–256, 1989.
95. Baden HP, Kvedar JC, Magro CM: Loose anagen hair as a cause of hereditary hair loss in children. Arch Dermatol 128:1349–1353, 1992.
96. *Physicians' Desk Reference,* 47th ed. Montvale, NJ, Medical Economics Data, 1993.
97. Cleveland CB, Francke DE, Heller WM, et al. (eds): *AHFS Drug Information.* Bethesda, MD, American Society of Hospital Pharmacists, 1992, p 497.
98. Dorr RT, Fritz WL (eds): *Cancer Chemotherapy Handbook.* New York, Elsevier Science Publishing, 1980.

Chapter

10

DIFFUSE ALOPECIA: TELOGEN HAIR LOSS

Virginia C. Fiedler and Abdul Hafeez

INTRODUCTION

Diffuse alopecia with excessive telogen hair shedding has been associated with a variety of hormonal and nutritional factors, ingestion of various drugs, exposure to certain chemicals, systemic and local cutaneous disease, and psychological stress. Some of these associations are well-documented; others are often quoted but less well established. Prognosis for hair regrowth is generally good if the cause of the telogen hair shedding can be found and eliminated and if the patient does not have associated androgenetic alopecia.

Determining the etiology of diffuse alopecia is usually time-consuming. Assessment includes a thorough history of the evolution of the loss, review of systems, review of exposure to drugs and chemicals, dietary history, history of recent illnesses, family history of hair loss (e.g., androgenetic alopecia), hair grooming procedures, and evaluation for psychological stress. Evaluation of a role for stress is complicated significantly by the fact that hair loss usually provokes at least a moderate stress reaction; therefore, establishing a causal role for stress is difficult and often impossible. Quickly dismissing the patient with the admonition that stress is probably the cause of the hair loss and/or prescribing tranquilizers or other similar agents is certainly to be avoided.

Examination of the density and distribution of scalp hair as well as body hair provides critically useful information. A comparative assessment of part width should be made at several sites on the scalp. The parts should also be observed from a tangential vantage point for evidence of short hairs of normal texture (e.g., regrowing hairs) vs. short hairs of visibly diminished shaft diameter (e.g., indeterminate hairs of androgenetic alopecia). Evidence of underlying scalp and/or other cutaneous or systemic disease should be sought. Evaluation of the nails should not be overlooked.

At times, the patient's concern may appear to be out of proportion to the extent of alopecia observed. In fact, many times the scalp hair density may appear to be well within normal limits, leaving the observer in doubt as to whether hair loss is real or is only perceived by the patient to be so. In such cases the light hair pull test, the hair pluck test, or daily hair counts may be useful.

The light hair pull test is accomplished by pinching approximately 20 hairs between the thumb and index finger and gently pulling. If any anagen hairs are extracted, then one can assume that an abnormal situation exists which needs further evaluation. Generally telogen hairs are extracted by the light pull test, which gives a crude assessment of the telogen count. Telogen counts obtained by plucking have been reported to vary widely, ranging from 4 to 37 percent and averaging 13 to 15 percent in healthy adults.[1,2] The data for telogen counts are conflicting concerning similarities vs. differences in men vs. women and changes with advancing age.[2,3] For practical purposes, Kligman[1] has defined telogen counts higher than 25 percent as being diagnostic of telogen effluvium, and counts above 20 percent as presumptively abnormal. If more than two telogen hairs are extracted by light pull from any site on the scalp, then further evaluation is warranted. The light hair pull test may be falsely negative if the patient's hair has recently been combed, brushed, or shampooed.

Daily hair counts may provide useful information. For the daily hair count, the patient is asked to record the number of hairs collected on the comb, brush, pillowcase, sink, shower, and collar. Each daily hair collection should be placed in a separate envelope and marked with the date, number of hairs collected, and whether or not the patient shampooed on that day. These hairs may be evaluated microscopically to determine if they are telogen or anagen hairs or if the hairs are broken. The structural appearance of the hair shafts should also be evaluated for defects and variability in diameter. Under normal circumstances, 50 to 100 telogen hairs are shed on average per day.

Hair plucking is sometimes suggested to be the most accurate measure of anagen-telogen ratios, but as we shall discuss, it may provide misleading results with regard to anagen hair morphology. Van Scott, Reinertson, and Steinmuller[2] described in 1957 a technique for plucking and examining hair roots. The grasping surfaces of surgical needle-holding forceps are covered with several layers of cellulose tape to ensure a tight closure and prevent slipping of hair shafts during the pulling procedure. Approximately 50 hairs are grasped simultaneously close to the scalp surface and extracted with a quick pull. Hair roots are hydrated, examined microscopically, and classified as anagen, catagen, or telogen. Although the act of plucking normal anagen hair may distort its fragile root,[4] plucking should not affect telogen hairs and can be a useful method for evaluation of diffuse hair loss associated with abnormal telogen shedding.

Shed telogen hairs are said to derive exclusively from follicles which are generating new anagen hairs.[1] Excessive telogen shedding (effluvium) begins 2 to 4 months after the inciting event has precipitated anagen follicles to enter catagen and subsequent telogen. Normally, telogen lasts 2 to 4 months and is followed by reentry of the follicle into anagen. The latency between the inciting event and the hair loss reflects the duration of the catagen and telogen phases.

Telogen hair shedding may be constant or intermittent. Apparent hair thickness, which depends on hair density, hair shaft width, and hair length, varies considerably among individuals. The objective observer, therefore, is often left with the dilemma as to whether or not hair loss has occurred. A decrease of at least 25 percent of scalp hairs may be necessary for an objective observer to consistently diagnose diffuse alopecia.[1] The patient's perception, therefore, is probably more valid than the physician's in making the assessment that a diffuse alopecia has occurred.

HORMONES AND ALOPECIA

Alterations in hormones (especially thyroid and sex hormones) influence the hair follicle and may alter the normal trichogram. The associated alopecia is usually reversible when hormonal homeostasis is reestablished unless it is superimposed on the evolution of androgenetic alopecia. Patients with androgenetic alopecia may report that although hair regrowth has occurred, the resulting scalp hair density is less than that prior to the episode of hair shedding (V. C. Fiedler, unpublished data).

Hypothyroidism

Diffuse scalp plus or minus body hair loss may be present as the only symptom of hypothyroidism. This is exemplified by the case of an 18-year-old woman who had unexplained hair loss for 3 years and was found to be hypothyroid.[5] The loss of the outer one-third of the eyebrows (Hertoghe's symptom) may be seen in about a quarter of patients with hypothyroidism.[6] Scalp hair loss has been reported to be present in 18 to 50 percent of myxedema patients.[6,7] Saito, Hori, and Kuribayashi[6] found no correlation between duration or severity of the myxedema and degree or extent of hair loss. Hypothyroid patients treated with thyroid hormone replacement generally begin to experience regrowth of hair within approximately 8 weeks.[8]

Deficiency of thyroid hormone, whether disease-associated or drug-induced, is apparently responsible for the alopecia which is characterized by a decrease in the anagen-telogen ratio.[8,9] Freinkel and Freinkel[8] reported cases in which the hypothyroidism had been induced by propylthiouracil or I^{131} therapy. The percentage of telogen hairs returned to normal with thyroid replacement therapy even during concurrent administration of propylthiouracil. Thyroid hormone deficiency in the rat results in delayed spontaneous eruption of hair and prolongation of the telogen phase.[10] In adult sheep, thyroidectomy decreases wool production.[11] In humans, cell kinetics of the hair bulb were assessed using DNA flow cytometry. Hypothyroid patients showed hair bulbs with decreased S and $G_2 + M$ phase and increased G_0 and G_1 phase cell percentages.[12]

Hypothyroidism as a cause of diffuse alopecia is clearly established, although no correlation between thyroid hormone levels and degree of alopecia has been made. Why some individuals are affected and others are not is unknown.

Hyperthyroidism

Hyperthyroidism as a cause of diffuse alopecia is less clearly substantiated. Hyperthyroid patients have been shown to have increased S and $G_2 + M$ phase and decreased G_0 and G_1 phase cell percentages in their hair bulbs.[12] Williams[13] reported subnormal amounts of axillary hair in about 60 percent of 102 patients with thyrotoxicosis. Short, scanty, or thin scalp hair was observed in about half of 40 cases of diffuse toxic and toxic multinodular goiter seen in a Nigerian hospital.[14] Further studies on the association of hyperthyroidism and alopecia need to be done.

Pregnancy

Postpartum alopecia is probably the most commonly recognized form of telogen hair shedding (Fig. 10-1). Pecoraro, Barman, and Astore[15] found a progressive increase in the percentage of anagen hairs during the second and third trimesters of pregnancy (90 percent and 94 percent) compared with 84 percent in nonpregnant women. Lynfield[16] found 95 percent anagen and 5 percent telogen hairs during both the second and third trimesters. Following delivery there is a rapid decrease in the percentage of anagen hairs, with an associated increase in the percentage of telogen hairs. Lynfield[16] reported postpartum telogen hair counts of 24 percent at 6 weeks, and Dawber and Connor[17] have reported telogen counts as high as 65 percent at 2 months. Hair shedding begins from less than a month to 4 months postpartum and may last as long as a year.[1,18] Typically the duration of shedding is less than 6

Figure 10-1 Postpartum telogen effluvium.

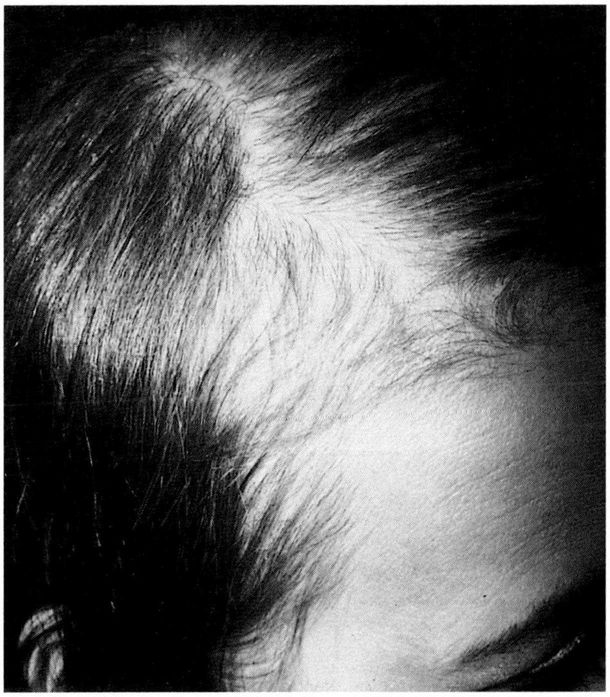

months.[1,19] Basal metabolic rate and 17-ketosteroid excretion have been measured in some patients and found to be normal.[19] Administration of thyroid hormone and local applications of estrogen or estrogen plus progesterone have not shown any consistent beneficial effect.[18] The majority of patients have a return to normal hair density[1,19] unless they have associated androgenetic alopecia, in which case regrowth may not return scalp hair density to prepregnancy levels (V. C. Fiedler, unpublished data).

It is widely thought that the high estrogen levels of pregnancy are responsible for prolongation of the anagen phase of the follicular cycle, accounting for the changes observed in the trichogram of the pregnant patient. Pecoraro's data[15] suggest an alternative explanation, i.e., a more rapid shedding of telogen hairs during pregnancy. Pregnant women in the first trimester showed anagen counts of 81 percent vs. 84 percent in nonpregnant women. During the second and third trimesters, when the anagen percentages were 90 percent and 94 percent, respectively, the hair counts were lower than those obtained in the first trimester. Hair density was significantly lower on the parietal scalp of pregnant patients during the second and third trimesters (166.3 and 195.8 hairs per cm^2) compared with their first-trimester values (246.7 hairs per cm^2). Pecoraro, Barman, and Astore also showed an increased percentage of thick hairs in pregnant vs. nonpregnant women and a slower rate of hair growth. Estradiol treatment of rats results in delayed initiation of anagen, retention of club hairs, shortened duration of anagen, and decreased hair growth rate.[20,21] These rat data are difficult to extrapolate to the human situation. Until scalp biopsy data are available to determine the actual follicular changes associated with pregnancy and the postpartum period, determination of an appropriate animal model and evaluation of hormonal effects is an impossible task. Additional factors which may be relevant to postpartum hair loss may include stress, blood loss, and other hormonal factors such as prolactin secretion with nursing.

Androgenetic Alopecia

Androgenetic alopecia is characterized by progressive follicular miniaturization, a shortened anagen cycle, and an increased percentage of telogen hairs.[22–24] Inflammation and, in later stages, follicular fibrosis are also seen.[23] Telogen percentages vary considerably in this process and may be quite high.[25,26]

Androgenetic alopecia usually manifests as a distinct pattern of scalp hair thinning (i.e., frontotemporal recession and vertex thinning in male-pattern hair loss and diffuse thinning over the frontovertical scalp in female-pattern hair loss). Diffuse alopecia over the entire scalp with increased telogen shedding may also be a manifestation of androgenetic alopecia in women and occasionally also in men (Fig. 10-2). It may be confused clinically with other causes of telogen hair shedding. A biopsy is sometimes necessary to clarify the diagnosis. In most instances, the diagnosis is made by exclusion of other causes, a positive family history of androgenetic alopecia, and microscopic hair assessment which reveals marked variability in hair shaft diameters.

The majority of women with androgenetic alopecia have no evidence of abnormal androgen production.[27,28] One is particularly unlikely to find endocrine abnormalities if mild alopecia is unassociated with hirsutism, acne, oligomenorrhea, amenorrhea, galactorrhea, or signs of Cushing's syndrome.

The *ovaries* and *abnormal androgen production:* Polycystic ovary (PCO) syndrome, as originally described by Stein and Leventhal[29] was defined as a syndrome consisting of obesity,

Figure 10-2 Diffuse androgenetic alopecia in a woman.

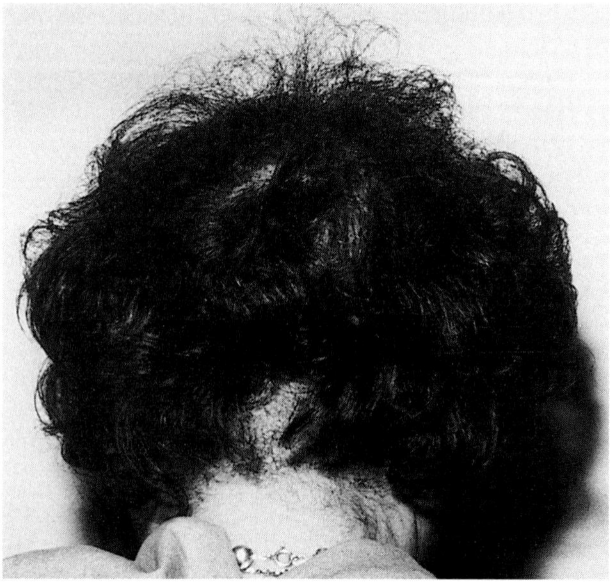

amenorrhea, hirsutism, and infertility associated with bilaterally enlarged polycystic ovaries. Modern imaging techniques have also shown similar ovarian changes in apparently normal women.[30] Using ultrasound visualization to diagnose PCO in a series of 556 patients, hirsutism was present in 61 percent, acne in 24 percent, alopecia in 8 percent, acanthosis nigricans in 2 percent, obesity in 35 percent, menorrhagia in 1 percent, oligomenorrhea in 45 percent, amenorrhea in 26 percent, and infertility in >29 percent.[31] Elevations of luteinizing hormone; of the ratio of luteinizing hormone to follicle-stimulating hormone; and of testosterone, androstenedione, and estradiol levels may occur.[32]

Virilizing ovarian tumors are rare. Hirsutism occurs in nearly 100 percent of such patients and alopecia in approximately 50 percent. The majority of these patients have elevated plasma testosterone levels.[33]

The *adrenals* and *abnormal androgen production:* Congenital adrenal hyperplasia (CAH) is usually obvious before early childhood. However, partial reduction in enzyme activity (most commonly 21-hydroxylase deficiency) may present as late-onset CAH and be associated with hirsutism and alopecia.[34] Cushing's syndrome is associated with hypertrichosis (generalized growth of fine hair due to increased cortisol) in 36 percent, hirsutism in 81 percent, and alopecia in 50 percent.[35] Testosterone levels may be markedly raised if a carcinoma is present.[36]

Hyperprolactinemia may be responsible for abnormal adrenal androgen production[37,38] or it may be associated with PCO.[39] In either case, hirsutism and, less commonly, alopecia may result. Amenorrhea and galactorrhea may be present. Elevations in prolactin levels have been associated with pituitary hypersecretion, the use of psychotropic drugs, and prolactinomas. Adrenal receptors for prolactin are present. Data suggest that prolactin may stimulate adrenal androgen production, resulting in elevations of DHEA(S).[37,38] DHEA has been shown to inhibit the activity of glucose-6-phosphate-dehydrogenase in isolated human hair follicles, which may interfere with anagen follicular development and hair growth.[40]

Low levels of sex hormone–binding globulin (SHBG) may result in increased free testosterone levels. It is this unbound fraction which is biologically active and may contribute to androgenetic alopecia.[41] High estrogen levels increase SHBG, thereby reducing available androgen. One might speculate that postmenopausal exacerbation of androgenetic alopecia may be related in part to the effects of decreased estrogen levels on SHBG and circulating free androgens.

Involutional Alopecia

Involutional (senescent, senile) alopecia occurs in both sexes and is defined as diffuse hair thinning occurring after the age of 50 years with a negative family history of male-pattern baldness.[42] The pattern often closely resembles androgenetic alopecia, and in my experience careful questioning may uncover female relatives with hair thinning historically consistent with androgenetic alopecia. The histology shows an increase in telogen follicles and usually decreased follicular size.[42] Follicles may or may not be diminished in number.[42,43] Much remains to be learned to further refine the concept of involutional alopecia.

Oral Contraceptives

Diffuse alopecia may occur in some women when they stop taking oral contraceptives. Other women may experience hair loss while using oral contraceptives.

Telogen hair percentages have been measured in a few patients with alopecia occurring after discontinuation of oral contraceptives. Some patients have had high telogen counts, while others have not. History of postpartum hair loss was variably present.[17,44] Suggestions that postcontraceptive hair loss is similar to postpartum hair loss are difficult to evaluate because so little is known about either process. Studies of the effects of oral contraceptives on the hair cycle have not shown consistent effects.[45–47]

Hair loss during oral contraceptive use has been documented.[44,48] Griffiths[48] described six such patients in whom no other etiologic factors could be found. Three of the six patients had hair loss 1 to 5 months after switching from one pill to another; the other three patients had been on treatment from 6 to 28 months prior to the onset of hair loss. The progestins in the contraceptives used in these six cases were predominantly of moderate androgenic potency, suggesting that the pill may have been exacerbating an underlying androgenetic alopecia. Scalp biopsies were performed on these six individuals, and no characteristic changes were seen. Zaun and collegues[45,46] showed increased telogen percentages in some women during the early months of oral contraceptive use.

Further studies are needed to document the role of contraceptive use in hair loss.

NUTRITION AND ALOPECIA

Weight Loss

Stringent dieting may result in diffuse hair shedding within 1 to 6 months after onset of the diet. Calorie deprivation associated with hair loss has been reported to vary from 0 to 1000 kcal per day.[49–52] Other experience suggests that diets as generous as 1200 kcal per day may be associated with this phenomenon (V. C. Fiedler, unpublished data). Hair loss may recur with subsequent diets.[51,52] Prognosis for regrowth after discontinuation of the diet is generally good.

It has been suggested that hair loss is seen only in those with negative nitrogen balance (i.e., loss of lean body mass). Increases in protein intake or refeeding have resulted in diminution or cessation of the loss.[53,54] In the mouse, a relatively modest 25 percent calorie restriction resulted in 57 percent inhibition of cellular proliferation in the skin.[55] Obese women were studied before and after a 15-day 329-kcal-per-day diet (62 g carbohydrate, 1.2 g lipid, 21 g protein). Basal metabolic rate dropped below levels that would be explained by loss of lean body mass. Significant reductions in T3 were noted in the patients. It was concluded that reduced thyroid activity contributed to the reduced metabolic rate.[56] It is possible that diet-related reduction of thyroid activity may also contribute to hair loss. Fasting has been shown to result in an increase in the biologic half-life of plasma dehydroepiandrosterone sulfate, which in theory could also contribute to an exacerbation of an underlying androgenetic alopecia.[57] Much remains to be learned about the pathogenesis of diet-related hair loss.

Protein-Calorie Malnutrition

Marasmus is a chronic deficiency of protein and calories which usually begins in the first year of life. Marasmus may be caused solely by poor nutrition or may become manifest after the stress of illnesses such as gastroenteritis, parasitic infections, or glomerulonephritis.[58] It results in hair which is thin, sparse, straight, lighter in color than normal, and easily plucked. Kwashiorkor may be either an acute or a chronic deficit of protein in an otherwise calorically adequate diet. With acute protein deficiency, dark hair may exhibit bands of red or white, the "flag sign" of kwashiorkor. Advanced protein deficiency results in fine, brittle, and sparse hair.

The rate of proliferation of hair root cells is one of the most rapid in the body. Regeneration of the mass of generative cells is reported to take about 23 hours.[59] Deficient protein intake has been shown to correlate positively with protein content of anagen roots.[60] During relative depletion of protein stores, impairment of hair root protein synthesis apparently occurs before a decrease in synthesis of serum albumin, which serves a more vital function.[60,61] Progressive bulb atrophy is the most consistent sign of early protein deprivation.[61] An increase of telogen hairs was found to occur in elderly individuals who were protein-deficient,[60] as well as in children with classic protein-calorie malnutrition.[62]

Johnson, Latham, and Roe[58] studied 55 children: group 1, 29 healthy children; group 2, 5 children with nutritional marasmus and 9 with kwashiorkor; and group 3, 12 children with depressed height and weight associated with diseases having a secondary effect on nutritional status. They measured percent anagen hairs, percent telogen hairs, percent atrophic bulbs, diameter of anagen bulbs, and hair shaft diameter. Significant decreases in percent anagen hairs and in hair shaft diameter and a significant increase in percent telogen hairs were found only in the severely malnourished children compared to the well-nourished. No significant differences in any of the hair root characteristics were found comparing children with marasmus and those with kwashiorkor. Assessment of these parameters was inadequate to reliably diagnose less severe forms of protein-calorie malnutrition. The data suggest that deficiency of protein or of protein and calories may have significant effects on hair growth. Those effects may show great individual variation except in individuals who are severely malnourished, in which case the findings are uniformly similar.

Essential Fatty Acid Deficiency

Hair and skin changes of essential fatty acid deficiency may occur after 2 to 4 months of inadequate intake. This situation is most likely to arise in those with inadequately supplemented parenteral alimentation.[63–65] Redness and scaling of the scalp and eyebrows are early symptoms and are followed by significant telogen hair shedding. The remaining hair is dry, unruly, and lighter in color.

High serum levels of eicosatrienoic acid 20:3,N-9) and low levels of arachidonic acid confirm the diagnosis. Topical linoleic acid (safflower oil) has been shown to reverse the scaling and redness within 3 weeks and the hair changes within 3 months.[65]

Lightening of black hair in essential fatty acid–deficient hooded rats has been reported,[66] suggesting a relationship between pigmentation and linoleic acid and its metabolites. Further studies are needed to clarify the causes of the changes occurring in essential fatty acid deficiencies.

Iron Deficiency

Iron deficiency with or without associated anemia has been reported to be present in as many as 72 percent of women with diffuse alopecia associated with an increased percentage of telogen hairs.[28] Hård[67] reported that 18.6 percent of his patients with diffuse hair loss had nonanemic iron deficiency. Oral iron therapy resulted in cessation of hair loss followed by regrowth and was associated with an increase of iron levels to normal. Patients who discontinued iron therapy noted a resumption of the hair loss and evidence of iron deficiency. Reinstitution of iron therapy was again followed by return of hair growth and iron levels to normal, suggesting that the hair loss in these patients was caused by iron deficiency. Rushton and Ramsay[68] suggest that ferritin levels of ≥ 40 µg/liter may be necessary for optimal hair growth.

It is thought that iron deficiency results in decreased depot iron and tissue iron much earlier than the anemia is manifest. Hård[67] suggested that hair loss is a prodromal symptom which appears when the serum iron level has declined but before anemia has become demonstrable. Iron is an essential requirement for the enzyme ribonucleotide reductase, the activity of which in turn is strongly correlated with the rate of DNA synthesis.[69] It is likely that iron availability limits DNA synthesis in proliferating cells.[70] It seems reasonable to expect that minor iron depletion might have an early effect on the rapidly multiplying cells of the follicular matrix prior to the development of an anemia.

Zinc Deficiency

Zinc deficiency may be hereditary or acquired. Symptoms of zinc deficiency include hair loss, acral and periorificial dermatitis, diarrhea, susceptibility to infection and altered cellular immunity, mood changes, anorexia, neurological disturbances, and growth retardation. The overall mortality rate in untreated children is approximately 20 percent.[71]

Hereditary zinc deficiency, acrodermatitis enteropathica, is an inborn error of metabolism resulting in zinc malabsorption and severe zinc deficiency. It is an autosomal recessive disorder which usually becomes manifest at the time of weaning. Spontaneous remission may occur at adolescence.[71] Occasionally the disease may remain undiagnosed until well into adulthood.[72] Diagnosis is usually established by reduced serum zinc levels. Zinc deficiency is thought to be associated with reduced absorption of unsaturated fatty acids and impaired desaturation of linoleic and alpha-linoleic acids to their long-chain metabolites. Perhaps essential fatty acid deficiency may account in part for some of the cutaneous changes associated with this disorder. Occasionally serum zinc levels may be normal. In such cases the clinical response to zinc supplementation (3–30 µmol zinc/kg per day) for 5 days, as well as seeing the expected increases in serum levels of essential fatty acids and their long-chain metabolites, will confirm the diagnosis.[71,73]

Acquired zinc deficiency was described in the past with parenteral alimentation.[74,75] It has also been described in association with pancreatitis and intestinal bypass surgery.[76] Symptoms and signs are similar to those seen in acrodermatitis enteropathica.

Dupré, Bonafé, and Carriere described the hairs in acrodermatitis enteropathica. Hairs are white, sparse, short, and brittle, and they appear defective when examined under polarization.

The ends of the hairs appear "spearlike"; the shafts show narrowing and "wavelike changes"; and mild trichonodosis or trichoschisis is present. Further studies need to be done to determine the nature of the hair growth abnormalities in zinc deficiency.

Biotin Deficiency

Biotin deficiency disorders may be congenital or acquired. Symptoms vary but may include dermatitis, alopecia, seizures, hypotonia, ataxia, sensorineural hearing loss, visual pathway defects, mental retardation, and recurrent infections.

Inherited disorders of each of the four biotin-dependent carboxylases have been reported.[78–81] Combined carboxylase deficiency is reported in many patients. The early-onset (neonatal) form is usually due to functional deficiency of holocarboxylase synthetase.[82] The late-onset (after 3 months) form is usually due to biotinidase deficiency.[83] In the neonatal form, defective biotinylation of apocarboxylase occurs because of a mutant holocarboxylase synthetase;[82] serum biotin levels are normal.[83] Characteristic organic aciduria (3-methylcrotonylglycine and 3-hydroxyisovalerate) is diagnostic.[84] In the late-onset form, biotinidase deficiency is caused by failure to recycle endogenous biotin and liberate dietary biotin; serum biotin levels may be low.[83] Treatment with biotin (10 mg per day) results in clinical and biochemical improvement, although patients may have residual neurological damage comprising sensorineural hearing loss, visual pathway defects, ataxia, and mental retardation. It is not certain why this residual damage occurs or if early treatment will prevent it.[84,85] Early hair regrowth may be noted between 2 to 4 weeks after starting treatment and has been reported to be complete after 2 months.[86]

Acquired biotin deficiency has been reported in association with parenteral alimentation[86] or excessive ingestion of raw egg white.[87] Symptoms and signs are similar to those observed in the congenital disorders.

Williams, Packman, and Cowan studied the hair in children affected with biotin-responsive multiple carboxylase deficiency[88]. Scalp hair was diffusely sparse and finely textured. No hair shaft irregularities were noted on light microscopy. Anagen-telogen ratios were not measured, and no scalp biopsy was performed. Much remains to be learned about the alopecia associated with biotin deficiency.

PHYSIOLOGICAL STRESS AND ALOPECIA

Fever

Postfebrile alopecia has been described as an increased telogen hair shedding beginning anywhere from 2 to 5 months after a febrile illness. In many instances, the patients were otherwise in poor health such that weight loss or malnutrition and perhaps other factors may have contributed to the alopecia.[1,89] It is reasonable to assume that fever, which augments metabolic demands, would be likely to impair the ability of the rapidly multiplying follicular matrix cells to proliferate normally in a nutritionally compromised host. It is also possible that fever itself via one of the endogenous pyrogens [interleukin I α or β, tumor neurosis factor, or interferon α or γ (IFN α or γ)][90] may directly downregulate follicular matrix cell proliferation. Interleukin I is an unlikely candidate in that it has been shown to protect against cytosine arabinoside–induced alopecia in the rat.[91] Interferons α and γ are more likely candidates to mediate direct follicular matrix effects. These two cytokines have been shown to decrease epithelial proliferation in tissue culture.[92,93] Alopecia has been reported to occur in individuals receiving parenteral IFN α or γ.[94,95]

Biopsies in four patients thought to have postfebrile alopecia showed an increased number of normal telogen follicles; no other histological changes were observed.[1] More studies are needed to document the occurrence of postfebrile alopecia and clarify the role of fever and/or other associated factors in the development of hair loss.

Systemic Illness

A variety of systemic illnesses have been reported to be associated with diffuse hair loss. Alopecia associated specifically with telogen hair shedding is less adequately documented.

Kligman[1] evaluated 28 hospitalized patients with debilitating chronic illnesses including terminal carcinoma, ulcerative colitis, leukemia, tuberculosis, and malnutrition. Only 6 of the 28 patients had telogen counts above 25 percent, and only 2 of the 6 had obvious hair thinning. Biopsies on those two were normal except for an increased number of telogen follicles. Kligman noted that telogen counts in the patients correlated with morbidity, i.e., the less "sick" patients had normal telogen counts. Other case reports suggest that true telogen hair shedding may herald the onset of some systemic diseases and that indeed the patients may not be "sick" at the onset of the hair loss.

Syphilis may present as diffuse telogen hair shedding. Histologically an increase in telogen follicles, absence of organisms, and inflammation resembling alopecia areata may be seen. Hair regrowth and decreased telogen counts have occurred 4 to 6 weeks after onset of treatment in the reported cases.[96,97]

Lymphoproliferative disorders have also been associated with telogen hair shedding.[98] Alopecia has been reported as the presenting sign in a patient who subsequently developed Hodgkin's disease. In that case the trichogram revealed 85 percent telogen hairs, and the biopsy showed no evidence of a lymphomatous infiltrate.[99]

Inflammatory bowel disease has been associated with chronic hair loss. Generally malabsorption or wasting are also present, suggesting that malnutrition and not the primary disease is responsible for the hair loss.[1,100] Diffuse hair loss as the presenting sign of Crohn's disease has been reported, although no trichogram nor biopsy data were given to define the nature of the alopecia.[100]

Hepatic disease has been reported to be associated with diffuse alopecia. Zaun, Müting, and Steinmann[101] studied 53 patients who had either hepatitis, cirrhosis, or fatty liver. They found increased telogen counts in 34 patients and evident hair loss in 11 of them. The liver is the major site of amino acid interconversion. It was suggested that disturbed liver metabolism of cystine and methionine may have been related to the hair loss.

Systemic amyloidosis has been reported to be associated with diffuse hair loss and/or loss of hair pigment.[102–104] In one patient sequential biopsies were performed to document the evolution of the loss. Perifollicular deposits of amyloid and increased telogen follicles were noted initially. Follow-up biopsy 7 months later showed persistent telogen structures (telogen germinal units); no telogen follicles and only sparse anagen follicles were observed. The authors concluded that the findings indicated a failure of anagen restoration.[104]

Eosinophilia-myalgia syndrome has been associated with hair loss in up to 18 percent of patients. Hair loss may have been the result of telogen effluvium in at least some of the cases.[105]

Surgery

Diffuse hair loss temporally consistent with postoperative telogen effluvium has been described.[106,107] The cause of hair loss in these instances is probably multifactorial and has not been well-studied to date. Postoperative localized pressure alopecia probably caused by pressure-induced ischemia may occur as well.[108]

PSYCHOLOGICAL STRESS AND ALOPECIA

Psychological stress is widely thought to be a common cause of hair loss. It must be remembered that hair loss itself is very stressful to the large percentage of persons who experience it. Determining which comes first, stress or hair loss, can often be difficult if not impossible. Personal observation (V. C. Fiedler, unpublished data) suggests that psychogenic alopecia does occur but only in a small minority of persons complaining of hair loss. Eckert[109] studied 32 women complaining of diffuse hair loss. Seven of the 32 women did have evidence of psychiatric disturbance, but they did not have evidence of greater daily hair loss or telogen counts than did those women with alopecia and no psychiatric disturbance. The literature does support the notion of psychogenic telogen effluvium,[1,110] but the paucity of reports suggests that it is uncommon.

DRUGS AND ALOPECIA

A large number of drugs have been reported to cause diffuse alopecia;[111] the incidence of hair loss is generally not well-documented. A cause-effect relationship is also not well-documented in many instances. To confirm an etiologic relationship, (1) one must see the hair loss resolve after stopping the medication and reappear after rechallenge, and (2) the patient must not have an active systemic illness for which the medication is prescribed that in itself could cause hair loss.

Drugs reported to cause or possibly cause telogen hair loss are listed in Table 10-1. Prognosis for hair regrowth is generally good after the drug is stopped unless the patient has associated androgenetic alopecia.

Allopurinol was reported in one case to be associated with telogen hair shedding 2 months after a 2-week course of Zyloprim.[112] The mechanism of hair loss is unknown. Allopurinol inhibits the action of xanthine oxidase, but it is not cytotoxic.[113]

Androgens and derivatives such as danazol given systemically will exacerbate androgenetic alopecia.[111]

Angiotensin-converting enzyme inhibitors which are useful in the treatment of hypertension include captopril and enalapril. Both of these drugs have been implicated as causes of diffuse hair loss which is temporally consistent with telogen effluvium.[114,115] Captopril contains a thiol group which may be a metal chelator. It complexes zinc, which may be one mechanism for hair loss with this agent. Zinc supplementation has reversed alopecia and returned serum zinc levels to normal despite continued captopril treatment.[116] Captopril-associated hair loss may also occur with normal zinc levels.[114] Enalapril has no thiol group, but it also is associated with alopecia.[115]

Table 10-1
DRUGS AND CHEMICALS REPORTED TO CAUSE OR POSSIBLY CAUSE TELOGEN HAIR LOSS

Allopurinol
Androgens (danazol)
Angiotensin-converting enzyme inhibitors (captopril, enalapril)
Anticholesterolemic drugs (clofibrate, triparanol)
Anticoagulants (coumarin, dextran, heparin, heparinoids)
Antimitotic agents (colchicine, methotrexate)
Antithyroid medications (carbimazole, methylthiouracil, propylthiouracil)
Benzimidazoles (albendazole, mebendazole)
Beta blockers (systemic: metoprolol, propranolol; topical ophthalmic: betaxalol, levobunolol, timolol)
Bromocriptine
Cimetidine
Gold
Immunoglobulin
Interferon (alpha, gamma)
Levodopa
Methysergide
Minoxidil
Oral contraceptives
Proguanil
Psychotropic medications (amphetamines, desipramine, dixyrazine, fluoxetine, imipramine, lithium, tranylcypromine, valproic acid)
Pyridostigmine bromide
Retinoids
Sulfasalazine
Terfenadine
Vitamin A

Anticholesterolemic drugs such as clofibrate and triparanol have been reported to cause dry skin, brittle hair, and alopecia.[111] Triparanol-associated alopecia was reported to occur in 5 of 19 treated patients;[117] this drug has subsequently been taken off the market. Cholesterol is utilized as a structural substance in cell membranes. These drugs reduce cholesterol biosynthesis and presumably may disrupt the normal process of keratinization.[118]

Anticoagulants of all kinds commonly produce telogen hair shedding.[111] The reported incidence of alopecia has varied from 4 to 100 percent.[119] Kligman[1] reported on the clinical and histological evaluation of telogen effluvium produced by the heparinoid Paritol C, documenting the sequence of follicular events resulting in hair shedding. Glycosaminoglycans such as heparin are thought to affect epithelial-mesenchymal interactions in general and probably play a role in follicular growth regulation in particular. Paus[120] studied the effects of intraperitoneal heparin administration on in vivo anagen induction in mice. He found that it inhibited the development of anagen follicles in a dose-dependent manner. In vitro heparin added to mouse skin (early anagen) organ culture showed dose-dependent inhibitory effects on dermal ^{3}H-thymidine incorporation, reflecting decreased hair bulb keratinocyte proliferation. Heparin added in vitro inhibited mouse epithelial (PAM) cell and dermal papilla cell proliferation. Much remains to be learned about the interesting phenomenon of anticoagulant-induced alopecia; useful information about hair biology will probably emerge from such studies.

Antimitotic agents given in high doses usually induce anagen hair loss; however, some follicles may later show a telogen effluvium.[111] Low-dose colchicine has been reported to cause alopecia associated with increased telogen counts. High doses may cause anagen effluvium.[121] Low-dose methotrexate has been reported to be associated with alopecia, affecting 1 to 27 percent of treated patients.[122–124] Telogen hair loss has not been documented, nor have other possible contributing factors, such as anemia or iron deficiency, been evaluated.

Antithyroid medications may cause hair loss by inducing a hypothyroid state.[8] They may also directly produce hair loss in euthyroid patients. Methylthiouracil, propylthiouracil, and carbimazole have all been reported to cause this effect.[125–127]

Benzimidazoles (albendazole and mebendazole) used to treat hydatid disease have been reported to cause telogen effluvium in approximately 50 percent of patients.[128,129]

Beta blockers [propranolol (Inderal) and metoprolol (Lopressor)] have been reported to cause telogen effluvium.[111,130,131] Hair loss is relatively common with these agents, but the true incidence is not well-documented. Topical ophthalmic beta blockers (timolol, betaxalol, and levobunolol) have all been reported to be associated with a diffuse, reversible alopecia.[132] The mechanism of hair loss is not known but may involve the reduction of cyclic adenosine monophosphate (cAMP), which is known to suppress epidermal mitosis.[133]

Bromocriptine is an ergot derivative which inhibits prolactin secretion. One report indicates that women, but not men, treated with this drug had increased hair shedding which was dose-dependent and stopped with interruption of treatment.[134]

Cimetidine has been reported to be associated with alopecia areata as well as diffuse scalp hair loss.[111,135,136] The significance of these associations needs further evaluation.

Gold therapy has been reported to be associated with partial or complete hair loss. Alopecia is stated to be rare and usually reversible following discontinuation of treatment.[137] The nature and incidence of gold-associated hair loss remains to be clarified.

Intravenous immunoglobulin treatment has very rarely been associated with presumed telogen hair shedding. Histology did not confirm an increase in telogen follicles. Immunopathology was not helpful. The alopecia resolved within 4 months.[138]

Interferon α or γ may cause diffuse scalp hair loss or exacerbation of androgenetic alopecia.[94,95] The incidence of effluvium with IFN α was reported as 23 percent.[95]

Levodopa has been associated with diffuse alopecia consistent with telogen effluvium in two patients being treated for Parkinson's disease.[139]

Methysergide has been reported to cause hair loss in at least one woman taking the medication for migraine prophylaxis.[140] The hair loss was reversed off therapy.

Minoxidil applied topically has been reported to be associated with increased telogen shedding.[141] Personal observation suggests that this is a relatively common phenomenon with either topical or oral administration of minoxidil to individuals with androgenetic alopecia. Increased telogen hair shedding occurs between 2 and 6 weeks after initiation of treatment and at at cyclic intervals during therapy. The early hair loss can probably be attributed to club hair shedding induced by anagen hair formation. The subsequent cyclic loss can probably be attributed to synchronization of follicular cycles. Experience shows that the hair shedding is rapidly followed by regrowth of hair if minoxidil treatment is continued (V. C. Fiedler, unpublished data).

Oral contraceptives have been previously discussed.

Proguanil-associated hair loss is controversial. Fleming[142] states he has never seen it in the thousands of patients he has treated. Hanson, Kuylen, and Bjakam[143] report alopecia in 10 of 2500 treated patients but do not document details except to correlate the severity of alopecia with the duration of therapy.

Among the psychotropic medications, amphetamines used for weight loss have been incriminated as a cause of hair loss temporally consistent with telogen effluvium.[144] Weight loss was a confounding factor in evaluating the causal connection between amphetamine drug usage and alopecia.[145] Antidepressants (imipramine [Tofranil], desipramine, and fluoxetine) may cause alopecia consistent with telogen effluvium.[133,146,147] Dixyrazine, a phenothiazine, has been associated with documented telogen hair loss as well as decreased pigmentation and brittleness of the hair. Ichthyosiform skin changes were also noted. All the changes resolved within 2 months after withdrawal of treatment in the four patients reported.[148]

Lithium has been reported to be associated with alopecia areata as well as diffuse scalp hair loss. Some form of alopecia has been reported in as many as 17 percent of patients treated with lithium.[133] Hair loss has been reported in children as well as adults.[149] Hair loss may subside even when the patient remains on drug but is generally reversible off drug.[150] Further studies to clarify the nature of the hair loss and the significance of the association are needed. Lithium-induced hypothyroidism must be ruled out in any patient who develops hair loss during treatment.[151] Lithium appears to act similarly to iodide; it prevents release of both hormonal and nonhormonal iodide from the thyroid gland.[152] Tranylcypromine (Parnate), a potent nonhydrazine monoamino oxidase inhibitor, was reported to cause hair loss consistent with telogen effluvium in 11 of 1000 treated patients. The hair regrew in all cases after many months off treatment.[153] Valproic acid is an anticonvulsant that has been found to be effective in the treatment of major affective and schizoaffective disorders. It has also been reported to produce a telogen effluvium, with hair loss reported in less than 1 percent of treated patients.[133,154,155]

Pyridostigmine bromide used to treat myasthenia gravis was reported in one case to cause telogen effluvium.[156]

Retinoids used systemically and chronic hypervitaminosis A are associated with varying degrees of telogen hair shedding.[111] In some cases the hair loss may be very dramatic. The smallest dose of vitamin A reported to produce symptoms was 50,000 U daily for 18 months.[157] Acitretin, etretinate, and isotretinoin have all been causally linked to alopecia. The incidence of acitretin-associated alopecia has been variously reported as 15 percent and 87.5 percent,[158,159] etretinate-associated alopecia as 4 to 76 percent,[160,161] and isotretinoin-associated alopecia as 8 to 10 percent.[160,162] Individuals with androgenetic alopecia may not have complete return of hair density to baseline levels following discontinuation of treatment (V. C. Fiedler, unpublished data). It is useful to forewarn such patients of that possibility prior to prescribing retinoid therapy. The mechanism for hair loss induction by these drugs is not known.

Sulfasalizine used to treat inflammatory bowel disease has rarely been reported to be associated with hair loss consistent with telogen effluvium. Rechallenge with the drug induced recurrent alopecia in some but not all patients. The underlying bowel disease may have played a role in the hair loss in some or all of the patients reported.[163–165]

Terfenadine (Seldane) has rarely been reported to be associated with presumed telogen hair loss. Since sales began in 1981, alopecia has been reported at a rate of 2/1 million patient-months of use.[166]

CONCLUDING REMARKS

In summary, diffuse telogen hair shedding may be associated with a variety of hormonal and nutritional factors, ingestion of various drugs, exposure to certain chemicals, systemic and local cutaneous disease, and rarely psychological stress. Prognosis for hair regrowth is generally good if the cause can be found and climinated and if the patient does not have associated androgenetic alopecia.

REFERENCES

1. Kligman AM: Pathologic dynamics of human hair loss. Arch Dermatol 83:175–198, 1961.
2. Van Scott EJ, Reinertson RP, Steinmuller R: The growing hair roots of the human scalp and morphologic changes therein following amethopterin therapy. J Invest Dermatol 29:197–204, 1957.
3. Barman JM, Astore I, Pecoraro V: The normal trichogram of the adult. J Invest Dermatol 44:233–236, 1965.
4. Maguire HC, Kligman AM: Hair plucking as a diagnostic tool. J Invest Dermatol 43:77–79, 1964.
5. Church RE: Hypothyroid hair loss. Br J Dermatol 77:661–662, 1965.
6. Saito R, Hori Y, Kuribayashi T: Alopecia in hypothyroidism. In Kobori T, Montagna W (eds): *Biology of Diseases of the Hair.* Tokyo, University of Tokyo Press, 1976, pp 279–285.
7. Watanakunakorn C, Hodges RE, Evans TC: Myxedema. Arch Intern Med 116:183–190, 1965.
8. Freinkel RK, Freinkel N: Hair growth and alopecia in hypothyroidism. Arch Dermatol 106:349–352, 1972.
9. Smith JG, Weinstein GD, Burr JM: Hair roots of the human scalp in thyroid disease. J Invest Dermatol 32:35–38, 1959.
10. Ebling FJ, Johnson E: The action of hormones on spontaneous hair growth cycles in the rat. J Endocrinol 29:193–201, 1964.
11. Comaish JS: The thyroid and hair growth. Semin Dermatol 4(1):4–8, 1985.
12. Schell H, Kiesewetter F, Seidel C, Hintzenstern JV: Cell cycle kinetics of human anagen scalp hair bulbs in thyroid disorders determined by DNA flow cytometry. Dermatologica 182:23–26, 1991.
13. Williams RH: Thyroid and adrenal interrelations with special reference to hypotrichosis axillaris in thyrotoxicosis. J Clin Endocrinol 7:52–57, 1947.
14. Famuyiwa OO, Bella AF: Thyrotoxicosis in Nigeria. Trop Geogr Med 42:248–254, 1990.
15. Pecoraro V, Barman JM, Astore I: The normal trichogram of pregnant women. Adv Biol Skin 9:203–210, 1967.
16. Lynfield YL: Effect of pregnancy on the human hair cycle. J Invest Dermatol 35:323–327, 1960.
17. Dawber RPR, Connor BL: Pregnancy, hair loss and the pill. Br Med J 4:234, 1971.

18. Skelton JB: Postpartum alopecia. Am J Obstet Gynecol 94:125–129, 1966.
19. Schiff BL, Pawtucket RI, Kern AB: Study of postpartum alopecia. Arch Dermatol 87:609–611, 1963.
20. Rook A: Endocrine influences on hair growth. Br Med J 1:609–614, 1965.
21. Hale PA, Ebling FJ: The effects of epilation and hormones on the activity of rat hair follicles. J Exp Zool 191:49–62, 1975.
22. Headington JT: Transverse microscopic anatomy of the human scalp. Arch Dermatol 120:449–456, 1984.
23. Abell E: Pathology of male pattern alopecia. Arch Dermatol 120:1607–1608, 1984.
24. Bergfeld WF: Etiology and diagnosis of androgenetic alopecia. Clin Dermatol 6(4):102–107, 1988.
25. Rassner B, Zaun H, Braun-Falco O: Zum Pathomechanismus der Männlichen Glatzenbildung. Arch Klin Exp Dermatol 216:307–318, 1963.
26. Vogelsburg H, Klarner W, Rupec M: Einige Beobachtungen zur Frage der Androgenetischen Alopezie der Frau. Z Hautkr 55(3):125–132, 1980.
27. Futterweit W, Dunaif A, Yeh H-C, Kingsley P: The prevalence of hyperandrogenism in 109 consecutive female patients with diffuse alopecia. J Am Acad Dermatol 19:831–836, 1988.
28. Rushton DH et al.: Biochemical and trichological characterization of diffuse alopecia in women. Br J Dermatol 123:187–197, 1990.
29. Stein IF, Leventhal MC: Amenorrhea associated with bilateral polycystic ovaries. Am J Obstet Gynecol 29:181–191, 1935.
30. Polson DW, Adams J, Wadsworth J, Franks S: Polycystic ovaries: A common finding in normal women. Lancet 1:870–872, 1988.
31. Conway GS, Honour JW, Jacobs HS: Heterogeneity of polycystic ovary syndrome—Clinical, endocrine and ultrasound features in 556 patients. Clin Endocrinol 30:459–470, 1989.
32. Coney P: Polycystic ovarian disease—Current concepts of pathophysiology and therapy. Fertil Steril 42:667–682, 1984.
33. Moltz L et al.: Ovarian and adrenal vein steroids in seven patients with androgen-secreting ovarian neoplasms—Selective catheterization findings. Fertil Steril 42:585–593, 1984.
34. Dewailly D et al.: Clinical and biological phenotypes in late-onset 21-hydroxylase deficiency. J Clin Endocrinol Metab 63:418–423, 1986.
35. Soffer LJ, Iannaccone A, Gabrilone L: Cushing's syndrome—A study of fifty patients. Am J Med 30:129–146, 1961.
36. Simpson NB, Borth JH: Hair patterns—Hirsuties and baldness. In Rook A, Dawber R (eds): *Diseases of the Hair and Scalp.* London, Blackwell Scientific Publications, 1991, p 96.
37. Carter JN et al.: Adrenocortical function in hyperprolactinemic women. J Clin Endocrinol Metab 45: 973–980, 1977.
38. Vermuelen A, Suy E, Rubens R: Effect of prolactin in plasma DHEA(S) levels. J Clin Endocrinol Metab 44: 1222–1225, 1977.
39. Lavic MV: Galactorrhea and amenorrhea with polycystic ovaries. Am J Obstet Gynecol 104:814–817, 1969.
40. Fazekas AG, Sandor T: Metabolism of androgens by isolated human hair follicles. J Steroid Biochem 3:485–491, 1972.
41. Miller JA et al.: Low sex-hormone binding globulin levels in young women with diffuse hair loss. Br J Dermatol 106:331–336, 1982.
42. Kligman AM: The comparative histopathology of male-pattern baldness and senescent baldness. Clin Dermatol 6(4):108–118, 1988.
43. Pinkus H: Alopecia—Clinopathologic correlations. Int J Dermatol 19:245–253, 1980.
44. Cormia FE: Alopecia from oral contraceptives. JAMA 201:635–637, 1967.
45. Zaun H, Gerber T: Die Wirkung Monophasischer Ovulationshemmer auf das Wachstum der Kopfhaare. Arch Klin Exp Dermatol 234:353–361, 1969.
46. Zaun H, Ruffing H: Untersuchungen über den Einfluβ Antikonzeptiver Zweiphasen-Hormonpräparate auf das Wachstum der Kopfhaare. Arch Klin Exp Dermatol 238:197–206, 1970.
47. Tronnier H: Dermatologische Nebenwirkungen von Ovulationshemmern. Arch Klin Exp Dermatol 237: 197–200, 1970.
48. Griffiths WAD: Diffuse hair loss and oral contraceptives. Br J Dermatol 88:31–36, 1973.
49. Goette DK, Odom RB: Profuse hair loss. Arch Dermatol 111:930, 1975.
50. Krusinski PA: Telogen effluvium secondary to weight loss and therapy with chorionic gonadotropin. Arch Dermatol 112:556, 1976.
51. Kaufman JP: Telogen effluvium secondary to starvation diet. Arch Dermatol 112:731, 1976.
52. Goette DK, Odom RB: Alopecia in crash dieters. JAMA 235:2622–2623, 1976.
53. Blackburn GL, Bistrian BR, Hoag C. Hair loss with rapid weight loss. JAMA 236:252, 1976.
54. Rooth G, Carlström S: Therapeutic fasting. Acta Med Scand 187:455–463, 1970.
55. Lok E et al.: Calorie restriction and cellular proliferation in various tissues of the female Swiss Webster mouse. Cancer Lett 51:67–73, 1990.
56. Cavallo E et al.: Resting metabolic rate, body composition and thyroid hormones. Horm Metab Res 22: 632–635, 1990.
57. Hendrikx A, Heyns W, Moor PD: Influence of a low-calorie diet and fasting on the metabolism of dehydroepiandrosterone sulfate. J Clin Endocrinol 28: 1525–1533, 1968.
58. Johnson AA, Latham MC, Roe DA: An evaluation of the use of changes in hair root morphology in the assessment of protein-calorie malnutrition. Am J Clin Nutr 29:502–511, 1976.
59. Van Scott EJ, Ekel TM, Auerbach R: Determinants of rate and kinetics of cell division in scalp hair. J Invest Dermatol 41:269–273, 1963.
60. Jordan VE: Protein status of the elderly as measured by dietary intake, hair tissue and serum albumin. Am J Clin Nutr 29:522–528, 1976.
61. Bradfield RB: Protein deprivation—Comparative response of hair roots, serum protein, and urinary nitrogen. Am J Clin Nutr 24:405–410, 1971.
62. Bradfield RB, Cordano A, Graham GG: Hair root adaptation to marasmus in Andean Indian children. Lancet 2:1395–1397, 1969.
63. Caldwell MD, Jonsson HT, Othersen HB: Essential fatty acid deficiency in an infant receiving prolonged parenteral alimentation. J Pediatr 81:894–898, 1972.
64. Riella MC, Broviac JW, Wells M, Scribner BH: Essential fatty acid deficiency in human adults during total parenteral nutrition. Ann Intern Med 83:786–789, 1975.
65. Skolnik P, Eaglstein WH, Ziboh VA: Human essential fatty acid deficiency. Arch Dermatol 113:939–941, 1977.
66. Sinclair HM: Essential fatty acids and the skin. Br Med Bull 14:258–262, 1958.
67. Hård S: Non-anemic iron deficiency as an etiologic factor in diffuse loss of hair of the scalp in women. Acta Derm Venereol 43:562–569, 1963.

68. Rushton DH, Ramsay ID: The importance of adequate serum ferritin levels during oral cyproterone acetate and ethinyl oestradiol treatment on diffuse androgen-dependent alopecia in women. Clin Endocrinol 36: 421–427, 1992.
69. Thelander L, Reichard P: Reduction of ribonucleotides. Annu Rev Biochem 48:133–158, 1979.
70. Laskey J, Webb I, Schulman HM, Ponka P: Evidence that transferrin supports cell proliferation by supplying iron for DNA synthesis. Exp Cell Res 176:87–95, 1988.
71. Wouwe JPV: Clinical and laboratory diagnosis of acrodermatitis enteropathica. Eur J Pediatr 149:2–8, 1989.
72. Graves K, Kestenbaum T, Kalivas J: Hereditary acrodermatitis enteropathica in an adult. Arch Dermatol 116:562–564, 1980.
73. Mack D et al.: Acrodermatitis enteropathica with normal serum zinc levels—Diagnostic value of small bowel biopsy and essential fatty acid determination. Gut 30:1426–1429, 1989.
74. Kay RG, Tasman-Jones C: Acute zinc deficiency in man during intravenous alimentation. Aust NZ J Surg 45:325–330, 1975.
75. Tucker SB, Schroeter AL, Brown PW, McCall JT: Acquired zinc deficiency. JAMA 235:2399–2402, 1976.
76. Weismann K et al.: Acquired zinc deficiency dermatosis in man. Arch Dermatol 114:1509–1511, 1978.
77. Dupré A, Bonafé JL, Carriere JP: The hair in acrodermatitis enteropathica—A disease indicator? Acta Derm Venereol 59:177–178, 1979.
78. Gravel RA, Robinson BH: Biotin-dependent carboxylase deficiencies (propionyl CoA and pyruvate carboxylases). Ann NY Acad Sci 447:225–234, 1985.
79. Leonard JV et al.: Inherited disorders of 3-methylcrotonyl CoA carboxylation. Arch Dis Child 56:53–59, 1981.
80. Blom W, Muinck Keizer SMPF, Scholte HR: Acetyl CoA carboxylase deficiency—An inborn error of de novo fatty acid synthesis. N Engl J Med 305:465–466, 1981.
81. Tang TT et al.: Pathogenesis of Leigh's encephalomyelopathy. J Pediatr 81:189–190, 1972.
82. Burri BJ, Sweetman L, Nyhan WL: Mutant holocarboxylase synthetase. J Clin Invest 68:1491–1495, 1981.
83. Wolf B, Heard GS, McVoy JRS, Grier RE: Biotinidase deficiency. Ann NY Acad Sci 447:252–262, 1985.
84. Nyhan WL: Inborn errors of biotin metabolism. Arch Dermatol 123:1696–1698, 1987.
85. Wastell HJ, Bartlett K, Dale G, Shein A: Biotinidase deficiency: A survey of 10 cases. Arch Dis Child 63: 1244–1249, 1988.
86. Mock DM et al.: Biotin deficiency complicating parenteral alimentation—Diagnosis, metabolic repercussions, and treatment. J Pediatr 106(5):762–769, 1985.
87. Sydenstricker VP et al.: Observations on the "egg white injury" in man. JAMA 118:1199–1200, 1942.
88. Williams ML, Packman S, Cowan MJ: Alopecia and periorificial dermatitis in biotin-responsive multiple carboxylase deficiency. J Am Acad Dermatol 9:97–103, 1983.
89. Bernstein GM, Crollick JS, Hassett JM: Postfebrile telogen effluvium in critically ill patients. Crit Care Med 16(1):98–99, 1988.
90. Dinarello CA, Cannon JG, Wolff SM: New concepts on the pathogenesis of fever. Rev Infect Res 10(1):168–189, 1988.
91. Jimenez JJ, Wong GHW, Yunis AA: Interleukin 1 protects from cytosine arabinoside-induced alopecia in the rat model. FASEB J 5:2456–2458, 1991.
92. Yaar M, Karassik RL, Schnipper LE, Gilchrest BA: Effects of alpha and beta interferons on cultured human keratinocytes. J Invest Dermatol 85:70–74, 1985.
93. Tabibzadeh SS, Satyaswaroop PG, Rao PN: Antiproliferative effect of interferon-γ in human endometrial epithelial cells in vitro—Potential local growth modulatory role in endometrium. J Clin Endocrinol Metab 67: 131–138, 1988.
94. Brown TD et al.: A phase I clinical trial of recombinant DNA gamma interferon. J Clin Oncol 5:790–798, 1987.
95. Olsen EA et al.: Interferon alfa-2a in the treatment of cutaneous T cell lymphoma. J Am Acad Dermatol 20:395–407, 1989.
96. Kennedy C: Syphilis presenting as hair loss. Br Med J 2:854, 1976.
97. Lee JYY, Hsu ML: Alopecia syphilitica, a simulator of alopecia areata: Histopathology and differential diagnosis. J Cutan Pathol 18(2):87–92, 1991.
98. Savoie JM, Moschella SL: Cutaneous manifestations of malignant lymphoproliferative diseases. Cutis 5:49–56, 1969.
99. Klein AW, Rudolph RI, Leyden JJ: Telogen effluvium as a sign of Hodgkin disease. Arch Dermatol 108:702–703, 1973.
100. Schattner A, Shanon Y: Crohn's ileocolitis presenting as chronic diffuse hair loss. J R Soc Med 82:303–304, 1989.
101. Zaun H, Müting D, Steinmann I: Wachstumsstörungen der Kopfhaare als Folge von Hepatopathien. Arch Klin Exp Derm 235:386–393, 1969.
102. Wheeler GE, Barrows GH: Alopecia universalis—A manifestation of occult amyloidosis and multiple myeloma. Arch Dermatol 117:815–816, 1981.
103. Hsieh SD et al.: Amyloidosis presented with whitening and loss of hair which improved after dimethylsulfoxide (DMSO) treatment. Jpn J Med 26(3):393–395, 1987.
104. Hunt SJ, Caserio RJ, Abell E: Primary systemic amyloidosis causing diffuse alopecia by telogen arrest. Arch Dermatol 127:1067–1068, 1991.
105. Benedict LM, Abell E, Jegasothy B: Telogen effluvium associated with eosinophilia-myalgia syndrome. J Am Acad Dermatol 25:112, 1991.
106. Desai SP, Roaf ER: Telogen effluvium after anesthesia and surgery. Anesth Analg 63:83–84, 1984.
107. Thompson JS: Alopecia after ileal pouch-anal anastomosis. Dis Colon Rectum 32:457–459, 1989.
108. Wiles JC, Hansen RC: Postoperative (pressure) alopecia. J Am Acad Dermatol 12:195–198, 1985.
109. Eckert J: Diffuse hair loss and psychiatric disturbance. Acta Derm Venereol 55:147–149, 1975.
110. Dahlin PA, George J, Nérette JC: Telogen effluvium—Hair loss after spinal cord injury. Arch Phys Med Rehab 65:485–486, 1984.
111. Brodin MB: Drug related alopecia. Dermatol Clin 5(3):571–579, 1987.
112. Auerbach R, Orentreich N: Alopecia and ichthyosis secondary to allopurinol. Arch Dermatol 98:104, 1968.
113. Lovatt GE: Allopurinol and drug induced alopecia. Br J Dermatol 91:115, 1974.
114. Leaker B, Whitworth JA: Alopecia associated with captopril treatment. Aust NZ J Med 14:866, 1984.
115. Ahmad S: Enalapril and reversible alopecia. Arch Intern Med 151:404, 1991.
116. Smit AJ, Hoorntje SJ, Donker AJM: Zinc deficiency during captopril treatment. Nephron 34:196–197, 1983.
117. Winkelmann RK, Perry HO, Achor RWP, Kirby TJ: Cutaneous syndromes produced as side effects of triparanol therapy. Arch Dermatol 87:140–146, 1963.
118. Flesch P: Inhibition of keratinizing structures by systemic drugs. Pharmacol Rev 15:653–671, 1963.
119. Miki Y: Alopecia from heparin. Med J Osaka Univ 11:315–323, 1960.
120. Paus R: Hair growth inhibition by heparin in mice: A model system for studying the modulation of epithelial cell growth by glycosaminoglycans. Br J Dermatol 124:415–422, 1991.

121. Malkinson FD, Lynfield YL: Colchicine alopecia. J Invest Dermatol 33:371–384, 1959.
122. Weinblatt ME: Toxicity of low dose methotrexate in rheumatoid arthritis. J Rheumatol 12 (suppl 12):35–39, 1985.
123. Weinblatt ME et al.: Long-term prospective trial of low-dose methotrexate in rheumatoid arthritis. Arthritis Rheum 31:167–175, 1988.
124. Scully CJ, Anderson CJ, Cannon GW: Long-term methotrexate therapy for rheumatoid arthritis. Semin Arthritis Rheum 20:317–331, 1991.
125. Levy LK: Loss of hair following use of propylthiouracil. JAMA 143:860, 1950.
126. Wilburne M: Hair loss and pigmentation due to thiouracil derivatives. JAMA 147:379–380, 1951.
127. Papadopoulos S, Harden RM: Hair loss in patients treated with carbimazole. Br Med J 2:1502–1503, 1966.
128. Steiger U, Cotting J, Reichen J: Albendazole treatment of echinococcosis in humans—Effects on microsomal metabolism and drug tolerance. Clin Pharmacol Ther 47:347–353, 1990.
129. Garcia-Muret MP, Sitjas D, Tuneu L, de Moragas JM: Telogen effluvium associated with albendazole therapy. Int J Dermatol 29:669–670, 1990.
130. Martin CM, Southwick EG, Maibach HI: Propranolol induced alopecia. Am Heart J 86(2):236–237, 1973.
131. Graeber CW, Lapkin RA: Metoprolol and alopecia. Cutis 28:633–634, 1981.
132. Fraunfelder FT, Meyer SM, Menacker SJ: Alopecia possibly secondary to topical ophthalmic β-blockers. JAMA 263(11):1493–1494, 1990.
133. Warnock JK: Psychotropic medication and drug-related alopecia. Psychosomatics 32:149–152, 1991.
134. Blum I, Leiba S: Increased hair loss as a side effect of bromocriptine treatment. N Engl J Med 303:1418, 1980.
135. Tullio CJ, Roberts MA: Cimetidine-induced alopecia. Clin Pharmacol 4:145, 1985.
136. Ahmad S: Cimetidine and alopecia. Ann Intern Med 91:930, 1979.
137. Rosenbaum EE, Rosenbaum RB: Chrysotherapy. Arch Intern Med 139:1316, 1979.
138. Chan-Lam D, Fitzsimons EJ, Douglas WS: Alopecia after immunoglobulin infusion. Lancet 1:1436, 1987.
139. Marshall A, Williams MJ: Alopecia and levodopa. Br Med J 2:47, 1971.
140. Sadjadpour K: Methysergide alopecia. JAMA 229:639, 1974.
141. Bardelli A, Rebora A: Telogen effluvium and minoxidil. J Am Acad Dermatol 21:572–573, 1989.
142. Fleming AF:Proguanil. Lancet 1:439, 1989.
143. Hanson SN, Kuylen K, Bjakam AB: Hair loss and scaling with proguanil. Lancet 1:225, 1989.
144. Eckert J, Church RE, Ebling FJ, Munro DS: Hair loss in women. Br J Dermatol 79:543–548, 1967.
145. Fiedler VC: Amphetamines and hair loss. JAMA 260(2): 184, 1988.
146. Jenike MA: Severe hair loss associated with fluoxetine use. Am J Psychiatry 148(3):392, 1991.
147. Ananth J, Elmishaugh A: Hair loss associated with fluoxetine treatment. Can J Psychol 36:621, 1991.
148. Poulsen J: Hair loss, depigmentation of hair, ichthyosis, and blepharoconjunctivitis produced by dixyrazine. Acta Derm Venereol 61:85–88, 1981.
149. Wagner KD, Teicher MH: Lithium and hair loss in childhood. Psychosomatics 32:355–356, 1991.
150. Brodin MB: Drug-related alopecia. Dermatol Clin 5(3):571–579, 1987.
151. Mortimer PS, Dawber RPR: Hair loss and lithium. Int J Dermatol 23:603–604, 1984.
152. Connors JM: Thyroid and antithyroid drugs. In Craig CR, Stitzel RE (eds): *Modern Pharmacology.* Boston: Little, Brown and Company, 1990, p 922.
153. Lesse S: Tranylcypromine (Parnate): A study of 1000 patients with severe agitated depressions. Am J Psychother 32:220–242, 1978.
154. Lewis JR: Valproic acid (Depakene). JAMA 240: 2190–2192, 1978.
155. Zaccara G et al.: Long-term treatment with sodium valproate: Monitoring of venous ammonia concentrations and adverse effects. Ther Drug Monitor 9:34–40, 1987.
156. Field LM: Toxic alopecia caused by pyridostigmine bromide. Arch Dermatol 116:1103, 1980
157. Stimson WH: Vitamin A intoxication in adults—Report of a case with a summary of the literature. N Engl J Med 265:369–373, 1961.
158. Lauharanta J, Kanerva L, Turjanmaa K, Geiger JM: Clinical and ultrastructural effects of acitretin in Darier's disease. Acta Derm Venereol (Stockh) 68:492–498, 1988.
159. Madhok R, Muller SA, Dicken CH: Treatment of psoriasis with etretin: A preliminary report. Mayo Clin Proc 62:1084–1089, 1987.
160. Windhorst DB, Nigra T: General clinical toxicology of oral retinoids. J Am Acad Dermatol 6:675–678, 1982.
161. Grekin RC, Ellis CN, Voorhees JJ: Retinoids in the treatment of psoriasis—Monotherapy and combinations. Dermatol Clin 2(3):439–451, 1984.
162. Peck GL et al.: Prolonged remissions of cystic and conglobate acne with 13-cis retinoic acid. N Engl J Med 300(7):1028–1038, 1979.
163. Attar A, Anuras S: Sulfasalazine and hair loss. Gastroenterology 80:1102, 1981.
164. Fich A, Eliakim R: Does sulfasalazine induce alopecia? J Clin Gastroenterol 10:466–470, 1988.
165. Codeluppi PL et al.: A complication of SASP therapy: Hair loss. Dig Dis Sci 32:221–222, 1987.
166. Olsen EA: Seldane associated hair loss (reply to letter to editor). NC Med Soc J 53: 390, 1992.

Chapter

11

ANDROGENETIC ALOPECIA

Elise A. Olsen

INTRODUCTION

Androgenetic alopecia is considered pathological by some physicians and most affected subjects but a normal variant of aging by others.[1,2] Certainly it is a common problem, affecting approximately 50 percent of men,[3] and perhaps as many women, over the age of 40. There is a genetically determined predisposition to androgenetic alopecia, but expression is quite variable.[4] Although women and men have much different clinical presentations of androgenetic alopecia as well as potential systemic influences, the underlying cellular mechanisms are presumably the same.

The purpose of this chapter is to define androgenetic alopecia at the clinical and cellular level and to discuss current and potential treatments based on the potential etiologic mechanisms involved.

CLINICAL PRESENTATION

Men

In men who develop androgenetic alopecia, the hair loss may begin any time after puberty when serum androgen levels rise above the low level seen in normal young boys. The first change is usually a bitemporal recession, which is seen in 96 percent of sexually mature Caucasian males, including those men not destined to progress to further hair loss.[3] Bitemporal recession, therefore, may be under different control mechanisms than the patterned loss seen in the vertex and top of the scalp of affected men.[5] We owe much to Hamilton, who, in the 1950s, subclassified the patterns of baldness based on frontoparietal and frontal recession and vertex thinning (Fig. 11-1). Norwood, more than 25 years later, improved on this pictorial classification of androgenetic alopecia. He eliminated Hamilton's type III (a "waste-

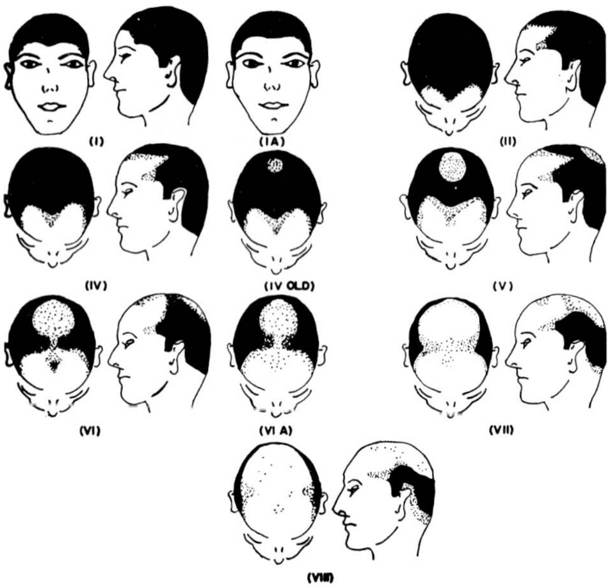

Figure 11-1 Hamilton's classification of male-pattern baldness. (*Reprinted with permission from Hamilton.*[3])

basket" for uncertain diagnoses) and type IV "old" and emphasized the progressive loss (1) in the "bridge" of hair over the midscalp in types IV through VI and (2) over the frontoparietal scalp that may occur independently of vertex loss[6] (Fig. 11-2).

Although the density of hair in a given pattern of loss tends to diminish with age, there is no way to predict what pattern of hair loss a young man with early androgenetic alopecia will eventually assume. In general, those who begin losing hair in the second decade are those in whom the alopecia will be the most progressive. In some men, initial male-pattern hair loss may be delayed until the late third to fourth decade.

There are racial as well as age-related differences in the incidence or pattern of hair loss in androgenetic alopecia. Sexually mature Oriental and Native American men are more likely to have preservation of the frontal hairline, later onset of baldness, and less extensive baldness.[3,7,8] African-American men may also have a lower incidence and extent of baldness[5,9] with decreased frequency of frontoparietal loss.[10]

Women

The literature is replete with alternative terms for androgenetic alopecia in women, including

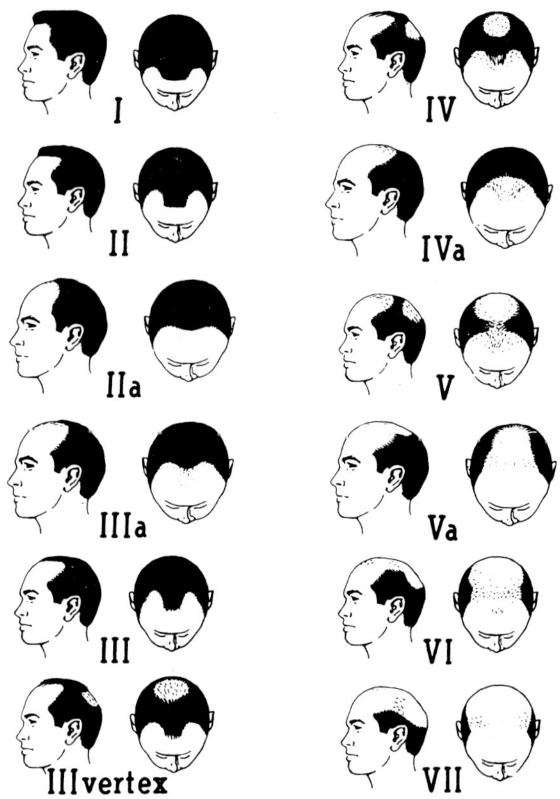

Figure 11-2 Norwood's classification of male-pattern baldness. (*Reprinted with permission from Olsen, et al: Topical minoxidil in early male pattern baldness. J AM Acad Dermatol* 13: 185–192, 1985.)

female-pattern alopecia, androgenic alopecia, common female baldness, and diffuse (hormonal) alopecia. The hair loss in women affected by androgenetic alopecia is much more likely to be first noticed in the late twenties through early forties compared to the late teens and twenties in men. It is particularly likely to be initiated at times of hormonal change, i.e., institution or discontinuation of oral contraceptive pills, the postpartum period, and the perimenopausal and early postmenopausal periods. Bitemporal recession occurs at sexual maturation in approximately 80 percent of females as well as most men but is generally much less prominent in women[3] (Fig. 11-3). Deep bitemporal recession in women, as in men, is more likely to be associated with the more obvious male phenotype of androgenetic alopecia.

In both sexes, the entire top of the scalp is the area at risk, but in women there is generally a diffuse decrease in density throughout the area vs. the vertex patterning seen in men. In approxi-

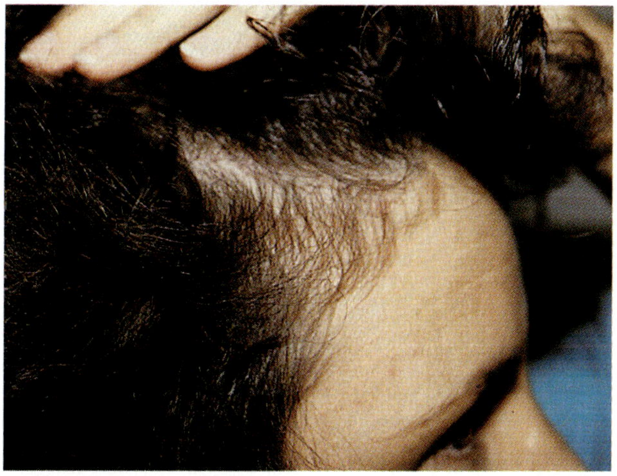

Figure 11-3 Bitemporal recession in a woman with androgenetic alopecia.

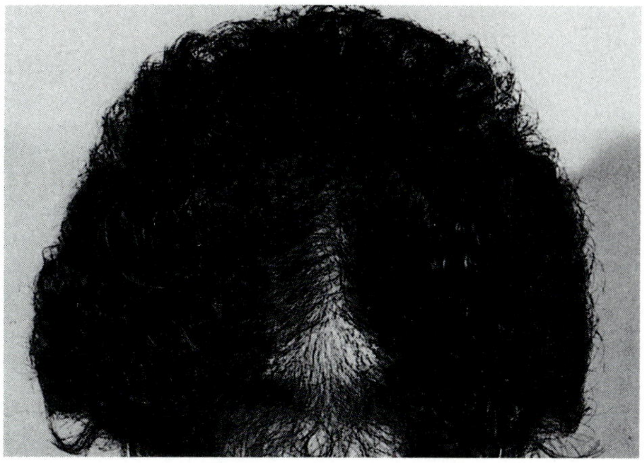

Figure 11-5 Prominent triangular diminution in hair density in frontal scalp in woman with androgenetic alopecia.

mately 5 percent of women with androgenetic alopecia, there is a global decrease in scalp hair density, although most prominent on top of the scalp (E. A. Olsen, unpublished data) (Fig. 11-4). In women with androgenetic alopecia, there may be a triangular diminution in hair density in the frontal scalp immediately behind a preserved frontal fringe (Fig. 11-5). This preservation of the frontal hairline is another phenotypic difference between androgenetic alopecia in women vs. men.

Ludwig arbitrarily divided female androgenetic alopecia into three subtypes based on hair density[11] (Figs. 11-6 through 11-10). Those with Ludwig pattern I make up the vast majority of affected women with androgenetic alopecia, but the hair loss may be discernable only by comparing the relative width of the part on the top of the scalp with that of the occipital scalp (Fig. 11-7*A* and *B*). Those women with Ludwig pattern III (Fig. 11-10) are rare and, like those premenopausal women who assume a male-type patterning with deep frontal recession, require an assessment for a potential hyperandrogen state.

Figure 11-4 Diffuse decrease in hair density in woman with androgenetic alopecia.

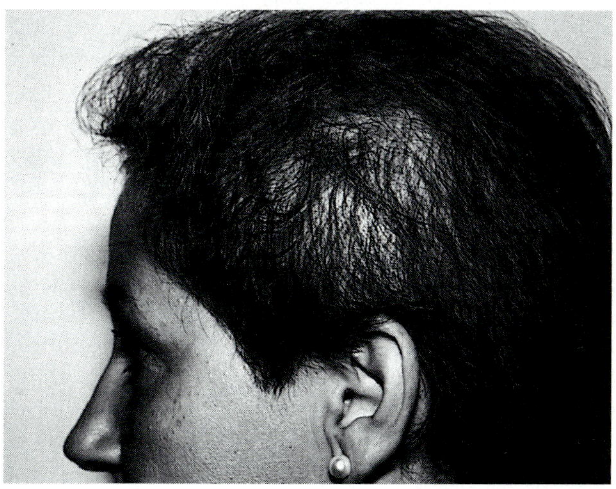

Sulzberger, Witten, and Kopf first noted some important associated clinical findings in women with "diffuse alopecia."[12] The hair, besides becoming finer and less dense, often is less manageable for the patient. Patients may also note increased oiliness and, often, symptoms of "tenderness, tingling, crawling, burning, itching, and uncomfortable awareness of the scalp."[12]

The incidence of androgenetic alopecia in women has been reported as 8 percent[13] to 25 percent,[14] but these studies may have excluded

Figure 11-6 Ludwig patterns of androgenetic alopecia in women. (*Reprinted with permission from Ludwig.*[11])

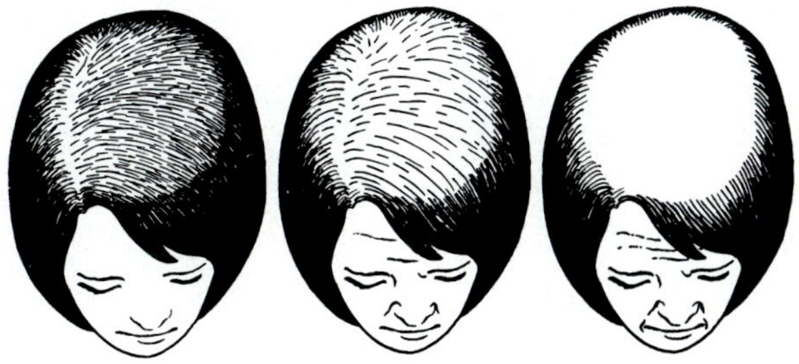

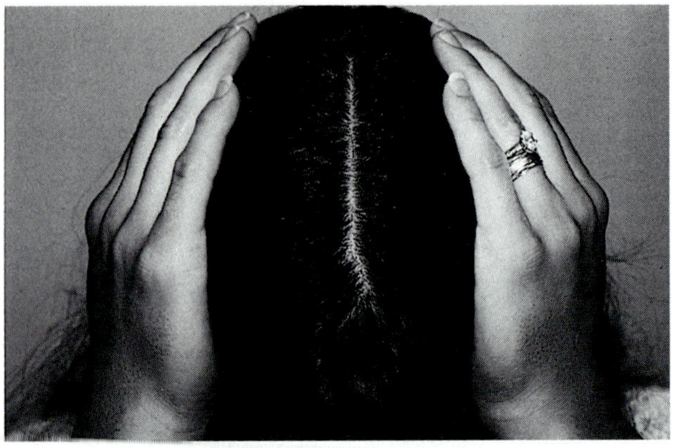

A

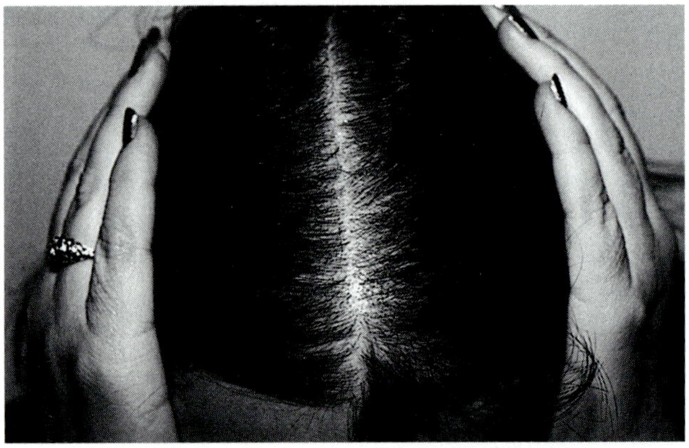

B

Figure 11-7 Comparison of scalp part width. (*A*) Normal scalp. (*B*) Ludwig pattern I androgenetic alopecia.

those women with mild degrees of hair thinning which are readily camouflaged. Venning and Dawber found that of 254 premenopausal women being seen in a dermatology clinic without hair loss as a complaint, 220, or 87 percent, had Ludwig pattern I–III hair loss and 34, or 13 percent, had Hamilton type II–IV alopecia.[15] Androgenetic alopecia appears to be as common in women as in men.

In women, a diminution in hair density becomes particularly notable at menopause and may include further bitemporal recession. In 310 postmenopausal women without a specific complaint of hair loss, 195 (63 percent) had Ludwig pattern I–III loss and 115 (37 percent) had Hamilton pattern II–V, i.e., frontal or frontoparietal, recession.[15] Whether this menopausal hair loss is related to androgenetic alopecia is as yet unclear. It would appear to be related to the hormonal changes seen with anovulation and inadequate physiological replacement of estrogen and/or progesterone. However, the adrenal gland independently undergoes androgen production changes in women in their fifties[16] and may play a role in this hair loss. How this all fits together remains to be determined.

Figure 11-8 Ludwig pattern I androgenetic alopecia.

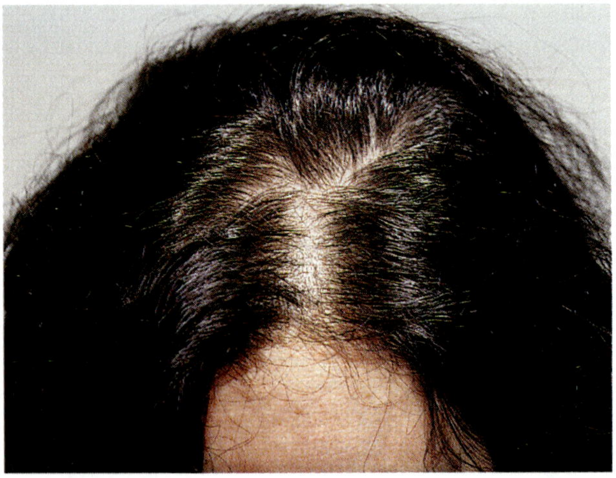

MORPHOLOGY

The hairs in androgenetic alopecia become progressively miniaturized with time, both the papilla and matrices, as well as the resulting hair shafts. In men with androgenetic alopecia, all the hairs in an affected area may eventually (but not necessarily) become involved in the process and may with time cover the region with fine vellus hair. Since the pigment production is also terminated with progressive miniaturization, the area may appear bald long before this vellus hair covering is finally lost. Involved areas in men *can* become devoid of hair over time.

Women, on the other hand, rarely become bald and, if they do, should be considered to have an underlying pathological hyperandrogen state. Instead, the process of miniaturization in women assumes more of a mosaic pattern in affected areas, with an exaggerated wide range in hair diameter in affected areas compared with normal.[17]

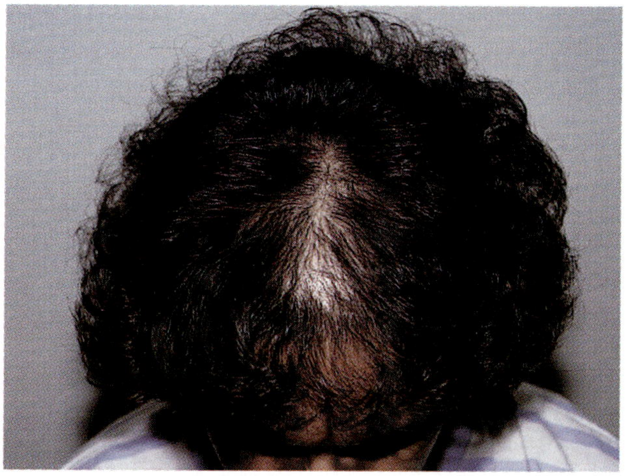
A

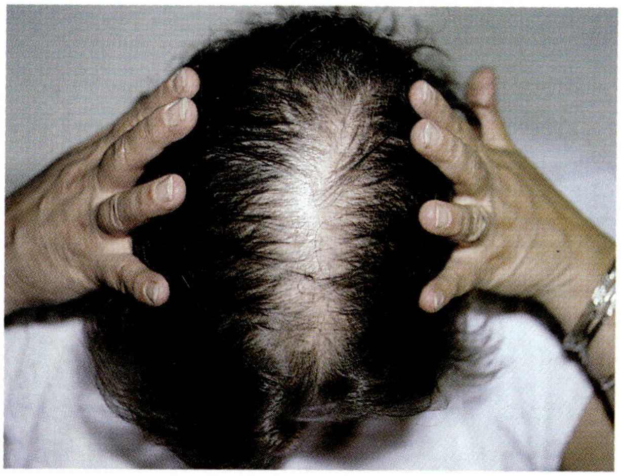
B

Figure 11-9 (*A,B*) Ludwig pattern II androgenetic alopecia.

Normal, thick terminal hairs are intermixed with finer, smaller-diameter hairs which may eventually become vellus hairs. The end result in women with androgenetic alopecia is a visual decrease in density of hair, rather than baldness, in the affected areas.

It should be remembered that this miniaturization is not unique to male-pattern baldness. In early fetal life, the forehead is covered with long lanugo hair like that on the scalp, but this hair begins to miniaturize and involute after the fifth month in utero. In children, vellus hairs are commonly found on the scalp, are rare in late puberty—possibly due to conversion to terminal hairs—and then reappear in the twenties. Both sexes have a progressive miniaturization and reduced terminal scalp hair density as a normal effect of aging. The density of terminal scalp hair is 615/cm^2 in the third decade and 485/cm^2 in the fourth decade.[18] Part of this may be due to the age-related increase in telogen hairs that is more pronounced in central areas.[2,19]

Figure 11-10 Ludwig pattern III androgenetic alopecia.

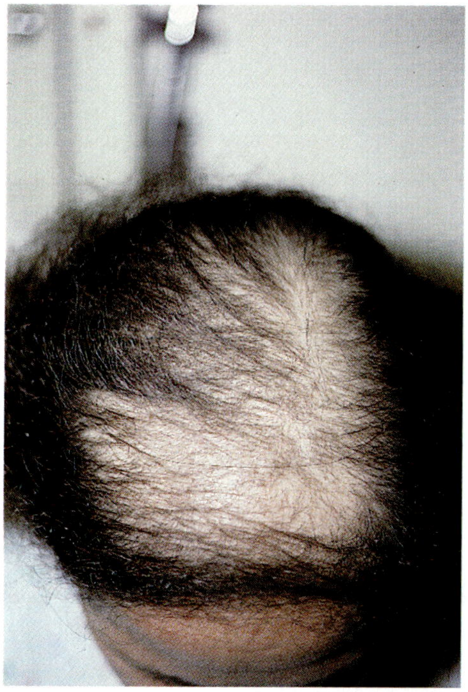

The cycle of scalp hairs is also affected by androgenetic alopecia. The percentage of hairs in anagen[20] and the duration of anagen diminish in affected areas of androgenetic alopecia, resulting in shorter hairs.[21] More hairs are in telogen for longer time periods,[1] and telogen hairs are much more subject to loss with daily trauma than anagen hairs: this affects the apparent density of the hair.

The blood flow in the scalp in early male-pattern baldness (Hamilton III vertex or IV), as measured by ^{133}Xe washout method, is diminished compared with that in controls.[22] Whether this is a primary phenomenon or is secondary to either the decreased skin temperature of balding vs. nonbalding scalp or to the relative percentage of hairs in anagen and telogen is unclear.

HISTOLOGY

The earliest, but relatively nonspecific, change in androgenetic alopecia appears to be a spotty perivascular degeneration of the lower one-third of the connective tissue sheath of affected anagen follicles.[23] This is recognized by a characteristic basophilic smudging in the otherwise pink and fibrillary connective tissue and by retention of elastic tissue stains in these foci. What then transpires is a progressive (over several cycles) miniaturization of affected terminal hair follicles, although not all follicles in a given area involute at the same rate.[24] Beneath the atrophic follicle lies a "streamer" representing the now-defunct portion of the associated connective tissue sheath. This pathological streamer, according to Maguire and Kligman, is pathognomonic for male-pattern baldness[23] (Fig. 11-11). There is an increased percentage of vellus hairs and of telogen hairs due to a shortened anagen cycle. The miniaturized follicles retain fragments of the arrector pili muscle in contradistinction to normal vellus hairs.[25] Maguire and Kligman noted no associated inflammation,[23] but Lattanand and Johnson noted a moderate chronic inflammatory infiltrate surrounding capillaries and adnexal structures in 50 percent of specimens from areas of balding.[26]

Figure 11-11 Scalp biopsy of patient with androgenetic alopecia. Two miniaturized hair follicles are seen in the dermis and a cross-section of a terminal hair is seen in the subcutaneous tissue. The arrow points to a "streamer" or involuted connective tissue sheath. (H&E, × 50). (*Photograph courtesy of Dr. David Whiting.*)

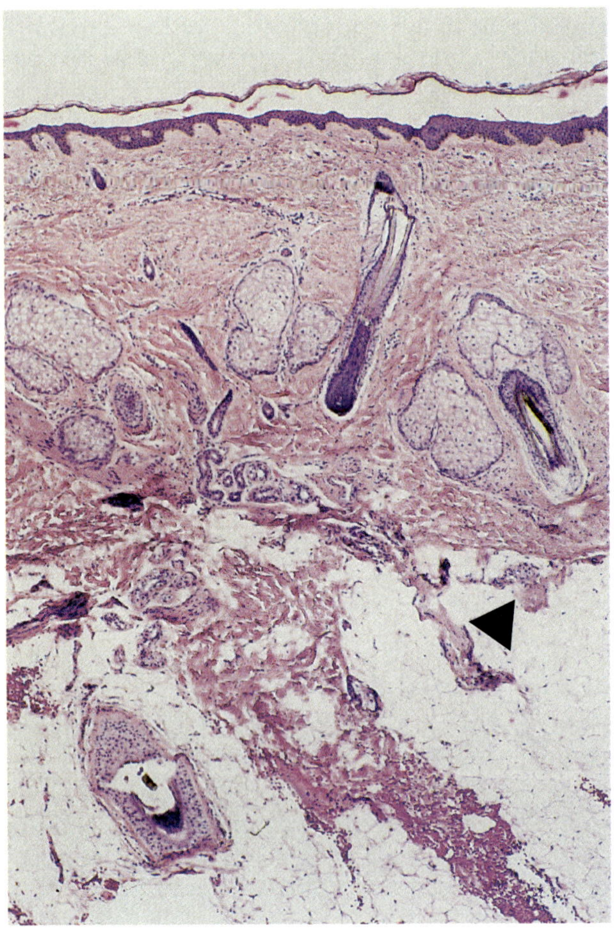

CONTROL

Inheritance

There has been much debate over the type of inheritance seen in androgenetic alopecia. Typically, it appears to be autosomal dominant, with a wide variation in penetrance and expression.[5] Inheritance may be polygenic in nature.[4] In women with androgenetic alopecia, a family history of male-pattern baldness is present in 54 percent of male and 23 percent of female first-degree relatives over 30 years of age.[5] Gene expression appears determined by follicle location, presumably imposed during embryonic differentiation.[27]

Local

The local vs. systemic control of hair growth in androgenetic alopecia was proved dramatically by the introduction of autografts in hair transplantation.[28] Punch grafts of hair removed from the occipital area of the scalp in men with male-pattern baldness and moved into recipient sites of androgenetic hair loss maintain the characteristics of the donor site after transplantation (donor dominance).

Androgens

PHENOTYPIC EXPRESSION OF ANDROGEN-DEPENDENT HAIR

Although Aristotle noted that eunuchs did not become bald,[29] it was not until 1942 that Hamilton, an anatomist, clearly proved the correlation between sexual immaturity and lack of patterned alopecia.[30] Hamilton studied 104 men with testicular insufficiency. In 20 of the subjects, the condition had developed before puberty, 34 of the subjects had been castrated during adolescence, and 50 of the subjects had been castrated after sexual maturation. Hamilton observed that in the men who had had testicular insufficiency since before puberty—and thus had failed to mature sexually—neither baldness nor hair recession at the temples or forehead had occurred. In the men who had been castrated during adolescence, little, if any, alopecia had developed. However, in the men castrated after puberty, variable loss of hair had occurred before castration, but none afterward. Hamilton further showed that androgens are necessary for the development of baldness: baldness was induced by administration of testosterone to sexually immature men and stopped on interruption of androgen therapy. No superphysiological dose of androgen was necessary to induce baldness. Androgens were the "incitants of common baldness" but the phenotypic expression of baldness was dependent on a genetic predisposition.[30]

More recent studies have shown that urinary androgen and plasma testosterone concentrations are similar in balding and nonbalding men[31] and that serum or plasma androgens do not correlate with the degree of male-pattern baldness.[31,32] Cipriani et al., however, noted elevation of the unbound, or active, fraction of testosterone,[33] and Pitts noted an increase in dehydroepiandrosterone (DHEA), a weak androgen,[34] in men with male-pattern baldness. Regardless, there is no relationship between male-pattern baldness and other androgen-related markers, including sebum excretion rate; body hair density; and bone, skin, or muscle thickness.[32]

Androgens variably affect different regions of hair growth. Androgens stimulate both the growth of hair (e.g., pubic, axillary, and beard and chest hair) and the loss of certain hair (scalp hair in genetically susceptible individuals). Different thresholds of androgens are necessary for the expression of certain patterns of hair growth and explain some of the differences in the secondary sex characteristics of men and women. Pubic, female escutcheon, and axillary hair is stimulated by female levels of androgens, but male escutcheon (i.e., upper pubic triangle), beard, ear hair, nasal tip hair, and coarse hair on the limbs and trunk require higher (male) levels of androgens.[27,35] Whether high levels of androgens in females genetically predisposed to androgenetic alopecia accelerate or accentuate the balding process is presumptive but speculative. Levels of androgen in men with male-pattern baldness do not correspond to the rapidity of hair loss.[30]

The phenotypic expression of syndromes affecting androgen action helps to define the various components of androgen control of hair growth. Males with complete testicular feminization are XY but lack functional androgen receptors: they have no scalp hair loss and no pubescent hair growth, not even a female escutcheon or axillary hair. Male patients with 5α-reductase deficiency have normal to increased testosterone but low dihydrotestosterone (DHT) at puberty. They develop a female escutcheon and axillary hair but no or sparse beard growth, bitemporal recession, or male-pattern baldness.[36] Whether the latter is reflective of the generic preponderance of audrogenetic alopecia in this population or secondary to local factors is unclear. Thus, not all androgen-sensitive hair growth is controlled by the same hormone: axillary and pubic hair are testosterone-dependent, whereas beard growth and male-pattern baldness are DHT-dependent. Clearly, male-pattern baldness is dependent on both functional androgen receptors and 5α-reductase (and its product, DHT) for full expression.

5α-REDUCTASE

5α-Reductase is the enzyme responsible for the metabolism of testosterone to DHT (Fig. 11-12). 5α-Reductase is not unique to androgen-sensitive tissue but is a ubiquitous property of skin fibroblasts and hair.[37,38] Studies using plucked hairs, which are generally devoid of dermal papillae and in which the major metabolite of testosterone is androstenedione,[27] have demonstrated an increased DHT production in balding vs. nonbalding scalps.[35] Studies using skin biopsies, which include the entire follicular unit, have also shown that the activity of 5α-reductase is higher in balding vs. nonbalding scalps.[39] Thus, regional differences in hair growth could be related to local differences in 5α-reductase.

The possibility of various forms of 5α-reductase or cofactors to explain these differences in 5α-reductase activity in different body areas was raised by Itami and coworkers.[37,38] They demonstrated that the Michaelis constant and optimum

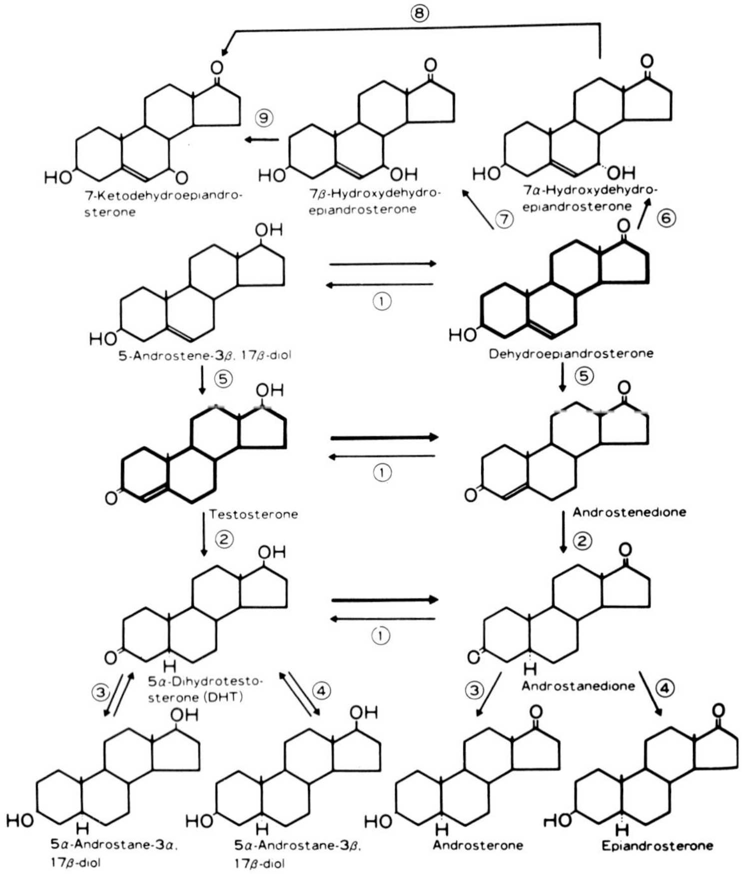

Figure 11-12 Metabolism of androgens in the skin. (1) 17β-hydroxysteroid dehydrogenase. (2) 5α-reductase. (3) 3α-hydroxysteroid dehydrogenase. (4) 3β-hydroxysteroid dehydrogenase. (5) $\Delta^{4,5}$-3β-hydroxysteroid dehydrogenase isomerase. (6) 7α-hydroxylase. (7) 7β-hydroxylase. (8) 7α-hydroxysteroid dehydrogenase. (9) 7β-hydroxysteroid dehydrogenase. (*Reprinted with permission from* Int J Dermatol *18:681–692, 1979.*)

pH activity of 5α-reductase in beard dermal papilla cells were similar to that of genital skin fibroblasts and that the 5α-reductase of both was located primarily in the crude nuclear fraction of the cells.[38] The 5α-reductase in occipital scalp dermal papillae cells, on the other hand, had a lower Michaelis constant; a broad and low-level pH activity of 6.5 to 9; and was more equally distributed in the nuclear, cytosolic, and microsomal fractions of the cells, much like that seen with the reticular dermal fibroblasts.[38]

Harris et al. subsequently confirmed at least two isoenzymes of 5α-reductase corresponding to the preceding that are distinguished by pH, Km for testosterone, and sensitivity to classes of 5α-reductase inhibitors.[40] Both isoenzymes were initially isolated in prostatic tissue and have been called 5α-reductase-1 and 5α-reductase-2. 5α-Reductase-1 has a broad pH optimum centered at pH 7, compared with a pH of 5.5 for 5α-reductase-2, and the Km for testosterone for 5α-reductase-1 is 25 times that of 5α-reductase-2. In the prostate, 5α-reductase-1 is present at only low levels in contrast to the abundance of 5α-reductase-2, but in the balding scalp of men with androgenetic alopecia, 5α-reductase-1 is the predominant isoenzyme.[40] It would appear, then, that 5α-reductase-1 may be necessary for the expression of male-pattern baldness. However, it has since been determined that those individuals demonstrating the phenotype of 5α-reductase deficiency with the typical lack of male-pattern baldness have a deficiency of only 5α-reductase-2.[40] Why these men, then, do not develop baldness is not clear: they may not demonstrate baldness because of racial or genetic infrequency of androgenetic alopecia rather than secondary to any 5α-reductase deficiency. Further delineation of the difference in 5α-reductase isoenzymes in balding vs. nonbalding scalp is necessary.

5α-Reductase is an NADPH-dependent enzyme and may, in certain locations, be regulated by androgens.[41] For example, the 5α-reductase of genital skin is androgen-independent, while the enzyme in pubic skin is androgen-dependent.[41] High levels of 5α-reductase are found in external genitalia at birth and throughout life in both sexes. However, pubic skin in prepubertal children of both sexes shows low levels of 5α-reductase, with a sharp rise in 5α-reductase evident at puberty in males as compared with females.[42] There is local positive feedback on 5α-reductase since DHT increases 5α-reductase activity in a dose-dependent fashion.[41,42]

INTERCONVERSION ANDROGENS

Although the level of DHT may be directly dependent on the activity of 5α-reductase, it is also obviously affected by both the supply of androgen precursors and the metabolism of DHT. Testosterone is the major precursor of DHT in men, but other weaker hormones such as DHEA are the major precursors of DHT in women. The skin is an active site of androgen metabolism where testosterone, androstenedione, and DHEA are metabolized extensively.[43] In both sexes, 17β-hydroxysteroid dehydrogenase (17β-HSD) assumes importance because of its conversion of 17-ketosteroids, which are weak androgens, to 17-hydroxysteroids, which are potent androgens. 17β-HSD also is responsible for the potential interconversion of both testosterone and DHT to less potent androgens (Fig. 11-12). Moreover, in plucked hair, the Vmax for the 17-oxidation pathway is four times that of 5α-reductase.[35] Hay and Hodgins demonstrated differences in the predominant direction of 17β-oxido-reduction in various androgen-sensitive tissues and hypothesized differences based on the relative tissue concentration of the oxidized and reduced coenzymes NAD and NADP.[44] Histochemically, 17β-HSD appears to be located primarily in the outer root sheath and bulb of hair follicles. The activity of 17β-HSD appears greater in anagen than in telogen but appears to diminish in the anagen follicle with progressive baldness.[42,45] Fazekas and Sandor showed that in plucked hairs from balding vs. nonbalding scalp there is diminished formation of 5-androstene-3β,17β-diol from DHEA secondary to decreased function of 17β-HSD and an increased formation of 4-androstene-3,17-dione[46] (Fig. 11-12).

3β-Hydroxysteroid dehydrogenase isomerase ($\Delta^{4,5}$ isomerase or 3β-HSD isomerase) is also important for the interversion of weak androgens to testosterone (Figs. 11-12 and 11-13). Sawaya, Honig, Garland, and Hsia have shown that there is increased activity of the cytosolic 3β-HSD isomerase in the sebaceous glands in balding vs. hairy scalp.[47] Whether the change in activity in sebaceous glands is equivalent to that of dermal papillae cells of balding scalp is undetermined.

Testosterone may bypass metabolism to DHT by being interconverted by the enzyme aromatase to estradiol. Sawaya, Price, and Harris have shown that aromatase is more abundant in the occipital vs. frontal scalp in women with androgenetic alopecia, and negligible in men.[48] This may help to explain the phenotypic differences of androgenetic alopecia in men and women.

The level of DHT is also affected by its metabolism to other weaker androgens. Almost all DHT is reduced in situ to 3α- and 3β-androstanediols by the NADH- and/or NADPH-dependent 3α- and 3β-ketoreductases (hydroxysteroid dehydrogenases)[49] (Fig. 11-12). These enzymes are present in both the cytosol and microsomes, and the relative predominance of one over the other appears to be cofactor-dependent. The reaction catalyzed by 3α-HSD is potentially reversible, whereas that of 3β-HSD is not, at least in pubic skin. Thus, local cofactors may again affect the cellular level of DHT. Schweikert and Wilson have shown that 5α-androstanediol formation is higher in balding frontal scalp vs. nonbalding scalp.[50] Clinically, urinary androstanediol is a far better measure of peripheral conversion of testosterone or androstenedione to DHT than is DHT itself.[51]

ANDROGEN RECEPTOR

Simplistically, androgens, like other steroids, diffuse across plasma membranes and combine with a cytosolic or nuclear receptor protein.[27,52] The androgen-receptor complex undergoes conformational changes in the nucleus, exposing sites that can interact with the relevant hormone response element in chromatin.[27] The steroid-binding domain of the androgen receptor is the carboxy-hydrophobic end of the androgen-receptor protein, and the DNA-binding domain is near the amino-terminal hydrophilic end.[53] The binding of the androgen-androgen receptor complex to DNA results in a change in DNA transcription and protein synthesis. Studies on preputial skin specimens of males of various ages show that although the total number of androgen receptor sites was fairly constant for all ages studied, the relative proportion of androgen receptor(s) in the cytosol vs. nucleus varied with age. Androgen receptors seemed to be predominantly

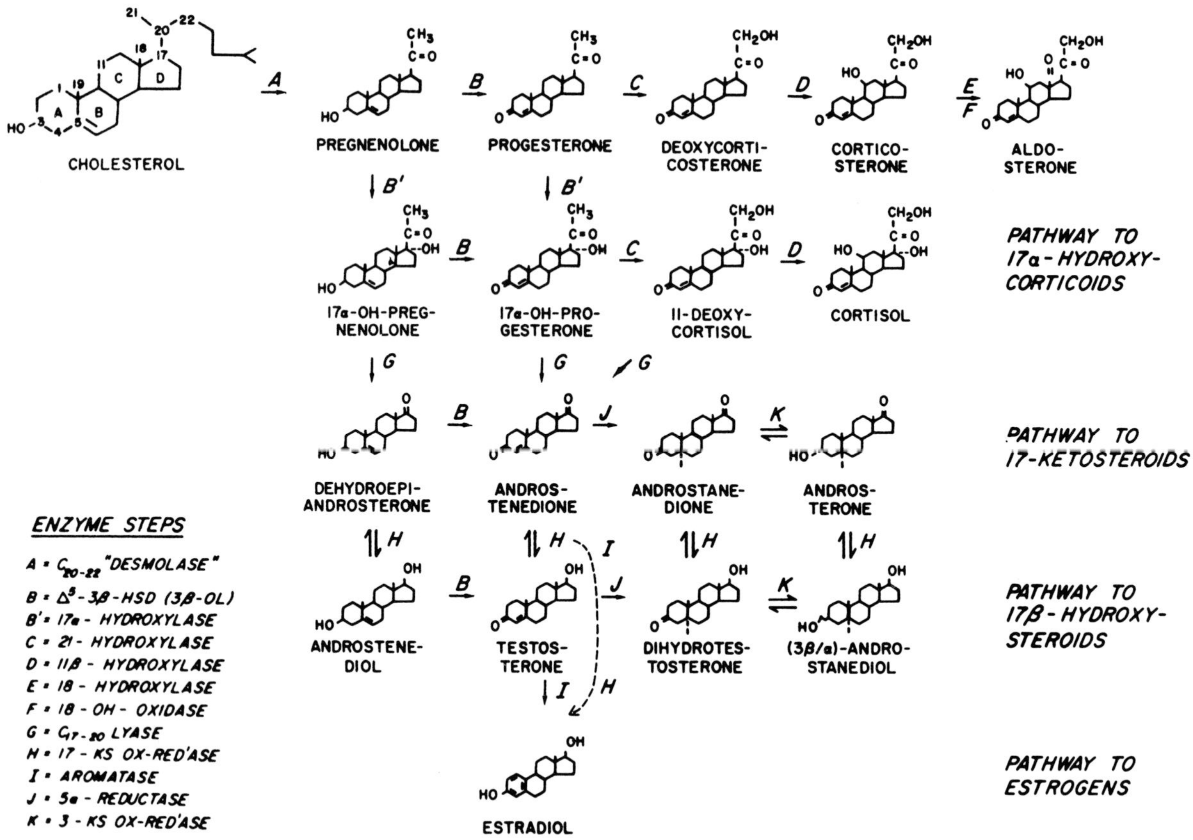

Figure 11-13 Steroid pathway. (*Reprinted with permission from Hatch, Rosenfield, Kim, and Treadway.*[69])

localized in the nuclear compartment at those developmental stages characterized by higher levels of circulating blood androgens.[41]

There appears to be one androgen receptor which binds the various steroid hormones in a rank order of affinity: DHT > testosterone > estrogen > progesterone.[27,53,54] The different effects of the bound steroid are potentially determined by the spatial effect on the hormone response element(s) in the chromatin or on regulatory transcription factors.[27] The DHT-androgen receptor complex has greater affinity for receptors in the nuclear chromatin than does the testosterone-androgen receptor complex.[55] The androgen receptor is not regulated by androgens, in contradistinction to 5α-reductase,[42] but has been reported in at least one study to be induced by estrogens.[56]

The androgen receptor is X-linked with the gene encoding the receptor near the centromere on the long arm of the X chromosome.[57] It spans at least 50 kb of genomic DNA and has eight coding exons. This gene gives rise to two principal species of androgen receptor mRNA that appear to encode the same protein.[57] The primary locations for the androgen receptor in hair appear to be the dermal papillae in both anagen and telogen hairs and the pilosebaceous duct keratinocytes.[37] The androgen receptor is absent in the bulge area and matrix.[58]

Randall, Thornton, and Messenger showed that the amount of specific high affinity, low-capacity androgen receptor is higher in cultured dermal papillae cells from androgen-dependent sites (e.g., beard, moustache) than in nonbalding scalp.[59] Sawaya, Honig, and Hsia reported a greater binding affinity and capacity for androgens in the cytosol androgen receptors isolated from the sebaceous glands of bald vs. hairy scalp.[60] Sawaya, Mendez, Lewis, and Hsia reported two forms of a cytosol androgen receptor: a monomer (67 Kd) and a tetramer (258 Kd).[61] The monomer androgen-binding affinity was higher and the monomer androgen receptor–androgen complex was preferentially incorporated in the nucleus vs. that of the tetramer. The monomer-tetramer ratio was noted to be higher in the hair follicles from bald vs. balding scalp. Further confirmation of the importance of these cytosolic androgen receptors and the differences in androgen binding in the various stages and areas of balding is necessary.

Although the target organ for DHT appears to be the dermal papilla,[27] androgens must affect epidermal tissue in order to maintain the constant size ratio between papilla and hair shaft.[27] Itami showed that the addition of testosterone to the culture of either outer root sheath cells or dermal papillae cells of beard hair follicles increased mitosis in either only slightly, whereas coculture of outer root sheath cells and dermal papillae cells increased DNA synthesis three times over either alone. Further addition of testosterone significantly increased DNA synthesis of the mixed cell culture.[38] They suggested that, although the primary target of the beard hair follicle responding to testosterone is the dermal papillae cells, the growth of these cells in turn stimulates, either directly or by diffusible factors, the secondary target, the epithelial cell.[38]

One potential control mechanism is through the second messenger, adenyl cyclase and cyclic adenosine monophosphate (cAMP).[62] Adachi and Kano demonstrated that DHT, but not testosterone, inhibits adenyl cyclase in plucked anagen hairs. Adenyl cyclase activity was strongly stimulated by estrone.[62] Estrone, by competition with DHT at adenyl cyclase sites, could then help regulate the effects of androgen on hair. Adachi et al. also showed that G6PD activity, which is stimulated by cAMP, increases during anagen.[63] This enzyme, which constitutes an important source of NADPH, is markedly inhibited by DHEA,[64] which, in turn, is dependent on 17β-HSD for metabolism. Fazekas and Sandor showed a marked decrease in the production of androstenediol from DHEA in the frontal scalp of balding men.[46] Metabolism of the weak androgen DHEA may thus play an important role in control of androgenetic alopecia.

ANDROGEN PRODUCTION IN WOMEN

Presumably, the peripheral mechanisms of androgen control of hair growth are the same in the two sexes. However, the type and proportion of the various androgens produced both centrally and peripherally are far different in the two sexes. In women, 50 to 60 percent of testosterone is produced by peripheral conversion of prehormones that are, in themselves, weak androgens.[65] Overall production of testosterone by the ovaries is far less than that of the testes, with the net result of a much lower plasma level of testosterone in women than in men. However, overproduction of androgens, either the potent 17-hydroxysteroids (androstenediol or testosterone) or the weaker 17-ketosteroids (DHEA or androstenedione) by the adrenal gland or ovary can lead to higher tissue levels of the active hair follicle androgen, DHT. The more potent androgens and estradiol are bound in the plasma to sex hormone–binding globulin (SHBG), although the binding affinities are quite different: DHT is three times that of testosterone and nine times that of estradiol.[66] The unbound or free testosterone appears to be the bioactive form. SHBG production is increased by estrogens and decreased by androgens, progestins, and glucocorticoids.[66] Thus, an increase in testosterone can lead to a decrease in SHBG and an increase in free testosterone, in addition to an increased activity of 5α-reductase.[67] Gonadal and adrenal overproduction of androgens in women, which can shift both the central and peripheral androgen levels to that approaching normal men, needs to be considered in women in whom potential clinical signs of androgen excess are present. These signs include androgenetic alopecia, acne, and hirsutism. Virilization is an absolute sign of androgen excess and should be considered separately.

Androgen excess has been evaluated most extensively in hirsutism: this is discussed in detail in Chapter 14. The ovary is the predominant source of androgen production in the majority of women with functional hyperandrogenism.[65,67,68] In the ovary, androgens are formed as obligate intermediates in the formation of estrogens and as metabolites of 17-hydroxyprogesterone secretion.[69] Androgens are produced predominantly by the theca and interstitial components of the ovary in response to luteinizing hormone (LH) and follicle-stimulating hormone (FSH).[69] There is a convoluted and multifactorial explanation for the ovarian overproduction of androgens which, in most cases, falls under the poorly defined condition of polycystic ovary syndrome (PCOS). In most women with ovarian hyperandrogenism, the pituitary is more sensitive to gonadotropin-releasing hormone (GnRH), and there is increased LH and decreased FSH secretion by the pituitary, which leads to increased androgen production and anovulation.[67] Deficiencies of two key enzymes for biosynthesis of estrogen may be present in PCOS: $\Delta^5$3β-HSD and aromatase.[66,69] The net result of this is the buildup of C_{19} androgens and the decreased production of estrogen by the ovaries.[69] Hyperinsulinemia may also contribute to ovarian hyperandrogenism by sensitizing the stroma to the stimulatory effects of LH.[67]

Androgen production in the adrenal gland is under a number of different controls. The adrenal cortex secretes androgens as by-products of cortisol biosynthesis, and thus androgen production is ACTH-dependent.[69] The unique population of cells which produce androgens (the zona reticularis) only comes to maturity at puberty.[69] Estrogens and possibly androgens alter the activity of the involved adrenal enzymes, and the pituitary hormone prolactin promotes adrenal androgenic function.[69]

Late-onset hirsutism related to overproduction of adrenal androgens has been well-documented for the hereditary deficiency of the following enzymes: 21-hydroxylase (21-OH), 11β-hydroxylase (11-OH), and $\Delta^5$3β-HSD.[69] Each of these genetic forms of congenital adrenal hyperplasia (CAH) presents most commonly in infancy and childhood along with other signs and symptoms. The most common enzyme deficiency is 21-OH, with an incidence of 1/14,000 (homozygotes)[70] and 1/35 to 1/50 incidence of carriers (heterozygotes) in the general population.[71] Female patients with any of these enzyme deficiencies may present with hirsutism, menstrual irregularities, and/or virilization[72] and presumably may have bitemporal recession of the hairline and, if genetically susceptible, an exaggerated androgenetic alopecia phenotype.

Since basal hormone levels may be normal in patients with mild defects in steroidogenesis[73] (presumably the scenario in late-onset CAH), ACTH stimulation tests are generally necessary for diagnosis. By examining the steroidogenesis pathway and ascertaining which hormones will be produced in overabundance because of a specific enzyme deficiency or block (Fig. 11-13), one can diagnose the specific problem. Baseline hormone levels are determined in the early morning before synthetic ACTH (Cortrosyn) 0.25 to 1 mg is given intravenously. Hormone tests are repeated 30 to 60 minutes later. Levels should be checked the first week of the menstrual cycle, since baseline values of these hormones (e.g., 17-OH progesterone) may be increased in the luteal phase.[74]

The following post-cortrosyn stimulation test results are seen in late-onset CAH:

1. In 21-OH deficiency, there is a marked increase in 17-hydroxyprogesterone[73] which, in turn, leads to increased secretion of androstenedione and testosterone.[70] Baseline 17-OH progesterone is > 6 nmol/liter (200 ng/dl), and post–cortrosyn values are > 36.3 nmol/liter (1200 ng/dl). Pregnanetriol is increased in the urine.[72]
2. In 3β-HSD deficiency, there is an incremental response (≥ 2 standard deviations over normal) of plasma 17-hydroxypregnenolone.[73] In the urine, 5-pregnanetriol is increased greater than pregnanetriol.[72] As opposed to an exaggerated "adrenarche" related to the zona reticularis, there is no increase of androstenedione after cortrosyn in patients with 3β-HSD deficiency.[71]
3. In 11β-hydroxylase deficiency, there is an incremental rise in plasma 11-deoxycortisol after Cortrosyn administration.

Although DHEA is primarily (95 percent) formed in the adrenal glands, and either DHEA or DHEAS has been thought to be a good marker for adrenal overactivity, this is not necessarily so. Thirteen of 19 women with abnormal ACTH testing had a normal baseline DHEAS, and 6 of 12 women with a normal response to ACTH had abnormal baseline DHEAS.[73] Only extremely high levels of DHEA, which would indicate adrenal tumor, are likely to be specific for an adrenal abnormality. Dexamethasone suppression is not specific for an adrenal source of androgens, as ovarian overproduction is also responsive to corticosteroids.[66]

Hyperprolactinemia is another cause of adrenal overproduction of androgens and should be considered in women with extensive or rapidly progressive androgenetic alopecia. Women with hyperprolactinemia have an increase in free testosterone (approximately 2× normal), decrease in SHBG, and a moderate increase in DHEAS.[75–77] Prolactin modifies ovulation by blocking the response of the gonads to LH and preventing the positive feedback of estrogen in promoting the ovulatory LH surge.[78] Consequently, less estradiol and more androstenedione are produced.[78] Hyperprolactinemia can occur without the presence of galactorrhea but, in women, is generally associated with amenorrhea and anovulatory or irregular bleeding.[79]

Studies of women with androgenetic alopecia have reported variable results on whether hyperandrogenism is a common occurrence. Most reports are of normal testosterone,[80,81] gonadotropins, and estradiol.[81] Part of the problem may be that testosterone, with relatively stable levels throughout the day, varies considerably from day to day.[78] The most reproducible abnormality appears to be a decrease in SHBG,[82–84] which can be reflective of either a decrease in estrogens or an increase in androgens and which would be expected to lead to an increase in free or unbound testosterone. Free testosterone and SHBG were measured in 308 women with androgenetic alopecia who had regular periods and were taking no exogenous hormones; only 40 of 308 (13 percent) had abnormal free testosterone and 33 (11 percent) had decreased SHBG (R. DeVillez, unpublished data). DHT is readily metabolized peripherally to androstanediol, and 3α-diol-G (3α-17β-androstanediol glucuronide) appears to be a better marker than DHT for androgen action in the skin.[69,85] DeVillez and Dunn found that a marked increase in the ratio of 3α-diol-G to SHBG was most indicative of female androgenetic alopecia,[82] reflecting an increased peripheral conversion of testosterone to DHT in affected women.

ANIMAL MODELS

Some nonhuman primates have patterned scalp hair loss that is age-related. This includes some chimpanzees, most adult stump-tailed macaques, and the South American red uacari.[86] The stump-tailed macaque is a reasonable animal model for male-pattern baldness with morphological and histological similarities. The hair loss, however, occurs in the frontal region of all postpubescent animals, somewhat more extensively in males than in females.[86] The hair loss begins at about age 3 to 4 years along with secondary sexual development, with the process well-advanced by the age of 6 years. The affected hairs undergo transformation from terminal to vellus follicles. The rate of incorporation and catabolism of testosterone is higher in follicles from the frontal scalp than those from the back.[87] Hair follicles in the frontal scalp of juveniles produce an increased amount of DHT relative to those in adults.[88] Vellus-like follicles in bald areas of mature macaques show decreased uptake and conversion of testosterone to DHT.[88]

CLINICAL CORRELATES

Men

The major clinical association with male-pattern baldness in men appears to be an increased risk of coronary artery disease.[10,89,90] The most compelling report is a case-controlled study of 655 men aged 21 to 54 admitted to the hospital with their first myocardial infarction who were compared to patients of similar age admitted for noncardiac diagnoses who did not have a history of prior myocardial infarction, cardiomyopathy, or cardiac surgery.[90] The incidence of frontal baldness was not associated with an increased risk of myocardial infarction, while vertex baldness was associated with a greater risk, which increased with the extent of vertex baldness. The age-adjusted relative risk of a myocardial infarction was 1.3 for mild-to-moderate vertex baldness and 3.4 for severe vertex baldness. The mechanism of the observed association is unclear. Other studies have not shown an association of male-pattern baldness with coronary artery disease.[91,92] Two British studies, one which evaluated 478 Caucasian hospital inpatients[91] and another of 48 male outpatients who had recovered from a myocardial infarc-tion,[92] failed to show any association with male-pattern baldness. The latter study excluded men with hypertension, diabetes mellitus, or hyper-cholesterolemia.

Women

In relation to the potential association of androgenetic alopecia and coronary artery disease, it is worthwhile to note that Hamilton reported a progressive decrease in the incidence of male-pattern baldness type IV (the highest pattern reported in women) and an increase in type I (no temporal recession) frontal hairline in women more than 50 years of age.[3] However, Venning and Dawber reported an increase in Hamilton pattern II–V hair loss in post- vs. premenopausal women.[15] No study has evaluated the risk of coronary artery disease in women with Ludwig pattern III or a male pattern of androgenetic alopecia.

Iron deficiency has been associated with hair loss[93] and may play a role in the response that women with male-pattern baldness have to treatment.[94]

TREATMENT

There are potentially several objectives in the medical treatment of androgenetic alopecia, including regrowth of the lost hair, maintenance of existing hair, and prevention of further hair loss. No single, current therapy can provide solutions to all of these objectives or complete fulfillment of even one objective. Treatment may target specifically (1) the disruption of production, transport, or metabolism of the androgen mediator (i.e., DHT); (2) production of the androgen receptor; or (3) the binding of the androgen receptor to either DHT or DNA. Promotion of mediators of follicular growth, dependent or independent of androgen stimulation, may also be utilized. There is no shortage of ideas or preparations to treat androgenetic alopecia, but few have been tested in any controlled fashion. The discussion here will focus on those therapies which have been found useful in controlled clinical trials or have shown some potential for efficacy in the hands of experienced investigators. The methodology used to assess efficacy of these agents will also be discussed.

Methodology

The large-scale clinical studies performed to evaluate topical minoxidil in the mid-1980s were the first ever performed for a hair growth promoter, and 10 years later the methodology used to evaluate efficacy is still evolving. The early studies primarily involved repetitive hair counts in a midvertex target area which was located at each visit by using physical landmarks. The target area of each individual was not exactly the same each time, but since it was located in the center of the annular balding vertex and since monthly independent assessments were made by the same observer, the reliability was acceptable.[95] Hair counts were performed by cutting the hair close to the scalp in the 1-in. target area and counting the hairs under low magnification. Patients and investigators were asked to assess the degree of regrowth, and global photography was used to document the physical results.[95]

Since then, several improvements in the methodology for assessment of potential hair growth promoters have occurred.[96] First, the target area is tattooed at baseline so the exact same target area may be examined at each visit. Second, the chosen target area generally is not the most developed area of baldness but rather on the leading edge. Third, the target area is photographed with standard lighting, and hair counts are performed from these standardized photographs by first marking each terminal or indeterminate hair on a transparent overlay and then either manually counting the dots or using image analysis to do the same. Fourth, standardized global photographs of the subject's scalp, with the hair combed identically at each visit, are used.

Other measures of in vitro assessment of efficacy of new hair growth promoters have been suggested. Clipping or shaving the hairs in a given area at regular intervals and weighing the hairs has been used for years in assessing the effect of various agents on hirsutism.[97] Price and Menefee modified this procedure for male-pattern baldness to include clipping, washing, weighing, and measuring the hairs in a given tattooed balding target area.[98] Subtle changes in hair growth can be identified by this means, and the total number of patients required, in order to observe a statistically significant difference between agents, is small. This may be a productive means to assess potential new agents without embarking on a large, more expensive clinical trial.

Topical Minoxidil

BACKGROUND

Minoxidil (Loniten) is a piperidinopyrimidine derivative that functions as a vasodilator in refractory hypertension.[99] When taken orally, about 15 percent of the parent compound is excreted in the urine while approximately 85 percent is metabolized by the liver and then excreted by the kidney, primarily as the glucuronide conjugate.[100] The half-life is about 4 hours, although the antihypertensive effect lasts longer due to retention by vascular smooth muscle.[100] Side effects of oral therapy include renal sodium retention, reflex activation of the adrenergic system with resultant tachycardia and increased cardiac output with secondary myocardial oxygen demand, and pericardial effusions.[100] Electrocardiographic changes are common, including flattening or inversion of T waves. In about 70 percent of patients, oral minoxidil treatment has been associated with hypertrichosis, which occurs most prominently on the face and extremities. A topical preparation was developed to exploit this hair growth promotion and has proven effective in treating androgenetic alopecia and alopecia areata.

The mechanism of action of topical minoxidil in promoting hair growth remains speculative. It does not appear to have any antiandrogen effect. In animal studies, minoxidil does not stimulate testosterone secretion or adrenal androgen secretion, or displace testosterone from the rat prostate cytosol androgen receptor.[101] In man, serum testosterone levels remain unchanged after therapy.[102] Not unexpectedly, given its vasodilating properties on oral administration, qualitative tests using laser Doppler velocimetry and photopulse plethysmography have shown an increased cutaneous blood flow for at least one hour after topical application of minoxidil.[103] However, a cause-and-effect relationship between increased perfusion and hair growth has not been proven.

Minoxidil has a direct mitogenic and morphological effect on epidermal cells,[104] prolongs the survival time of cultured epithelial cells, and prolongs the time cultured keratinocytes can be passed after confluence.[105] Minoxidil treatment of mouse vibrissae follicles in culture resulted in normalization of follicular morphology, decreased necrosis, and proliferation of both matrix and inner root sheath cells.[106] In vitro studies of the follicles of the stump-tailed macaque have shown a significant increase in DNA synthesis in follicular and perifollicular cells, but not in epidermal keratinocytes, following minoxidil therapy.[107] Hair bulbs with intact outer root sheath from plucked anagen hairs of men with male-pattern baldness treated with topical minoxidil were evaluated by DNA flow cytometry and found to have a significant increase in proliferation index.[108] These studies all suggest a direct effect of topical minoxidil on the hair follicle cells.

Minoxidil sulfate appears to be the active metabolite responsible for hair growth stimulation.[109] Although minoxidil appears to work in vascular smooth muscle by opening potassium channels, this is still a speculative mechanism of action in hair follicles. Minoxidil appears to act on at least two sites in the hair follicle, causing proliferation at the base of the bulb and differentiation above the dermal papilla.[106]

In vivo studies in the stump-tailed macaque show that topical minoxidil can reverse and prevent the balding process.[110] Four adult animals with mild to advanced baldness and four preadolescent animals that were either nonbald or showed only early baldness were treated with 5% topical minoxidil 5 days per week for ≥ 10 months. Two animals in each age-group served as controls. Those adult animals treated with topical minoxidil had increased regrowth, and preadolescents on minoxidil showed no signs of incipient baldness, whereas the control animals all had advancing baldness.[110] Histologically, the response to minoxidil corresponded to an increase in the length and size of follicles and an increase in the number of follicles in mid to late anagen.[110]

CLINICAL TRIALS

EFFICACY

Multicenter studies involved 2294 men with male-pattern baldness, Hamilton patterns III-VI, between the ages of 18 and 50 years.[102] Men were treated with 1 ml of 2% or 3% topical minoxidil vs. placebo twice daily and both target area hair counts and clinical assessments were used to assess efficacy as noted previously. Hair regrowth was not visually apparent until after 4 to 6 months of continuous use[102] and tended to plateau for most men at about 1 year. After 1 year of therapy, Olsen, Weiner, DeLong, and Pinnell showed that the mean target area terminal hair counts of patients treated with 2% topical minoxidil had increased 218 ± 158 per 1-inch-diameter circle over the baseline mean of 126 ± 104 per 1-in. target circle.[99] While this $2^1/_2$-times increase in terminal hairs was fairly dramatic, the mean hair count was still far below the normal density of terminal hairs seen in an occipital area unaffected by male-pattern baldness ($1346/in^2$).[110a] Not surprisingly, then, fewer than 5 percent of patients were noted to have dense regrowth, but approximately 25 to 30 per-

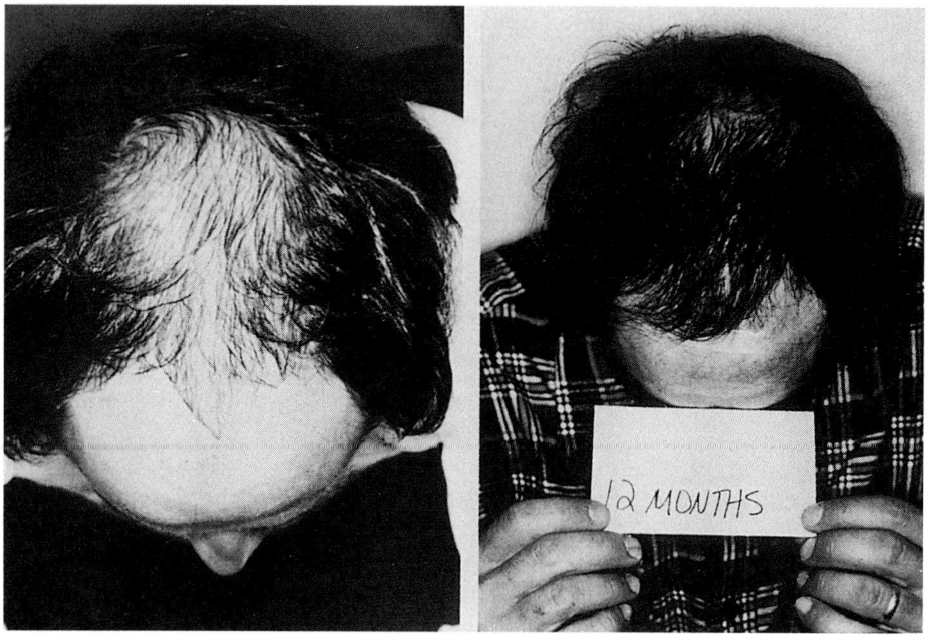

Figure 11-14 Patient treated with 2% topical minoxidil for 12 months, with excellent response (*Reprinted with permission from Olsen et al: Topical minoxidil in early male pattern baldness.* J Am Acad Dermatol. 13:185-192, 1985.)

cent had moderate regrowth of hair with the use of topical minoxidil (Fig. 11-14).[102]

Continued use of 2% minoxidil twice daily is necessary to maintain regrowth: those using a lower frequency of applications do not fare as well as those who persist with the b.i.d. treatment plan.[111] The mean terminal hair growth in patients continuously treated over a 5-year evaluation (as followed by this author) declined slightly from the 1-year level but did not fall below baseline.[112] Those patients who stop using topical minoxidil generally experience a loss of the regrown hair within 3 to 4 months.[113] Restarting the drug will usually recapture the prior growth.

The results in women with androgenetic alopecia have been similar to results in men with androgenetic alopecia. Two hundred fifty-six women, ages 18 to 45, with Ludwig I or II patterns of androgenetic alopecia, were treated with 2% topical minoxidil or placebo twice daily for 32 weeks. Nonvellus hair counts in a 1-cm^2 target area on the top of the scalp showed a mean increase of 14 percent over baseline after 9 months of therapy (140.4 ± 3.9 to 163.1 ± 4.7) compared with 7.3 percent for those on placebo (138.6 ± 3.3 to 148.7 ± 3.6). The investigators felt that 50 percent of the patients had minimal regrowth and 13 percent had moderate hair growth on 2% topical minoxidil compared with 33 percent and 6 percent, respectively, of patients on placebo (The Upjohn Company, unpublished data).

SAFETY

The side effects of 2% topical minoxidil are few and include allergic contact dermatitis in < 1 percent of patients and irritant dermatitis or folliculitis in 3 to 5 percent.[102] Hair growth on the forehead or cheeks is occasionally seen and represents either inadvertent transfer or spreading of the drug from the scalp or local intravascular spread by the generous scalp blood supply. The total amount of the drug absorbed is less than 2 percent. No relevant hemodynamic effects have been observed in normotensive or hypertensive patients using topical minoxidil (Upjohn Company, unpublished data). Although there were many men on the topical minoxidil trials who developed electrocardiographic changes, these changes occurred both in men on active drug and men on placebo; some abnormalities reversed while on drug.[99,114] No cardiac problems were definitively linked to topical minoxidil; instead, the background cardiac "noise" may have been associated with the underlying coronary artery disease linked to vertex baldness.[90]

CLINICAL USE

Rogaine (2% topical minoxidil) was the first, and is currently the only drug approved by the Food and Drug Administration for audrogenetic alopecia. The indication for men states for "male pattern baldness of the vertex," implying that the drug is efficacious only for that particular area of the balding scalp. In fact, the drug works equally well on the balding frontal area, but since the pivotal clinical trials did not directly address the hair growth in this area, this area was excluded from claims of efficacy in men.

This author approaches treatment of patients with androgenetic alopecia with Rogaine as follows. At the initial visit, a history and blood pressure are taken (as for any new patient); if one of these is abnormal, an ECG or further physical examination may be performed. Efficacy and expected side effects (cost, time), as well as potential risks of Rogaine (see previous text), are discussed. Any patient expressing interest in Rogaine treatment is asked to make a 1-year commitment to twice-daily therapy: anything less is not worth the patient's time, effort, and money. Photographs are taken of the scalp and a return appointment is scheduled in 6 months; compliance is not necessarily increased by more frequent visitation, and hair growth will be negligible before 6 months. A request for a dropper top with a 1-ml measure is made on the prescription. The existing commercially-packaged "dab-o-matic" and spray applicator tips waste too much drug on the hair rather than delivering the drug directly to the scalp. Patients are told to part their hair at approximately 2-mm intervals across the top of the scalp and vertex and to apply the topical minoxidil to the scalp along the part, rubbing each drop in carefully.

There was no statistically significant difference between the results for 2% and 3% topical minoxidil solution in the early clinical trials[99] and there was less efficacy with concentrations of topical minoxidil below 2%.[114] Higher concentrations of topical minoxidil resulted in higher blood levels and, thus, for both safety and efficacy reasons, the 2% topical minoxidil prepartion was chosen for FDA approval. However, the improved efficacy of 5% over 1% or 2% topical minoxidil in alopecia areata raises the question of a potential overlooked dose effect in androgenetic alopecia.[115] Several current studies are evaluating higher concentrations of topical minoxidil in the treatment of androgenetic alopecia; the preliminary results look very promising.

Topical Tretinoin

In one study of 36 men with male-pattern baldness treated with a topical mixture of 0.025% tretinoin and 0.5% minoxidil 1 ml twice daily for a mean of 8 to 10 months, 44 percent (16 out of 36) of the subjects had a "good" (≥ 46 percent increase in target area hairs) response to therapy.[116] This was compared with a "good" response in 2 of 12 (16 percent) subjects on 0.025% topical tretinoin alone, none of 3 on placebo, and none of 3 on 0.5% topical minoxidil alone.[116] A second study compared once-daily topical application of 0.05% tretinoin and once daily 2% minoxidil with twice-daily application of 2% topical minoxidil in men with male-pattern baldness. There was a marginal, but not statistically significant, increased effectiveness of the combination regimen over minoxidil alone. Minoxidil blood levels clearly did increase with the concomitant use of tretinoin (R. DeVillez, personal communication). Further studies have not been published.

The potential side effects of topical tretinoin are irritation and photosensitivity (not an insignificant consideration in a balding patient). The potential side effects of topical minoxidil are as noted earlier.

Topical Diazoxide

Diazoxide is a nondiuretic benzothiazide which is a potent but rarely used antihypertensive agent.[117] Diazoxide is also a potent hyperglycemic agent that inhibits insulin release and promotion of glycolysis, and is used to treat idiopathic hypoglycemia of infancy.[118] Oral diazoxide can induce hypertrichosis in a distribution similar to that caused by minoxidil but with far less frequency. A topical formulation of diazoxide was reported in 1989 to show efficacy in male-pattern baldness. Nineteen men with "early to mid-stage" androgenetic alopecia were treated with 3% diazoxide solution twice daily for 2 to 11 months (mean 5.7 months). Four had "dense" growth (abundant new hair), seven had moderate growth ("some new terminal hairs"), one had vellus hair growth, and seven had no regrowth. Local irritation occurred in one patient.[119]

The potential mechanism of action of diazoxide in hair growth may be through inhibition of phosphodiesterase, the enzyme that metabolizes cAMP. An increase in cAMP leads to promotion of glycolysis by stimulating glycogen phosphorylase and inhibiting glycogen synthetase.[118]

Antiandrogens

BACKGROUND

Hamilton noted that castration after male-pattern baldness had begun prevented further progression of hair loss and that the hair loss in eunuchs treated with testosterone abated when the testosterone was stopped.[30] Although it would appear feasible that employment of an antiandrogen would halt male-pattern baldness, this has not previously been evaluated in any concerted fashion (studies ongoing). A second issue to be addressed is whether an antiandrogen can reverse the hair loss in androgenetic alopecia.

The term *antiandrogen* as defined by Dorfman implies prevention of expression of androgen activity at target sites[120] and does not include other mechanisms of decreasing androgen action, such as a decrease in production of androgens, interference with androgen metabolism, or change in androgen plasma protein binding. These will all be discussed here, however, since the end result on hair growth may be similar.

Antiandrogens may be weak agonists, which compete less well than endogenous hormones and dissociate rapidly from the androgen receptor, or potent agonists, which form a complex with the receptor molecule and dissociate slowly.[121] The true antagonists of endogenous or exogenous androgens are the weak agonists, which rely only on a continuous supply of the compound to achieve full inhibition.[121]

Antiandrogens may have a steroidal structure (spironolactone, cyproterone acetate) or no steroidal structure (flutamide, cimetidine) (Fig. 11-15). Most steroidal antiandrogens not only have potent antiandrogen activity but also have associated hormonal properties, particularly progestational activity.[122] The progestin activity of steroidal antiandrogens suppresses gonadotropin secretion at the pituitary level. Normally, androgens decrease the sensitivity of the pituitary to luteinizing hormone–releasing hormone (LHRH), thus decreasing luteinizing hormone (LH) release.[122] Antiandrogens without a steroidal structure may inhibit the negative feedback of the gonadal steroids so that more gonadotropins are released by the hypophysis and more testosterone and estradiol are produced by the gonads.[121] These nonsteroidal antiandrogens, then, require a concomitant antigonadotropin to prevent an increase in androgen load which could neutralize their inherent antiandrogen effect.

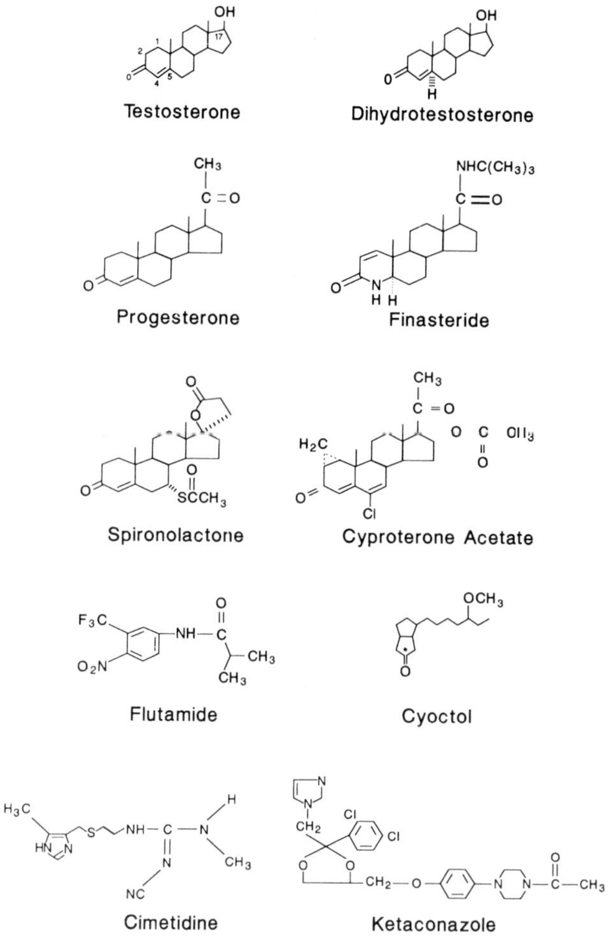

Figure 11-15 Structure of androgens and antiandrogens.

The potency of antiandrogens is evaluated by a variety of in vitro measures, the most reliable being the measure of relative binding affinity (RBA).[121] The most recent tests estimate the RBA of an antiandrogen in either rat prostatic cytosol or dispersed human genital skin fibroblasts.[121] These assays have shown that spironolactone has an ability to compete for androgen receptors which is greater than that of cyproterone acetate and flutamide.[121] These in vitro techniques, however, cannot evaluate those compounds that require biotransformation for activity (such as flutamide). Moreover, these screening tests only distinguish between compounds interacting with high or low affinity with the androgen receptor but do not discriminate agonists from all classes of antagonists.[122] One direct means of quantitatively measuring antiandrogen activity, although not in general use, is through the use of stable cell lines containing high levels of human androgen receptor by transfection of the receptor cDNA linked to an expression vector.[122] In vivo, antagonist and agonist activity of a compound is still most frequently determined by the effect of the antiandrogen on testosterone (or other androgen)-stimulated increase in the weight of the prostate and seminal vesicles in castrated rats.[122] The hamster flank organ, which is androgen-dependent sebaceous tissue, is frequently used to screen compounds for local antiandrogen activity.[122]

Most of the clinical studies of antiandrogens have been conducted with patients who have acne or hirsutism; few have included women with androgenetic alopecia.

TOPICAL ANTIANDROGENS

CYOCTOL

Cyoctol, or 6-(5-methoxy-1-heptyl)-bicyclo (3,3,0) octan-3-one) (Fig. 11-14), is a nonsteroid antiandrogen with neither estrogenic nor progestogenic activity.[123] It competitively inhibits DHT receptor binding,[123] and is completely metabolized in the skin after topical application.[124]

Only one study has been reported utilizing topical cyoctol in the treatment of androgenetic alopecia. Men with type IIIv, IV, or V Hamilton pattern male-pattern baldness applied 0.01% cyoctol, 0.05% cyoctol, or placebo 1 ml twice daily to the balding vertex. Ninety patients entered the study but only 40 completed 40 to 48 weeks; 25 of the 54 patients originally assigned to cyoctol completed this time span. Based on computerized counting of hairs in tattooed target areas, those patients on 0.05% cyoctol had an 11.3 percent increase in mean nonvellus target area hair counts vs. approximately 4 percent in the 0.01% group and a decrease of 8.9 percent in the placebo-treated group.[124a] (Strick RA, Burnison C, Orenberg EK: Treatment of androgenetic alopecia with cyoctol—A topical antiandrogen. American Academy of Dermatology presentation, December 1989). Only one patient on cyoctol experienced any local reaction (scalp dryness). There were no systemic side effects.

TOPICAL PROGESTERONE

Progesterone (Fig. 11-14) is a competitive inhibitor of DHT for 5α-reductase[125] and for binding to the cytosol androgen receptor.[126] It also inhibits the formation of 5α metabolites from androstenedione.[125] Progesterone is rapidly metabolized in most tissues (including skin) to relatively nonandrogenic substances.[127] One milliliter of a 2% solution applied topically twice daily appears to be well-tolerated in women, with higher doses leading to menstrual irregularities.[128] Topical progesterone has been used widely, but results are mostly anecdotal. Price and Ettinger utilized topical progesterone (concentration and vehicle unspecified) for 10 to 48 months in 12 men, ages 18–39 years, with male-pattern baldness. None of the 12 grew hair, one-half developed further thinning, and one-half remained with the same hair density.[129] Topical 11α-hydroxyprogesterone was used to treat 5 men and 9 women with male-pattern baldness.[130] Fifteen milliliters of 0.5% solution was applied twice daily to the scalp for 2.4 to 4 years. All 14 patients had a "positive" response. A second study with 11α-hydroxyprogesterone used a 1% lotion in young men with androgenetic alopecia. Ten patients were treated for 1 year with active medication, and 8 were left untreated as controls. The treated group had increased numbers of anagen hairs in the treated scalp, and 9 of 10 saw improvement, compared with a decrease in anagen hairs and worsening hair loss in 7 of the 8 controls.[131]

TOPICAL ESTROGEN

Estrogens are indirect antiandrogens, increasing the production of SHBG and, thus, leading to a decrease in the bioactive free testosterone. Although more than 70 percent of a topically applied preparation is metabolized to weak nonandrogenic by-products, the absorption of topical estrogen can lead to decreased libido in men. Reports of use of a topical estrogen preparation in subjects with androgenetic alopecia have been mostly anecdotal. However, one double-blind, controlled, 6-month trial of 0.025% 17α-estradiol was performed with 51 subjects (males and females) who had androgenetic alopecia. There was a significant reduction in the percentage of telogen hairs along with stabilization of the hair loss.[132]

SYSTEMIC ANTIANDROGENS

SPIRONOLACTONE

Spironolactone (Fig. 11-15) is an aldosterone antagonist employed in clinical practice as a potassium-sparing diuretic and antihypertensive agent. Spironolactone is rapidly absorbed, with maximum plasma levels reached in 30 to 60 minutes. Excretion is through both urine and feces, the biliary route primarily related to the elimination of metabolites.[121] The major metabolites are canrenone and potassium canrenoate. The half-life of canrenone is approximately 20 hours.[133]

Spironolactone is a potent antiandrogen, working both to decrease production and to block the effect of androgens at the cellular level.[134] Spironolactone appears to decrease testosterone production in the adrenal gland by depleting microsomal cytochrome P_{450} and by affecting the cytochrome P_{450}–dependent enzymes 17α-hydroxylase and desmolase[134,135] (Fig. 11-13). The destruction of microsomal cytochrome P_{450} by spironolactone may be limited to those tissues in which microsomal 17-hydroxylase activity is high:[136] the binding of spironolactone to 17-hydroxylase–cytochrome P_{450} may convert spironolactone to a metabolite that destroys the heme portion of cytochrome P_{450}, thereby decreasing steroid 17-hydroxylation.[136] Spironolactone is also a competitive inhibitor of DHT-receptor binding and interferes with the translocation of this complex into the nucleus.[134,137] Spironolactone, a strong competitor for the androgen receptor, is a potent agonist, while canrenone, a weak competitor, is a potent antagonist.[121] The antiandrogen effect of spironolactone may be produced by the parent compound on the adrenal gland and the metabolite on the receptor site.

Doses of spironolactone used in clinical practice vary from 50 to 300 mg per day. The minimum threshold for effective treatment of androgenetic alopecia appears to be 100 mg daily, similar to that seen in hirsutism.[121,138] The drug is available only in 25-mg tablets and can be given as a single dose or divided doses. At doses of 100 mg a day, minimal changes in circulating androgens are observed.[121] At ≥ 300 mg, plasma testosterone decreases significantly,[121] but the higher dose offers little advantage clinically and is more likely to be accompanied by side effects.

There are few reports in the literature regarding the use of spironolactone in androgenetic alopecia. Since there is no topical preparation available, all studies have been performed in women only. In one study, twelve patients with androgenetic alopecia, six on spironolactone 75 to 100 mg per day and six untreated controls, were followed for 12 months.[139] Both groups showed a mean decrease in target area nonvellus hairs: 197/cm^2 to 189/cm^2 for those on spironolactone, and 191/cm^2 to 169/cm^2 for those on the control drug, but only the decrease in the control group was statistically significant. Enhanced nonvellus growth was noted in two patients who had their spironolactone dose doubled after 12 months from the 75 or 100 mg per day used during the first year.[139] In a second study, six of seven patients with androgenetic alopecia treated with 200 mg spironolactone daily were "pleased" at the end of 6 months with a mean improvement of 41 percent.[140]

Potential side effects of spironolactone are hyperkalemia and, in women, breast tenderness, irregular menses, and mood swings. Decreased libido, impotence, and gynecomastia can occur in men treated with spironolactone,[136] thus far limiting the systemic use to women. Women of childbearing potential who are treated with spironolactone should probably use a concomitant oral contraceptive pill and certainly should be forewarned of the potential for feminization of a male fetus if pregnancy occurs while on spironolactone.

CYPROTERONE ACETATE

Oral cyproterone acetate is poorly absorbed (5–30 percent), with maximum plasma levels achieved in a few hours.[121,141] The half-life of cyproterone acetate is 1.5 ± 0.6 days, and excretion is via bile (58 percent) and urine (30 percent).[121] Cyproterone acetate has been shown to block DHT-androgen receptor binding.[142] Cyproterone, given its steroidal structure (Fig. 11-15), is antigonadotropic and is also a strong progestogen.[141] Estrogens are given in conjunction with cyproterone acetate in order to ensure regular menses, to increase SHBG levels, and to reinforce the antigonadotropic action.[121] Because of the depot effect of cyproterone in adipose tissue, the combination with estrogen is usually delivered in a reverse sequential regimen termed *cyclical an-*

tiandrogen therapy (CAT). The dose of CAT is 100 mg cyproterone acetate on days 5 to 15 and 0.05 mg ethinyl estradiol on days 5 to 25 of the menstrual cycle.[121,141] A low-dose combined formulation of 2 mg cyproterone acetate and 50 μg ethinyl estradiol given on days 5 to 25 (Diane) is also utilized in patients with mild acne or hirsutism or for maintenance doses in the same conditions.[141] Side effects with CAT include nausea, headache, asthenia, increased weight, and decreased libido, and are similar to those of oral contraceptive pills.[141] Breast discomfort and depression have been reported in more than 5 percent of cases treated with CAT.[141]

There have been no large, well-controlled studies of cyproterone acetate use in female androgenetic alopecia.[143–147] One study compared 29 women with androgenetic alopecia treated with CAT to 20 women without specific treatment (duration unspecified).[145] Eighteen of the 29 patients treated with CAT subjectively improved, and 21 of 29 had objective improvement including decreased shedding, increased diameter of hairs, and/or decreased telogen counts in affected areas. Seven of the 20 patients without therapy also subjectively improved, but no note was made of an objective improvement in these patients.[145] Two reports each of fewer than 11 patients treated with CAT showed decreased shedding and/or an increased density of nonvellus hair with therapy.[143,144] In one series, 40 percent of women with androgenetic alopecia treated with CAT showed "improvement."[148]

The results with the lower doses of cyproterone in Diane have apparently been less dramatic than with CAT, although in one series of 101 hirsute women, 85 percent of those with concomitant androgenetic alopecia had a "satisfactory" response to Diane.[146] In another study, 14 of 17 women with androgenetic alopecia had maintenance of hair growth while on Diane.[145]

FLUTAMIDE

Flutamide (Eulexin) (Fig. 11-15) is currently approved for the treatment of prostate cancer. Flutamide is rapidly absorbed, reaching maximum plasma levels after 4 to 6 hours.[121] The drug is rapidly metabolized to at least 10 plasma metabolites, one of which (2-hydroxy-flutamide) presumably is responsible for its biologic activity.[149,150] Excretion is primarily renal.[149] Five milligrams of a topical preparation of flutamide in 50% propylene glycol and 50% ethanol showed at least 16 percent systemic absorption.[151] The same metabolites are present in urine and plasma after oral and topical doses, although the rate of metabolism is slower with the topical route.[151]

Flutamide, or most likely 2-hydroxy-flutamide, inhibits the tissue uptake and retention of testosterone and also the formation of the nuclear steroid-androgen receptor complex.[121] Flutamide inhibits the negative feedback of gonadal steroids at the hypothalamic-pituitary level.[121]

Doses of flutamide for metastatic prostatic carcinoma are 250 mg three times daily. Side effects are primarily gastrointestinal, chiefly diarrhea.[152] Increased liver function tests, usually reversible with a decrease in dose or discontinuation of therapy, have been reported. Combination with an oral contraceptive pill is recommended in women of childbearing potential in order to avoid the risk of pregnancy and to inhibit the expected gonadotropin rise.

There are no published controlled studies of the use of flutamide in male-pattern baldness. Twenty premenopausal women with hirsutism refractory to oral contraceptive pills, spironolactone, or dexamethasone were treated with flutamide 250 mg twice daily and, in those 18 women without tubal ligation, a concomitant oral contraceptive pill (Ortho 1/35). Seventeen of the 18 women treated with combination therapy had a rapid and marked reduction in their hirsutism score. Fifteen of the 18 women had associated acne, seborrhea, and hair loss, and the total "score" for these signs decreased by 84 percent by the end of 6 months of treatment. One woman with androgenetic alopecia showed remarkable improvement.[153] This author has also seen hair regrowth in a woman with androgenetic alopecia unresponsive to topical minoxidil and oral spironolactone who was treated with flutamide.

CIMETIDINE

Cimetidine is an H_2 antihistamine approved for the treatment of peptic ulcer disease. It is both a competitive inhibitor of DHT[154] and an inhibitor of the oxidative metabolism of estradiol, specifically the 2-hydroxylation, thus raising estradiol levels.[155,156] It does not appear to affect gonadotropins.[157] Hepatic metabolism is the principle pathway of elimination of the drug.[155] Cimetidine also increases serum concentration of prolactin, which may contribute to the symptoms of breast swelling and galactorrhea in women and gynecomastia in men. Impotence and loss of libido have been reported in men, and whether these symptoms in men are related to hyperprolactinemia, decreased androgen action, increased estrogen levels, or a combination thereof is uncertain.[155]

One small study has addressed the use of cimetidine in androgenetic alopecia. Ten women with advanced androgenetic alopecia were treated with 300 mg of cimetidine five times a day for 1½ to 9 months. Seven of the 10 demonstrated "good" to "excellent" hair regrowth based on serial photography and subjective evaluation by the patient and investigator.[158]

KETOCONAZOLE

Ketoconazole is an imidazole derivative that is an effective oral antimycotic agent for a variety of fungi. It interacts with cytochrome P_{450} at the heme iron site in several organs, including gonads and adrenals, but much higher concentrations are necessary to affect cytochrome P_{450}–dependent enzymes in mammals compared with those in fungi.[159] In the adrenal gland and gonads, ketoconazole inhibits C_{17-20}-lyase and 17α-hydroxylase (leading to a decrease in testosterone and androstenedione), 11β-hydroxylase, 18-hydroxylase, and cholesterol side-chain cleavage.[159] Patients on ketoconazole have a significant elevation of the estradiol-testosterone ratio, but the percentage of bound and free fractions of both hormones are not significantly altered.[159] There are only anecdotal reports of ketoconazole use in hirsutism,[159] and none in male-pattern baldness.

5α-REDUCTASE INHIBITORS

Finasteride is a 4-azasteroid compound that is a potent 5α-reductase inhibitor without any androgenic, antiandrogenic, or other steroid hormone activities.[160] The deficiency of 5α-reductase activity induced by finasteride is not specific for androgen metabolism but is a general deficiency in steroid metabolism affecting C_{19} and C_{21} steroids metabolized by both hepatic and extrasplanchnic 5α-reductase. Oral finasteride at doses of 5 mg per day causes a marked (~ 80 percent) suppression of circulating DHT without any change in circulating testosterone, cortisol, prolactin, SHBG, thyroxine, estradiol, or glucose tolerance.[160] Increases of approximately 10 percent are observed in LH and FSH levels with finasteride treatment, but they remain within normal range.[152]

Maximum plasma levels of finasteride are achieved 1 to 2 hours after oral dosing, with a mean plasma half-life of 6 hours.[152] Approximately 40 percent of the drug is excreted in the urine and 60 percent in the feces, most as monocarboxylic acid.[152] Metabolites possess ≤ 20 percent of the 5α-reductase inhibitory activity compared with finasteride. The prostate gland, being a DHT-dependent organ, undergoes a reduction in volume in those men with benign prostatic hypertrophy (BPH) treated with finasteride, and all treated men have a decrease in ejaculate volume. In studies of men with BPH, decreased libido and impotence occurred in fewer than 4 percent of the patients treated with finasteride compared with fewer than 2 percent of the patients on placebo.[152] Administration of the drug to pregnant women would be expected to cause ambiguous genitalia in any male fetus. No studies have been performed to date on women.

That 5α-reductase inhibitors can prevent baldness was shown in the following study. A related 5α-reductase inhibitor, N,N-diethyl-4-methyl-3-oxo-4-aza-5α-androstane-17β-carboxamide (4-MA), in DMSO was applied topically to three preadolescent stump-tailed macaques, and topical DMSO alone was applied to three macaques.[161] After 27 months, the control monkeys had varying degrees of hair loss, whereas the monkeys treated with 4-MA preserved their juvenile pattern of growth. Furthermore, the percentage of anagen hairs remained constant in the 4-MA–treated animals but significantly dropped in the controls. A second study in adult stump-tailed macaques evaluated four different treatments: 2% topical minoxidil ($n = 5$), minoxidil vehicle ($n = 6$), oral 0.5 mg finasteride with topical minoxidil vehicle ($n = 5$), and oral 0.5 mg finasteride plus 2% topical minoxidil ($n = 5$).[162] Each medication was given once daily for 20 weeks. Using shaved scalp hair weight as the objective measure, those animals treated with the vehicle had a decrease, those on topical minoxidil or oral finasteride had augmentation of similar degree, and those on combination therapy had a marked increase (> 2× single-treatment results) in hair weight. These data support the use of finasteride in potentially reversing established baldness. However, it should be noted that the

N-4-methyl-azasteroids are better inhibitors of 5α-reductase-1, the apparent principal 5α-reductase in the balding scalp, than are the 4-azasteroids (of which finasteride is one example).[40]

Combination of a topical 5α-reductase inhibitor (progesterone) with a topical competitive inhibitor of DHT binding to the cytoplasmic androgen receptor protein (spironolactone) has been shown to have synergistic antiandrogen activity on the Syrian hamster sebaceous gland.[163] A similar relationship was observed between spironolactone and 4-MA on cultured interstitial cells from immature rat testes.[164]

ORAL CONTRACEPTIVE PILLS

Progesterone is a potent inhibitor of 5α-reductase activity and androgen receptor binding but is quickly metabolized. The synthetically produced progestins in marketed oral contraceptive pills are more closely related structurally to testosterone and estrogen than to progesterone and have inherent and variable androgenic, estrogenic, and/or antiestrogenic activity. A progestin can compete with testosterone and DHT for androgen receptor binding and, depending on its inherent androgenic properties, can be an antagonist or agonist. Combination estrogen-progestin oral contraceptive pills may have an additional effect on decreasing central androgen production in the adrenals and ovaries. Combination oral contraceptive pills have demonstrated alterations of adrenal steroidogenesis similar to those seen with estrogen alone, namely, an increase in plasma levels of 17-hydroxycorticosteroids, a decrease in cortisol excretion rate, and an increase in plasma transcortin,[165] the net result being a decrease in adrenal androgen production. Oral contraceptive pills also suppress ovulation and thus diminish the production of androgens by the ovaries. Estrogens increase SHBG and thus further decrease the amount of free testosterone.

CONCLUDING REMARKS

The clinical presentation, etiology, and current therapy of androgenetic alopecia in both men and women have been presented in this chapter. Further directed treatment of androgenetic alopecia will depend on specific knowledge of hormonal interactions at the cellular level in affected tissue.

REFERENCES

1. Montagna W: Baldness: A disease? J Am Med Wom Assoc 28:447–458, 1973.
2. Barman JM, Pecoraro V, Astore I: Biological basis of the inception and evolution of baldness. J Gerontol 24:163–168, 1969.
3. Hamilton JB: Patterned loss of hair in man: Types and incidence. Ann NY Acad Sci 53:708–728, 1951.
4. Küster W, Happle R: The inheritance of common baldness: Two B or not two B? J Am Acad Dermatol 11:921–926, 1984.
5. Smith MA, Wells RS: Male-type alopecia, alopecia areata, and normal hair in women: Family histories. Arch Dermatol 89:95–98, 1964.
6. Norwood OT: Male pattern baldness: Classification and incidence. South Med J 68:1359–1365, 1975.
7. Muller SA: Alopecia: Syndromes of genetic significance. J Invest Dermatol 60:475–492, 1973.
8. Hamilton JB: Age, sex, and genetic factors in the regulation of hair growth in man: A comparison of Caucasian and Japanese populations. In Montagna W, Ellis RA (eds): *The Biology of Hair Growth.* New York, Academic Press, 1958, pp 399–433.
9. Setty LR: Hair patterns of the scalp of white and Negro males. Am J Phys Anthropol 33:49–55, 1970.
10. Buechner HA, Brown M, Tretola RJ: Baldness and emphysema. J La State Med Soc 116:329–332, 1964.
11. Ludwig E: Classification of the types of androgenetic alopecia (common baldness) occurring in the female sex. Br J Dermatol 97:247–254, 1977.
12. Sulzberger MB, Witten VH, Kopf AW: Diffuse alopecia in women. Arch Dermatol 81:556–560, 1960.
13. Snyder LH, Yingling HC: Studies in human inheritance: XII. The application of the gene frequency method of analysis to sex-influenced factors, with especial reference to baldness. Hum Biol 7:608–615, 1935.
14. Muller SA: Common baldness. Minn Med 57(10):809–812, 1974.
15. Venning VA, Dawber RPR: Patterned androgenic alopecia in women. J Am Acad Dermatol 18:1073–1077, 1988.
16. Crilly RG, Marshall DH, Nordin BEC: Effect of age on plasma androstenedione concentration in oophorectomized women. Clin Endocrinol 10:199–201, 1979.
17. Jackson D, Church RE, Ebling FJ: Hair diameter in female baldness. Br J Dermatol 87:361–367, 1972.
18. Giacometti L: The anatomy of the human scalp. In Montagna W (ed): *Advances in Biology of Skin,* vol. 6. Oxford, Pergamon Press, 1965, pp 97–120.
19. Pecoraro V, Astore I, Barman JM: The pre-natal and post-natal hair cycles in man. In Baccaredda-Boy A, Moretti G, Frey JR (eds): *Biopathology of Pattern Alopecia.* Basel/New York, Karger, 1968, pp 29–38.
20. Rushton DH, Ramsay ID, Norris MJ, Gilkes JJH: Natural progression of male pattern baldness in young men. Clin Exp Dermatol 16:188–192, 1991.
21. Rushton H, James KC, Mortimer CH: The unit area trichogram in the assessment of androgen-dependent alopecia. Br J Dermatol 109:429–437, 1983.
22. Klemp P, Peters K, Hansted B: Subcutaneous blood flow in early male pattern baldness. J Invest Dermatol 92:725–726, 1989.
23. Maguire HC Jr, Kligman AM: The histopathology of common male baldness. Excerpta Medica Foundation 55:1438–1439, 1962.
24. Maguire HC Jr, Kligman AM: Common baldness in women. Geriatrics 18:329–334, 1963.

25. Allegra F: Histology and histochemical aspects of hair follicles in pattern alopecia. In Baccaredda-Boy A, Moretti G, Frey JR (eds): *Biopathology of Pattern Alopecia.* Basel/New York, Karger, 1968, pp 107–128.
26. Lattanand A, Johnson WC: Male pattern alopecia: A histopathologic and histochemical study. J Cutan Pathol 2:58–70, 1975.
27. Randall VA, Thornton MJ, Hamada K, Messenger AG: Mechanism of androgen action in cultured dermal papilla cells derived from human hair follicles with varying responses to androgens *in vivo.* J Invest Dermatol 98:86S–91S, 1992.
28. Orentreich N: Autografts in alopecias and other selected dermatological conditions. In St. Whitelock OV, Furness FN, White EW, Lubowe II (eds): *Hair Growth and Hair Regeneration.* Ann NY Acad Sci 83:463–479, 1959.
29. Ludwig E: The role of sexual hormones in pattern alopecia. In Baccaredda-Boy A, Moretti G, Frey JR (eds): *Biopathology of Pattern Alopecia.* Basel/New York, Karger, 1968, pp 50–60.
30. Hamilton JB: Male hormone stimulation is prerequisite and an incitant in common baldness. Am J Anat 71:451–480, 1942.
31. Phillipou G, Kirk J: Significance of steroid measurements in male pattern alopecia. Clin Exp Dermatol 6:53–56, 1981.
32. Burton JL et al.: Male pattern alopecia and masculinity. Br J Dermatol 100:567–571, 1979.
33. Cipriani R et al.: Sex hormone-binding globulin and saliva testosterone levels in men with androgenetic alopecia. Br J Dermatol 109:249–252, 1983.
34. Pitts RL: Serum elevation of dehydroepiandrosterone sulfate associated with male pattern baldness in young men. J Am Acad Dermatol 16:571–573, 1987.
35. Schweikert HU, Wilson JD: Regulation of human hair growth by steroid hormones: I. Testosterone metabolism in isolated hairs. J Clin Endocrinol Metab 38:811–819, 1974.
36. Imperato-McGinley J, Guerrero L, Gautier R, Peterson RE: Steroid 5α-reductase deficiency in man: An inherited form of male pseudohermaphroditism. Science 186:1213–1215, 1974.
37. Itami S, Kurata S, Takayasu S: 5α-Reductase activity in cultured human dermal papilla cells from beard compared with reticular dermal fibroblasts. J Invest Dermatol 94:150–152, 1990.
38. Itami S, Kurata S, Sonoda T, Takayasu S: Mechanism of action of androgen in dermal papilla cells. Ann NY Acad Sci 642:385–395, 1991.
39. Bingham KD, Shaw DA: The metabolism of testosterone by human male scalp skin. J Endocrinol 57:111–121, 1973.
40. Harris G et al.: Identification and selective inhibition of an isozyme of steroid 5α-reductase in human scalp. Proc Natl Acad Sci USA 89:10787–10791, 1992.
41. Mauvais-Jarvis P: Regulation of androgen receptor and 5α-reductase in the skin of normal and hirsute women. Clin Endocrinol Metab 15:307–317, 1986.
42. Mowszowicz I, Melanitou E, Kirchhoffer M-O, Mauvais-Jarvis P: Dihydrotestosterone stimulates 5α-reductase activity in pubic skin fibroblasts. J Clin Endocrinol Metab 56:320–325, 1983.
43. Fazekas AG, Lanthier A: Metabolism of androgens by isolated human beard hair follicles. Steroids 18:367–379, 1971.
44. Hay JB, Hodgins MB: Metabolism of androgens *in vitro* by human facial and axillary skin. J Endocrinol 59:475–486, 1973.
45. Crovato F, Moretti G, Bertamino R: 17-Beta-hydroxysteroid-dehydrogenases in hair follicles of normal and bald scalp: A histochemical study. J Invest Dermatol 60:126–133, 1973.
46. Fazekas AG, Sandor T: The metabolism of dehydroepiandrosterone by human scalp hair follicles. J Clin Endocrinol Metab 36:582–586, 1973.
47. Sawaya ME, Honig LS, Garland LD, Hsia SL: Δ^5-3β-Hydroxysteroid dehydrogenase activity in sebaceous glands of scalp in male-pattern baldness. J Invest Dermatol 91:101–105, 1988.
48. Sawaya ME, Price VH, Harris KA: Human hair follicle aromatase activity in females with androgenetic alopecia. J Invest Dermatol 94(4):575, 1990.
49. Wright F, Giacomini M: Reduction of dihydrotestosterone to androstanediols by human female skin *in vitro.* J Steroid Biochem 13:639–643, 1980.
50. Schweikert HU, Wilson JD: Regulation of human hair growth by steroid hormones: II. Androstenedione metabolism in isolated hairs. J Clin Endocrinol Metab 39:1012–1019, 1974.
51. Kuttenn F, Mowszowicz I, Schaison G, Mauvais-Jarvis P: Androgen production and skin metabolism in hirsutism. J Endocrinol 75:83–91, 1977.
52. Keenan BS et al.: Syndrome of androgen insensitivity in man: Absence of 5α-dihydrotestosterone binding protein in skin fibroblasts. J Clin Endocrinol Metab 38:1143–1146, 1974.
53. King RJB: Structure and function of steroid receptors. J Endocrinol 114:341–349, 1987.
54. Eil C, Edelson SK: The use of human skin fibroblasts to obtain potency estimates of drug binding to androgen receptors. J Clin Endocrinol Metab 59:51–55, 1984.
55. Metcalf BW, Levy MA, Holt DA: Inhibitors of steroid 5α-reductase in benign prostatic hyperplasia, male pattern baldness and acne. Trends in Pharm Sci 10:491–495, 1989.
56. Moore RJ, Gazak JM, Wilson JD: Regulation of cytoplasmic dihydrotestosterone binding in dog prostate by 17β-estradiol. J Clin Invest 63:351–357, 1979.
57. McPhaul MJ, Marcelli M: Molecular defects in the androgen receptor causing androgen resistance. J Invest Dermatol 98:97S–99S, 1992.
58. Choudhry R et al.: Localization of androgen receptors in human skin by immunohistochemistry: Implications for the hormonal regulation of hair growth, sebaceous glands and sweat glands. J Endocrinol 133:467–475, 1992.
59. Randall VA, Thornton MJ, Messenger AG: Cultured dermal papilla cells from androgen-dependent human hair follicles (e.g., beard) contain more androgen receptors than those from non-balding areas of scalp. J Endocrinol 133:141–147, 1992.
60. Sawaya ME, Honig LS, Hsia SL: Increased androgen binding capacity in sebaceous glands in scalp of male-pattern baldness. J Invest Dermatol 92:91–95, 1988.
61. Sawaya ME, Mendez AJ, Lewis LA, Hsia SL: Two forms of androgen receptor protein in human hair follicles and sebaceous glands: Variation in transitional and bald scalp (abstract). J Invest Dermatol 90:606, 1988.
62. Adachi K, Kano M: Adenyl cyclase in human hair follicles: Its inhibition by dihydrotestosterone. Biochem Biophys Res Commun 41(4):884–890, 1970.
63. Adachi K et al.: Human hair follicles: Metabolism and control mechanisms. J Soc Cosmet Chem 21:901–924, 1970.
64. Fazekas AG, Sandor T: Metabolism of androgens by isolated human hair follicles. J Steroid Biochem 3:485–491, 1972.

65. Kirschner MA, Zucker IR, Jespersen D: Idiopathic hirsutism: An ovarian abnormality. N Engl J Med 294:637–640, 1976.
66. Yen SSC: The polycystic ovary syndrome. Clin Endocrinol 12:177–208, 1980.
67. Barbieri RL, Smith S, Ryan KJ: The role of hyperinsulinemia in the pathogenesis of ovarian hyperandrogenism. Fertil Steril 50:197–212, 1988.
68. Ehrmann DA et al.: Detection of functional ovarian hyperandrogenism in women with androgen excess. N Engl J Med 327:157–162, 1992.
69. Hatch R, Rosenfield RL, Kim MH, Tredway D: Hirsutism: Implications, etiology, and management. Am J Obstet Gynecol 140:815–830, 1981.
70. Cutler GB Jr, Laue L: Congenital adrenal hyperplasia due to 21-hydroxylase deficiency. N Engl J Med 323:1806–1813, 1990.
71. Lucky AW et al.: Adrenal androgen hyperresponsiveness to adrenocorticotropin in women with acne and/or hirsutism: Adrenal enzyme defects and exaggerated adrenarche. J Clin Endocrinol Metab 62:840–848, 1986.
72. Bongiovanni AM: Acquired adrenal hyperplasia: With special reference to 3β-hydroxysteroid dehydrogenase. Fertil Steril 35:599–608, 1981.
73. Siegel SF, Finegold DN, Lanes R, Lee PA: ACTH stimulation tests and plasma dehydroepiandrosterone sulfate levels in women with hirsutism. N Engl J Med 323:849–854, 1990.
74. Azziz R, Zacur HA: 21-Hydroxylase deficiency in female hyperandrogenism: Screening and diagnosis. J Clin Endocrinol Metab 69:577–584, 1989.
75. Glickman SP, Rosenfield RL, Bergenstal RM, Helke J: Multiple androgenic abnormalities, including elevated free testosterone, in hyperprolactinemic women. J Clin Endocrinol Metab 55:251–257, 1982.
76. Vermeulen A, Andó S, Verdonck L: Prolactinomas, testosterone-binding globulin, and androgen metabolism. J Clin Endocrinol Metab 54:409–412, 1982.
77. Serafini P, Lobo RA: Prolactin modulates peripheral androgen metabolism. Fertil Steril 45:41–46, 1986.
78. Edwards O, Rook A: Androgen-dependent cutaneous syndromes. In Rook A, Savin J (eds): *Recent Advances in Dermatology.* Edinburgh, Churchill Livingstone, 1980, pp 159–183.
79. Thorner MO, Besser GM: Hyperprolactinaemia and gonadal function: Results of bromocriptine treatment. In Crosignani PG, Robyn C (eds): *Prolactin and Human Reproduction.* London, Academic Press, 1977, pp 285–301.
80. Kasick JM, Bergfeld WF, Steck WD, Gupta MK: Adrenal androgenic female-pattern alopecia: Sex hormones and the balding woman. Cleve Clin Q 50:111–122, 1983.
81. Schmidt JB: Endokrine Konstellation bei der Androgenetischen Alopezie der Frau. Wien Klin Wochenschr 99:21–24, 1987.
82. DeVillez RL, Dunn J: Female androgenic alopecia: The 3α, 17β-androstanediol glucuronide/sex hormone binding globulin ratio as a possible marker for female pattern baldness. Arch Dermatol 122:1011–1015, 1986.
83. Miller JA et al.: Low sex-hormone binding globulin levels in young women with diffuse hair loss. Br J Dermatol 106:331–336, 1982.
84. Georgala G, Papasotiriou V, Stavropoulos P: Serum testosterone and sex hormone binding globulin levels in women with androgenetic alopecia. Acta Derm Venereol (Stockh) 66:532–534, 1986.
85. Rittmaster RS et al.: Effect of MK-906, a specific 5α-reductase inhibitor, on serum androgens and androgen conjugates in normal men. J Androl 10:259–262, 1989.
86. Uno H: Nonhuman primate model of baldness: Premature aging of hair follicle and hormones. Int J Dermatol 21:21–23, 1982.
87. Takashima I, Adachi K, Montagna W: Studies of common baldness in the stumptailed macaque. J Invest Dermatol 55:329–334, 1970.
88. Adachi K: The metabolism and control mechanism of human hair follicles. Curr Probl Dermatol 5:37–78, 1973.
89. Cotton SG, Nixon JM, Carpenter RG, Evans DW: Factors discriminating men with coronary heart disease from healthy control. Br Heart J 34:458–464, 1972.
90. Lesko SM, Rosenberg L, Shapiro S: A case-control study of baldness in relation to myocardial infarction in men. JAMA 269:998–1003, 1993.
91. Cooke NT: Male pattern alopecia and coronary artery disease in men. Br J Dermatol 101:455–458, 1979.
92. Halim MMB et al.: Myocardial infarction, androgen and the skin. Br J Dermatol 98:63–68, 1978.
93. Comaish S: Metabolic disorders and hair growth. Br J Dermatol 84:83–86, 1971.
94. Rushton DH, Ramsay ID: The importance of adequate serum ferritin levels during oral cyproterone acetate and ethinyl oestradiol treatment of diffuse androgen-dependent alopecia in women. Clin Endocrinol 36:421–427, 1992.
95. Olsen EA, DeLong E, Weiner MS: Effect of time on male pattern baldness (reply). J Am Acad Dermatol 16:393–394, 1987.
96. Olsen EA, DeLong E: Transdermal viprostol in the treatment of male pattern baldness. J Am Acad Dermatol 23:470–472, 1990.
97. Casey JH, Moxham A, Nabarro JDN: Idiopathic hirsutism: Seasonal variation of hair-growth and response to estrogen administration. Lancet 1:587–588, 1964.
98. Price VH, Menefee E: Quantitative estimation of hair growth: I. Androgenetic alopecia in women: Effect of minoxidil. J Invest Dermatol 95:683–687, 1990.
99. Olsen EA, Weiner MS, DeLong ER, Pinnell S: Topical minoxidil in early male pattern baldness. J Am Acad Dermatol 13:185–192, 1985.
100. Linas SL, Nies AS: Minoxidil. Ann Intern Med 94:61–65, 1981.
101. Parker LN, Lifrak ET, Odell WD: Lack of a gonadal or adrenal androgenic mechanism for the hypertrichosis produced by diazoxide, phenytoin and minoxidil. Biochem Pharmacol 31:1948–1950, 1982.
102. Olsen EA: Treatment of androgenetic alopecia with topical minoxidil. Res Staff Phys 35:53–69, 1989.
103. Wester RC, Maibach HI, Guy RH, Novak E: Minoxidil stimulates cutaneous blood flow in human balding scalps: Pharmacodynamics measured by laser Doppler velocimetry and photopulse plethysmography. J Invest Dermatol 82:515–517, 1984.
104. Cohen RL et al.: Direct effects of minoxidil on epidermal cells in culture. J Invest Dermatol 82:90–93, 1984.
105. Baden HP, Kubilus J: Effect of minoxidil on cultured keratinocytes. J Invest Dermatol 81:558–560, 1983.
106. Buhl AE, Waldon DJ, Kawabe TT, Holland JM: Minoxidil stimulates mouse vibrissae follicles in organ culture. J Invest Dermatol 92:315–320, 1989.
107. Uno H, Cappas A, Brigham P: Increased DNA Synthesis of the hair follicular and perifollicular cells by topical minoxidil in the macaque scalp. J Invest Dermatol 84:358, 1985.
108. Kiesewetter F, Langer P, Schell H: Minoxidil stimulates mouse vibrissae follicles in organ culture (letter). J Invest Dermatol 96:295–296, 1991.
109. Buhl AE: Minoxidil's action in hair follicles. J Invest Dermatol 96:73S–74S, 1991.

110. Uno H, Cappas A, Schlagel C: Cyclic dynamics of hair follicles and the effect of minoxidil on the bald scalps of stumptailed macaques. Am J Dermatopathol 7:283–297, 1985.

110a. Olsen EA, Pinnell SR, Weiner MS, DeLong MS: Evaluation technics for male pattern baldness (Reply). J AM Acad Dermatol 14:850–851, 1986.

111. Olsen EA, DeLong ER, Weiner MS: Long-term follow-up of men with male pattern baldness treated with topical minoxidil. J Am Acad Dermatol 16:688–695, 1987.

112. Olsen EA, Weiner MS, Amara IA, DeLong ER: Five-year follow-up of men with androgenetic alopecia treated with topical minoxidil. J Am Acad Dermatol 22:643–646, 1990.

113. Olsen EA, Weiner MS: Topical minoxidil in male pattern baldness: Effects of discontinuation of treatment. J Am Acad Dermatol 17:97–101, 1987.

114. Olsen EA, DeLong ER, Weiner MS: Dose-response study of topical minoxidil in male pattern baldness. J Am Acad Dermatol 15:30–37, 1986.

115. Fiedler-Weiss VC: Topical minoxidil solution (1% and 5%) in the treatment of alopecia areata. J Am Acad Dermatol 16:745–748, 1987.

116. Bazzano GS, Terezakis N, Galen W: Topical tretinoin for hair growth promotion. J Am Acad Dermatol 15:880–883, 1986.

117. Burton JL, Schutt WH, Caldwell IW: Hypertrichosis due to diazoxide. Br J Dermatol 93:707–711, 1975.

118. Moore PF: The effects of diazoxide and benzothiadiazine diuretics upon phosphodiesterase. Ann NY Acad Sci 150:256–260, 1968.

119. Wei C-T, Wong C-K, Hashimoto K: A clinical trial of 3% diazoxide solution for androgenetic alopecia. Dermatologica Sinica 7(7):209–212, 1989.

120. Dorfman RI: Biological activity of antiandrogens. Br J Dermatol 82(suppl 6):3–8, 1970.

121. Sciarra F, Toscano V, Concolino G, Di Silverio F: Antiandrogens: Clinical applications. J Steroid Biochem Mol Biol 37:349–362, 1990.

122. Moguilewsky M, Bouton MM: How the study of the biological activities of antiandrogens can be oriented towards the clinic. J Steroid Biochem 31:699–710, 1988.

123. Ford LC et al.: Determination of estrogen and androgen receptors in *Trichomonas vaginalis* and the effects of antihormones. Am J Obstet Gynecol 156:1119–1121, 1987.

124. Wiechers JW, Herder RE, Drenth BFH, de Zeeuw RA: Percutaneous absorption, disposition, metabolism, and excretion of ^{14}C-labelled cyoctol in humans after a single dermal application. Int J Pharmacol 65:77–84, 1990.

124a. Strick RA, Burnison C, Orenberg EK: Treatment of androgenic alopecia with cyoctol—a topical antiandrogen. American Academy of Dermatology presentation. December, 1989.

125. Vermorken AJM, Goos CMAA, Roelofs HMJ: A method for the evaluation of the local antiandrogenic action of 5α-reductase inhibitors on human skin. Br J Dermatol 102:695–701, 1980.

126. Wright F, Kirchhoffer M-O, Mauvais-Jarvis P: Antagonist action of dihydroprogesterone on the formation of the specific dihydrotestosterone-cytoplasmic receptor complex in rat ventral prostate. J Steroid Biochem 10:419–422, 1979.

127. Rittmaster RS: Topical antiandrogens in the treatment of male-pattern baldness. Clin Dermatol 6:122–128, 1988.

128. Orentreich N, Durr NP: Biology of scalp hair growth. Clin Plast Surg 9:197–205, 1982.

129. Frieden IJ, Price VH: Androgenetic alopecia. In Thiers BH, Dobson RL (eds): *Pathogenesis of Skin Disease.* New York, Churchill Livingstone, 1986, pp 41–55.

130. Tamm J, Seckelmann M, Volkwein U, Ludwig E: The effect of the antiandrogen 11α-hydroxyprogesterone on sebum production and cholesterol concentration of sebum. Br J Dermatol 107:63–70, 1982.

131. van der Willigen AH, Peereboom-Wynia JDR, van Joost T, Stolz E: A preliminary study of the effect of 11α-hydroxyprogesterone on the hair growth in men suffering from androgenetic alopecia. Acta Derm Venereol (Stockh) 67:82–85, 1987.

132. Orfanos CE, Vogels L: Lokaltherapie der Alopecia Androgenetica mit 17α-Östradiol. Dermatologica 161:124–132, 1980.

133. Tremblay RR: Treatment of hirsutism with spironolactone. Clin Endocrinol Metab 15:363–371, 1986.

134. Lobo RA et al.: The effects of two doses of spironolactone on serum androgens and anagen hair in hirsute women. Fertil Steril 43:200–205, 1985.

135. Menard RH, Guenthner TM, Kon H, Gillette JR: Studies on the destruction of adrenal and testicular cytochrome P-450 by spironolactone. J Biol Chem 254:1726–1733, 1979.

136. Loriaux DL et al.: Spironolactone and endocrine dysfunction (NIH conference). Ann Intern Med 85:630–636, 1976.

137. Corvol P et al.: Antiandrogenic effect of spirolactones: Mechanism of action. Endocrinology 97:52–58, 1975.

138. Namer M: Clinical applications of antiandrogens. J Steroid Biochem 31:719–729, 1988.

139. Rushton DH et al.: Quantitative assessment of spironolactone treatment in women with diffuse androgen-dependent alopecia. J Soc Cosmet Chem 42:317–325, 1991.

140. Burke BM, Cunliffe WJ: Oral spironolactone therapy for female patients with acne, hirsutism or androgenic alopecia (letter). Br J Dermatol 112:124–125, 1985.

141. Hammerstein J et al.: Use of cyproterone acetate (CPA) in the treatment of acne, hirsutism and virilism. J Steroid Biochem 6:827–836, 1975.

142. Takayasu S: Effect of antiandrogens on the binding of androgen to cytosol and nuclei of hamster sebaceous glands. Arch Dermatol Res 264:49–54, 1979.

143. Mortimer CH, Rushton H, James KC: Effective medical treatment for common baldness in women. Clin Exp Dermatol 9:342–350, 1984.

144. Ekoe JM, Burckhardt P, Ruedi B: Treatment of hirsutism, acne and alopecia with cyproterone acetate. Dermatologica 160:398–404, 1980.

145. Dawber RPR, Sonnex T, Ralfs I: Oral anti-androgen treatment of common baldness in women. Br J Dermatol 107(suppl 22):20, 1982.

146. Moltz L, Meckies J, Hammerstein J: Die Kontrazeptive Betreuung Androgenisierter Frauen mit Einem Niedrig Dosierten Cyproteronacetathaltigen Einphasenpräparat. Dtsch Med Wochenschr 104:1376–1382, 1979.

147. Braendle W et al.: Wirkung und Nebenwirkung der Cyproteronacetatbehandlung. Arch Gynäk 216:335–345, 1974.

148. Neumann F: Pharmacology and potential use of cyproterone acetate. Horm Metab Res 9:1–13, 1977.

149. Tindall DJ, Chang CH, Lobl TJ, Cunningham GR: Androgen antagonists in androgen target tissues. Pharmacol Ther 24:367–400, 1984.

150. Radwanski E, Perentesis G, Symchowicz S, Zampaglione N: Single and multiple dose pharmacokinetic evaluation of flutamide in normal geriatric volunteers. J Clin Pharmacol 29:554–558, 1989.

151. Katchen B, Dancik S, Millington G: Percutaneous pene-

tration and metabolism of topical [^{14}C] flutamide in men. J Invest Dermatol 66:379–382, 1976.
152. *Physicians' Desk Reference.* Medical Economics Data, Montvale, NJ, 1993.
153. Cusan L et al.: Treatment of hirsutism with the pure antiandrogen flutamide. J Am Acad Dermatol 23:462–469, 1990.
154. Strauss JS, Kligman AM: The effect of progesterone and progesterone-like compounds on the human sebaceous gland. J Invest Dermatol 36:309–319, 1961.
155. Feldman M, Burton ME: Histamine$_2$-receptor antagonists: Standard therapy for acid-peptic diseases. N Engl J Med 323:1672–1680, 1990.
156. Galbraith RA, Michnovicz JJ: The effects of cimetidine on the oxidative metabolism of estradiol. N Engl J Med 321:269–274, 1989.
157. Winters SJ, Banks JL, Loriaux DL: Cimetidine is an antiandrogen in the rat. Gastroenterology 76:504–508, 1979.
158. Aram H: Treatment of female androgenetic alopecia with cimetidine. Int J Dermatol 26:128–130, 1987.
159. Sonino N: The use of ketoconazole as an inhibitor of steroid production. N Engl J Med 317:812–818, 1987.
160. Stoner E: The clinical development of a 5α-reductase inhibitor, finasteride. J Steroid Biochem Mol Biol 37:375–378, 1990.
161. Rittmaster RS et al.: The effects of N,N-diethyl-4-methyl-3-oxo-4-aza-5α-androstane-17β-carboxamide, a 5α-reductase inhibitor and antiandrogen, on the development of baldness in the stumptail macaque. J Clin Endocrinol Metab 65:188–193, 1987.
162. Diani AR et al.: Hair growth effects of oral administration of finasteride, a steroid 5α-reductase inhibitor, alone and in combination with topical minoxidil in the balding stumptail macaque. J Clin Endocrinol Metab 74:345–350, 1992.
163. Matias JR, Malloy VL, Orentreich N: Synergistic antiandrogenic effects of topical combinations of 5α-reductase and androgen receptor inhibitors in the hamster sebaceous glands. J Invest Dermatol 91:429–433, 1988.
164. Verhoeven G, Cailleau J: Inhibition by a 4-methyl-4-aza-steroid of NADPH: Δ^4-3-oxosteroid-5α-oxido-reductase activity in cultured interstitial cells derived from immature rat testis. J Steroid Biochem 18:365–367, 1983.
165. Mestman JH, Anderson GV, Nelson DH: Adrenal-pituitary responsiveness during therapy with an oral contraceptive. Obstet Gynecol 31:378–386, 1968.

Chapter

12

CICATRICIAL ALOPECIA (AND OTHER CAUSES OF PERMANENT ALOPECIA)

*MAJ Dirk M. Elston, MC, USA, and Wilma F. Bergfeld**

INTRODUCTION

The evaluation of permanent alopecia is commonly a source of frustration for the physician. In this chapter, the authors will guide the physician through the maze of clinical entities which may eventuate in permanent alopecia. Particular emphasis will be placed on histological findings, because biopsy is often key to the diagnosis.

Biopsy should be an early step in the evaluation of any case suspected to represent scarring alopecia. A 4-mm punch biopsy generally provides a sufficient number of hair follicles for examination. It is also relatively easy for the dermatopathology technician to orient a 4-mm punch specimen (as compared to a 3-mm punch). Smaller specimens may prove unsatisfactory. Ideally, in straight-haired patients, the biopsy punch should be placed diagonally on the scalp to follow the direction of the hair fiber. In curly haired individuals, the punch is placed perpendicular to the skin surface. In most cases of inflammatory hair loss, the biopsy should be performed in an area of active hair destruction (e.g., a boggy plaque or toward the edge of the alopecic patch). In cases of noninflammatory alopecia, a biopsy anywhere within the alopecic patch is generally adequate.

In general, biopsies should be submitted for routine microscopy and immunofluorescent studies. The formalin-fixed, paraffin-embedded tissue should be stained with hematoxylin and eosin (H&E) and an elastic tissue stain. An elastic tissue stain is necessary to evaluate the presence or absence of a true scar. A periodic acid–Schiff (PAS) stain will highlight basement membrane thickening, fungal organisms, and apoptotic cells in catagen follicles and is particularly useful to perform in suspected cases of lu-

*The opinions expressed are those of the authors and are not to be construed as official or as representing those of the United States Army or the Department of Defense.

pus erythematosus, tinea capitis, and trichotillomania.

Specimens may be sectioned vertically or horizontally. The major advantage of horizontal sections is that many follicles can be examined in a single section. If multiple levels are examined, however, vertical sections can yield the same information. Although horizontal sections are being used more and more, many dermatologists remain less comfortable with horizontal sections. Therefore, for teaching purposes, the histology of vertical sections of scalp biopsies will be presented here.

Many practitioners regard the evaluation and classification of hair disorders as one of the more confusing areas of dermatology. One source of confusion is the term *scarring alopecia* itself. Some conditions destroy the hair follicle and surrounding connective tissue, producing a true scar. However, other conditions, traditionally grouped under the heading "*scarring* alopecia," may produce permanent alopecia without a true histological scar (see later text). In these cases, it is better to replace the term *scarring alopecia* with the descriptive clinical term *permanent alopecia.*

A scar results when tissue is destroyed and replaced with collagen (reparative fibrosis). True scars differ from hyalinizing processes such as scleroderma, in which collagen bundles become thickened and hyalinized but connective tissue is not destroyed. Elastic tissue stains easily differentiate true scarring alopecia from hyalinizing alopecia. In true scars, elastic tissue is absent (Fig. 12-1). Areas of hyalinized dermis may appear similar to true scars in H&E-stained sections, but an elastic tissue stain will demonstrate a normal number and distribution of elastic fibers.

Recent evidence suggests that hair follicle stem cells (the cells responsible for regrowth of the anagen follicle) reside in the bulge area of the hair follicle. The bulge area is located in the midportion of the follicle at the arrector pili attachment site (the lower end of the "permanent portion of the follicle"). Ultrastructural studies have demonstrated that the cells in this area are relatively undifferentiated.[1] The bulge area represents a slow-cycling population of cells which can be stimulated to proliferate by a variety of physical and chemical stimuli.[1] Cell proliferation in the bulge area at the onset of anagen phase has been demonstrated by tritiated thymidine labeling.[2] *Middermal scarring or hyalinization with destruction of the bulge area is the histological hallmark of permanent alopecia.*

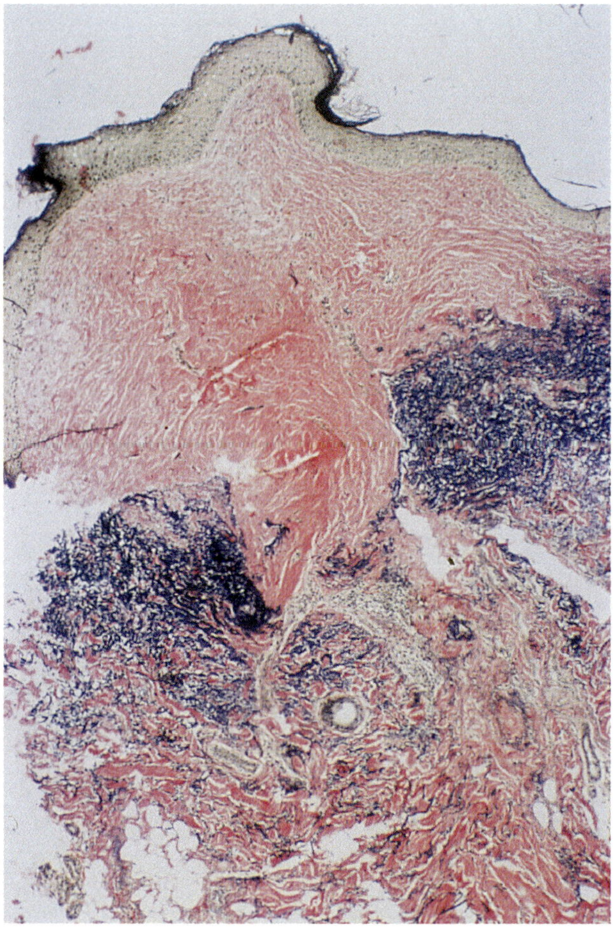

Figure 12-1 True histological scar: absence of elastic fibers in the upper dermis. (Scalp biopsy, elastic stain ×100)

A classification of the causes of permanent alopecia is offered in Table 12-1. Included are causes of true scarring alopecia, conditions which result in a hyalinized dermis and involution of the hair follicle, and genetic disorders resulting in permanent alopecia. Permanent alopecia may be divided into inflammatory and noninflammatory types. Causes of inflammatory alopecia include chronic cutaneous lupus erythematosus, lichen planopilaris, inflammatory pseudopelade, and infectious disorders. Noninflammatory causes of permanent alopecia include developmental, hereditary, and neoplastic conditions. The clinical and histological presentation and treatment of these and unclassified

Table 12-1
CAUSES OF PERMANENT ALOPECIA

Inflammatory	*Noninflammatory*
NONINFECTIOUS	AUTOIMMUNE
Autoimmune bullous disorders	Pseudopelade
Cicatricial pemphigoid	DEVELOPMENTAL/HEREDITARY
Epidermolysis bullosa acquisita	Alopecia triangularis
Chemical and physical agents	Aplasia cutis congenita
Mechanical trauma	Baraitser's syndrome
Chemical and thermal burns	Darier's disease
Radiation injury	Ectodermal dysplasia
Dermatomyositis	Epidermal nevi*
Eosinophilic cellulitis	Epidermolysis bullosa
Lichen planopilaris	Facial hemiatrophy*
Graham-Little syndrome	Follicular atrophoderma/BCC (Bazex)
Lichen sclerosus et atrophicus	Follicular keratoses syndromes*
Lupus erythematosus	Hair follicle hamartomas (see also neoplastic)
Mixed inflammatory destructive alopecia	Hallermann-Streiff syndrome
Necrobiosis lipoidica	Ichthyosis
Perifolliculitis capitis abscedens et suffodiens	Incontinentia pigmenti*
Pseudopelade	Pachyonychia congenita
Pyoderma gangrenosum	Polyostotic fibrous dysplasia
Sarcoidosis	Porokeratosis
Scleroderma variants	Rothmund-Thomson syndrome
Traction	NEOPLASTIC
Trichotillomania	Benign
Vasculitis	Adnexal tumors
INFECTIOUS	Hair follicle hamartomas
Bacterial folliculitis	Syringoma
Fungal infections	Angiomas
Tinea/kerion	Keloid
Favus	Malignant
Herpetic folliculitis	Angiosarcoma
Protozoan infections (leishmaniasis)	Basal cell carcinoma
Syphilis	Metastatic disease
HYPERSENSITIVITY-RELATED PUSTULAR DISORDERS	Mycosis fungoides
Erosive pustular dermatosis	Follicular mucinosis
Folliculitis decalvans	Squamous cell carcinoma
	UNCLASSIFIED
	Unclassified alopecia seen in black women (including the follicular degeneration syndrome)

*May also demonstrate inflammatory infiltrates.

causes of alopecia such as the recently described "follicular degeneration syndrome" will be discussed.

CLINICAL AND HISTOLOGICAL PRESENTATION

Lupus Erythematosus

Chronic cutaneous lupus erythematosus (Fig. 12-2) accounts for about 30 to 40 percent of cases of inflammatory, true scarring alopecia. The condition occurs more frequently in females than in males and is more common in adults than in children. Associated systemic lupus erythematosus may or may not be present. Occasionally, subacute cutaneous lupus erythematosus may produce a permanent alopecia.

Patients with systemic lupus erythematosus (SLE) may have discoid lesions of the scalp, resulting in patches of true scarring alopecia, as well as short frontal "lupus hairs."[3] The generalized hair loss seen in systemic lupus erythematosus is usually the result of a telogen effluvium. Occasionally, however, patients with severe sys-

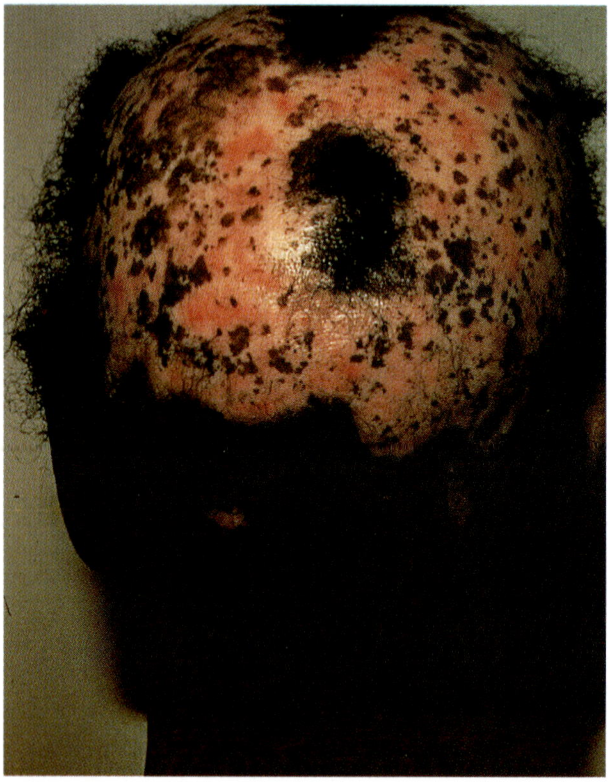

Figure 12-2 Lupus erythematosus.

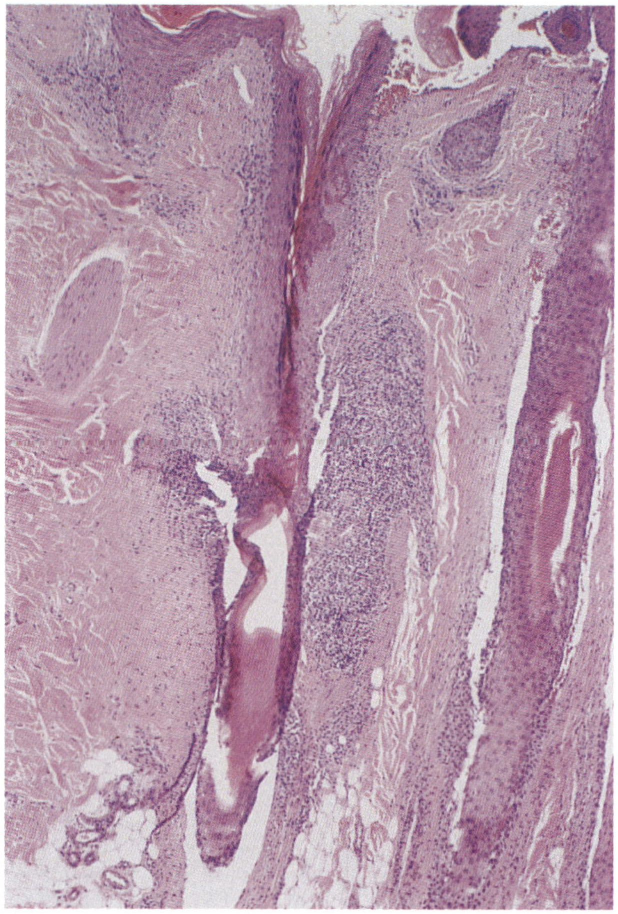

Figure 12-3 Lupus erythematosus. Perifollicular lymphoid aggregates. (Scalp biopsy, H&E stain ×100)

temic lupus will experience an anagen effluvium (W. Bergfeld, D. Elston, unpublished data). In anagen effluvium, episodes of severe illness result in a temporary shutdown of the hair matrix, producing a narrowed segment of hair shaft (similar to a Beau's line of the nail). This narrowed segment is prone to fracture. The mechanisms which produce generalized hair loss in systemic lupus do not result in scarring.

Scalp lesions of chronic cutaneous lupus erythematosus may be red, pink, or violaceous, with variable atrophy and mottled areas of hyper- and hypopigmentation. Keratin plugging of follicular orifices may be noted clinically. Alopecic patches without clinically appreciable inflammation may also occur. These "clinically noninflammatory" patches may resemble alopecia areata or pseudopelade. The presence of other, more typical lesions of cutaneous lupus erythematosus may suggest the diagnosis of lupus in these cases.

As with most causes of permanent alopecia, biopsy is often critical in establishing a diagnosis. Histological features include vacuolar degeneration of the basal cell layer and a moderate to dense perivascular and periadnexal lymphoid infiltrate (Fig. 12-3). Lymphocytes may be present within follicular epithelium. An increase in dermal mucin may be noted. In some cases, a lichenoid dermatitis may be observed at the skin surface. Colloid bodies may be seen, although generally in smaller numbers than in lichen planus[4] (see Table 12-2). Rarely, changes of leukocytoclastic vasculitis or lymphocytic panniculitis (lupus profundus) may be present. Clinically *"noninflammatory"* alopecic patches fail to demonstrate superficial inflammation (interface dermatitis). Deeper inflammation is present, however. Generally, perifollicular lymphoid infiltrates or infiltrates within fibrous tracts are present.* Hair fiber granulomas may be noted in

*Fibrous tracts represent the connective tissue associated with follicular epithelium. During the normal telogen phase, and in alopecia, fibrous tracts mark the location where an anagen follicle once resided.

Table 12-2
HISTOLOGICAL FEATURES OF SOME PERMANENT ALOPECIAS

	Early	*Late-Stage*	*True Scarring*
Lupus Erythematosus	Basilar vacuolopathy; perifollicular infiltrate; perivascular infiltrate; +/– dermal mucin; BMZ thickening; *linear/granular IgG/C3*	+/– Hair fiber granulomas; decreased number of follicles; fibrosis	Present
Lichen Planopilaris	Lichenoid interface change; perifollicular infiltrate; *globular immunoreactants adjacent to follicles**	+/– Hair fiber granulomas; decreased number of follicles; fibrosis	Present
Mixed Inflammatory	Vacuolar/lichenoid change; infiltrate in fibrous tracts; *granular/linear and globular immunoreactants*	+/– Hair fiber granulomas; decreased number of follicles; fibrosis	Present
Pseudopelade	+/– Inflammation, perifollicular and within fibrous tracts	Decreased number of follicles; hyalinized dermis	Absent*
Morphea	Perivascular infiltrate deep dermis/panniculus	Decreased number of follicles; hyalinized dermis	Absent

* See text.

the deeper portion of the fibrous tracts. Hair fiber granulomas may be seen in any destructive alopecia (Fig. 12-4). Late-stage, "burned-out" lesions demonstrate absence of hair follicles and reparative fibrosis with an absence of elastic fibers (i.e., true scar formation). The PAS stain is helpful in demonstrating the thickening of the basement membrane zone which may occur in chronic lesions.

Direct immunofluorescent studies most commonly demonstrate granular deposits of IgG and C3 at the dermoepidermal junction of the surface epithelium and at the junction of the dermis and follicular epithelium (Fig. 12-5).[4–6] Occasionally, globular deposits of IgM, corresponding to colloid bodies seen on light microscopy, may be found at the dermoepidermal junction but never deep in the dermis adjacent to hair follicles. In contrast to lichen planopilaris, when globular immune deposits are seen in lupus, they tend to be few in number and are not grouped.[4] Occasionally, in a clinically "noninflammatory" lesion, a telogen follicle may be present which demonstrates linear deposition of immunoreactants.

The results of histological and immunofluorescent studies should always be interpreted in the context of the clinical presentation and the results of serological evaluation. One cannot overemphasize the importance of a global evaluation. Especially when differentiating lupus from lichen planopilaris, reliance on an H&E-stained biopsy alone may result in misdiagnosis. Elastic tissue and PAS stains, immunofluorescent studies, and serological studies will generally allow for a specific diagnosis even in cases with "ambiguous" H&E histology.

Lichen Planopilaris

Lichen planopilaris accounts for approximately 30 to 40 percent of inflammatory alopecia with true scarring (W. Bergfeld, D. Elston, unpublished data). It generally presents as a patchy alopecia in a middle-aged adult. Individual follicular papules or follicular hyperkeratosis may be present (Fig. 12-6). The condition tends to be progressive, and individual patches expand and coalesce. The end stage may be similar in appearance to lupus erythematosus. Any hair-bearing area may be affected.

In some cases of lichen planopilaris, cutaneous or mucosal lesions of lichen planus are present. In the absence of such lesions, the diagnosis may be more challenging. As both clinical and histological features may overlap with those of lupus erythematosus, the diagnosis is best established by the combination of routine histolog-

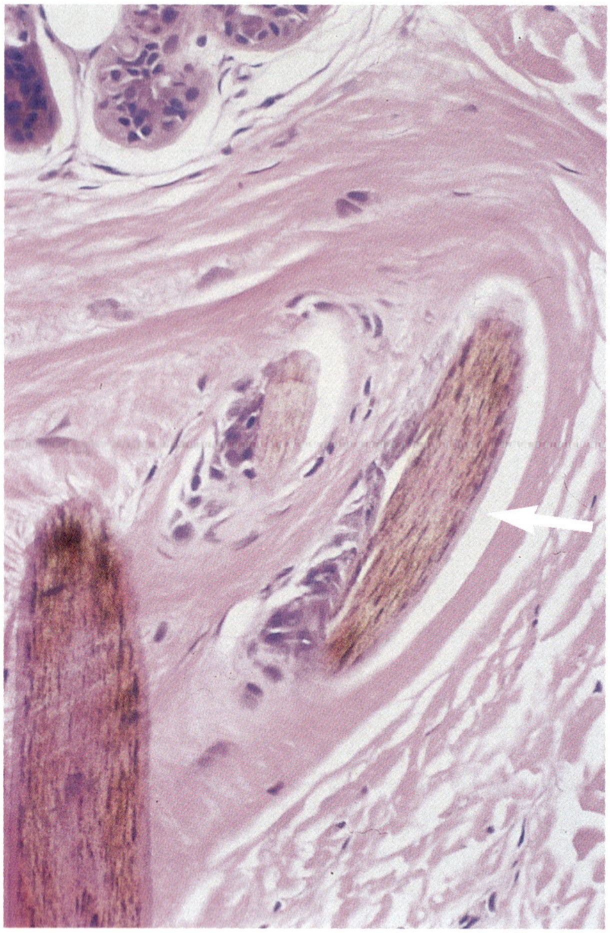

Figure 12-4 Hair fiber granuloma (arrow). (Scalp biopsy, H&E stain ×400)

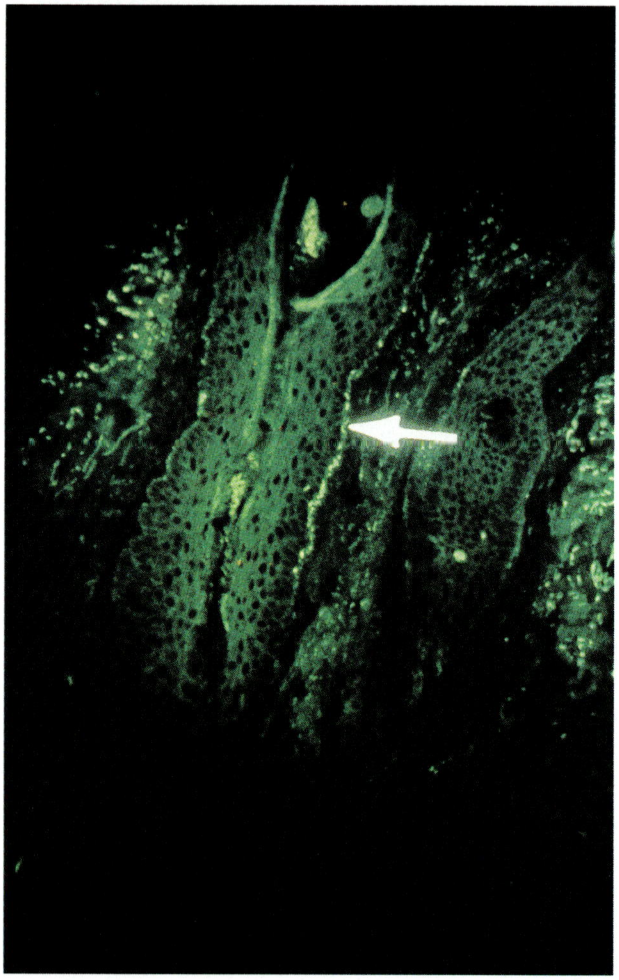

Figure 12-5 Lupus erythematosus. Linear immunofluorescence, IgG at BMZ. (×200)

ical examination and direct immunofluorescent studies. Screening serological tests to help exclude connective tissue disease are recommended.

Histological features of lichen planopilaris include a perifollicular lymphoid infiltrate, often bandlike, with interface changes involving the follicular epithelium (Fig. 12-7).[7] Colloid bodies may be seen adjacent to the follicular epithelium. Although the changes tend to occur in the upper portion of the dermis (top-heavy), deeper infiltrates may occur. Occasionally, overlying epidermal changes of lichen planus (interface dermatitis, sawtooth rete ridges, hypergranulosis, and Civatte bodies) may be seen (Fig. 12-8). Later, hair fiber granulomas may be present. End-stage lesions demonstrate reparative fibrosis with absence of elastic fibers—changes similar to those seen in end-stage lupus erythematosus (see

Figure 12-6 Lichen planopilaris.

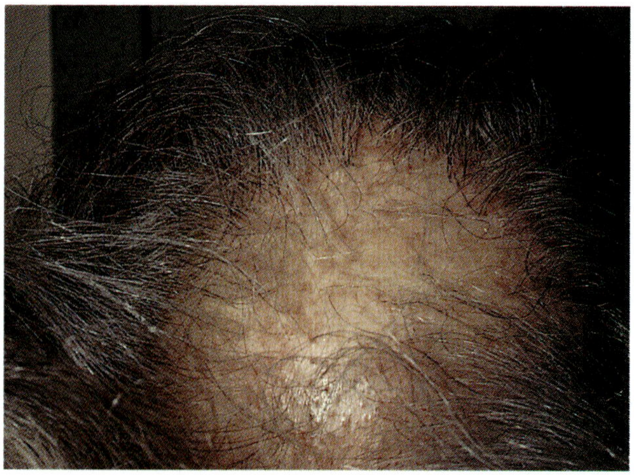

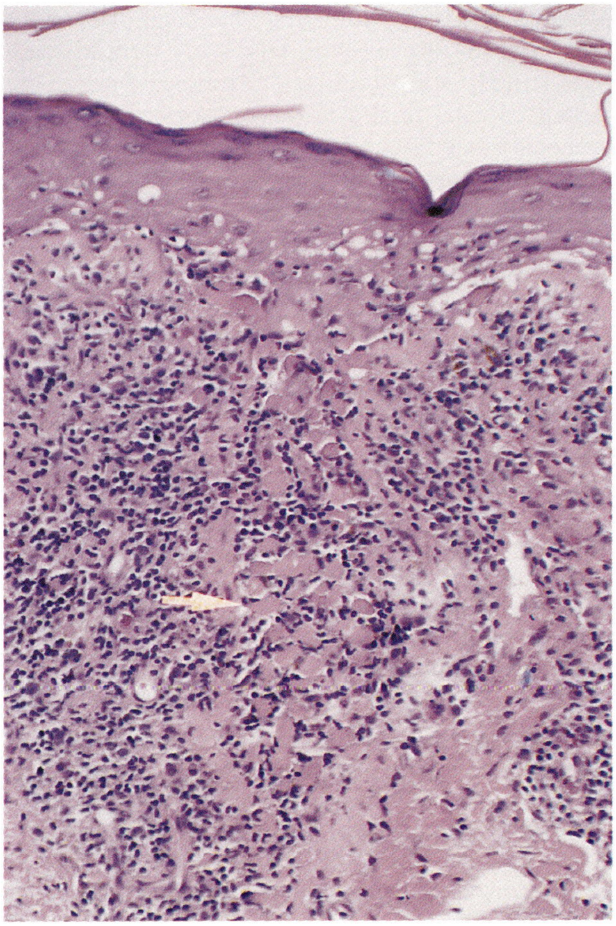

A

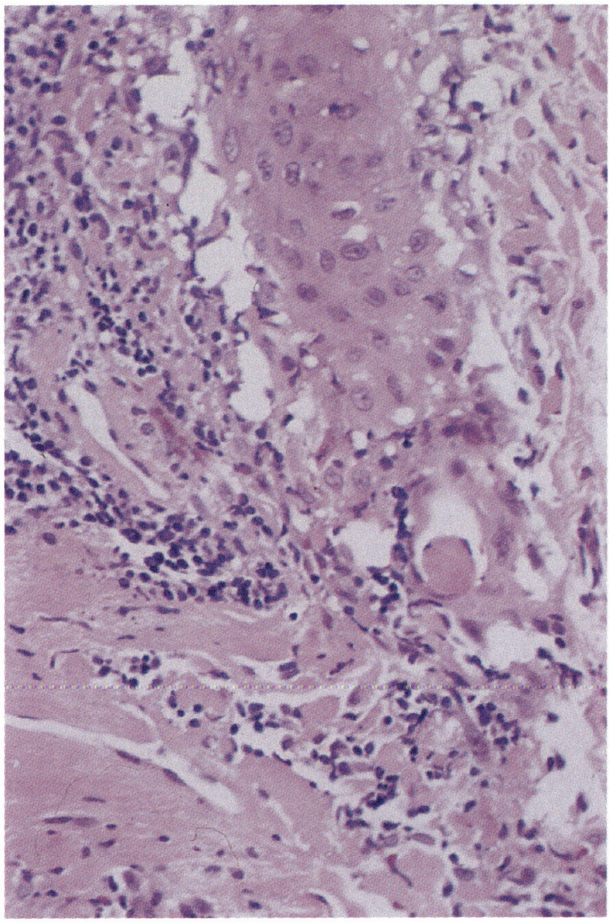

B

Figure 12-7 Lichen planopilaris. (*A*) Arrow points to numerous Civatte bodies in the region of a destroyed follicle. (Scalp biopsy, H&E stain ×200) (*B*) Follicular interface dermatitis. (Scalp biopsy, H&E stain ×400)

Table 12-2). A PAS stain may be helpful in confirming the absence of basement membrane changes.

The most characteristic immunofluorescent finding in cases of lichen planopilaris consists of globular deposits of IgM adjacent to follicular epithelium (Fig. 12-9).[4,5,8] Cases with superficial interface changes of lichen planus demonstrate similar globular deposits at the dermoepidermal junction. Globular deposits deeper within the dermis, adjacent to follicular epithelium, are more specific for lichen planopilaris.[4]

Recently, Ioannides and Bystryn reported linear immunoglobulin deposits restricted to the basement membrane zone of hair follicles in seven of seven patients believed to have lichen planopilaris.[9] Their findings differ from previous observations.[4,5,8] It is tempting to speculate that

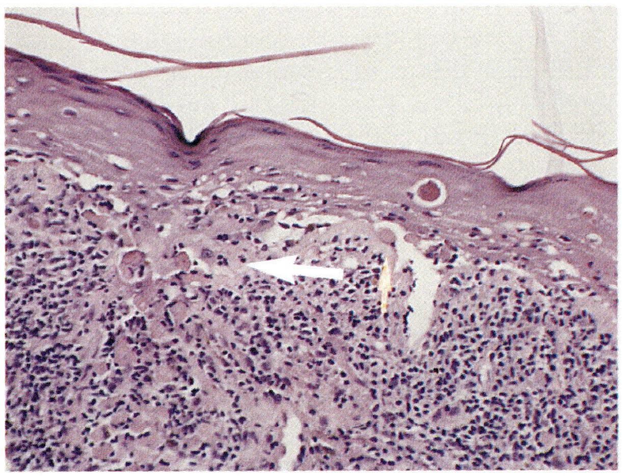

Figure 12-8 Overlying epidermis (lichen planopilaris). Interface dermatitis, many Civatte bodies (arrow). (Scalp biopsy, H&E stain ×200)

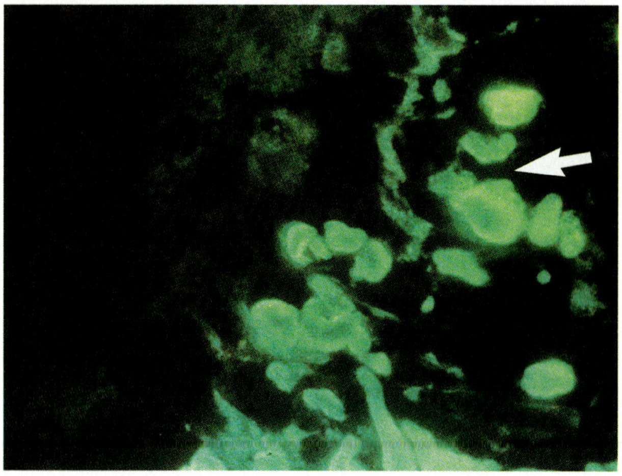

Figure 12-9 Lichen planopilaris. Globular immunofluorescence, IgM (arrow) at follicular-dermal interface (×200)

some (and possibly all) of their cases actually represent cases of lupus erythematosus. The clinical and histological findings in their patients are certainly compatible with lichen planopilaris, i.e., areas of scarring alopecia associated with violaceous to brownish keratotic follicular papules and histological findings of a bandlike infiltrate around follicles, compact orthokeratosis, and zones of hypergranulosis. However, it has been our experience that some cases of lupus can demonstrate considerable clinical and histological overlap with lichen planopilaris. Smith, Grabski, McCollough, and Davis recently published their experience with immunofluorescent findings in seven patients with lichen planopilaris.[10] Four of their seven patients demonstrated cytoid bodies in the upper dermis. Only one demonstrated linear perifollicular C3 and fibrin in addition to cytoid bodies. Of interest, three of four black patients had negative findings on direct immunofluorescence (DIF). One could speculate as to the effects of race, sex, and lesion duration on the DIF results. It is possible that these series distinguish two real and distinct subsets of lichen planopilaris. Further investigation is necessary.

For the present, grouped globular immunofluorescence, especially when seen adjacent to follicular epithelium, is regarded as the characteristic immunofluorescent pattern in lichen planopilaris. It is important to remember that lupus can present with clinical features and histology similar to lichen planopilaris, but with linear immunoreactants: long-term follow-up of such patients generally confirms the diagnosis of lupus. Those rare individuals who demonstrate *both* linear and globular immuno*globulins* are classified as "mixed inflammatory destructive alopecia" (see later text). This separate classification will allow for further study of this most interesting group of patients.

Again, one must stress the importance of a global evaluation. Ideally, such an evaluation should include a good history and physical examination together with evaluation of H&E-, PAS-, and elastic tissue–stained sections, and immunofluorescent and serological studies.

GRAHAM-LITTLE SYNDROME

The Graham-Little syndrome includes scarring alopecia of the scalp, follicular horny papules, and, in some cases, alopecia of the pubic region, eyebrows, or axillae. The syndrome occurs mostly in adult women. Although in the past this condition has been grouped with pseudopelade,[11] histological and immunofluorescent changes more commonly suggest lichen planopilaris.[7,12–14] The authors prefer to group the Graham-Little syndrome together with lichen planopilaris and use the term *Graham-Little syndrome* to denote the clinical appearance of progressive permanent scalp alopecia associated with horny follicular papules and loss of pubic and/or axillary hair.

Mixed Inflammatory Destructive Alopecia

Occasionally, patients present with overlapping clinical, histological, and immunologic features of lupus erythematosus, lichen planopilaris, and inflammatory pseudopelade. These patients demonstrate negative serological testing for lupus and generally present with small alopecic patches without follicular plugging. The patches, which expand and coalesce, may appear clinically inflammatory or noninflammatory. No other cutaneous lesions are present.

In the acute stage, histological examination reveals a patchy lymphoid infiltrate within the fibrous tracts. Epidermal and follicular epithelium may demonstrate an interface dermatitis with prominent vacuolar degeneration of the basal layer. Hair fiber granulomas may occasionally be seen. End-stage lesions demonstrate widening of the fibrous tracts. True scarring, with absence of elastic fibers, may be seen. Direct immunofluorescent studies demonstrate a mixed pattern with both globular and linear deposits of immunoglobulins.

Mixed inflammatory destructive alopecia may represent a distinct entity, or it may represent cases of lupus erythematosus and lichen planopilaris with indeterminate histological and immunologic features. In the absence of a test which can provide definitive diagnosis, it may be best to group these patients separately. Mixed inflammatory destructive alopecia is relatively uncommon.

Pseudopelade of Brocq

Pseudopelade is a rare disorder which primarily affects adult females. Childhood cases have been reported but are uncommon (incidence 3–4 percent).[15–18] Characteristically, pseudopelade presents with small, flesh-colored patches of alopecia involving primarily the parietal and vertex areas of scalp (Fig. 12-10).[19] The condition is generally self-limited and may involve relatively small areas of scalp. The natural course of pseudopelade is slow progression over a number of years. Eventually the condition "burns itself out," leaving patches of permanent alopecia. Figure 12-11 illustrates an unusually extensive case.

There has been considerable debate as to whether pseudopelade constitutes a single entity or whether it represents an end stage of several well-recognized disorders. In the past, histological studies have centered on the presence or absence of light-microscopic features of lichen planopilaris or lupus erythematosus. Such studies have concluded that as many as 90 percent or as few as 15 percent of cases could be attributed to lichen planopilaris.[11,20] Some authorities have chosen to define pseudopelade as a clinical syndrome in which destruction of hair follicles is not accompanied by clinically evident folliculitis and individual hairs are often spared. This defini-

Figure 12-10 Pseudopelade.

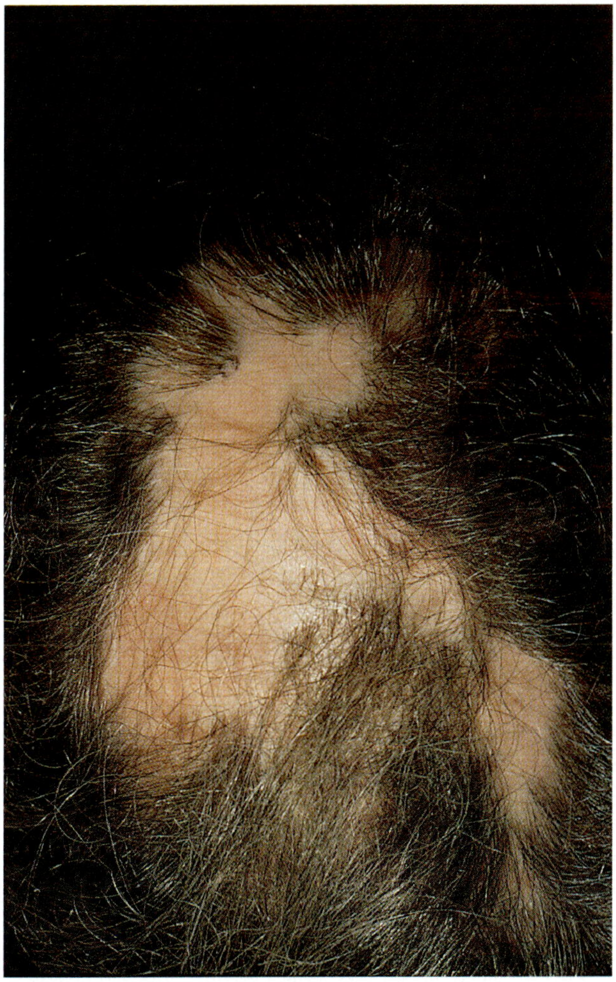

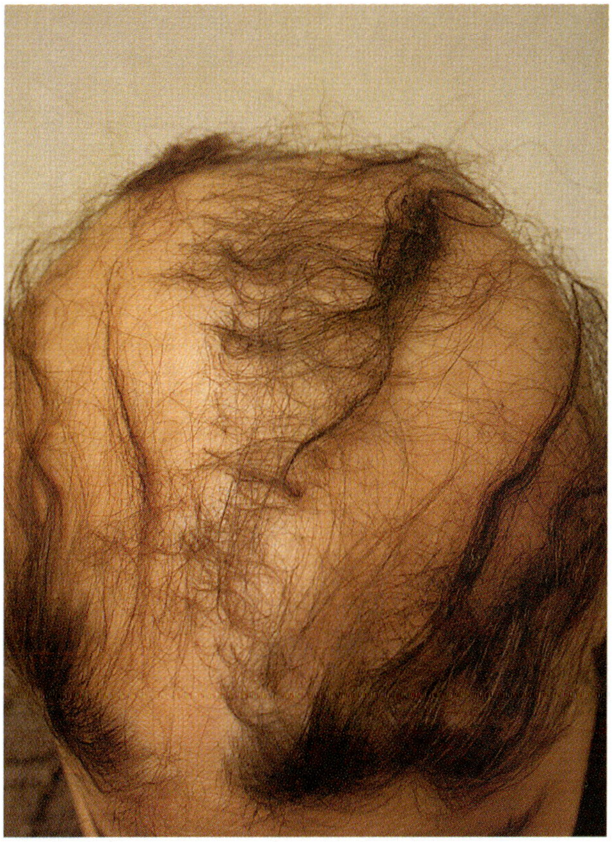

Figure 12-11 Pseudopelade, late stage.

tion of pseudopelade would include "clinically noninflammatory" cases of lupus and lichen planopilaris.[7,11,14,21] Other authors distinguish between true idiopathic pseudopelade and a "pseudopeladic stage or state" that occurs as an end stage of cutaneous diseases such as lupus and lichen planopilaris.[17,18]

To determine the presence or absence of true scarring, elastic tissue stains are essential when evaluating patients in whom the clinical presentation suggests pseudopelade. Central to this argument is a landmark study of elastic tissue–stained sections in scarring and nonscarring alopecia.[22] Among patients with a clinical presentation suggestive of pseudopelade, those who actually represented cases of lupus and follicu- lar lichen planus demonstrated true scarring (fibrosis with an absence of elastic fibers) in the area of the destroyed follicles. In contrast, a subset of patients (those that we regard as having *true idiopathic pseudopelade*) demonstrated a heavy elastic fiber component in the area of the destroyed follicles.

We propose that the term *pseudopelade* be restricted to cases characterized by the clinical presentation of skin-colored (i.e., not erythematous) patchy areas of permanent alopecia in which scalp biopsy fails to demonstrate features of lichen planopilaris or lupus. Biopsy of end-stage lesions generally demonstrates a normal or increased number of elastic fibers in the areas of destroyed follicles. This definition would tend to exclude "clinically noninflammatory" cases of lupus erythematosus and lichen planopilaris from overlap with pseudopelade.

The following histological features are based on the authors' experience and published series which attempt to exclude "pseudopeladic" patches of lupus and lichen planopilaris.[18,22–24] Scalp biopsy in early stages of pseudopelade may demonstrate no infiltrate or a patchy lymphoid infiltrate within fibrous tracts and surrounding follicular epithelium, often around the upper portion of the follicle. In later stages, hyalinized connective tissue and the loss of follicles are noted (Fig. 12-12). "Orphaned" arrector pili muscles may be noted.[18] A common and characteristic finding is the loss of sebaceous gland lobules.[22,23] Although characteristic, the loss of sebaceous glands is not specific for pseudopelade and may be seen in most types of permanent alopecia. True scarring (fibrosis with absence of elastic tissue) is not generally seen in the areas of destroyed follicles (Fig. 12-13). Small, very superficial areas of true scarring may, however, be noted. The epidermis generally remains normal, with well-developed rete ridges.[22] Some cases have been characterized by massive apoptosis of follicular epithelial cells, associated with a dense lymphoid infiltrate.[24]

Cases characterized by patchy lymphoid infiltrates may be referred to as *inflammatory pseudopelade,* a histological term that does not imply the presence of clinical signs of inflammation. The term *noninflammatory pseudopelade* is used to describe cases with hyalinized connective tissue and loss of follicles and sebaceous

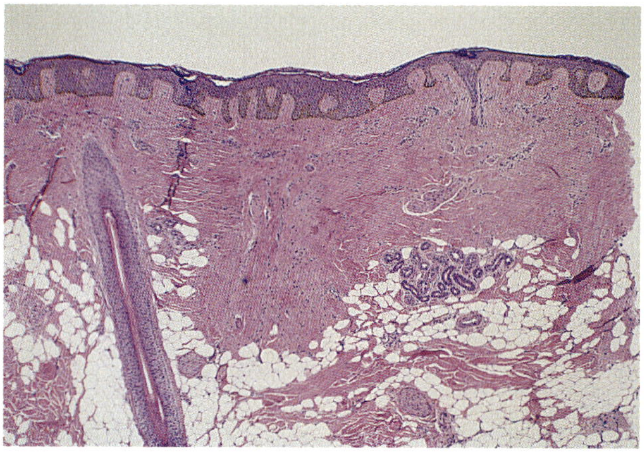

Figure 12-12 Pseudopelade: A single terminal hair is present. The thick hyalinized dermis may mimic true scar in H&E-stained sections. (Scalp, H&E stain, ×40)

Figure 12-13 Pseudopelade. Elastic stain reveals intact elastic fibers throughout most of hyalinized dermis. Only small focal subepidermal areas of true scarring exist. (Scalp, elastic stain, ×100)

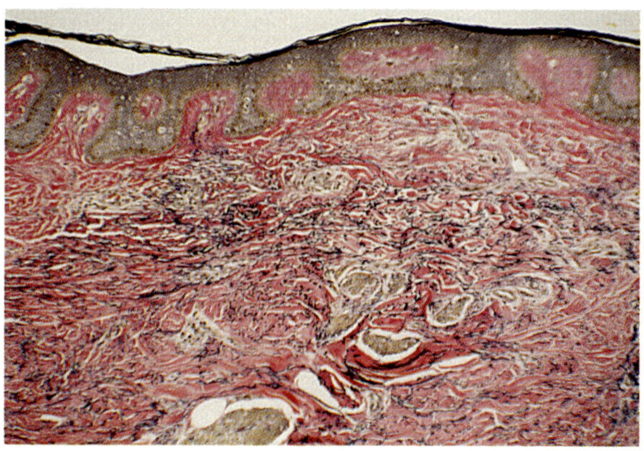

glands but with no identifiable inflammatory phase in histological sections.

Using this definition of pseudopelade, histological differentiation from lichen planopilaris and lupus erythematosus (two causes of true scarring alopecia) generally poses little difficulty. Pseudopelade shares many histological features with scleroderma/morphea variants. Both pseudopelade and morphea cause permanent alopecia with hyalinization of the dermis but without true scarring. Morphea may be distinguished from pseudopelade in histological sections by the presence of more diffuse thickening and homogenization of collagen bundles, often replacing the superficial subcutaneous tissue. Another distinguishing feature of morphea is the presence of perivascular lymphoid infiltrates at the dermal-subcutaneous junction and within subcutaneous fibrous septa (see Table 12-2).[25]

Scleroderma Variants (Including Morphea)

Scleroderma variants, especially the linear type, may affect the scalp. Cutaneous changes of scleroderma, including the "en coup de sabre" presentation, are generally readily recognized by the dermatologist (Fig. 12-14). Cases with less obvious cutaneous changes also occur. The hair loss tends to be slowly progressive. Clinically, it generally appears to be "noninflammatory" (not associated with erythema or induration).

Biopsy generally reveals dermal changes characteristic of scleroderma. Early lesions demonstrate a perivascular lymphoid infiltrate within the dermis and subcutaneous septa. End-stage lesions demonstrate a thick dermis with hyalinized collagen bundles.[25] Hair follicles are decreased in number or absent, but elastic tissue stains demonstrate a normal number and distribution of elastic fibers. This is not a true scarring alopecia. The dermis is hyalinized, and follicles atrophy or involute, but true scarring does not occur (see Table 12-2).

Sarcoidosis

The alopecia of sarcoidosis represents a true scarring alopecia. It is commonly seen in black women with evidence of intrathoracic sarcoidosis.[26] In addition to the alopecic patches, cutaneous involvement is generally seen at other sites. Clinically, the alopecic areas may appear as

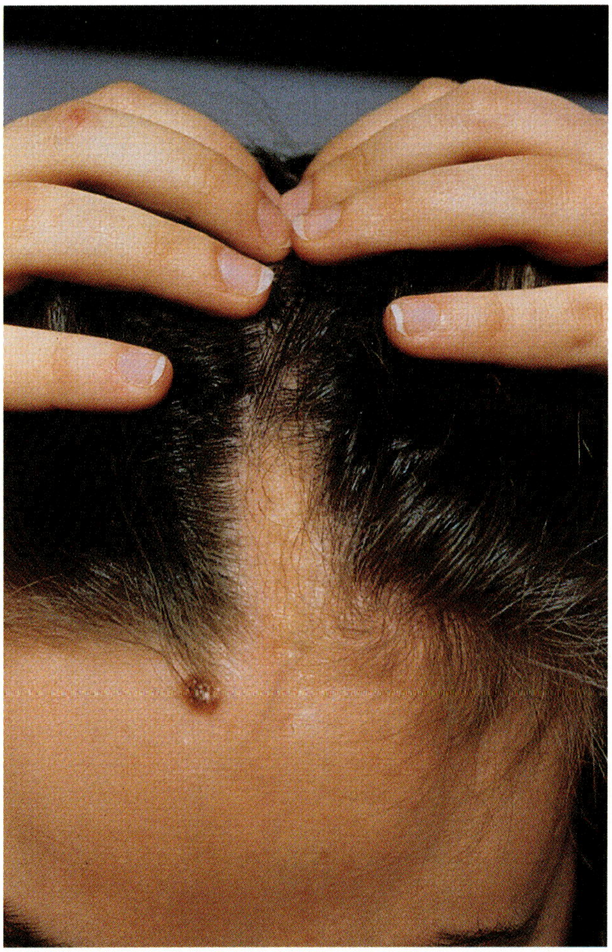

Figure 12-14 Linear morphea.

Figure 12-15 Sarcoidosis.

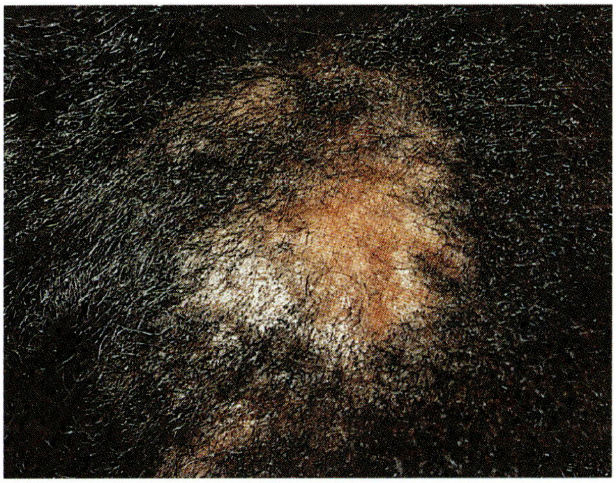

papules, plaques, or atrophic patches (Fig. 12-15). The lesions may suggest a clinical diagnosis of necrobiosis lipoidica or discoid lupus erythematosus. Histological examination reveals noncaseating granulomas composed of epithelioid and giant cells with a variable number of lymphoid cells. Foamy histiocytes have been reported overlying typical sarcoidal granulomas.[26]

Erosive Pustular Dermatosis and Folliculitis Decalvans

Erosive pustular dermatosis occurs in both sexes and at all ages but particularly in the elderly.[27] Other disorders which are closely related to, or synonymous with, erosive pustular dermatosis include folliculitis decalvans, cicatrizing seborrheic eczema, atrophic folliculitis in seborrheic dermatitis, folliculite epilante, lupoid sycosis, ulerythema sycosiforme, and folliculitis depilans.[28–32] All of these conditions are characterized by round or oval patches of alopecia with or without overlying erosion, scale, or crust.[27] Around these patches, follicular pustules occur in successive crops. Each crop of pustules results in expansion of the alopecic patch (Fig. 12-16). Many patients also have evidence of seborrheic dermatitis. *Staphylococcus aureus* is often isolated from the follicular pustules, and patients may respond to long-term treatment with antistaphylococcal antibiotics. It is unlikely that the condition merely represents recurrent staphylococcal folliculitis. Rather, an abnormal immune response (perhaps directed at staphylococcal antigens) may be involved. Case reports have described abnormal cell-mediated immune responses, abnormal neutrophil chemotaxis, increased immunoglobulins, and hypocomplementemia.[33–35]

Figure 12-16 Folliculitis decalvans.

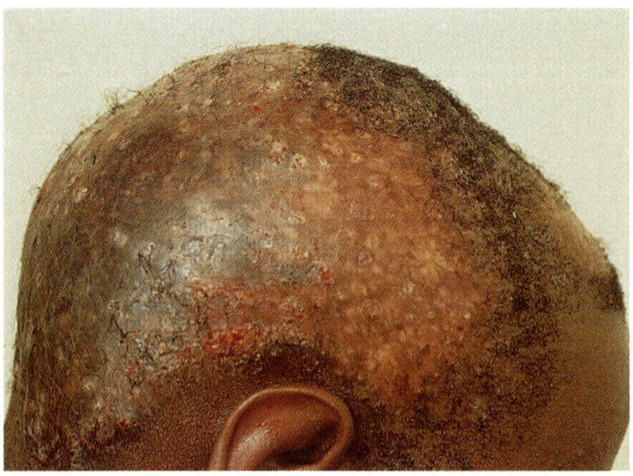

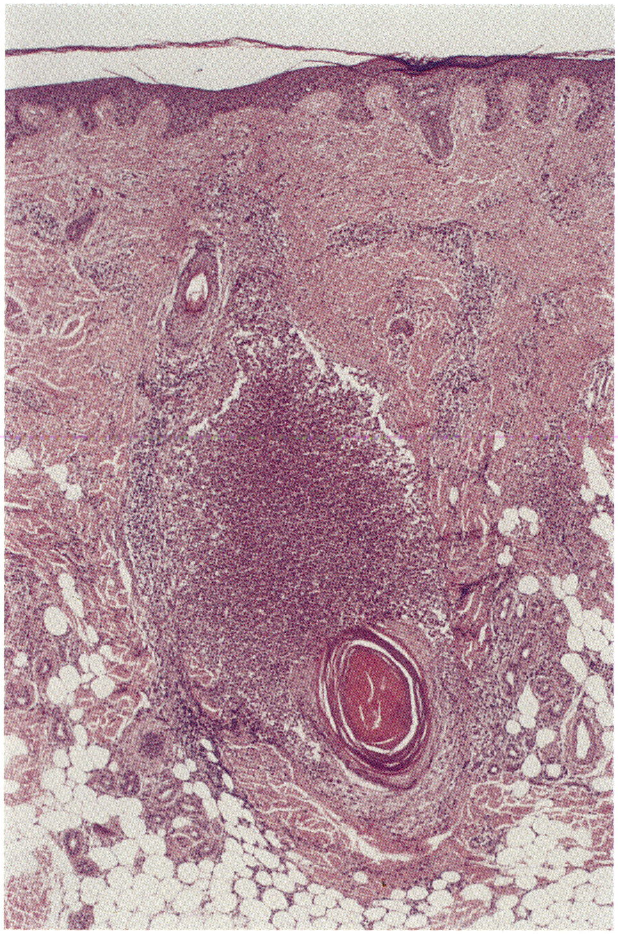

Figure 12-17 Folliculitis decalvans, acute suppurative folliculitis. (Scalp biopsy, H&E stain ×200)

In the acute stage of erosive pustular dermatosis, biopsy demonstrates acute suppurative folliculitis (Fig. 12-17). Typically, a neutrophilic follicular pustule is seen. Occasionally, eosinophils are noted within the inflammatory infiltrate. This is consistent with the idea that erosive pustular dermatosis represents a hypersensitivity disorder. The late stage is characterized by reparative fibrosis (true scarring).

Perifolliculitis Capitis Abscedens et Suffodiens (Hoffman)

Perifolliculitis capitis abscedens et suffodiens of Hoffman, also known as *dissecting folliculitis* or

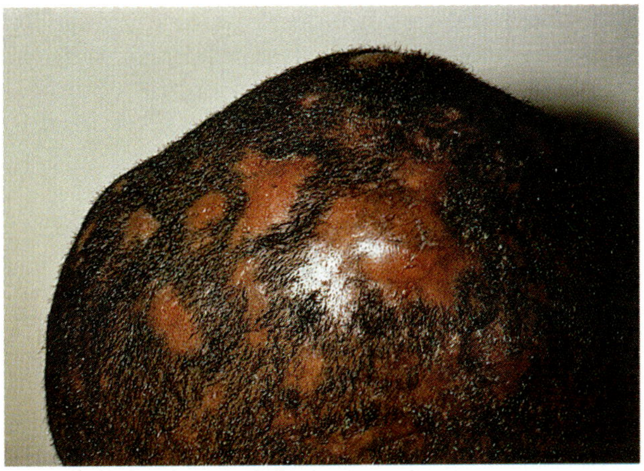

Figure 12-18 Dissecting cellulitis.

dissecting cellulitis of the scalp, is often grouped with acne conglobata and hidradenitis suppurativa (Fig. 12-18). The term *follicular occlusion triad* has been used to refer to these three conditions. The condition begins with isolated deep inflammatory nodules, then progresses to extensive confluent boggy plaques. Sinus tracts may form and discharge purulent material. Progressive scarring with permanent alopecia occurs. It has been suggested that the pathogenesis of this disorder may include an abnormal host response to bacterial antigens,[36] suggesting a possible relationship to folliculitis decalvans. *S. aureus* is the most commonly isolated organism.[37] Further studies are needed to define the spectrum of scalp disorders related to abnormal host immune responses.

The histological features vary according to the stage of the disease. Early lesions are characterized by follicular plugging, suppurative folliculitis, or perifollicular abscesses. The infiltrate may include neutrophils, lymphoid and plasma cells, and eosinophils. As the lesions evolve, foreign body giant cells and granulation tissue may be present. Late-stage lesions include scarring and sinus tracts.[37,38]

The diagnosis of noninfectious pustular conditions of the scalp requires consideration of potential infectious causes. Bacterial and fungal culture, Gram's stain, and potassium hydroxide (KOH) examination should be performed. Bear in mind that lesions of both erosive pustular dermatosis and perifolliculitis capitis abscedens et suffodiens may yield positive bacterial cultures. The diagnosis is based on the clinical and histological appearance and the clinical course.

Infectious Agents

Bacterial folliculitis may present as superficial follicular pustules or deep furuncles. Hair loss is generally a late phenomenon and is permanent only in extreme cases, generally in the absence of treatment. The diagnosis of bacterial folliculitis should be confirmed by Gram's stain. Cultures may also be employed, especially in the evaluation of bacterial sensitivities.

In contrast, hair loss is generally an early finding in fungal infections of the scalp. In fact, hair loss and a mild seborrhea-like scale may be the only signs of fungal infection: this does not generally result in permanent alopecia. The lesions of a kerion are tender, boggy, erythematous, and sometimes studded with pustules. Fortunately, with adequate treatment, permanent alopecia is unusual, even in cases of extensive kerion. The diagnosis of fungal scalp infection should be confirmed by KOH examination or fungal culture. A useful technique is to rub the affected area of scalp with a moist gauze pad (in the case of kerion, rub *gently*). The broken hair fragments which adhere to the pad are ideal for KOH examination or culture.

Herpes zoster may involve the scalp and may eventuate in scarring and alopecia (Fig. 12-19). Zoster may present as grouped vesicles, ulcers, or crusts, or as edematous plaques. Pain is usually a prominent symptom. The diagnosis is usu-

Figure 12-19 Herpes zoster.

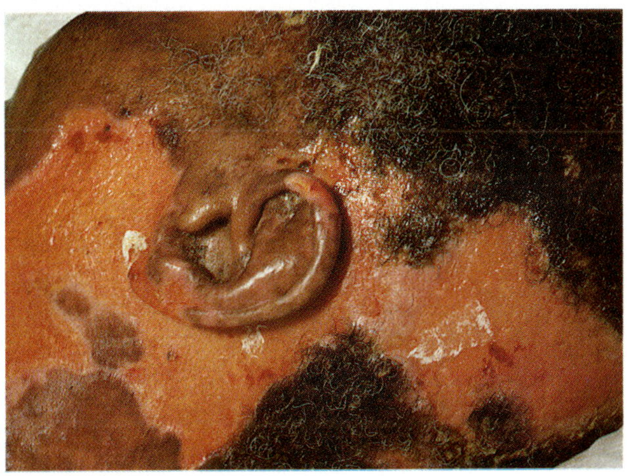

ally based on clinical findings, but Tzanck preparation, immunolabeling, and viral culture may be used to confirm the diagnosis. Early treatment with acyclovir may reduce the incidence of scarring.

Although Herpes simplex can also involve the scalp, it is less likely to result in scarring. In other anatomic sites, scarring may result from chronic ulcerative Herpes simplex infections or, rarely, as a result of secondary bacterial infection.

Acne Keloidalis Nuchae (Dermatitis Papillaris Capillitii)

Acne keloidalis nuchae presents with grouped papules and keloidal plaques on the nape of the neck (Fig. 12-20). Severe or long-standing cases may be associated with pustules or sinus tracts. This condition is seen most commonly in black males. Acne keloidalis nuchae represents a foreign body reaction to hair fibers with resulting hypertrophic scar. Histological sections demonstrate disrupted follicles with acute and/or chronic granulomatous inflammation and hypertrophic scarring. Sinus tracts may be evident, but true keloid formation would be exceptional.

Pityriasis Amiantacea

Pityriasis amiantacea is a clinical syndrome characterized by thick, adherent silvery scales which surround and bind down tufts of hair. It most commonly presents in the occipital scalp and represents a chronic eczematous dermatitis. Some patients also have seborrheic dermatitis, psoriasis, or a superimposed bacterial or fungal infection. Scarring alopecia has been reported in some cases of pityriasis amiantacea.[39]

Figure 12-20 Acne keloidalis nuchae.

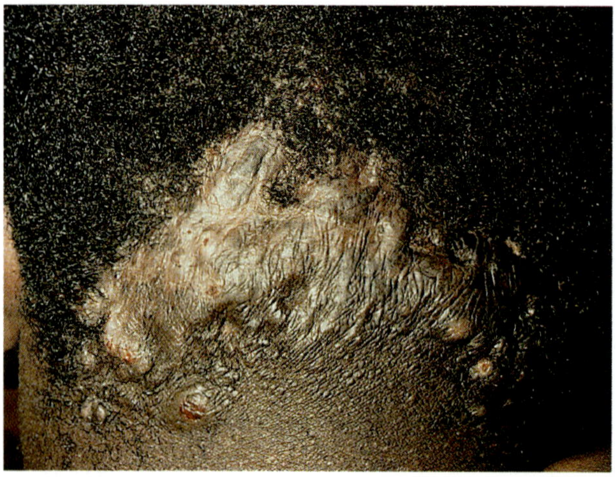

Lipedematous Alopecia

The term *lipedematous alopecia* has been applied to a syndrome characterized by thickened, indurated subcutaneous scalp tissue associated with diffuse scalp hair loss. Palpation of the scalp may give the impression that it is "underlayed with soft cotton batting."[40] Pruritus or soreness is sometimes noted. Biopsies in some cases have demonstrated hyperkeratosis, follicular plugging, follicular atrophy, and a marked increase in the subcutaneous fat with or without fibrosis.[41,42] Associated trichorrhexis nodosa has been reported.[41] Short scalp hairs with normal morphology have also been reported, suggesting a shortened hair cycle or decreased rate of hair growth.[42] Curtis and Heising reported a case associated with skin hyperelasticity and loose joints.[41]

Developmental and Hereditary Disorders

A wide variety of developmental and hereditary conditions are associated with permanent alopecia.[36,43,44] Some of these entities produce true scarring alopecia (reparative fibrosis with absent elastic fibers). Others are associated with permanent alopecia on the basis of dysgenesis or atrophy of the follicular unit. Most dermatologists are quite familiar with a large number of these conditions, but as the list of recognizable syndromes continues its rapid growth, it is frequently advisable for the dermatologist to work closely with a medical geneticist. The importance of accurate diagnosis and proper genetic counseling cannot be overemphasized. Some of the more fascinating developmental or hereditary disorders associated with permanent alopecia are discussed below.

ALOPECIA ICHTHYOTICA

The term *alopecia ichthyotica* has been used to describe alopecia associated with congenital ichthyosis.[44] Inflammatory scarring alopecia has been described in cases of autosomal recessive ichthyosis congenita (congenital ichthyosiform erythroderma).[44] The clinical descriptions given are incomplete, but at least some of these patients appear to have had lamellar ichthyosis. The authors have seen additional cases of permanent alopecia associated with lamellar ichthyosis.

The X-linked dominant form of the Conradi-Hünermann chondrodysplasia punctata is notable for ichthyosiform erythroderma at birth and the development of follicular atrophoderma and scarring alopecia.[45] An adult male with scarring alopecia and features suggestive of the Conradi-Hünermann syndrome has also been described.[46]

Dorfman, Hershko, Eisenberg, and Sagher described four patients with ichthyosis (resembling nonbullous ichthyosiform erythroderma) and systemic lipidosis.[47] Lipid accumulations were found in granulocytes, in granulocyte precursors (marrow), and in the liver. One patient demonstrated alopecia "reminiscent of pseudopelade." Histological features of the alopecia were not presented.

The keratitis, ichthyosis, and deafness (KID) syndrome may be associated with scalp crusting, pustules, and permanent alopecia.[48] Eyebrows and eyelashes may be affected. The alopecia may be related to preceding suppurative folliculitis, since follicular pustules are seen clinically. Keratotic follicular plugging is also present. Nails may also be dystrophic or absent.

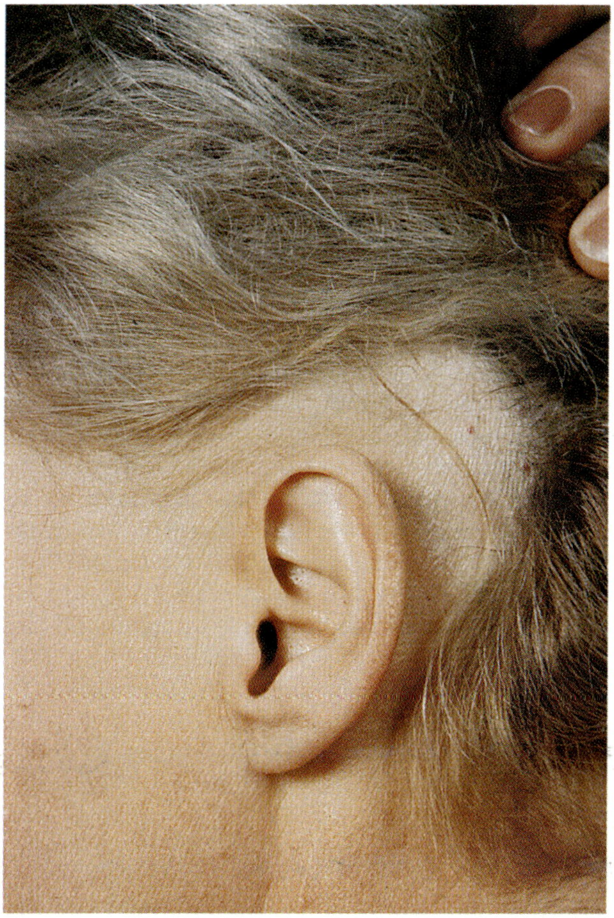

Figure 12-21 Alopecia triangularis: unusual location.

ALOPECIA TRIANGULARIS

Alopecia triangularis (Fig. 12-21) is probably more common than the small number of reported cases might suggest.[49] The characteristic shape of the alopecic patch and a history suggesting that the patch has not undergone change help to distinguish this disorder from alopecia areata. The base generally is at the junction of the frontal and temporal hairline. Histological examination reveals an absence of terminal hairs but the presence of vellus hair follicles. Follicular keratin plugs may be present.[50]

APLASIA CUTIS CONGENITA

Aplasia cutis congenita generally presents as a small, solitary lesion near the vertex of the scalp. The affected areas may be circular, oval, triangular, or stellate. The lesions generally heal with atrophic scarring and alopecia. Major, deep lesions may be associated with hemorrhage or meningitis. Aplasia cutis congenita has been associated with a variety of congenital abnormalities, including trisomy 13, congenital heart disease, genitourinary abnormalities, cleft lip and palate, and mental retardation. Proposed etiologies include intrauterine trauma, defective neural tube closure, and vascular occlusion with subsequent skin necrosis.[51,52]

BARAITSER'S SYNDROME

Alopecia, mental and physical retardation are components of this syndrome. Inheritance appears to be autosomal recessive.[53]

DARIER'S DISEASE

Darier's disease (keratosis follicularis) is an autosomal dominant genodermatosis characterized by brownish-colored keratotic papules in a seborrheic distribution. Although nail changes are characteristic of the disorder, significant alopecia is not a common manifestation. However, alopecia may occur in this disorder and may be quite extensive. Histological evaluation of a patient with Darier's disease and almost total alopecia revealed typical corps ronds and grains in the epidermis. Signs of Darier's disease were also noted within the abortive follicular epithelium. Cystic degeneration of sebaceous glands was noted.[54]

ECTODERMAL DYSPLASIAS

The ectodermal dysplasias are a complex group of hereditary conditions involving the skin and its appendages. More than 137 distinct syndromes have been described. A classification scheme proposed by Freire-Maia subdivides the syndromes based on which skin appendages are involved.[55] Group A conditions feature at least two of the following: (1) trichodysplasia, (2) dental defects, (3) onychodysplasia, or (4) abnormal sweating. The syndromes are subgrouped by combinations of these findings (example: 1–2, 1–2–4, 1–3–4, etc.). Group B conditions feature only one of these signs along with at least one other ectodermal defect. This scheme includes several genodermatoses which dermatologists do not always group with the other ectodermal dysplasias, such as Rothmund-Thomson syndrome and incontinentia pigmenti.[56] KID syndrome (grouped here with the ichthyoses), dyskeratosis congenita, and some of the keratosis pilaris–like syndromes (see later text) would also fit into Freire-Maia's classification of ectodermal dysplasias. Solomon and Keuer have suggested restricting the term *ectodermal dysplasia* to disorders that (1) are congenital, (2) have diffuse involvement of the epidermis with at least one appendage involved, and (3) are *not progressive.*[57]

The type A ectodermal dysplasias are presented in detail in Chapter 7. Two of the more recently described type B ectodermal dysplasias associated with permanent alopecia are presented here. One has alopecia, an elevated frequency of chromosomal breaks, normal dentition, normal sweating, and an associated immunodeficiency. It is probably inherited as an autosomal-recessive trait.[58] Another ectodermal dysplasia also has a type of immunodeficiency associated with an elevated frequency of chromosomal breaks but with normal teeth, normal sweating, mental and growth retardation, congenital atrichia, and papular lesions of the forearms. The latter presents sporadically.[59]

EPIDERMAL NEVI

Epidermal nevi, including linear epidermal nevus and nevus sebaceus, are commonly associated with permanent alopecia. Linear epidermal nevus is characterized histologically by varying degrees of hyperkeratosis, acanthosis, papillomatosis, and occasionally epidermolytic hyperkeratosis. An inflammatory variant exists. Nevus sebaceus generally begins as a flat, hairless patch which becomes raised, yellowish, and cerebriform around the time of puberty. Histological examination before puberty may demonstrate a hairless area with basaloid buds resembling the primary epithelial germ. After puberty, sebaceous and apocrine glands are generally prominent. Both linear epidermal nevus and nevus sebaceus may be associated with neurocutaneous syndromes.[52,60]

EPIDERMOLYSIS BULLOSA

The term *epidermolysis bullosa* refers to a group of inherited disorders characterized by blistering of the skin. The recessive dystrophic type is most commonly associated with scarring alopecia.[61,62] The junctional and simplex types have also been associated with permanent alopecia.[63]

FIBROUS DYSPLASIA

Permanent alopecia has been reported as a feature of polyostotic fibrous dysplasia (Albright's disease).[64] Scalp, pubic, and axillary hair, as well as eyelashes, are affected. Biopsy demonstrated thick, fibrous "coils" with increased cellularity and vascularity along with haphazard arrangement of fibrocytes. Underlying hyperplasia of the panniculus was noted. Small osteomas were present in the skin, usually associated with follicular fibrous tracts. Elastic tissue was absent or poorly developed within the connective tissue tracts. Where follicular structures were still present, elastic tissue was "clumped in tight opposition to the follicular epithelium, with loss of fibers in the surrounding connective tissue sheath."[64]

Fibrodysplasia (myositis) ossificans progressiva is a rare autosomal disorder characterized by malformations of the big toe, reduction defects of all digits, deafness, baldness, mental retardation, and ectopic calcification.[65] Hair thinning tends to be diffuse, with sparing of single terminal hairs or small groups of hairs.

KERATOSIS PILARIS AND ASSOCIATED DISORDERS

Conditions characterized by follicular keratosis are often accompanied by permanent alopecia. In some cases, the alopecia may be related to a secondary bacterial or fungal infection. In others, the alopecia appears to be related to the keratinizing disorder itself.[66] Some cases have been associated with abnormalities of the teeth or nails and could be grouped with the ectodermal dysplasias. The histological feature common to all of these conditions is the presence of follicular keratotic plugging. The clinical presence of perifollicular inflammation and scarring varies from case to case. The presence or absence of true histological scarring has not been sufficiently consistent to be used to differentiate between these entities (Table 12-3). Absent or atrophic sebaceous glands have been reported in cases of atrophoderma vermiculata, ichthyosis follicularis with alopecia and photophobia, and atrichia with papular lesions.[67] Further study is needed to determine whether sebaceous gland changes are really a consistent feature of these entities.

INCONTINENTIA PIGMENTI

Incontinentia pigmenti is a rare, X-linked dominant genodermatosis. Skin lesions begin in infancy or in utero as linear arrays of vesicles. Lesions progress through verrucous and hyperpigmented stages. Scarring alopecia has been estimated to occur in about 30 percent of cases[56] (Fig.12-22).

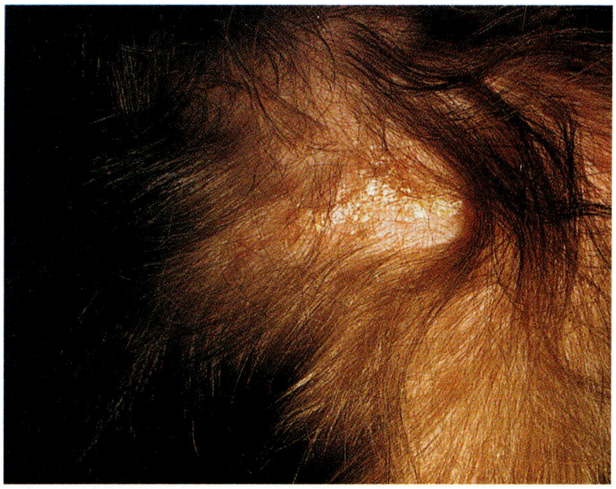

Figure 12-22 Incontinentia pigmenti.

POROKERAÏTOSIS

Porokeratosis of Mibelli presents as an annular, expanding lesion with a keratotic rim. The central portion of the lesion is typically atrophic. The expanding edge is characterized by a column of parakeratosis which lies at about a 45-degree angle and "points" to a focus of dyskeratotic cells (the cornoid lamella). This expanding edge is thought to represent a mutant clone of cells. Porokeratosis of the scalp may result in alopecia.[62,63]

ROTHMUND-THOMSON SYNDROME

The Rothmund-Thomson syndrome is an autosomal recessive syndrome characterized by poikiloderma, light sensitivity, dwarfism, and skeletal defects. Diffuse hypotrichosis may be evident.[63]

TUFTED HAIR FOLLICULITIS

Tong and Baden described a patient with two circumscribed, inflamed areas of scalp with residual tufted hairs[68] (Fig. 12-23). Each tuft consisted of 10 to 15 hairs, each arising from its own follicle but all converging toward a single orifice in the epidermis. The early inflammatory phase seemed to involve the papillary and middermis with sparing of the deep portion of the follicles. The authors suggested that the areas of tufting represented a nevoid malformation. Dalziel,

Figure 12-23 Tufted hair folliculitis. (*Reprinted with permission from Tong and Baden;[68] Photo courtesy of Dr. Howard Baden.*)

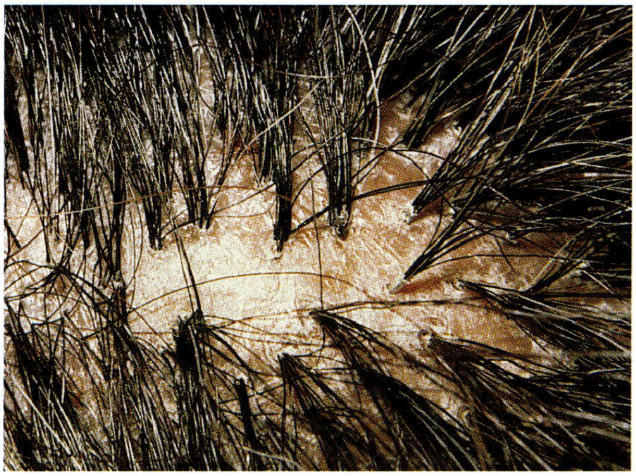

Table 12-3
KERATOSIS PILARIS AND RELATED CONDITIONS

Synonyms	*Clinical Features*	*Associations*
Keratosis pilaris atrophicans faciei[43,114,115] [ulerythema ophryogenes, keratosis pilaris rubra atrophicans faciei (KPRAF)]	Follicular keratotic papules initially restricted to the eyebrow region. Typically, the lateral portion of the eyebrow is involved first, with slow inward progression. Individual papules are surrounded by an erythematous halo. Scarring alopecia of eyebrows. Cases called KPRAF may involve temples or cheeks first. Probably AD inheritance.	May be associated with Noonan's syndrome, atopy, later development of keratosis pilaris elsewhere on body.
Atrophoderma vermiculata (acne vermiculata, folliculitis ulerythematosa reticulata, honeycomb atrophy)[43,66]	Honeycomblike atrophic scarring of the cheeks. Generally begins in childhood, with follicular plugs which shed, leaving atrophic scarring. Scarring alopecia of scalp[66] Probably AD inheritance.	Cardiac abnormalities[116]
Keratosis pilaris decalvans (keratosis follicularis spinulosa decalvans, follicular ichthyosis)[43,115]	Keratosis pilaris with inflammation and atrophy resulting in permanent alopecia. Begins on face in infancy. Often involves trunk and extremities by childhood. Permanent alopecia of scalp and eyebrows often starts during childhood/teens. Most likely represents a group of related disorders, rather than a single entity. Some cases may be X-linked dominant, others AD.	Hyperkeratosis of palms, soles. Atopy, photophobia, corneal abnormalities, abnormal nails.
Ichthyosis follicularis with alopecia and photophobia[67]	Widespread alopecia, photophobia. Generalized thorn-like spiny follicular projections. Hyperkeratosis over extensor surfaces. May be a subset of keratosis pilaris decalvans. The absence of true scarring has been used as a differentiating feature, but similar cases have been reported in which some family members have scarring, while others do not.[117]	Natal teeth
Atrichia with papular lesions[43]	Born hairless or hair lost early in life. Follicular, sometimes horny papules, follicular cysts. Possible AR inheritance.	
Alopecia, premature cataracts, widespread keratosis pilaris and psoriasis[118]	Patchy scarring alopecia beginning in childhood. Features of both keratosis follicularis spinulosa decalvans and ichthyosis follicularis. Probable AD inheritance with variable penetrance. The relationship of psoriasis to the syndrome is uncertain, as psoriasis also existed in other members of the family. May be a subset of keratosis pilaris decalvans.	Abnormal teeth/nails

Telfer, Wilson, and Dawber reported histological findings in four patients with similar clinical findings.[69] *S. aureus* was cultured from all four patients. Perifollicular inflammation was present around the upper portions of the follicles, and neutrophils were consistently present in the infiltrate. Disruption of the follicular wall with granulomatous inflammation was present in some sections. The tufts of hair consisted of a central anagen hair surrounded by telogen hairs which converged toward a common dilated infundibulum. It remains to be determined whether tufted hairs represent a nevoid malformation or an acquired phenomenon. Tufted hairs differ from compound hairs (2–3 anagen hairs emerging from a single infundibulum), which occur normally in the occipital scalp.[70] Compound hairs may also be associated with folliculitis.[70]

OTHER SYNDROMES

Other syndromes[43,63,71,72] associated with permanent alopecia include the Hallermann-Streiff syndrome (dyscephaly, dwarfism, mandibular aplasia), in which sparse hair and patchy alopecia have been reported, and pachyonychia congenita (thick nails, oral white sponge nevus, palmoplantar keratoses), which may demonstrate hypotrichosis in 10 percent of cases. Porphyria (including erythropoietic porphyria and porphyria cutanea tarda) and Bazex's follicular atrophoderma syndrome (follicular atrophoderma, basal cell carcinoma) have been associated with sparse fine hair.

Neoplastic Disorders

Many neoplastic conditions may produce permanent alopecia. The alopecia results from encroachment upon or replacement of follicles by the tumor and may not represent a true scarring alopecia. Primary adnexal tumors, such as *syringoma*, and *hair follicle hamartomas* have been associated with permanent alopecia.[73–76] In the case of syringoma, the diagnosis may not be suspected prior to biopsy.[77] Syringoma-like sweat duct proliferations may also occur as a secondary phenomenon in both scarring and nonscarring alopecia (including alopecia areata and female-pattern alopecia).[78] Therefore, caution must be exercised in attributing hair loss to syringomas, based on a single biopsy.

Generalized hair follicle hamartoma may present with progressive permanent alopecia involving most of the body, including the scalp, eyebrows, and pubic region. In some areas, infiltrated plaques may be evident. Histological examination reveals islands of basaloid cells related to abnormal pilosebaceous follicles. The abnormal follicles fail to produce hairs. Empty follicles and follicular plugging are characteristic. Associated clinical findings may include myasthenia gravis and aminoaciduria.[75,76] Basaloid follicular hamartoma may present as a localized plaque of alopecia on the scalp. The histology is similar to that of generalized hair follicle hamartoma.[74]

Primary and metastatic malignancies may

Figure 12-24 Lymphoma.

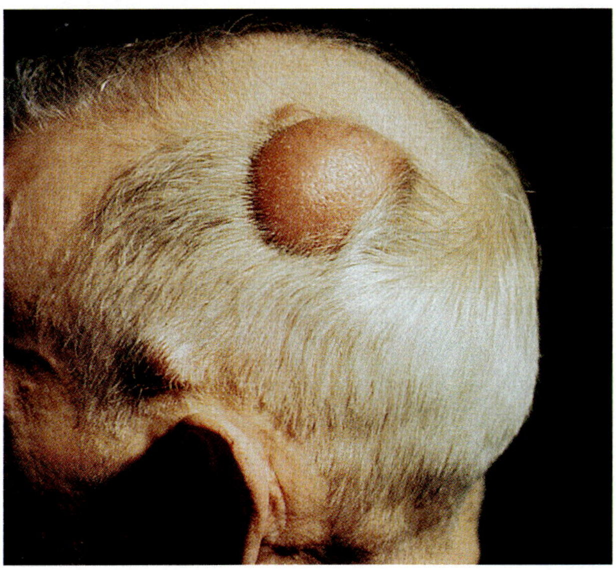

Figure 12-25 Alopecia mucinosa.

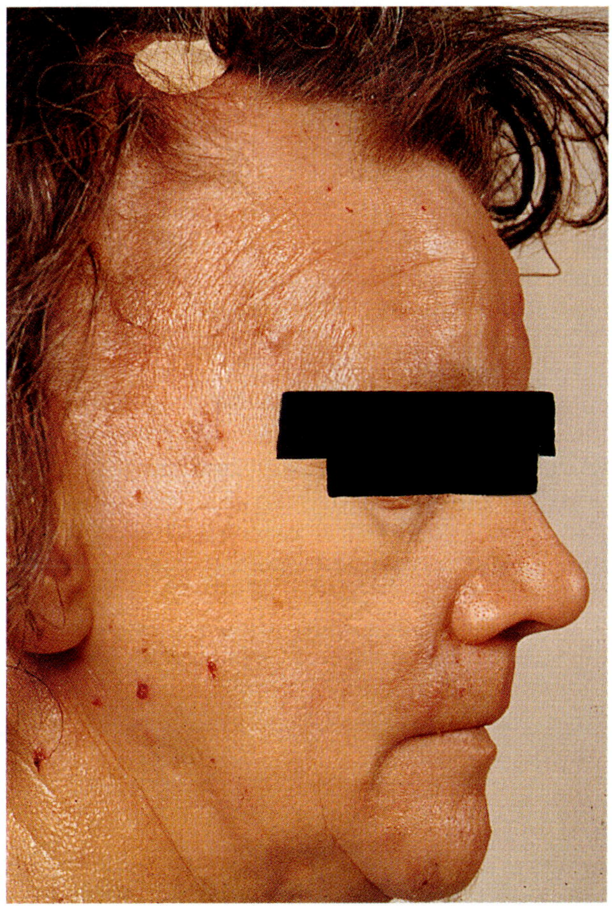

produce alopecia. The diagnosis rests on the results of a biopsy. Renal, breast, and lung tumors are the most common sources of scalp metastases. Occasionally, the primary tumor is not suspected prior to biopsy of the scalp metastasis. Lymphoma (both B-cell and cutaneous T-cell lymphoma) may present in the scalp (Fig. 12-24). Cutaneous T-cell lymphoma (CTCL) may demonstrate "folliculotropism" and may be accompanied by alopecia mucinosa. Alopecia mucinosa not associated with CTCL may also occur in the scalp (Fig. 12-25). Primary alopecia mucinosa may present with progressive diffuse alopecia in a normal-appearing scalp.[79] Histological examination demonstrates degeneration of the follicular epithelium with the accumulation of acid mucopolysaccharide (hyaluronic acid) (Fig. 12-26). The mucin is well-demonstrated in sections stained with colloidal iron. Although the alopecia seen with alopecia mucinosa is likely to be permanent, no true histological scar exists.

Chemical and Physical Agents

TRAUMATIC, THERMAL, CHEMICAL, AND ISCHEMIC ALOPECIA

A variety of chemical (corrosive) and physical agents can cause permanent alopecia of the scalp. In general, any thermal, physical, or chemical injury sufficient to cause scalp necrosis can produce a permanent alopecia. In the acute stage, necrosis with crusting, an adherent eschar, or ulceration may be present. Later, the scalp heals by reparative fibrosis. The result is usually an atrophic alopecic patch. Ischemic necrosis of the scalp produces a similar clinical picture. Ischemic scalp necrosis may be seen after prolonged anesthesia. The necrosis generally involves the occipital scalp and represents a pressure phenomenon. Ischemic necrosis may also occur as a result of vasoconstriction related to the infusion of pharmacologic agents such as vasopressin.

In the acute stage, crusting, necrosis, and/or ulceration are present. End-stage lesions are characterized histologically by alopecia and fibrosis, with an absence of elastic fibers (true scarring alopecia).

RADIATION

Radiation injury may cause transient nonscarring alopecia (epilating dose). Higher doses produce permanent alopecia with scarring. Histological changes in anagen hair follicles can be noted as early as 4 days following radiation.[80] Similar effects are noted with x-rays and electron beam radiation. The earliest change is thinning of the hair bulb, especially in the area of the matrix. Two to 3 weeks following irradiation, hairs with tapered shafts are apparent. The number of follicles showing radiation effects is roughly proportional to the dose of radiation.[80] Various units have been used to measure radiation dose. Currently, the gray (Gy) is used as an international standard (1 Gy = 1 J/Kg = 100 rads). Older studies often reported doses in roentgens (1 R = .893 rad). Maguire has stated that a dose as low as 400 roentgens (Hvl, 0.5-mm Al filter) can cause transient nonscarring alopecia, and single doses above 1200 roentgens can produce permanent

Figure 12-26 Alopecia mucinosa. Mucinous degeneration of follicular epithelium (arrow). (Scalp biopsy, H&E stain ×200)

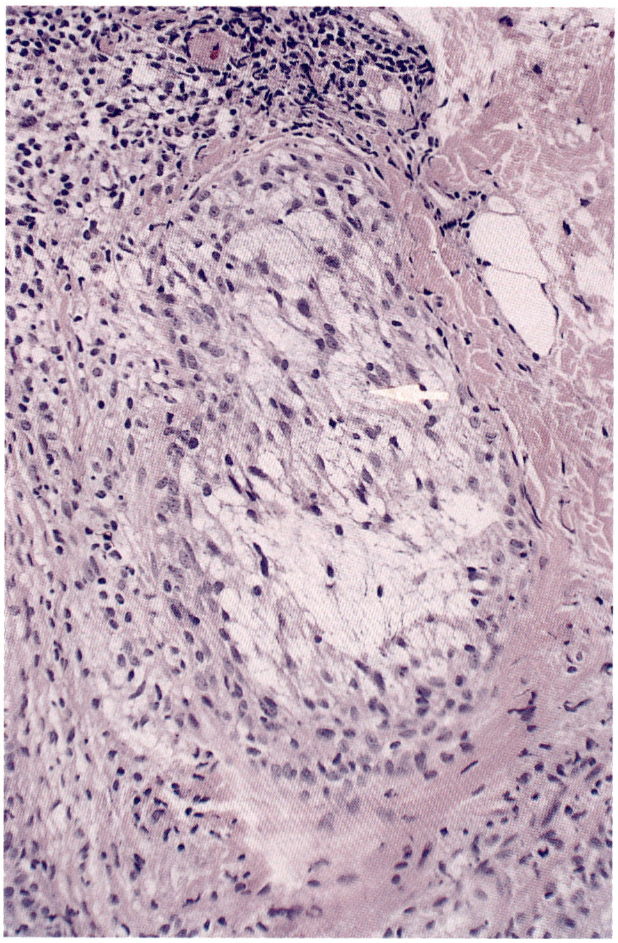

alopecia.[81] The Kienböck-Adamson technique for treating tinea capitis involved an epilating dose of about 400 roentgens in each of five fields of exposure. Not only the total dose but also the penetration of the radiation used, the fraction per session, and the frequency of treatments are important in determining the effect on follicular epithelium. Radiation scarring can occur with 5000 to 6000 cGy (rads) of soft x-rays (50 kV, 1-mm Al filter) or 300 cGy of deep x-rays (180–200 kV, 0.5–0.1-mm Cu filter).[62]

For practical purposes, in the setting of the current practice of radiation therapy for malignancy with standard treatment schedules, *a dose of 3000 cGy will generally cause a transient alopecia,* whereas *doses in excess of 5000 cGy will generally cause permanent alopecia.* These doses generally hold for the treatment of mycosis fungoides with 3 to 5 MeV electron-beam radiation as well as for the treatment of brain metastases with radiation. In the latter case, the fractions can vary from 180 to 300 cGy per treatment (if a surgical procedure has been performed, the lower dose per treatment is often preferred). With a total dose of 3000 cGy, temporary alopecia can be expected in those treated with both the 180- and 300-cGy dose fractions. In the group receiving the smaller dose per treatment, the onset of alopecia is delayed.

DRUGS

Para-aminosalicylic acid has been reported to cause a lichenoid eruption with permanent alopecia.[82] The eruption is widespread and poikilodermatous and associated with fever and severe hepatitis. Quinacrine hydrochloride can produce a lichenoid dermatitis which may be associated with widespread alopecia.[83] Drugs should be considered in the evaluation of patients with permanent alopecia, especially those with lichenoid eruptions.

TRACTION ALOPECIA AND TRICHOTILLOMANIA

Traction alopecia and trichotillomania are types of physical trauma that can lead to alopecia. Traction alopecia is seen most commonly in black females. It is often associated with tight braiding or cornrow hairstyles. Alopecia is generally evident along the hairline. Follicular papules are sometimes present. Trichotillomania is a traction alopecia related to a compulsive disorder. Patients pull on and pluck hairs, often resulting in bizarre patterns of alopecia. Frequently, the peripheral hairline is spared. Patients may ingest the hairs, resulting in a trichobezoar. Chronic cases may mimic androgenetic alopecia or an inflammatory "scarring alopecia." Any hair-bearing area may be involved, including the scalp, eyebrows, and lashes. The peak incidence has a bimodal distribution, occurring frequently in both young and older women. In long-term cases of trichotillomania, permanent alopecia may occur.

Biopsy specimens from acute lesions of trichotillomania may demonstrate perifollicular hemorrhage and fractured fibers. Later stages of trichotillomania characteristically demonstrate the presence of normal follicles surrounded by empty follicles in a noninflammatory dermis. Numerous catagen follicles (characterized by numerous apoptotic cells and a wavy surrounding vitreous membrane) and pigment casts within the upper segments of the follicle may be noted. Trichomalacia (the presence of wavy amorphous, sometimes corkscrewlike hairs) is a less common but highly characteristic finding. Chronic cases of trichotillomania may demonstrate scarring.[84–87]

HOT-COMB ALOPECIA

Hot-combing (oiling the hair and pulling it under tension through a "hot comb") is not practiced as commonly today as it once was. At one time, it was a popular method of hair straightening. Hot-combing has been implicated as a cause of permanent alopecia in black women. Severe thermal burns resulting from careless hot-combing may certainly result in scarring alopecia. Frequent hot-combing also has the potential to create a traction alopecia. The oils used during the treatments may cause a chemical folliculitis. Although true hot-comb alopecia does exist, the diagnosis is probably overused. It has become a "wastebasket" diagnosis for any poorly defined alopecia in a black female. This issue is discussed further in the following section.

Unclassified Alopecia in Black Women

It is not uncommon for black women to develop permanent alopecia which defies classification. In the past, such cases were attributed to the use of hot-combs and hair cosmetics. Recently, Sperling and Sau studied 10 black women with clinical findings suggestive of "hot-comb alopecia"[88].

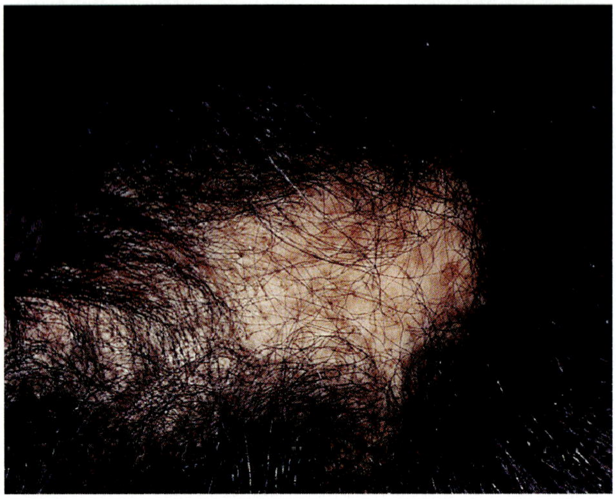

Figure 12-27 Follicular degeneration syndrome. (*Courtesy of Dr. Leonard Sperling.*)

(Fig. 12-27). They noted poor correlation between the usage of a hot-comb and the onset and progression of hair loss. In transverse sections, biopsies demonstrated premature desquamation of the inner root sheath, followed by premature keratinization of the outer root sheath. In the upper portion of the follicular isthmus, the outer root sheath thinned to a few flattened cells, and a mononuclear infiltrate and onion skin fibrosis were noted. In the infundibulum, the hair fiber often returned to its central portion, accompanied by less inflammation and fibrosis. In later stages, there was progressive degeneration of the follicular epithelium, most pronounced in the follicular isthmus (Fig. 12-28*A* and *B*). Eventually, the epithelium degenerated altogether, leaving the hair fiber free in the dermis. At this stage, hair fiber granulomas could be seen. The end stage was characterized by replacement of the follicle with a thick fibrous tract. The authors proposed the term "*follicular degeneration syndrome*" for this disorder. Further research is needed to determine whether these findings are universal in black women with "unclassified permanent alopecia." Ideally, future studies should include elastic tissue stains and immunofluorescent studies.

TREATMENT

Treatment of permanent alopecia can be divided into (1) treatments effective in the acute stage of specific disorders and (2) treatments applicable to any "burned-out" end-stage alopecia. Specific treatment for the acute stage of a destructive alopecia depends on proper diagnosis. Biopsy should be an early step in the evaluation of scarring alopecia since a rational choice for therapy can be made only after the diagnosis is firmly established. Accurate diagnosis often depends on careful correlation of the clinical presentation, histology, immunofluorescent findings, and serological findings.

Figure 12-28 Follicular degeneration syndrome. Transverse section skin of scalp. (*A*) Asymmetrical thinning of follicular epithelium at level of isthmus. Secondary granulomatous response to exposed hair fiber. (H&E stain ×100) (*B*) Asymmetrical thinning of follicular epithelium. (H&E stain ×200)

A

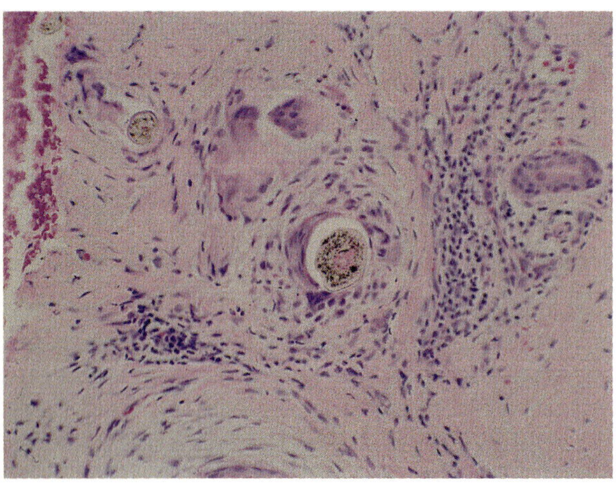

B

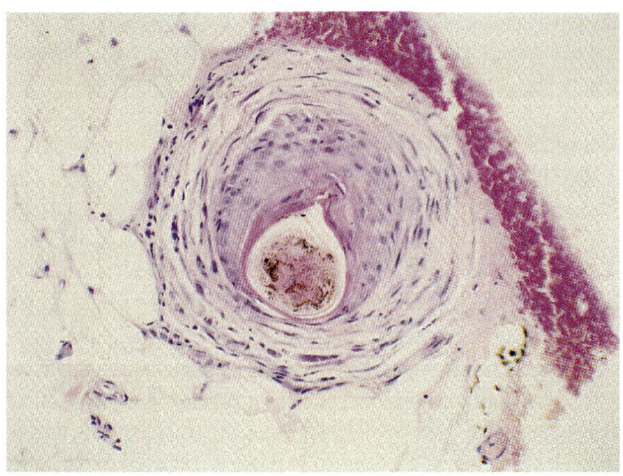

The inflammatory, true scarring alopecias (including lupus erythematosus and lichen planopilaris) are often progressive and disfiguring. The goal of treatment in the active phase of the disorder is to minimize further permanent hair loss. The treatments appropriate for the active phase will have no effect on scarred areas. When no active disease remains, "burned-out" areas of scarring may be treated surgically (see later text).

Lupus Erythematosus

Corticosteroids are a mainstay of treatment for active lesions of cutaneous lupus. Topical corticosteroids, especially class I (ultrapotent) and class II (superpotent) steroids may be effective. Ultrapotent topical steroids should be used judiciously, as they may result in adrenal suppression. In general, each course of application should not exceed 2 weeks. Intralesional corticosteroids may be effective and are a good choice in localized lesions refractory to topical agents. Concentrations of 3 to 10 mg/ml of triamcinolone are injected using a 30-gauge needle. Overuse of intralesional or topical steroids may result in atrophy (although the scarring and atrophy caused by discoid lupus generally outweigh the risks of local steroid-induced atrophy). Oral corticosteroids are often effective. The initial dosage of 1 mg/kg per day is adjusted according to the clinical response. Once initial control has been achieved, it is often best to switch to topical or intralesional steroids (or possibly an antimalarial agent) for maintenance therapy. If prolonged treatment with oral corticosteroids is required, alternate-day dosing may reduce the associated risks. Aseptic bone necrosis, cataracts, and glucose intolerance are a few of the many possible steroid complications.

Alternative therapies include the use of antimalarials, retinoids, dapsone, and thalidomide. Hydroxychloroquine (Plaquenil), chloroquine (Aralen), and quinacrine (Atabrine) have all been used effectively for the treatment of chronic cutaneous lupus erythematosus.[89] The authors generally begin treatment with hydroxychloroquine, 200 to 400 mg per day. Patients should be monitored for side effects, especially ocular toxicity (corneal deposits and retinal damage).[90] Other potential side effects of antimalarials include hematologic effects (including thrombocytopenia and agranulocytosis), gastrointestinal disturbances, pruritus, lichenoid dermatitis, yellow discoloration (with quinacrine), and toxic psychosis.[89,91,92] Regular eye examinations (at approximately 3- to 4-month intervals), hematologic studies, and routine blood chemistries should be performed. Quinacrine, although associated with skin discoloration, appears to have the advantage of a reduced potential for ocular toxicity.[93] If a 3-month trial of hydroxychloroquine proves ineffective, chloroquine, quinacrine, or a combination may be used.[91] Once a favorable response has been achieved, the dose is tapered to the lowest effective dose.

Isotretinoin, a retinoid, has been effective in some cases of discoid lupus refractory to other treatments.[89,94] Doses of 80 mg daily, 40 mg daily, and 40 mg every other day have been used. One approach would be to begin with 1 mg/kg per day, and then taper the dose once improvement has been achieved or side effects dictate a reduction in dosage. ***CAUTION:*** *Retinoids are teratogenic. Numerous abnormalities have been reported in infants exposed to the drug in utero. Pregnancy is an absolute contraindication to the use of this class of drugs. The use of retinoids in women of childbearing potential has been a subject of controversy. Any practitioner prescribing these agents should be thoroughly familiar with their effects, current labeling, and current guidelines for care.* Retinoids may produce changes in serum lipids, and patients should be monitored for elevations in triglycerides. Elevated liver enzymes and a possible association with inflammatory bowel disease have also been reported. Long-term administration of retinoids has been associated with skeletal abnormalities resembling diffuse idiopathic skeletal hyperostosis. In view of the potential for side effects, it may be best to use a retinoid to establish initial control, then switch to another agent for maintenance therapy.

Dapsone, 100 mg daily, may be an effective treatment in some cases of discoid lupus refractory to other drugs. In one study, 9 of 11 patients with cutaneous lupus demonstrated improvement with dapsone.[95] Patients should first be screened for G-6-PD deficiency. Potential side effects include hemolysis, methemoglobinemia, and neuropathy.

Thalidomide has been used effectively for the treatment of discoid lesions of lupus erythematosus. Doses in the range of 100 to 300 mg per day have been used initially, with maintenance doses of 50 mg per day.[96] The teratogenic effects of thalidomide are well known. Peripheral neuropathy may also develop as a side effect of therapy. In this country, thalidomide is available only on a compassionate basis (usually for the treatment of erythema nodosum leprosum).

Patients with cutaneous lupus may respond to a single agent, but those who do not may respond to combination therapy. In fact, in a referral practice it is common for a large proportion of patients to be treated with combination therapy. Once a response is achieved, the agents with a less favorable safety profile can be tapered. There continues to be a need for the development of new effective regimens. Cytotoxic agents, cyclosporin, and cimetidine are some of the agents that may be valuable additions to the medical armamentarium for cutaneous lupus erythematosus.

Lichen Planopilaris

Corticosteroids are the mainstay of treatment for lichen planopilaris. Corticosteroids are used in much the same way that they would be for the treatment of discoid lupus erythematosus (discussed previously). Dosing, routes of administration, and side effects are similar.

Retinoids have demonstrated some effect in the treatment of lichen planus.[97] They provide a possible alternative to corticosteroids in the treatment of lichen planopilaris (refer to earlier discussion of teratogenic potential and other side effects).

Griseofulvin, 1 g per day, has been found to be effective in some cases of lichen planopilaris (W. F. Bergfeld, unpublished data).

Mixed Inflammatory Alopecia

Mixed inflammatory alopecia generally responds to corticosteroid treatment. Further study is needed in order to define the pathogenic mechanisms in this group of disorders. In refractory cases, consideration may be given to alternative therapies effective in lupus erythematosus and lichen planopilaris.

Graham-Little Syndrome

No treatment is uniformly effective for Graham-Little syndrome. Topical, intralesional, and systemic corticosteroids may be used, as they would be used for the treatment of lichen planopilaris. Follicular papules may respond to topical retinoic acid preparations. End-stage patches of alopecia may be treated surgically.

Pseudopelade

During the active phase, this condition may respond to hydroxychloroquine[16] or corticosteroids.[17] These drugs should be used as in the treatment of cutaneous lupus. The response is highly variable. "Pseudopeladic states" may result from lichen planopilaris or lupus erythematosus. Treatment for these conditions has been discussed previously.

Scleroderma Variants (Including Morphea)

Scleroderma variants respond poorly to most therapeutic interventions. Intralesional corticosteroids have been used in the acute phase, sometimes with good results. The role of antimalarial agents requires further study. Another question which deserves further study is the relationship between morphea and spirochetes (in particular, the Lyme spirochete). It is unclear what role antibiotics should have in the treatment of morphea.

Nonscarring "hyalinizing" alopecias (including morphea and scleroderma variants and pseudopelade) are often self-limited. This is fortunate, as they may respond poorly to therapy. Because the conditions may affect only limited areas of the scalp, end-stage lesions are particularly amenable to scalp reduction.[98] Hair transplantation should also be considered as an option.

Erosive Pustular Dermatosis and Folliculitis Decalvans

Erosive pustular dermatosis and the closely related condition folliculitis decalvans often respond poorly to treatment, although some patients improve with courses of antibiotics.[30,31] Topical corticosteroids are sometimes effective. As there is some evidence that this condition represents an abnormal immune response to bacterial antigens, prolonged suppressive treatment with antistaphylococcal agents is recommended. Erythromycin, 500 mg b.i.d., may prove adequate, but cephalosporins and semisynthetic penicillins are other alternatives. Single-drug therapy with rifampin has been reported as effective in a case of folliculitis decalvans refractory to other agents,[99] but because of the potential for emergence of resistant strains, rifampin probably should not be used as single-agent therapy. In refractory cases, combination therapy with rifampin plus dicloxacillin could be considered. Topical antimicrobial agents may be used as adjunctive therapy.

Zinc appears to have a role in modulating cutaneous inflammation.[100] Zinc sulfate (30–60 mg t.i.d.) has been used successfully in the treatment of a reported case of erosive pustular dermatosis of the scalp.[101]

Perifolliculitis Capitis Abscedens et Suffodiens

Perifolliculitis capitis abscedens et suffodiens responds unpredictably to treatment. Antibiotics and oral, topical, or intralesional corticosteroids may be helpful. Effective treatment may require combination therapy, such as a combination of incision and drainage, corticosteroids, antibiotics, and isotretinoin.[102] Isotretinoin and oral zinc are promising as single-agent therapies.[103–106] Isotretinoin therapy may be started at a dose of 1 mg/kg per day and the dose tapered once an effect has been achieved or side effects dictate a reduction in dosage. Retinoids are teratogenic. The dose of zinc used in the treatment of a case of perifolliculitis capitis abscedens et suffodiens was 90 mg of zinc (corresponding to 400 mg of zinc sulfate) three times daily.[106] A response was noted within 3 weeks, with complete healing after 12 weeks. Other treatments that have been used successfully include x-ray epilation[37] and surgical scalping with grafting.[107]

Infectious Disorders

Treatment of infectious disorders should be directed at the responsible microorganism. For staphylococcal folliculitis, a cephalosporin or semisynthetic penicillin is recommended, as erythromycin-resistant staphylococci are being encountered with increasing frequency.[108]

Fungal scalp infections should be treated with a systemic agent. Griseofulvin is the drug of choice. Ketoconazole may also be effective. Newer oral antifungals are becoming available and will no doubt have a place in the armamentarium of agents for fungal scalp infections. Topical treatment with selenium sulfide may reduce the risk of contagion and should be considered as adjunctive therapy. Markedly inflamed lesions may respond more quickly if an oral corticosteroid is given during the first few days of systemic antifungal therapy:[52,89] prednisone (about 1 mg/kg per day) for 3 to 5 days may be useful.

Viral infections of the scalp, including Herpes simplex and zoster may be treated with appropriate doses of acyclovir (Zovirax). In adults, Herpes simplex infections usually respond to acyclovir 200 mg given five times daily for 5 to 10 days. Immunosuppressed patients may not respond to this therapy. Other agents, such as Foscarnet, are being evaluated as alternative treatments. In adults, zoster generally responds to acyclovir 800 mg given five times daily for 10 days. Patients should be advised to maintain adequate hydration as acyclovir demonstrates limited solubility at higher doses.

Sarcoidosis

Sarcoidosis of the scalp may respond to intralesional, potent topical, and oral corticosteroids. Local atrophy, dyspigmentation, and systemic steroid effects must be monitored. Antimalarial agents may be of benefit in refractory cases.

Acne Keloidalis Nuchae

Acne keloidalis nuchae (dermatitis papillaris capillitii, keloidal folliculitis) often presents a real therapeutic challenge. Mild cases may respond to intralesional and topical corticosteroids. Generally, class I or class II (ultrapotent and superpotent) topical steroids are needed. Treatment should be continued until the papules flatten or hypopigmentation of the surrounding skin occurs. The physician must remain alert to the possibility of cutaneous atrophy. Ultrapotent (class I) topical steroids may cause adrenal suppression and are not suitable for long-term use: these should be limited to 1 to 2 weeks of continual use. A less potent corticosteroid such as fluocinonide gel (class II) works well to produce initial clearing (over a 1- to 2-month period) and is also suitable for intermittent use as maintenance therapy.

For advanced cases of acne keloidalis nuchae with secondarily infected sinus tracts, antibiotic therapy may be of use. These can be combined with topical or intralesional corticosteroids. Tetracyclines are often helpful, but it is often best to obtain sensitivity studies before choosing an antibiotic, especially if infected sinus tracts are present. Good results have been obtained with chloramphenicol 500 mg compounded in 30 g of fluocinonide cream, applied t.i.d. (H. Minus, personal communication). This preparation is not available commercially and has not been evaluated by the Food and Drug Administration. Bone marrow effects are possible with topically applied chloramphenicol. Surgery may be of value in individual cases and may be the only effective therapy in some cases.

Unclassified Alopecia in Black Females, Including the Follicular Degeneration Syndrome

No effective treatment has been documented. Further study is needed to define the mechanisms involved. Specific treatment for the acute phase of the follicular degeneration syndrome in black women awaits further study of the pathogenesis of this disorder.

Surgical Treatment of End-Stage Permanent Alopecia

Treatments which may be used in end-stage permanent alopecia, regardless of the cause, include scalp reduction and hair transplantation.[98,109] In general, these treatments should be reserved for "burned-out" cases of permanent alopecia, when no active lesions remain. The use of tissue-expansion techniques has significantly expanded the role of scalp reduction in the treatment of permanent alopecia.[110] The implantation of artificial fibers has been associated with severe complications and is not considered an acceptable approach to treatment.[111–113] Hair transplantation, scalp reduction, and tissue expansion should be performed only by individuals skilled in these techniques.

CONCLUDING REMARKS

Proper diagnosis in cases of permanent alopecia relies on a global evaluation of the patient, including a thorough history and physical examination, biopsy for routine and immunofluorescent microscopy, and serological evaluation. Often, multiple histological sections must be examined to establish the correct diagnosis. This is particularly true if vertical sections are used. Elastic tissue and PAS stains may be of great value, in addition to the routine H&E-stained sections. Elastic tissue stains are particularly helpful in differentiating "hyalinizing" alopecia from true scarring alopecia.

We use the clinical term *permanent alopecia* because it encompasses true scarring alopecia as well as hyalinizing conditions such as morphea and pseudopelade. Histological evidence of destruction of the bulge region of the hair follicle appears to be the best marker for true permanent alopecia.

Surgical techniques such as scalp reduction, tissue expansion, and hair transplantation are of immense value in the treatment of end-stage permanent alopecia. Specific treatment in the acute stage depends on accurate diagnosis. Biopsy should be considered early in the evaluation of any scarring alopecia.

REFERENCES

1. Cotsarelis G, Sun T, Lavker RM: Label-retaining cells reside in the bulge area of pilosebaceous unit: Implications for follicular stem cells, hair cycle, and skin carcinogenesis. Cell 61:1329–1337, 1990.
2. Lavker RM, Fryer E, Margolis-Fryer J, Ostad M: Cells in the bulge region of mouse hair follicle undergo transient proliferation during onset of anagen and in response to physical and chemical stimuli (abstract). J Invest Dermatol 98(4):581, 1992.
3. Armas-Cruz R et al.: Clinical diagnosis of systemic lupus erythematosus. Am J Med 25:409–419, 1958.
4. Jordan RE: Subtle clues to diagnosis by immunopathology: Scarring alopecia. Am J Dermatopathol 2:157–159, 1980.
5. Harrist TJ, Mihm MC: Cutaneous immunopathology: The diagnostic use of direct and indirect immunofluorescence techniques in dermatologic disease. Hum Pathol 10:625–653, 1979.
6. Valenzuela R, Bergfeld WF, Deodhar SD: Lupus erythematosus: Immunohistopathology. In *Interpretation of Immunofluorescent Patterns in Skin Diseases.* Chicago, American Society of Clinical Pathologists Press, 1984, pp 66–79.
7. Silver H, Chargin L, Sachs PM: Follicular lichen planus (lichen planopilaris). Arch Dermatol 67:346–354, 1953.
8. Valenzuela R, Bergfeld WF, Deodhar SD: Lichen planus. In *Interpretation of Immunofluorescent Patterns in Skin Diseases.* Chicago, American Society of Clinical Pathologists Press, 1984, pp 127–131.
9. Ioannides D, Bystryn JC: Immunofluorescence abnormalities in lichen planopilaris. Arch Dermatol 128:214–216, 1992.

10. Smith WB, Grabski WJ, McCollough ML, Davis TL: Immunofluorescent findings in lichen planopilaris: A contrasting experience (letter). Arch Dermatol 128:1405–1406, 1992.
11. Gay Prieto J: Pseudopelade of Brocq: Its relationship to some forms of cicatricial alopecia and to lichen planus. J Invest Dermatol 24:323, 1955.
12. Horn RT et al.: Immunofluorescent findings and clinical overlap in two cases of follicular lichen planus. J Am Acad Dermatol 2:203–207, 1982.
13. Spier HW, Kellig W: Lichen Ruber Follicularis Decalvans (Graham-Little Syndrom) und Seine Beziehungen zur Pseudopelade Brocq. Hautarzt 4:457–467, 1953.
14. Waldorf DS: Lichen planopilaris. Arch Dermatol 93:684–691, 1966.
15. Bulengo-Ransby SM, Headington JT: Pseudopelade of Brocq in a child. J Am Acad Dermatol 23:944–945, 1990.
16. Bulengo-Ransby SM, Headington JT: Pseudopelade of Brocq (reply—letter). J Am Acad Dermatol 25:865–866, 1991.
17. Bergner T, Braun-Falco O: Pseudopelade of Brocq (letter). J Am Acad Dermatol 25:865, 1991.
18. Braun-Falco O, Bergner T, Heilgemeir GP: Pseudopelade Brocq—Krankheitsbild oder Krankheitsentitat. Hautarzt 40:77–83, 1989.
19. Brocq L, Lenglet E, Ayrignac J: Recherches sur l'alopecie atrophiante, variete pseudopelade. Ann Dermatol Syphil 6:97, 1905.
20. Kaminsky A, Kaminsky CA, de Kaminsky AR, Abulafia J: Liquen folicular alopeciante. Med Cutan 2:135, 1967.
21. Ronchese F: Pseudopelade. Arch Dermatol 82:336, 1960.
22. Pinkus H: Differential patterns of elastic fibers in scarring and non-scarring alopecias. J Cutan Pathol 5:93–104, 1978.
23. Braun-Falco O et al.: Pseudopelade of Brocq. Dermatologica 172:18–23, 1986.
24. Pierard-Franchimont C, Pierard GE: Massive lymphocyte-mediated apoptosis during the early stage of pseudopelade. Dermatologica 172:254–257, 1986.
25. Reed RJ, Clark WH, Mihm MC: The cutaneous collagenoses. Hum Pathol 4:165–186, 1973.
26. Golitz LE, Shapiro L, Hurwitz E, Stritzler R: Cicatricial alopecia of sarcoidosis. Arch Dermatol 107:758–760, 1973.
27. Caputo R, Veraldi S: Erosive pustular dermatosis of the scalp. J Am Acad Dermatol 28:96–98, 1993.
28. Laymon CW: The cicatricial alopecias. J Invest Dermatol 8:99, 1947.
29. Binazzi M: In Tema di Folliculiti Decalvanti. Annali Italiani di Dermatologia e di Sifiligrafi 9:325, 1954.
30. Bogg A: Folliculitis decalvans. Acta Derm Venereol 43:14, 1963.
31. Loewenthal LJA: A case of lupoid sycosis or ulerythema sycosiforme, beginning in infancy. Br J Dermatol 69:443, 1957.
32. Miller RF: Epilating folliculitis of the glabrous skin. Arch Dermatol 83:115, 1961.
33. Frazer NG, Grant PW: Folliculitis decalvans with hypocomplementemia. Br J Dermatol 107(suppl 22):88, 1982.
34. Shitara A, Igareshi R, Morohashi M: Folliculitis decalvans and cellular immunity—Two brothers with oral candidiasis. Jpn J Dermatol 28:113, 1974.
35. Wheeland RG, Thurmond RD, Gilmore WA, Blackstock R: Chronic blepharitis and pyoderma of the scalp: An immune deficiency state in a father and son with hypercalcemia and decreased intracellular killing. Pediatr Dermatol 1(2):134–142, 1983.
36. Ebling FJG, Dawber R, Rook A: The hair. In Rook A et al. (eds): *Textbook of Dermatology*, 4th ed. Oxford, Blackwell Scientific Publications, 1986, pp 1937–2037.
37. McMullan FH, Zeligman I: Perifolliculitis capitis abscedens et suffodiens: Its successful treatment with x-ray epilation. Arch Dermatol 73:256–263, 1956.
38. Moyer DG, Williams RM: Perifolliculitis capitis abscedens et suffodiens. Arch Dermatol 85:378–384, 1962.
39. Langtry JAA, Ive FA: Pityriasis amiantacea, an unrecognized cause of scarring alopecia, described in four patients. Acta Derm Venereol (Stockh) 71:352–353, 1991.
40. Cornbleet T: A case for diagnosis: Cutis verticis gyrata? Lipoma? Arch Dermatol 32:688, 1935.
41. Curtis JW, Heising RA: Lipedematous alopecia associated with skin hyperelasticity. Arch Dermatol 89:819–820, 1964.
42. Coskey R, Fosnaugh RP, Fine G: Lipedematous alopecia. Arch Dermatol 84:619–622, 1961.
43. Birnbaum PS, Baden HP: Heritable disorders of hair. Dermatol Clin 5(1):137–153, 1987.
44. Traupe H, Happle R: Alopecia ichthyotica: A characteristic feature of congenital ichthyosis. Dermatologica 167:225–230, 1983.
45. Happle R: X-linked dominant chondrodysplasia punctata: Review of the literature and report of a case. Hum Genet 53:65–73, 1979.
46. Crovato F, Rebora A: Acute skin manifestations of Conradi-Huenermann syndrome in a male adult. Arch Dermatol 121:1064–1065, 1985.
47. Dorfman M, Hershko C, Eisenberg S, Sagher F: Ichthyosiform dermatosis with systemic lipidosis. Arch Dermatol 110:261–266, 1974.
48. Rycroft RJG, Moynahan EJ, Wells RS: Atypical ichthyosiform erythroderma, deafness and keratitis. Br J Dermatol 94:211–217, 1976.
49. Tosti A: Congenital triangular alopecia. J Am Acad Dermatol 16:991–993, 1987.
50. Minars N: Congenital temporal alopecia. Arch Dermatol 109:395–396, 1974.
51. Levin DL, Nolan KS, Esterly NG: Congenital absence of skin. J Am Acad Dermatol 2:203–206, 1980.
52. Levy ML: Disorders of the hair and scalp in children. Pediatr Dermatol 38:905–919, 1991.
53. Baraitser M, Carter C, Brett EM: A new alopecia/mental retardation syndrome. J Med Genet 20:64–75, 1983.
54. Welton DG: Keratosis follicularis with unusual involvement of the scalp. Arch Dermatol Syphilol 47:398–404, 1943.
55. Freire-Maia N: Ectodermal dysplasia revisited. Acta Genet Med Gemellol 26:121–131, 1977.
56. Pinheiro M, Pereira LC, Freire-Maia N: A previously undescribed condition: Tricho-odonto-onycho-dermal syndrome. A review of the tricho-odonto-onychial subgroup of ectodermal dysplasias. Br J Dermatol 105:371–382, 1981.
57. Solomon LM, Keuer EJ: The ectodermal dysplasias:

Problems of classification and some newer syndromes. Arch Dermatol 116:1295–1299, 1980.
58. Kuklik M: Ectodermal dysplasia with alopecia, elevated frequency of chromosomal breaks and normal dentition. Cas Lek Cesk 129:1266–1270, 1990.
59. Christodorescu D, Nedelcu EF, Popovici F: Mental and growth retardation with congenital atrichia and papular lesions. Rev Roum Med—Neurol Psychiatr 22:163–165, 1984.
60. Moynahan EJ, Wolff OH: A new neuro-cutaneous syndrome (skin, eye and brain) consisting of linear nevus, bilateral lipo-dermoid of the conjunctiva, cranial thickening, cerebral cortical atrophy and mental retardation. Br J Dermatol 79:651–652, 1967.
61. Wagner W: Alopezia und Nagelveranderungen bei Epidermolysis Bullosa Hereditaria. Z Hautkr Geshlechtskr 20:278–284, 1956.
62. Goerz G, Kind R, Lehmann P: Cicatricial alopecias. In Orfanos CE, Happle R (eds): *Hair and Hair Diseases.* Berlin, Springer-Verlag, 1990, pp 611–639.
63. Dawber RPR, Ebling FJG, Wojnarowska FT: Disorders of hair. In Champion RH, Burton JL, Ebling FJG (eds): *Textbook of Dermatology,* 5th ed. Oxford, Blackwell Scientific Publications, 1992, pp 2533–2613.
64. Shelley WB, Wood MG: Alopecia with fibrous dysplasia and osteomas of the skin. Arch Dermatol 112:715–719, 1976.
65. Connor JM, Evans DAP: Fibrodysplasia ossificans progressiva. J Bone Joint Surg 64:76–83, 1982.
66. Barber HW: Folliculitis erythematosa reticulata combined with lichen spinulosus, epidermal cysts, and folliculitis decalvans. Br J Dermatol 40:24–26, 1928.
67. Eramo LR et al.: Ichthyosis follicularis with alopecia and photophobia. Arch Dermatol 121:1167–1174, 1985.
68. Tong AKF, Baden HP: Tufted hair folliculitis. J Am Acad Dermatol 21:1096–1099, 1989.
69. Dalziel KL, Telfer NR, Wilson CL, Dawber RPR: Tufted folliculitis: A specific bacterial disease? Am J Dermatopathol 12:37–41, 1990.
70. Loewenthal LJA: "Compound" and grouped hairs of the human scalp: Their possible connection with follicular infections. J Invest Dermatol 8:263–273, 1947.
71. Falls HF, Schull WJ: Hallermann-Streiff syndrome: A dyscephaly with congenital cataracts and hypotrichosis. Arch Ophthalmol 63:409–420, 1960.
72. Clementi M et al.: Pachyonychia congenita Jackson-Lawler type: A distinct malformation syndrome. Br J Dermatol 114:367–370, 1986.
73. Dupre A, Bonafe JL, Christol B: Syringomas as a causative factor for cicatricial alopecia (letter). Arch Dermatol 117:315, 1981.
74. Mehregan AH, Baker S: Basaloid follicular hamartoma. J Cutan Pathol 12:55–65, 1985.
75. Brown AC, Crounse RG, Winkelmann RK: Generalized hair-follicle hamartoma associated with alopecia, aminoaciduria, and myasthenia gravis. Arch Dermatol 99:478–493, 1969.
76. Ridley CM, Smith N: Generalized hair follicle hamartoma associated with alopecia and myasthenia gravis: Report of a second case. Clin Exp Dermatol 6:283–289, 1981.
77. Shelley WB, Wood MG: Occult syringomas of the scalp associated with progressive hair loss. Arch Dermatol 116:843–844, 1980.
78. Mehregan AH, Mehregan DA: Syringoma-like sweat duct proliferation in scalp alopecias. J Cutan Pathol 17:355–357, 1990.
79. Snyder RA, Crain WR, McNutt NS: Alopecia mucinosa: Report of a case with diffuse alopecia and normal-appearing scalp skin. Arch Dermatol 120:496–498, 1984.
80. Van Scott EJ, Reinertson RP: Detection of radiation effects on hair roots of the human scalp. J Invest Dermatol 29:205–212, 1957.
81. Maguire HC Jr, Hanno R: Diseases of the hair. In Moschella SL, Hurley HJ (eds): *Dermatology,* 2d ed. Philadelphia, W. B. Saunders, 1985, pp 1369–1397.
82. Pinol Aguade J et al.: Grave dermatitis liquenoide con alopecia irreversible y beta-alaninuria en pacientes tratados con tuberculostaticos. Med Cutan 3:27–42, 1968.
83. Bauer F: Quinacrine hydrochloride drug eruption (tropical lichenoid dermatitis). J Am Acad Dermatol 4:239–248, 1981.
84. Lachapelle JM, Pierard GE: Traumatic alopecia in trichotillomania. J Cutan Pathol 4:51–67, 1977.
85. Mehregan AH: Trichotillomania. Arch Dermatol 102:129–133, 1970.
86. Muller SA: Trichotillomania: A histologic study in sixty-six patients. J Am Acad Dermatol 23:56–62, 1990.
87. Muller SA, Winkelmann RK: Trichotillomania. Arch Dermatol 105:535–540, 1972.
88. Sperling LC, Sau P: The follicular degeneration syndrome in black patients. Arch Dermatol 128:68–74, 1992.
89. Newton RC, Hebert AA, Freese TW, Solomon AR: Scarring alopecia. Dermatol Clin 5:603–618, 1987.
90. Shearer RV, Dubois EL: Ocular changes induced by long-term hydroxychloroquine (Plaquenil) therapy. Am J Ophthalmol 64:245–252, 1967.
91. Tuffanelli DL: Lupus erythematosus. J Am Acad Dermatol 4:127–142, 1981.
92. Ward WQ, Walter-Ryan WG, Shehi GM: Toxic psychosis: A complication of antimalarial therapy. J Am Acad Dermatol 12:863–865, 1985.
93. Zuehlke RL, Lillis PJ, Tice A: Antimalarial therapy for lupus erythematosus: An apparent advantage of quinacrine. Int J Dermatol 20:57–61, 1981.
94. Rubenstein DJ, Huntley AC: Keratotic lupus erythematosus: Treatment with isotretinoin. J Am Acad Dermatol 14:910–914, 1986.
95. Coburn PR, Shuster S: Dapsone and discoid lupus erythematosus. Br J Dermatol 106:105–106, 1982.
96. Hasper MJ, Klokke AH: Thalidomide in the treatment of chronic discoid lupus erythematosus. Acta Derm Venereol (Stockh) 62:321–324, 1982.
97. Mahrle G, Meyer-Hamme S, Ippen H: Oral treatment of keratinizing disorders of skin and mucous membranes with etretinate. Arch Dermatol 118:97–100, 1982.
98. Stegman SJ, Tromovitch TA: Cosmetic dermatologic surgery. Arch Dermatol 118:1013–1016, 1982.
99. Brozena SJ, Cohen LE, Fenske NA: Folliculitis decalvans—Response to rifampin. Cutis 42:512–515, 1988.
100. Norris D: Zinc and cutaneous inflammation. Arch Dermatol 121:985–989, 1985.

101. Ikeda M, Arata J, Isaka H: Erosive pustular dermatosis of the scalp successfully treated with oral zinc sulphate. Br J Dermatol 106:742–743, 1982.
102. Shaffer N, Billick RC, Srolvitz H: Perifolliculitis capitis abscedens et suffodiens: Resolution with combination therapy. Arch Dermatol 128:1329–1331, 1992.
103. Bjellerup M, Wallengran J: Familial perifolliculitis capitis abscedens et suffodiens in two brothers successfully treated with isotretinoin. J Am Acad Dermatol 23:752–753, 1990.
104. Taylor AEM: Dissecting cellulitis of the scalp: Response to isotretinoin (letter). Lancet 2:225, 1987.
105. Schewach-Millet M, Ziv R, Shapira D: Perifolliculitis capitis abscedens et suffodiens treated with isotretinoin (13-cis-retinoic acid) (letter). J Am Acad Dermatol 15:1291–1292, 1986.
106. Berne B, Venge P, Ohman S: Perifolliculitis capitis abscedens et suffodiens (Hoffman): Complete healing associated with oral zinc therapy. Arch Dermatol 121:1028–1030, 1985.
107. Moschella SL, Klein MH, Miller RJ: Perifolliculitis capitis abscedens et suffodiens: Report of a successful therapeutic scalping. Arch Dermatol 96:195–197, 1967.
108. Feldman P, Lynfield Y: Antibiotic choice for pyodermas (letter). J Am Acad Dermatol 17:859–860, 1987.
109. Schultz BC, Roenigk HH: Scalp reduction for alopecia. J Dermatol Surg Oncol 5:808–811, 1979.
110. Roenigk RK, Wheeland RG: Tissue expansion in cicatricial alopecia. Arch Dermatol 123:641–646, 1987.
111. Hanke CW, Bergfeld WF: Fiber implantation for pattern baldness. JAMA 241(2):146–148, 1979.
112. Hanke CW, Ceilley RI, Bergfeld WF: Complications of fiber implantation for baldness. Am Fam Physician 24(1):115–118, 1981.
113. Hanke CW, Norins AL, Pantzer JG Jr: Hair implant complications. JAMA 245(13):1344–1345, 1981.
114. Rand R, Baden HP: Keratosis follicularis spinulosa decalvans: Report of two cases and literature review. Arch Dermatol 119:22–26, 1983.
115. Davenport DD: Ulerythema ophryogenes. Arch Dermatol 89:74–80, 1964.
116. Kooij R, Venter J: Atrophodermia vermiculata with unusual localization and associated congenital anomalies. Dermatologica 118:161–167, 1959.
117. Manson M: Three cases of ichthyosis follicularis. Br J Dermatol 33:20–22, 1921.
118. Appell ML, Sherertz EF: A kindred with alopecia, keratosis pilaris, cataracts, and psoriasis. J Am Acad Dermatol 16:89–95, 1987.

Chapter

13

Elise A. Olsen

HYPERTRICHOSIS

INTRODUCTION

The medical literature is replete with case reports of patients whose excess hair is erroneously termed *hirsutism* when *hypertrichosis* is the correct term. Both words infer excessive hair, but *hirsutism* is best defined as excessive hair growth in women in anatomic sites where such growth is considered to be a secondary male characteristic.[1] Women with hirsutism have excess hair primarily in the beard, moustache, chest, and linea alba areas where hair growth is under androgen control. The term *hypertrichosis* implies only hair density or length beyond the accepted limits of normal for a particular age, race, and sex,[2] and does not imply a particular distribution of hair.

Hypertrichosis may be generalized or localized and of lanugo, vellus, or terminal hairs. The first hair to form in utero (third through seventh month) is lanugo hair, which covers the entire fetus with generally unpigmented, unmedullated fine hair that may grow several centimeters in length.[3,4] This hair is normally shed in utero at 7 to 8 months, to be replaced by vellus hair on the body and terminal hair on the scalp. Although lanugo hair may be seen on the limbs and shoulders of full-term, normally developed, healthy newborns, it is not normally seen beyond the first or second month of life. Vellus hair is also unmedullated, unpigmented, or lightly pigmented, generally growing to a maximum of < 2 cm.[5] Terminal hair is usually pigmented, although age or heredity may lead to loss of pigment in terminal hair. Terminal hair is best defined by its size relative to vellus hair ($\sim 2\times$ diameter), medullation (although this may be intermittent), and length of anagen, with the possibility of length far surpassing 2 cm. Most cases of localized hypertrichosis involve terminal hair, whereas generalized hypertrichosis may be of lanugo, vellus, or terminal hair. The fact that individual hairs, even in adult life, may express any of the three phenotypes and may metamor-

Table 13-1
CAUSES OF HYPERTRICHOSIS

- Generalized hypertrichosis
  - Congenital or hereditary
    - Congenital hypertrichosis lanuginosa[2,6,9,11]
    - Congenital hypertrichosis lanuginosa with gingival fibromatosis ± breast fibroadenoma[12,13,154]
    - Cornelia de Lange's syndrome[18–20,23,24,155,156]
    - Hurler's syndrome[28,157]
    - Coffin-Siris syndrome[158–161]
    - Gorlin's syndrome[162,163]
    - Hyperkinetic circulatory disorder[164]
    - Schinzel-Giedion syndrome[165,166]
    - Lawrence-Seip syndrome[167,168]
    - Generalized smooth muscle hamartoma[115]
      - Michelin-Tire Syndrome
    - Osteochondrodysplasia with hypertrichosis[169]
  - Acquired
    - Acquired hypertrichosis lanuginosa (malignancy)[31,32,40–42]
    - Drugs
      - Minoxidil[43–45]
      - Diazoxide[53,56,57]
      - Phenytoin sodium[59–62]
      - Cyclosporine[63–67]
      - PUVA[71–73]
      - Topical steroids[74,170]
      - Streptomycin[75,76]
      - Acetazolamide[77]
      - Oxadiazolopyrimidine[78]
      - Fenoterol[79]
    - Porphyria
      - Porphyria cutanea tarda[80,82,86,88]
      - Variegate porphyria[89]
      - Erythropoietic porphyria[91,92]
    - POEMS syndrome[94–96]
    - Hypothyroidism[97–99]
    - Acrodynia[76]
    - Malabsorption syndromes[76]
    - CNS-related problems or trauma
      - After encephalitis[31]
      - Multiple sclerosis[31]
      - Schizophrenia[31]
      - Head injury[31,62]
      - Hyperostosis interna[31]
      - Anorexia nervosa[31]
- Localized hypertrichosis
  - Congenital or hereditary
    - Middorsum hypertrichosis with underlying neuroectodermal abnormality
      - Spina bifida occulta[100,102]
      - Spina bifida[100,102]
      - Traction (e.g., meningocoele manque)[100,102,103]
      - Diastematomyelia[101]
    - Hairy elbows[105,106]
    - Hairy pinna[109–111]
    - Trichomegaly[114]
    - Congenital smooth muscle hamartoma[116,117,127]
    - Winchester syndrome[118]
    - Pigmented nevus[2]
  - Acquired
    - Becker's[122]
    - Melorheostatic scleroderma[130]
    - Post morphea[121]
    - Osteosclerotic myeloma[93]
    - Drugs
      - Interferon[131]
      - Sodium tetradecyl sulfate[135]
    - Under casts[120,171,172]
    - Irritants (topical)[121,171]
    - Repeated trauma
      - Pressure (e.g., sack bearers)[173]
      - Lichen simplex chronicus[171]
      - Biting[171]
      - Insect bites[174,175]
    - Stasis/lymphedema[120,175]
    - Congenital A-V fistula[171,175,176]
    - Denervated areas[8,175]
    - Chronic osteomyelitis[175]
    - Sympathetic dystrophy[177]
    - Site of immunizations
      - Smallpox[178]
      - Diphtheria-tetanus[179]
    - Chickenpox[179]
    - HIV (eyelashes)[134]
    - Periphery burned area[121,180]

phose one into the other should not be overlooked.

To simplify the assessment and diagnosis of disorders of hypertrichosis, the author has developed an outline based on division first into generalized or localized hypertrichosis (Table 13-1) and then into congenital or hereditary vs. acquired hypertrichosis. Generalized hypertrichosis here includes multiple areas of excess growth as well as a diffuse distribution of excess hair, whereas localized hypertrichosis implies excess hair limited to a single area or to a few areas clearly associated with either physical trauma or abnormalities of the underlying skin. Since the type of excess hair often changes with time, this will not be used to further subclassify hypertrichosis.

GENERALIZED HYPERTRICHOSIS

Congenital or Hereditary Hypertrichosis

There are few conditions in which hypertrichosis is truly generalized and confluent; most of these conditions are associated with overgrowth of lanugo hair. In *congenital hypertrichosis lanuginosa,* the excessive hair growth may be present at birth or may develop within the first few months of life. The excess hair may involve the

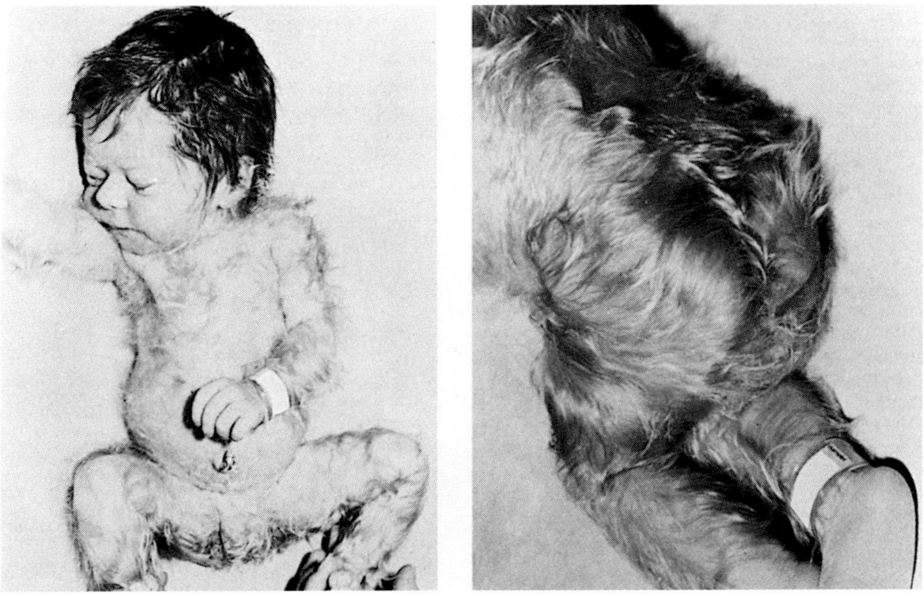

Figure 13-1 Congenital hypertrichosis lanuginosa. (*Reprinted with permission from Partridge J.W.*[6]

entire body surface except the palms, soles, lips, glans penis, and distal phalanges,[6,7] and may be up to 4 to 10 inches in length. The hair is usually silvery gray to blond in color[7] and grows in a direction away from the midline[8] (Figs. 13-1 and 13-2). The hypertrichosis may persist, diminish, or increase with age.[6] Inheritance of congenital hypertrichosis lanuginosa is generally considered to be autosomal dominant with variable expressivity,[6,9] although one family with X-linked dominant inheritance has been noted.[10] The incidence is only 1/1000 million.[6,9]

Because of the rarity and arresting appearance of people with this condition, affected individuals have been frequently exploited in sideshows

Figure 13-2 Congenital hypertrichosis lanuginosa.

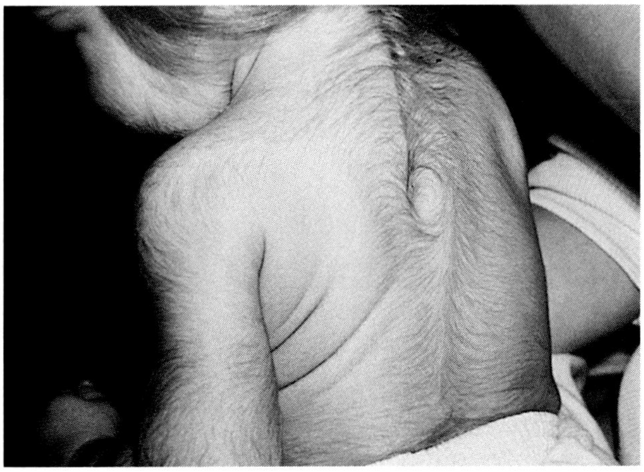

or royal courts and termed "dog men," "ape men," or "human werewolves."[2,9] An illustration of one of the more famous individuals with congenital hypertrichosis lanuginosa is shown in Figure 13-3. In most cases of congenital hypertrichosis lanuginosa, patients are generally otherwise normal except for possible anomalous dental eruptions[6] and thus may be categorized as a form of tricho-odonto ectodermal dysplasia.[11]

Hereditary gingival fibromatosis associated with generalized hypertrichosis can mimic congenital hypertrichosis lanuginosa. Gingival fibromatosis, in which the gingival tissue hypertrophies and buries the emerging teeth in redundant tissue,[12] is generally autosomal dominant or sporadic in nature, with an incidence of 1/175,000.[13] As the presence of teeth is necessary for the development of gingival hypertrophy, gingival fibromatosis usually appears with the emergence of the primary or secondary teeth.[12,14] In the cases associated with hypertrichosis (uncommon), in which the affected persons frequently also have findings of epilepsy and oligophrenia, the gingival fibromatosis almost always either is present at birth or appears within the first year of life,[14] although it can appear as late as puberty.[13] The hypertrichosis is usually not as extreme as that seen with congenital hypertrichosis lanuginosa and mainly involves the eyebrows, face, limbs, and midback.[13] Most cases associated with gingival fibromatosis have noted black vs. light-colored hair,[14] at least by adult life.[13]

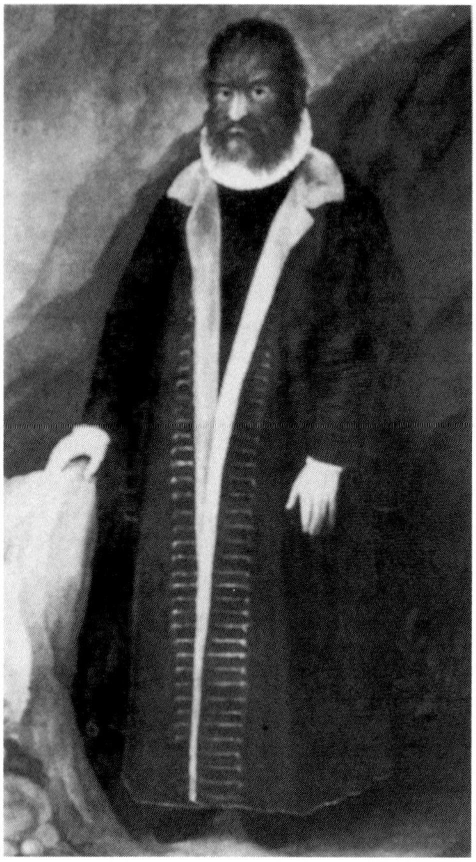

Figure 13-3 Peter Gonzales, valued member of the sixteenth-century French court of King Henry II, famous for his congenital hypertrichosis lanuginosa. (*Reprinted with permission from Ravin and Hodge*[7] *and* from the *Kunsthistorisches Museum, Vienna, Austria.*)

Hereditary gingival fibromatosis associated with hypertrichosis probably represents a unique syndrome. Gingival fibromatosis can occur as a part of many other syndromes, most of which do not involve hypertrichosis. The exception is the case report of a generalized but not confluent hypertrichosis with congenital macrogingivae and giant fibroadenomas of the breast leading to breast hypertrophy.[14,15] Although this was termed "Cowden's" syndrome,[14] the case did not include the usual cutaneous stigmata of Cowden's syndrome, i.e., tricholemmomas, angiomas, and lipomas.[16]

Congenital hypertrichosis lanuginosa, while dramatic and seemingly obvious in its fully developed form, may be difficult in infancy to distinguish from other syndromes that include a generalized but not necessarily confluent hypertrichosis. The alert clinician will seek out and catalog all other abnormalities in affected children to determine if another syndrome is present. Often it is only after publication of a single case or group of cases that recognition of a syndrome and determination of its critical features take place. Table 13-2 lists associations with congenital or hereditary generalized hypertrichosis: only selected conditions will be discussed further here.

The hypertrichosis in *Cornelia de Lange's syndrome* is nowhere as confluent or generalized as in the fully developed syndrome of congenital hypertrichosis lanuginosa, but there may be some overlap in amount of excess hair growth in infancy. The affected infants with Cornelia de Lange's syndrome, however, have a very characteristic and constant clinical appearance which facilitates recognition. First described by a Dutch pediatrician in 1933,[17] affected patients have distinctive facies secondary to a low hairline, bushy confluent eyebrows, long eyelashes, antepalpebral slant, thin lips, long philtrum, and flat nasal bridge with upturned tip[17–19] (Fig. 13-4). These patients have many other relatively constant abnormalities including mental and growth retardation, microbrachiocephaly, micromelia, and phocomelia, oligodactyly (ulnar), syndactyly of the second and third toes, and a low-pitched, growling cry. Excess lanugo hair occurs at birth or infancy over the forehead, nape of the neck, lateral face and back, shoulders, and extremities, and tends to be persistent.[17,20] Patients with Cornelia de Lange's syndrome have hyperglutamicacidemia, hypoaminoaciduria, and, more specifically, an increase in serum α-ketoglutarate.[21] Hypogammaglobulinemia, but with normal IgG, IgA, and IgM subgroups, has been noted[21] and may account for the increased susceptibility to infection seen in these patients.[20] A complete list of associated clinical abnormalities is given in Table 13-3.

Cornelia de Lange's syndrome is usually sporadic but may be familial.[22] As the risk of recurrence in affected families is low at 2 to 5 percent, the most commonly suggested mode of inheritance, autosomal recessive, would need to be accompanied by variable penetrance or multigenic inhibitors.[18,21] Chromosomal analysis has usually been normal.[18,23] Two reports of translo-cation of chromosomal fragments suggest a partial trisomy, but each report involved different chromosomes and nonsatellited acentric

Table 13-2
GENERALIZED CONGENITAL OR HEREDITARY HYPERTRICHOSIS

Condition	*Onset Abnormal Hair*	*Type Excess Hair/ Distribution*	*Associated Abnormalities*	*Course of Hair Growth*	*Inheritance*	*References*
Congenital hypertrichosis lanuginosa	Birth or early infancy	Lanugo/generalized	Anomalous dental eruptions frequent; occasional ear malformations; one case pyloric stenosis	Persistent, increase or decrease with time	AD	2,6,9,11
Hereditary hypertrichosis lanuginosa with gingival fibromatosis	Birth to puberty	Lanugo/generalized and bushy eyebrows that meet in center	Gingival fibromatosus with delayed eruption teeth; may include mental retardation, convulsions, characteristic nose and ears	Develop terminal hair; may increase or decrease with time	AD	12,13,154
Cornelia de Lange's syndrome	Birth to infancy	Lanugo hair low on forehead and neck; lanago hair shoulder, back, extremities; bushy eyebrows that meet in center; long eyelashes	Severe growth and mental retardation, microbrachycephaly, micromelia +/− phocomelia +/− clinodactyly, oligodactyly upper extremities, syndactyly 2d and 3d toes; characteristic facies with flat nasal bridge and upturned tip and low-set ears; high arched or cleft palate; unusual cry; +/− deafness, simian creases, and hypoplastic dermal ridges, hypertonicity; +/− delayed eruption dentition, increased susceptibility to infection, ocular abnormalities, especially pupillary abnormalities, cutis marmorata, and transient facial "cyanosis"	Persistent	Sporadic or partial trisomy	18–20,23,24,155, 156
Hurler's syndrome	Birth to early infancy	Trunk and extremities covered with dense lanugo hair	Disproportionate dwarfism; skeletal abnormality; hepatosplenomegaly; tendency to formation umbilical and inguinal hernias; clouding of cornea; mental retardation; ↑ chondroitin sulfate B and heparitin monosulfate	Unknown	AR or sex-linked recessive	28,157
Coffin-Siris syndrome	Birth to infancy	Variable face and body hair; eyelash and eyebrow hypertrichosis with synophrys; sparse scalp hair	Postnatal growth and mental retardation; microcephaly; psychomotor retardation, hypotonia; coarse facies with thick lips; hypoplasia or aplasia distal phalanges, fingers and toes; aplasia or hyoplasia nails, especially of 5th digits; lax joints; delayed eruption teeth or microdontia	Unknown	? AR, ? AD	158–161,163
Gorlin's syndrome	Unknown	Coarse scalp and body hair, especially arms, legs, back; low hairline	Craniofacial dysostosis; patent ductus arteriosus; hypoplasia of labia majora; dental and ocular abnormalities; mild bilateral conductive hearing loss; short stature	Persistent	Unknown	162,163

Table 13-2 (*Continued*)
GENERALIZED CONGENITAL OR HEREDITARY HYPERTRICHOSIS

Condition	*Onset Abnormal Hair*	*Type Excess Hair/ Distribution*	*Associated Abnormalities*	*Course of Hair Growth*	*Inheritance*	*References*
Hyperkinetic circulatory disorder	Birth to infancy	Low hairline; lanugo hair all over face, extremities, back	Persistent patent ductus arteriosus with hyperkinetic circulatory disorder s/p closure; peculiar facies with prognathism, thick lips, flat nose, and hypertelorism; ? relationship to Gorlin's syndrome	Persistent	Unknown	164
Schinzel-Giedion syndrome	Birth to infancy	Generalized hypertrichosis, especially over shoulders and upper arms	Midface retraction; mesomelic brachymelia; clubfeet; radiological skeletal abnormality of skull, ribs, hands, feet; mental and growth retardation, seizures; hydronephrosis, hypoplastic dermal ridges; congenital heart block; abnormal nails (± triangular or hyperconvex)	Early infant death secondary to cardiorespiratory abnormalities	? AR	164–166
Lawrence-Seip syndrome	Birth to childhood	Hypertrichosis of face, neck, extremities; curly scalp hair with low-set hairline	Acanthosis nigricans; loss of subcutaneous tissue with gaunt facies and marked prominence of musculature and protuberant abdomen; dolichocephaly; insulin-resistant diabetes mellitus; cutaneous xanthomata; corneal opacities; renal, cardiac, and ovarian anomalies; hepatosplenomegaly; simian creases; increased bone relative to chronological age; clitoral or penile enlargement; mental retardation	Increases with age	AR	167,168
Generalized smooth muscle hamartoma	Birth to infancy	Hypertrichosis of extremities and buttocks at birth or infancy	Excessive skin folds; biopsy = smooth muscle hamartoma	↓ with time	Sporadic	115
Osteochondrodysplasia with hypertrichosis	Birth	Generalized, including thick eyebrows and lashes	Coarse facial features; dental diastemata; clinodactyly 5th fingers; skeletal abnormalities including narrow thorax, wide ribs, and platyspondylia; cardiomegaly and associated cardiac abnormalities	May be persistent or decrease with puberty	AR	169

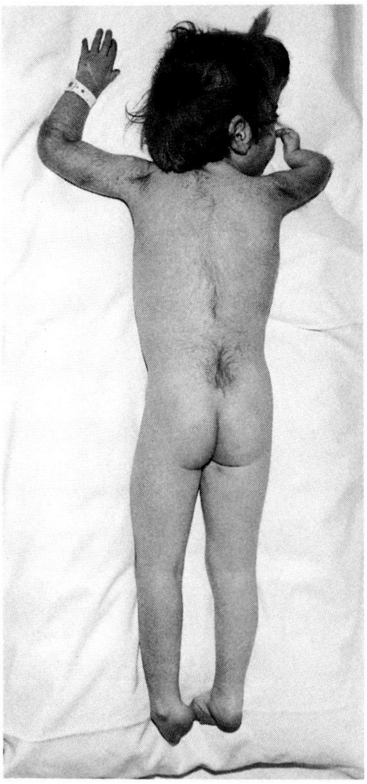
A

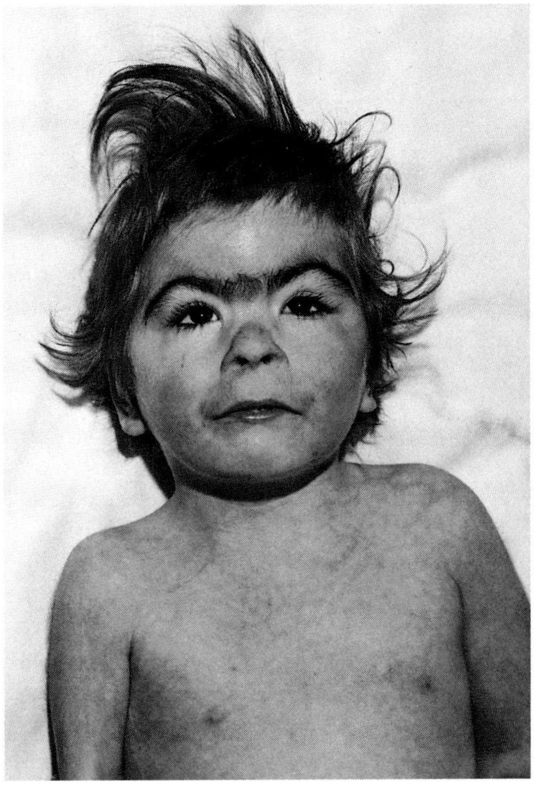
B

Figure 13-4 Cornelia de Lange's syndrome. (*Photo courtesy of Dr. Louis J. Ptacek. Reprinted with permission from Ptacek et al.*[20])

fragments which do not usually perpetuate themselves.[18,24,25] The exact nature of the genetic inheritance in Cornelia de Lange's syndrome remains to be determined.

There are several other hereditary syndromes with physical and/or mental retardation and hypertrichosis that may cause confusion with Cornelia de Lange's syndrome. The affected infants with *Rubinstein-Taybi syndrome* share with those of Cornelia de Lange's syndrome thick and highly arched eyebrows (but not fused in the midline), long eyelashes, and microcephaly, but they do not have diffuse hypertrichosis. Moreover, these individuals have characteristic facies with retrognathia, a beaked nose with a broad bridge and septum below the alae, deformed ears, and typically broad thumbs and great toes.[26] Patients with *Seckel's syndrome* ("bird-headed dwarfs") also have severe microcephaly and characteristic facies with receding forehead and chin, prominent curved nose, and large eyes with antimongoloid slant to the palpebral fissures along with various skeletal abnormalities.[27] Although "hirsutism" has been noted in up to 3 out of 10 cases of Seckel's syndrome, no further description of the excess hair is given, and hypertrichosis does not appear to be a prominent component of the syndrome. The facial features of Cornelia de Lange's syndrome may be confused with *Hurler's syndrome,* in which affected individuals are said to resemble "gargoyles."[28] In Hurler's syndrome, an autosomal recessive inherited condition, the trunk and extremities are covered with dense lanugo hair.

Not all cases of congenital hypertrichosis are hereditary in nature: some may be related either to in utero exposure to toxins or to birth defects. In most cases, the only description of the accompanying excess hair is "hirsutism" or "hypertrichosis" without note of the type or distribution of excess hair. "Hirsutism" has been reported in at least 5 percent of infants with fetal alcohol syndrome.[29] Children with holoprosencephaly, in which the defect also involves the diencephalon, are frequently born with "hypertrichosis."[14] "Hypertrichosis" was reported in one case of globoid leukodystrophy (Krabbe's disease), an autosomal recessive demyelinating dis-

Table 13-3
CLINICAL FEATURES OF CORNELIA DE LANGE'S SYNDROME

General
Primordial growth failure
Mental retardation
Initial muscular hypertonia
Characteristic facies
Low-pitched growling cry
Skeletal
Micromelia, phocomelia, and/or oligodactyly
Absence of ulnar digits
Flexion contractures of elbows
Proximally placed thumbs
Partial syndactyly 2d, 3d toes
Flat occiput
Arched palate
Micrognathia
Widely spaced teeth
Clinodactyly 5th digits hands
Simian creases
Short neck
Long philtrum and nose
Cutaneous
Generalized hirsutism
Low hairline
Thick eyebrows meeting in midline (synophrys)
Long, curly eyelashes
Cyanotic hue about eyes, nose, and mouth
Prominent veins in temporal area
Cutis marmorata
Hypoplastic nipples
Hypoplasia of hypothenar dermal ridges
Transverse palmar crease (simian line)
Capillary hemangiomas
Recurrent skin infections
Prominent veins lateral aspects forehead
Other
Congenital heart disease
Hypoplastic genitals
Pyloric stenosis, malrotation, and duplication of bowel
Ocular abnormalities
Blue sclera

Source: Modified from Soderquist and Reed.[19]

ease presenting in infancy and characterized by globular distended multinucleated bodies on histopathology.[30]

Acquired Hypertrichosis

Acquired generalized hypertrichosis may rarely be lanugo but more commonly is vellus hair. The association of lanugo hypertrichosis and malignancy was first noted by Turner in 1865 and is now a well-established paraneoplastic sign.[31] This *acquired hypertrichosis lanuginosa,* or "malignant down," is a late manifestation of malignancy and usually occurs in patients with widely disseminated or advanced disease.[31–33] However, the hypertrichosis may be the first clue to the diagnosis of an underlying cancer. In one series of affected patients, acquired hypertrichosis lanuginosa appeared in 15 out of 34 patients before the diagnosis of malignancy was made.[31] The potential latent period, almost 2 years in two reported cases,[31,34] between presentation of acquired hypertrichosis lanuginosa and diagnosis of cancer probably accounts for the rare case reports of acquired hypertrichosis lanuginosa without malignancy:[35] careful follow-up has generally revealed an unsuspected cancer.[36] Many cases of acquired hypertrichosis lanuginosa have been accompanied by tongue abnormalities, including burning or painful tongue, hypertrophied papillae, pronounced furrows, and/or oral pigmentation.[32,34–39] The presence of acquired hypertrichosis lanuginosa alone and especially with subjective or objective tongue abnormalities should be considered pathognomonic for malignancy and should signal repeated investigations for a source. There is no one particular type of cancer associated with acquired hypertrichosis lanuginosa (Table 13-4).

The hair growth in acquired hypertrichosis lanuginosa is generalized and pale or colorless[31] (Fig. 13-5). Most affected persons do not achieve the length of hair exhibited in cases of congenital hypertrichosis lanuginosa, although there are exceptions.[40] A histological investigation of the hair in acquired hypertrichosis lanuginosa re-

Table 13-4
TYPES OF CANCER REPORTED IN PATIENTS WITH ACQUIRED HYPERTRICHOSIS LANUGINOSA[31,42]

Type of Malignancy
Bladder
Breast
Colon
Gallbladder
Liver—adenocarcinoma
Lung—anaplastic, clear cell carcinoma, undifferentiated small cell, poorly differentiated squamous cell carcinoma, adenocarcinoma, polygonal cell
Lymphoma/leukemia—CLL; small cell follicular, diffuse histiocytic
Ovary
Pancreas
Rectum
Uterus

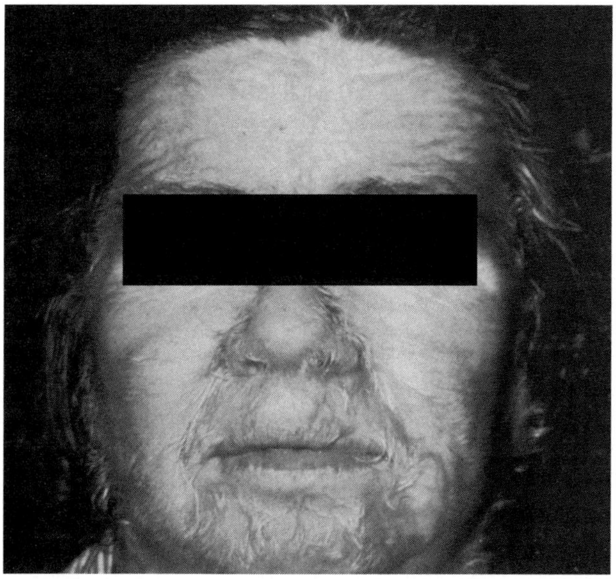

Figure 13-5 Acquired hypertrichosis lanuginosa.

vealed that almost all hair follicles are enlarged "mantle" hairs with an apronlike sheath of undifferentiated epithelial cells extending inferiorly from the isthmus like a mantle.[32] No consistent endocrine abnormalities have been noted in affected patients.[32] A hair growth factor produced by the cancer has been hypothesized, and endocrine-type membrane-bound secretory granules were noted on electron microscopy of the tumor in one case of carcinoid of the colon.[41] The tumor tested negative, however, for epidermal growth factor. Carcinoembryonic antigen has been noted to be elevated in several cases, but whether this is in any way related to the acquired hypertrichosis lanuginosa is unclear.[42] Of note, carcinoembryonic antigen is produced in fetal intestine, liver, and pancreas during the third through seventh months of gestation, at the time lanugo hair is also being produced.[38] In cases of acquired hypertrichosis lanuginosa, successful surgical removal of the underlying cancer has resulted in regression of the excess hair growth.[42]

DRUGS

Several drugs have regularly been associated with acquired hypertrichosis. Minoxidil, a piperidinopyrimidine derivative, is a vasodilator used to treat severe refractory hypertension.[43] Hypertrichosis occurs in more than 80 percent of patients treated with the oral medication, generally within weeks to months after beginning treatment.[43,44] The effect is apparently not dose-related.[45] Hair growth primarily involves the face, shoulders, arms, and legs, and affects men more than women[43] (Fig. 13-6). The hypertrichosis generally regresses within several months of stopping minoxidil therapy.[44]

A topical preparation of minoxidil was developed to exploit this side effect of systemic therapy and has given insight into the mechanism of hair growth induction with minoxidil. Both in men with androgenetic alopecia and in stumptailed macaques with a variant of male-pattern baldness, topical application of minoxidil stimulates miniaturized follicles to enter anagen and increases the diameter of the hair shafts.[46,47] Certainly blood flow is increased with local application of minoxidil,[48] but minoxidil has effects on cellular promotion as well. Culture of mouse vibrissae with minoxidil stimulates proliferation of the hair matrix and internal root sheath cells.[49] In macaques, minoxidil increases cell proliferation in the bulb and outer root sheath.[50] Minoxidil prolongs the survival and enhances the growth potential of confluent cultures of keratinocytes.[51] It may effect cell growth through opening cellular potassium channels.[52]

Diazoxide is another vasodilator associated with hypertrichosis but it is chemically unrelated to minoxidil. It is a benzothiadiazine which causes hyperglycemia, due in part to inhibition of insulin secretion and in part to inhibition of phosphodiesterase, causing increased cyclic adenosine monophosphate (cAMP) and promotion of glycolysis.[53,54] Because of this, diazoxide

Figure 13-6 Facial hypertrichosis of a woman on oral minoxidil for hypertension.

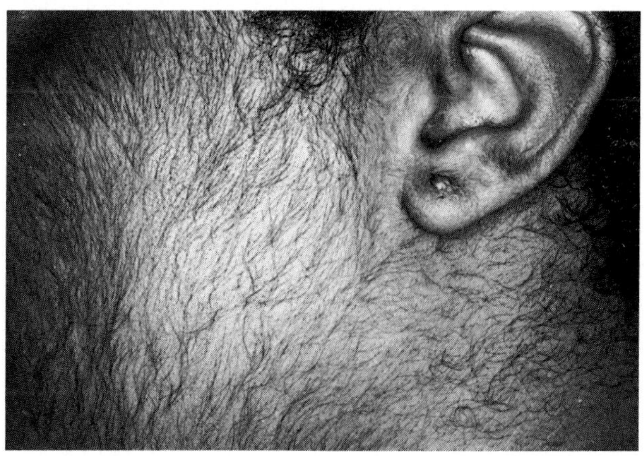

is used to treat idiopathic hypoglycemia of infancy. Hypertrichosis is seen frequently in children treated with diazoxide but occurs less frequently in adults (< 1 percent to 20 percent in two series), for whom the drug is used for refractory hypertension.[53,55] Hair growth occurs as early as 6 weeks after beginning the drug and is distributed predominantly over the forehead, nape of the neck, eyebrows, eyelashes, and the dorsum of the trunk and limbs.[53,56] The hair is generally lanugolike but may be pigmented.[53,57] In children, persistent growth has been reported for at least a year after stopping diazoxide, but usually the hypertrichosis regresses within 2 to 5 months after discontinuing the drug.[53,55] Infants born to women given diazoxide during pregnancy have a high incidence of hair abnormalities, including the potential for congenital hypertrichosis lanuginosa or focal alopecia.[58]

Phenytoin sodium (Dilantin) is associated with increased hair growth in approximately 5 to 12 percent of cases,[59,60] apparently unrelated to dosage or serum concentration of the drug.[60,61] The excess hair is particularly apparent on the extremities but also occurs on the trunk and face.[60] The hair growth generally regresses within a year off drug[61] but may persist to some degree well after drug withdrawal.[62] This latter fact has led to speculation that in many cases where hypertrichosis occurs after head trauma and the use of phenytoin sodium for secondary seizures, the excess hair may be secondary to the neurological damage itself and not to the drug.[62] Generalized hypertrichosis may occur 4 to 12 weeks after brain injury even without the use of phenytoin.[62]

Hypertrichosis has been reported in 44 to 60 percent[63,64] of patients with organ transplants,[65] 80 percent of patients with graft-versus-host disease after bone marrow transplant,[66] and 95 percent of patients with insulin-dependent diabetes mellitus treated with cyclosporine.[67] Hair growth is diffuse, primarily involving the shoulders, back, upper extremities, face, scalp, eyebrows, and earlobes[65–67] (Fig. 13-7). The density of the hair increases as well as transforms from vellus to pigmented terminal hair.[67] Hair growth generally begins within 2 to 4 weeks after commencement of drug[65] and increases rapidly over the first 3 months: it is rare to develop hypertrichosis after this time.[67] Children and adolescents are at the greatest risk of developing moderate to severe hypertrichosis.[67] Most patients lose the excess hair in a telogen effluvium beginning 1 to 2 months after discontinuing the drug, although a few patients may experience a 2- to 3-month delay in diminution of hair growth.[65,67]

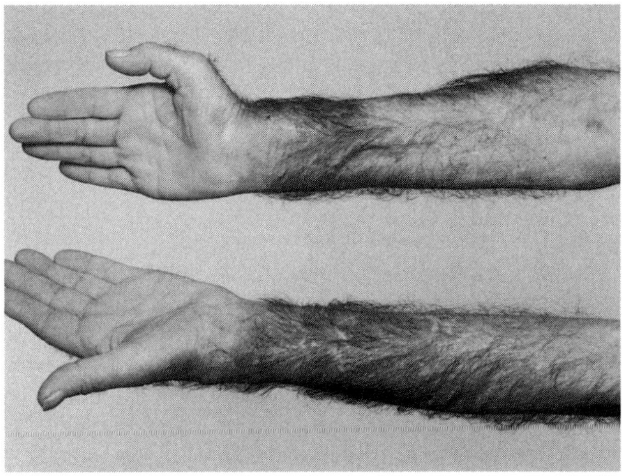

Figure 13-7 Cyclosporine-induced hypertrichosis. (*Photo courtesy of Dr. Peter S. Mortimer. Reprinted with permission from* J R Soc Med *76:786–787, 1983.*)

The mechanism for hair growth stimulation with cyclosporine is unclear. In nude mice, cyclosporine may transform hair follicles from lanugo to vellus or even terminal hairs,[68] and in the C57 B1-6 mouse, cyclosporine induces a switch from telogen to anagen.[69] The rate of anagen induction in mice is dependent on the dose, time course, and method of administration of cyclosporine.[69] In humans, there is no correlation between serum concentration of cyclosporine (within the therapeutic range) and degree of hair growth.[67] There are many similarities in the clinical side effects of phenytoin sodium and cyclosporine which may help unravel a common mechanism of action: both drugs may induce gingival hyperplasia, hypertrichosis, and a coarsening of facial features.[70]

Treatment with psoralen in combination with ultraviolet light has been reported to cause hypertrichosis. Four out of 27 patients with vitiligo in one retrospective series and 3 out of 100 in another utilizing systemic methoxsalen plus either sunlight or a General Electric R.S. Sunlamp developed a transient local hypertrichosis.[71,72] In a prospective study, 15 out of 23 women patients with vitiligo treated with psoralen plus ultraviolet A light (PUVA) and 2 out of 14 women patients with vitiligo treated with ultraviolet A light (UVA) alone for 208 months developed hypertrichosis.[73] The hair growth was most marked on the face and extremities, and began within 6 to 12 weeks after commencement of PUVA therapy.

A patient with psoriasis who applied 0.25% desoximetasone (a class II steroid) every day (~ 30 g qd) for 5 years developed Cushing's syndrome with increased hair growth on the upper lip, forehead, and back.[74] Certainly, patients on superphysiological doses of systemic steroids may also develop increased hair growth, but this is generally in an androgen-dependent pattern and, hence, is hirsutism rather than hypertrichosis.

Generalized hypertrichosis with pigmented hair 1 to 3 cm in length has been reported to occur within 2 months after streptomycin therapy for miliary tuberculosis or tubercular meningitis.[75] Fono reported an incidence of hypertrichosis in 22 out of 27 such cases.[75] However, in one of these cases, the hypertrichosis persisted for at least 1 year after discontinuing treatment, raising the question of whether the hypertrichosis was secondary to the medication or the disease.[75] Certainly, hypertrichosis has appeared coincidentally with miliary tuberculosis or tubercular meningitis in patients who never received any therapy.[76]

Acetazolamide (Diamox), a carbonic anhydrase inhibitor used for glaucoma, has been reported to cause growth of long, dark hair on the back and lower legs of women 12 to 16 months after commencement of drug with regression within 1 year off drug.[77]

In an open crossover study of carprazidil (oxadiazolopyrimidine) and minoxidil, both vasodilators used to treat hypertension, hypertrichosis prominent on the face and extremities was seen in "most patients."[78] It was not possible to ascribe the side effect to one drug or the other.

Twenty-eight out of 30 pregnant women who received a long-term intravenous infusion of Fenoterol for tocolysis had intensive generalized hair growth.[79]

SYSTEMIC DISEASE

PORPHYRIA

Patients with one of several types of porphyria may show hypertrichosis. *Porphyria cutanea tarda,* the most common type of porphyria, presents as a mechanobullous eruption, most prominent in sun-exposed areas, that heals with milia and variable hyperpigmentation.[80] Hypertrichosis is common (63 percent in one series) and most prominent along the temples, cheeks, eyebrows, and hairline, but may involve the trunk and extremities.[80] Porphyria cutanea tarda may be secondary to an inherent deficiency in uroporphyrin decarboxylase that, depending on the extent and distribution of the deficient enzyme, may either cause symptoms de novo or require a provoking agent such as alcohol or estrogen.[80] Certain chemicals, notably hexachlorobenzene and chlorinated phenols, can cause porphyria cutanea tarda in all exposed persons.[80,81] Hypertrichosis was particularly prominent in Turkish children who ate wheat grain treated with the fungicide hexachlorobenzene and who developed porphyria cutanea tarda: some were termed "monkey children." In these cases, the cutaneous manifestations of porphyria cutanea tarda, including hypertrichosis, generally disappeared within a month of discontinuing exposure to the chemical.[81,82] Porphyria cutanea tarda may also be a manifestation of benign or malignant hepatic tumors.[83]

The diagnosis of porphyria cutanea tarda is confirmed in all these conditions by finding increased urine uroporphyrins and a urine uroporphyrin-to-coproporphyrin ratio > 3:1. A porphyria cutanea tarda–like bullous eruption may be induced in patients with chronic renal failure on hemodialysis or in those taking nalidixic acid, furosemide, or tetracycline. Hypertrichosis is not usually a part of this spectrum of porphyria cutanea tarda, and urine porphyrins are generally normal.[84–87] However, there is a subset of patients who, after hemodialysis, develop a full clinical spectrum of porphyria cutanea tarda, including hypertrichosis, and these patients generally have abnormal porphyrins.[86,88]

The cutaneous features of porphyria cutanea tarda, including hypertrichosis, are also present in *variegate porphyria.*[89,90] This inherited condition, which is very prevalent in South African whites, is also characterized by acute intermittent porphyria (AIP)–like attacks (gastrointestinal, neuropsychological symptoms) after exposure to provoking medications such as barbiturates or sulfonamides. Diagnosis is by finding urine coproporphyrin greater than uroporphyrin with increased stool protoporphyrin and coproporphyrin,[89] increased urine δ-aminolevulinic acid (ALA) and porphobilinogen during AIP–like attacks, and increased hepatic ALA synthetase.[90]

Erythropoietic porphyria is a rare genetic disturbance (autosomal recessive) in porphyrin metabolism that primarily affects the hematopoietic system. Severe photosensitivity is the rule, with pain on sun exposure and vesiculobullous lesions that lead to scarring, hyperpigmentation, and hypopigmentation.[91] Hypertrichosis, which generally appears by age 5 or 6, is common and often widespread: the limbs and trunk are likely to be more involved than the face.[91] The hair may be either soft and downy or coarse and is generally pigmented; density is generally sparse.[91] Urine is pink due to increased excretion of uroporphyrin, and bones and teeth, which are brown in color, fluoresce red under Wood's light.[91,92] The exact porphyrin defect is unclear.

OTHER SYSTEMIC ILLNESSES

In the 1970s, a constellation of clinical findings including diffuse hyperpigmentation, hypertrichosis, edema, polyneuropathy, and dysglobulinemia was noted.[93] We now recognize this as *POEMS syndrome,* an acronym for the major constellation of signs including peripheral neuropathy, organomegaly, endocrine dysfunction, monoclonal gammopathy, and skin changes.[94] The hypertrichosis is most common on the extensor surfaces, malar areas, and forehead.[95,96]

Other systemic illnesses have rarely been associated with hypertrichosis. There have been several reports of children with hypothyroidism developing hypertrichosis over the back and extremities which has resolved after therapy.[97–99] Two patients diagnosed with acrodynia, with typical symptoms of sweating, acrocyanosis, and hypotonia, were noted to have long, downy hair over the face, back, thorax, and extremities that came and went with the acute illness.[76] Three children with malabsorption, one with celiac disease and two with "infantile steatorrhea," were reported to have developed hypertrichosis on the face and extremities. Another with "failure to thrive" but no obvious disease developed diffuse lanugolike hair growth.[76] Hypertrichosis is not a general feature of malnutrition.

LOCALIZED HYPERTRICHOSIS

Congenital or Hereditary Localized Hypertrichosis

Hypertrichosis may be localized and either acquired or related to congenital or hereditary problems (Table 13-1). It is of most concern when it serves as a marker for underlying occult neural abnormalities, as is frequently the case with midline hair on the back. The separation of the neuroectoderm from the epithelial ectoderm occurs in the third to fifth week in utero and is initiated along the midline posteriorly.[100] The cleavage can be incomplete at any phase so that a defect may appear in the skin, vertebrae, spinal cord, and/or central nervous system.[100] The term *faun tail* is often used to describe the hair growth observed by Darier, who stated in 1923, "Sometimes the hypertrichosis is predominant at the sacral region forming a mass of hair growth which the ancients have attributed to a 'faun tail' "[101] (Fig. 13-8).

A faun tail is frequently associated with one of a handful of underlying spinal defects including spina bifida occulta (vertebral defect without exposure of neural tissue), spina bifida, traction bands, and diastematomyelia.[100–103] Fibrous bands may tether the spinal cord or cauda equina to bone or skin directly or through attachment to the meninges or through a tight filum terminale. A meningocele manque refers to aberrant nerve roots, fibrous bands, and adhesions that tether the spinal cord, nerve roots, and filum terminale within the meninges and may continue through the dura to the skin:[103] 11 of 45 (24 percent) of such cases have overlying hypertrichosis.

Diastematomyelia is duplication or splitting of a portion of the spinal cord through which a bony spur or fibrous band passes and attaches to

Figure 13-8 Faun tail. (*Reprinted with permission from Thursfield and Ross.*[101])

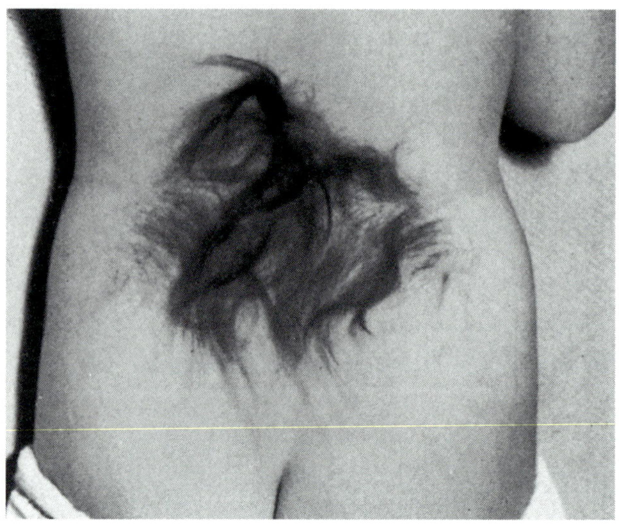

the vertebral body anteriorly and/or to the neural arch posteriorly[101] (Fig. 13-9). More than 40 percent of persons with diastematomyelia have patches of hair overlying the neural-bony abnormality.[100] These abnormalities may not cause neurological problems in infancy, but symptoms generally do eventually appear from toddlerhood to early adulthood.[101] Symptoms appear because there is a normally occurring dissimilar growth of the spinal cord and vertebral column with the spinal cord "ascending" in the vertebral column over the first 5 years of life.[102] The traction on the cord, either directly or by the cord being "hung up" by the bony or fibrous spur in diastematomyelia, will eventually cause a neurological deficit. Recognition of the process will allow prophylactic surgery.[101]

Faun tails are usually evident by early infancy and appear more frequently (4:1) in females than in males.[101] It should be noted, however, that the hair may not be at the level of the neural defect itself but will be in the general region.[104] Midback hypertrichosis is most common in the sacral or lumbar region occuring less frequently as one moves cephalad.

Midback hypertrichosis may accompany other cutaneous abnormalities that also signal underlying neurocutaneous abnormalities or that may secondarily cause damage to underlying neurological structures. Dermal sinuses, usually 1 to 2 mm in diameter and close to or at the dorsal midline, often are associated with local pigmentation, port-wine discoloration, or protrusion of hair from the sinus.[100] These sinuses can extend

Figure 13-9 Diastematomyelia commonly associated with overlying patch of hair. (*Reprinted with permission from Perret.*[104])

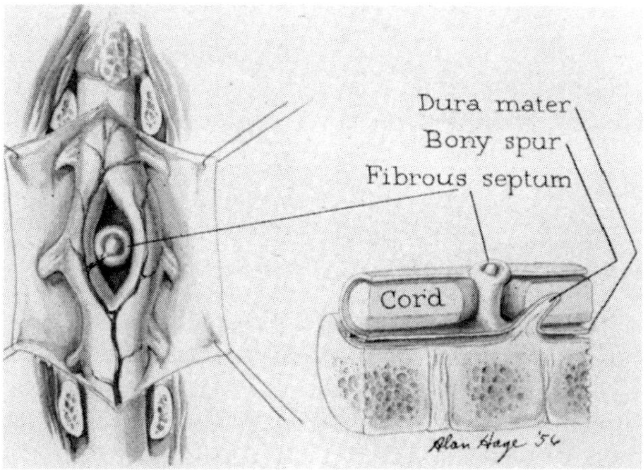

into the spinal canal and serve as a portal of infection or can expand into an epidermoid or dermoid cyst;[100] this can lead to neurological deficits secondary to pressure on the cord with tumor growth. Midline lipomas are frequently attached to the cord or cauda equina, filum terminale, or conus medullaris: excision or manipulation may lead to meningitis or central nervous system infection.

Midline dorsal patches of hypertrichosis should lead one to look for neurological deficits and underlying bony abnormalities. The absence of a neurological deficit at the time of examination does not rule out an underlying neurological abnormality. Invasive procedures such as myelography are potential sources of infection and should be avoided if noninvasive techniques such as MRI are available. Manipulation or excision of midline dorsal cutaneous structures should not be done without a thorough evaluation of the underlying cord and spinal column and without prior neurosurgical consultation.

Congenital hair on the elbows usually presents at birth as lanugo hair, becomes terminal hair and more dense during early childhood, and then usually regresses.[105,106] It is familial but not usually indicative of any underlying or associated problem.

Congenital hair on the external ears is common among some populations of the Pacific Islands as well as among babies with XYY syndrome.[107] Congenital hair on the pinna may, however, be a hallmark of offspring born to diabetic mothers,[107,108] its presence independent of the degree of diabetic control.[109] There has been one reported case of acquired hypertrichosis of the ears and brows in a patient with AIDS: no drugs could be implicated in this case.[110] Hairy pinnae may also be a Y-linked and androgen-dependent trait, with the excess hair not appearing until after puberty and increasing in frequency and amount with age[111,112] (Fig. 13-10). The incidence will vary depending on the definition of a "hairy pinna" and on the population screened. Slatis defined a hairy pinna as one with at least several hairs on the top or side of the ears and excluded hair around the external auditory meatus and lobe.[113] Using this definition, the incidence of hairy pinnae is 26 percent in Israel; 50 percent in Madras, India; and 10 percent in Bengal, India.[111,113] Hairy ears are not markers for other associated abnormalities.

Isolated excessive growth of only eyelash

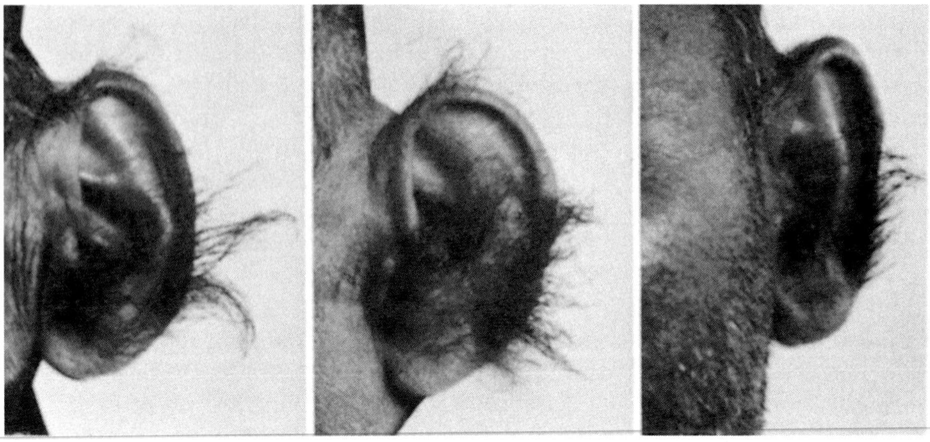

Figure 13-10 Y-linked hairy pinnae in three brothers. (*Reprinted with permission from Stern, Centerwall, and Sarkar.*[111])

and/or eyebrow hair may be familial but is usually extreme only in adult males. In infants, extremely long eyebrows can occur as a localized process, but the combination of extremely long eyelashes and eyebrows has been reported only in children with other anomalies. These include Cornelia de Lange's syndrome, Rubinstein-Taybi syndrome, congenital hypertrichosis lanuginosa, and congenital trichomegaly associated with dwarfism, mental retardation, and pigmentary degeneration of the retina.[114] In the one case report of the latter, the eyelashes were 4 cm in length.[113]

Congenital smooth muscle hamartomas are characterized by congenital indurated patches that are usually pigmented and have focal hypertrichosis: the hypertrichosis may take several months to develop.[115,116] With rubbing, the areas may become raised transiently (pseudo Darier's sign) secondary to local piloerection.[116] Histologically these lesions show smooth muscle bundles similar to arrectores pilorum which vary in size, shape, and orientation. There may be slight elongation of the rete ridges, focal acanthosis, and slight basal hypermelanosis, but no hyperkeratosis or papillomatosis. The hyperpigmentation, induration, and excessive hair tend to diminish with time.[115,117] Congenital smooth muscle hamartomas may be single or multiple. A generalized smooth muscle hamartoma associated with more extensive hypertrichosis and excessive skin folds has been reported under the term *Michelin-Tire syndrome*[115] (see Table 13-2).

Winchester syndrome may also present with irregular patches of thickened skin associated with mild hyperpigmentation and hypertrichosis. Affected infants also have multiple bony abnormalities (including generalized osteoporosis, osteolysis of carpal and tarsal bones, and periarticular and intraarticular joint erosions) leading eventually to short stature. The histology is different from congenital smooth muscle hamartomas in that there is fibroblastic proliferation with homogenized bundles of collagen.[118]

The occurrence of localized patches of hair follicles on the palms and soles inherited in an autosomal dominant fashion has been reported in two separate families.[119] These areas had variable associated pigmentation and textural changes. Histologically there was an increase in and disarray of the elastin fibers in the underlying dermis.[119] This appears to be another example of a congenital hamartoma.

Congenital pigmented hairy nevi, or *nevi pilorum,* are probably the most common cause of localized hypertrichosis in infants. The nevi are not indurated, do not become raised on stroking, and usually have prominent local hyperpigmentation. Biopsy confirms the diagnosis, and excision is generally done to prevent the development of melanoma more than for cosmetic purposes. The increase in the number of hairs in acquired nevi generally never reaches the confluence seen in congenital lesions. Hair in nevi is not a prognostic indicator of potential malignancy.

Acquired Localized Hypertrichosis

A wide range of types of physical insults may cause transient localized hypertrichosis (Table 13-1). Repeated trauma, irritation, or inflammation may lead to local transformation of vellus hairs to terminal hairs (Fig. 13-11). Localized hy-

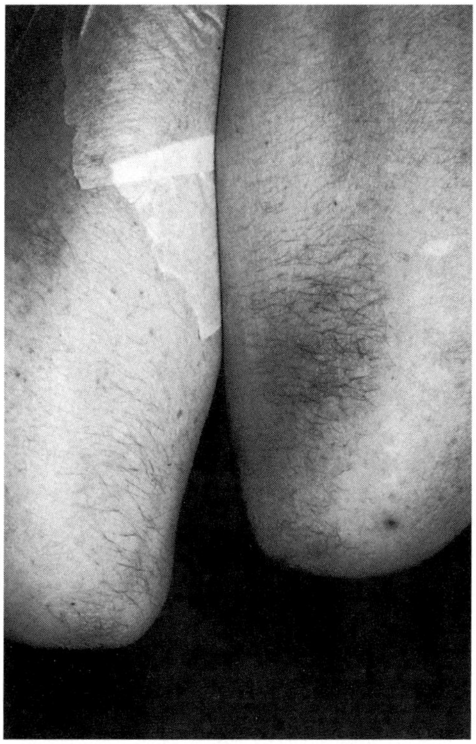

Figure 13-11 Localized hypertrichosis secondary to lichen simplex chronicus.

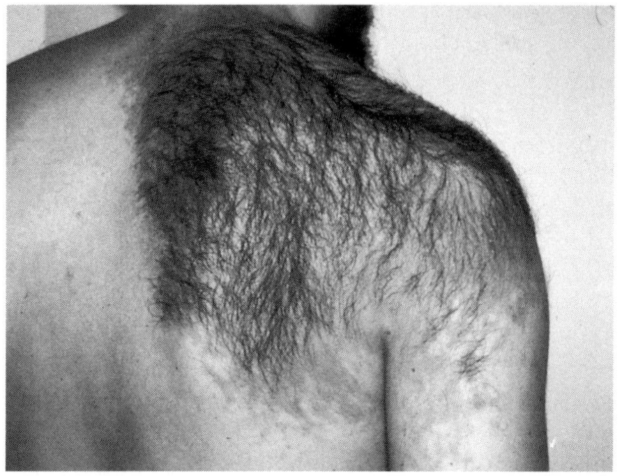

Figure 13-12 Becker's nevus. (*Photo courtesy of Dr. Robert A. Briggaman.*)

pertrichosis often follows occlusion of a limb by a cast, either plaster of Paris or the newer fiberglass casts.[120]

In 1949, Becker described two cases of adolescents who following a severe sunburn, developed first local hyperpigmentation and later hypertrichosis over the upper back.[121] Histologically, there was melanosis but no nevus cells, and he termed this "melanosis and hypertrichosis in the distribution of a nevus unius lateris."[121] There have been multiple reports of *Becker's nevus* (a misnomer, but accepted terminology) since then, generally characterized by a solitary area of pigmentation and hypertrichosis, usually greater than palm-sized but occasionally small enough to be confused with nevi[122,123] (Fig. 13-12). These lesions usually appear around the shoulders, although they can occur elsewhere and multiple lesions have been reported.[122,123] The hypertrichosis may be absent on initial presentation and can take several years to appear.[122,124] The pigmentation may fade with time.[122,125] Most cases occur in adolescence, but onset can be from infancy to middle age.[123] Familial and congenital cases have been described but are uncommon.[123] Males are predominantly affected.[123]

Histologically, Becker's nevi are characterized by slight acanthosis, variable hyperkeratosis, and marked hyperpigmentation in the basal layers with varying amounts of melanophages in the papillary dermis.[123,124] There is only a slight increase in the number of melanocytes but increased activity of the melanocytes and complexing of melanosomes. Hair follicles are normal[125] or enlarged.[123,124] By electron microscopy, the changes are indistinguishable from UVB-stimulated normal skin.[123]

An increase in smooth muscle bundles has been noted in some cases[124] of Becker's nevus and, in these situations, appears to be associated clinically with lesional perifollicular papules.[126] Becker's nevus has been hypothesized to be one end of the spectrum of a local hamartoma (literally "mass of tissue gone wrong"),[116] with congenital smooth muscle hamartomas at the other end.[127] Androgen cytosol receptors in involved areas are similar to genital skin but negative in surrounding uninvolved skin.[128] Together with the pubertal onset and occasional acne in lesions, this raises the speculation that Becker's nevus is an androgen-mediated process.[128]

Most patients with Becker's nevus are otherwise healthy, but there have been reports of hypoplasia of the ipsilateral breast and arm, hyperplasia of the ipsilateral leg, pectus carinatum, spina bifida[123] (these associations are mainly in women), and accessory scrotum.[129] A screen for associated bony and soft tissue abnormalities in patients with Becker's nevus, especially in affected women, may be important.

Several types of focal acquired sclerodermatous skin changes are associated with lesional hypertrichosis.[94,121,130] *Melorheostatic scleroderma,* another misnomer, is a rare condition that usually presents with joint pain, stiffness, contractures, and localized scleroderma-like changes with or without local hypertrichosis.[126] The hallmark is a unique radiographic appearance of the affected joints with hyperostosis likened to "melted wax dripping down the sides of a candle." This is a pseudoscleroderma, as biopsy of the involved skin reveals downward proliferation of normal-appearing collagen into the subcutaneous fat. Patients may also have proliferation or malformation of cutaneous blood vessels.[121] Localized hypertrichosis also has been reported with morphea. POEMS syndrome is commonly associated with a rare variant of myeloma (osteosclerotic myeloma) and sclerodermatous skin changes.[96] The localized hypertrichosis in osteosclerotic myeloma appears linked to the presence of polyneuropathy and thickened skin.[94]

Hypertrichosis of the eyelashes alone was reported in a patient with chronic granulocytic anemia on alpha interferon (IFN) and hydroxyurea and was ascribed to the IFN.[131] However, the IFN was suspended 3 months prior to the note of increased eyelashes, and the excess hair growth disappeared after another 3 months: proof of a cause and effect for IFN and hypertrichosis was clearly not proved in this case.[131] However, two other patients with lymphoma treated with alpha interferon developed hypertrichosis of the eyelashes.[132] Three patients with renal or hepatic allografts and one patient with systemic lupus erythematosus (SLE) noted trichomegaly 3 to 4 months after beginning cyclosporine: they were also on systemic steroids.[133] Hypertrichosis of the eyelashes was noted in three patients with acquired immunodeficiency syndrome (AIDS) and various infections, including pneumocystic carinii and hepatitis.[1] There did not appear to be one drug common to all three patients which could be implicated as the cause.[134] Whether the hypertrichosis in these cases is related to a disease process or a concomitant medication is not clear.

Injection of sodium tetradecyl sulfate into small venous varicosities for the purpose of sclerosis has been associated with hair growth at the injection site or along the course of the vein.[135]

TREATMENT

In cases of acquired hypertrichosis, a search for the potential underlying etiology should be sought and treatment instituted, if possible. In the absence of a potentially reversible process, one must consider the psychological debilitation of the patient with excess hair and whether physical treatment is necessary, acceptable, and affordable.

The simplest way to remove excess hair is shaving, which does not alter the coarseness, thickness, or growth rate or cycle of the shaved hair.[136] However, the process is extremely transient and many women reject it because of both the razor stubble and "five-o'clock shadow," as well as the defeminizing assumption of a male ritual. With kinky hairs, shaving may incite a pseudofolliculitis, with the cut hairs turning in on the perifollicular skin. Plucking certainly leaves a more cosmetically appealing result but is tedious and painful and is impractical if there is a large surface area involved. Moreover, plucking encourages a change from telogen to anagen and thus may actually encourage more active growth in the treated area. Repeated plucking can cause erythema, pigmentation, folliculitis, pseudofolliculitis, follicular distortion, and scarring.[137] "Electronic" tweezers offer no improvement over nonelectrified tweezers.* Wax epilation is a glorified method of plucking that epilates large amounts of hair at the same time. A wax of low melting point (or adhesive semisolid applied on a backing material) is applied to the hairy area, rapidly solidifies, and is then pulled off in a fast motion that removes the wax, stratum corneum, and hairs in the treated area. Results may last 1 month or more, but the procedure is painful and may be associated with folliculitis caused by some anagen hairs breaking off in the hair follicle; allergic reactions to the adhesive can occur. Hair must be at least 1 mm long to be properly "grasped" by the wax.[138]

Chemical depilatories are easy to use, are painless during the procedure, and can have ex-

* Willis J: Some basics on hair removal products. FDA Consumer 13(7):23–25, 1979.

cellent cosmetic results that last up to 2 weeks. Most depilatories are variants of the thioglycolates used to perm hair and work under similar principles: they disrupt disulfide bonds, primarily between cysteine molecules. Increasing osmotic pressure within the hair fiber results in swelling and deterioration of the hair to a soft plastic mass.[138] Since cysteine forms 15 percent of the keratin in hair and 2 percent of the keratin in skin, the thioglycolates preferentially hydrolyze hair keratin vs. skin keratin.[139] The depilatories are either aqueous 2 to 6% mixtures of the alkali NaOH (Neet cream) or CaOH (Nair aerosol, Gold Magic Shaving Powder, Surgex cream, Neet lotion with aloe vera), or a mixture of the two alkalis (Neet lotion with cocoa butter) along with 2 to 10% mercaptan calcium or sodium thioglycolate.[138] The calcium salt of thioglycolate is the least irritating salt form, and a concentration greater than 4% does not work appreciably faster than lower, less-irritating concentrations.[140] The alkali is added to increase the pH to 10 to 12.5, the level at which thioglycolate is the most active and still safe on the underlying skin.[141] The chemical depilatory is then left on the hair for variable time periods (3–15 minutes) depending on the thickness of the hair and the concentration and vehicle of the depilatory. The depilatory and the resulting jellylike mixture of dissolved hair is then wiped away with a spatula.

The main potential side effect of chemical depilatories is an irritant dermatitis (1–5 percent) secondary to the alkalinity or inherent action of the depilatory on skin keratin. Certain areas of the body are more prone to irritation than others, such as the perioral region.[141–144] A small test site outside the treatment area should be treated first and potential reactions monitored for 24 to 48 hours prior to use on large surface areas. Depilatories should not be used more often than every other day secondary to irritation, and the area must be thoroughly rinsed and an emollient (preferably acidic) or 1% hydrocortisone should be applied afterward to prevent irritation. Pastes, creams, and lotions are easier to apply and remove and are less variable in concentration and less irritating than powders that must be mixed prior to use.[141] Allergic contact dermatitis is rare but can be related to either the mercaptan or an added fragrance.

Strontium, calcium, or barium sulfide depilatories (Magic Shaving Powder, Royal Crown Shaving Powder are examples) act two to three times faster than thioglycolates and thus are more effective on thicker terminal hair, such as beard hair.[138] The enhanced speed of these powders is partly explained by some of the fatty ingredients in the cream and aerosol preparations interfering with the chemical process and by enhanced degradation of active ingredients by the increased water content in creams vs. powders.[145] However, these sulfide chemical depilatories give off an objectionable odor of hydrogen sulfide gas and tend to be more irritating than the thioglycolates,[139] and barium sulfide is poisonous if ingested.[140] Fragrances are usually used to help mask the odor.

Electrolysis offers the only potentially permanent form of epilation. The term *electrolysis* was first used to describe the destruction of germinative cells of the hair follicle by galvanic current.[146] With galvanic current, a direct electrical current passed down a needle into the hair follicle causes the production of NaOH (lye) and H_2 gas, the former of which is caustic to the surrounding tissue. Today, high-frequency electrocoagulation is used to accomplish hair destruction, a process termed *thermolysis.* It is faster than the original galvanic electrolysis and depends on alternating current to elicit local heat that secondarily damages surrounding tissue. In some locales, the "blend," which employs a combination of galvanic and low-intensity, high-frequency current to destroy hair, is used: it is useful for more resistant coarse hairs.

The term *electrolysis* has come now, by common usage, to describe the general process of electrochemical destruction of the hair follicle. Electrolysis employs use of either a rigid or a flexible probe that functions as an electrode when inserted into the hair follicle and an alternating current is applied. The frequency of the current of the electrolysis machines, regulated by the Food and Drug Administration, is usually 13.56 MHz. The current may be either a low-intensity current employed for 3 to 20 seconds or a higher-intensity current applied for less than 1 second, the so-called "flash" technique. The oscillating current of thermolysis causes a transformation of electrical energy into heat, which coagulates the surrounding tissue. The conducted heat is responsible for the pain as well as the tissue destruction of electrolysis, which can be minimized with the shorter pulses of the "flash" technique. Forceps are used to remove the hair from the treated follicular tract. Hairs are removed easily if sufficient tissue destruction has occurred to separate the hair shaft from the attached follicular sheaths.

The regrowth after electrolysis has been noted to be as much as 15 to 50 percent but appears to be dependent on a number of factors.[146,147] Operators of electrolysis machines are generally nonmedical personnel and subject to a wide variety of training practices. In many states, there are no standards for electrologists, whereas other states require as little as 100 hours to be certified and may or may not have a qualifying examination.[146] Electrolysis machines vary widely in amount and type of current and pulse timing. Probes are of variable length, diameter, flexibility, and insulation, which may affect the level of follicular insertion and subsequent follicular destruction. Part of the "regrowth" may be subsequent growth of untreated telogen hairs or, in the case of hirsutism, conversion of fine vellus hairs to terminal hairs by the continued presence of androgens.[137] Telogen hairs are also less likely than anagen hairs to respond to electrolysis.[137] This has been ascribed to the fact that the papillae in telogen vs. anagen hairs is separated from the distal end of the hair shaft. However, in light of the following information, this may not be a satisfactory explanation.

The classic concept prior to the late 1970s was that destruction of the dermal papillae led to abolition of hair regrowth. However, Oliver demonstrated in 1966 that rats in whom the whisker papillae and lower portion of the hair follicle were removed were capable of whisker regeneration as long as the upper two-thirds of the hair follicle was preserved.[148] Inaba, Anthony, Ezaki, and McKinstry reported in 1978 on regeneration of axillary hair after subcutaneous tissue shaving in the treatment of axillary bromhidrosis or excess odor.[149] The special shaving device removed the subcutaneous tissue, deep dermis, and adnexal tissues contained therein. The researchers concluded that hair could regrow from the outer root sheath if the upper portion of the follicular isthmus and sebaceous glands were intact.[149,150] In a subsequent study of selective destruction of various parts of the follicle by electrolysis, McKinstry, Inaba, and Anthony found that only when the isthmus and adjacent sebaceous glands were destroyed did permanent epilation occur and speculated that hair was regrowing from the region where the sebaceous duct opens into the isthmal portion of the hair follicle.[151] This area is analogous to the constant vs. transient portion of the "bulge" area opposite the insertion of the arrector pili muscle identified by Montagna and Parakkal:[152] this area has recently been shown by Cotsarelis, Sun, and Lavker to indeed have pleuripotential capabilities.[153] Permanent destruction of the follicle may then require destruction of this bulge area, at least in telogen.

Complications of electrolysis include immediate transient swelling and erythema, as well as the potential for folliculitis, infection, and postinflammatory hyperpigmentation and hypopigmentation. There has been no reported spread of hepatitis, herpes, or AIDS by electrolysis, but neither is there a standard of practice for using disposable vs. reusable probes or uniform standards of sterilization of the latter.

CONCLUDING REMARKS

Both congenital and acquired forms of diffuse hypertrichosis should trigger a search for other signs or symptoms of a hereditary syndrome, systemic disease, or causative medication. Localized hypertrichosis usually signals a malformation of the underlying skin or neural structures, or external trauma. The hypertrichosis may be ablated by removing or treating the underlying etiology. If this is not possible, the unwanted hairs may be removed by safely using physical, chemical, or electrical means.

REFERENCES

1. Kuttenn F, Mowszowicz I, Mauvais-Jarvis P: Androgen metabolism in human skin. In Mauvais-Jarvis P, Vickers CFH, Wapierre P (eds): *Percutaneous Absorption of Steroids.* London, Academic Press, 1980, pp 99–121.
2. Danforth CH: Studies on hair. Arch Dermatol Syphilol 12:380–401, 1925.
3. Barth JH: Normal hair growth in children. Pediatr Dermatol 4(3):173–184, 1987.
4. Danforth CH: Studies on hair. Arch Dermatol Syphilol 11:804–821, 1925.
5. Price ML, Griffiths WAD: Normal body hair: A review. Clin Exp Dermatol 10:87–97, 1985.
6. Partridge JW: Congenital hypertrichosis lanuginosa: Neonatal shaving. Arch Dis Child 62:623–625, 1987.
7. Ravin JG, Hodge GP: Hypertrichosis portrayed in art. JAMA 207(3):533–535, 1969.

8. Jackson GT, McMurty CW: *A Treatise on Diseases of the Hair.* Philadelphia, Lea & Febiger, 1912, p 144.
9. Beighton P: Congenital hypertrichosis lanuginosa. Arch Dermatol 101:669–672, 1970.
10. Macias-Flores MA et al.: A new form of hypertrichosis inherited as an X-linked dominant trait. Hum Genet 66:66–70, 1984.
11. Freire-Maia N et al.: Hypertrichosis lanuginosa in a mother and son. Clin Gen 10:303–306, 1976.
12. Laband PF, Habib G, Humphreys BS: Hereditary gingival fibromatosis: Report of an affected family with associated splenomegaly and skeletal and soft-tissue abnormalities. Oral Pathol 17(3):339–351, 1964.
13. Winter GB, Simpkiss MJ: Hypertrichosis with hereditary gingival hyperplasia. Arch Dis Child 49:394–399, 1974.
14. Witkop CJ Jr: Heterogeneity in gingival fibromatosis. Birth Defects: Original Article Series 7(7):210–221, 1971.
15. Byars LT, Jurkiewicz M: Congenital macrogingivae and hypertrichosis with subsequent giant fibroadenomas of the breasts. Plast Reconstr Surg 27:608–612, 1961.
16. Salem OS, Steck WD: Cowden's disease (multiple hamartoma and neoplasia syndrome). J Am Acad Dermatol 8:686–696, 1983.
17. De Lange C: Memoires Originaux: Sur un Type Nouveau de dégénération (Typus Amstelodamensis). Arch de Méd d enf 36:713–719+, 1933.
18. Pashayan H, Whelan D, Guttman S, Fraser FC: Variability of the de Lange syndrome: Report of 3 cases and genetic analysis of 54 families. J Pediatr 75(5):853–858, 1969.
19. Soderquist NA, Reed WB: Cornelia de Lange syndrome. Cutis 4:1333–1335, 1968.
20. Ptacek LJ et al.: The Cornelia de Lange syndrome. J Pediatr 63(5):1000–1020, 1963.
21. Daniel WL, Higgins JV: Biochemical and genetic investigation of the de Lange syndrome. Am J Dis Child 121:401–405, 1971.
22. Beck B: Familial occurrence of Cornelia de Lange's syndrome. Acta Paediatr Scand 63:225–231, 1974.
23. Milot J, Demay F: Ocular anomalies in de Lange syndrome. Am J Ophthalmol 74:394–399, 1972.
24. Falek A, Schmidt R, Jervis GA: Familial de Lange syndrome with chromosome abnormalities. Pediatrics 37(1):92–101, 1966.
25. Opitz JM, Segal AT, Lehrke R, Nadler H: Brachmann/De Lange syndrome. Lancet 2:1019, 1964.
26. Selmanowitz VJ, Stiller MJ: Rubinstein-Taybi syndrome: Cutaneous manifestations and colossal keloids. Arch Dermatol 117:504–506, 1981.
27. Majewski F, Goecke T: Studies of mirocephalic primordial dwarfism I: Approach to a delineation of the Seckel syndrome. Am J Med Genet 12:7–21, 1982.
28. Hambrick GW Jr, Scheie HG: Studies of the skin in Hurler's syndrome. Arch Dermatol 85:455–470, 1962.
29. Hanson JW, Jones KL, Smith DW: Fetal alcohol syndrome. JAMA 235:1458–1460, 1976.
30. Taori GM, Martin KC, Bhaktaviziam A, Bachhawat BK: Globoid leukodystrophy (Krabbe's disease). Indian J Med Res 58:993–1001, 1970.
31. Hovenden A: Acquired hypertrichosis lanuginosa associated with malignancy. Arch Intern Med 147: 2013–2018, 1987.
32. Hegedus SI, Schorr WF: Acquired hypertrichosis lanuginosa and malignancy. Arch Dermatol 106:84–88, 1972.
33. Fretzin DF: Malignant down. Arch Dermatol 95:294–297, 1967.
34. Wadskov S, Bro-Jorgensen A, Sondergaard J: Acquired hypertrichosis lanuginosa: A skin marker of internal malignancy. Arch Dermatol 112:1442–1444, 1976.
35. Delfino M et al.: Acquired hypertrichosis lanuginosa: A case report. Dermatologica 170:207–209, 1985.
36. Goodfellow A, Calvert H, Bohn G: Hypertrichosis lanuginosa acquisita. Br J Dermatol 103:431–433, 1980.
37. Price ML, Hall-Smith SP: Hypertrichosis lanuginosa acquisita. Clin Exp Dermatol 10:255–257, 1985.
38. Ikeya T, Izumi A, Suzuki M: Acquired hypertrichosis lanuginosa. Dermatologica 156:274–282, 1978.
39. van der Lugt L, de Wit CD: Hypertrichosis lanuginosa acquisita. Dermatologica 146:46–54, 1973.
40. Hensley GT, Glynn KP: Hypertrichosis lanuginosa as a sign of internal malignancy. Cancer 24:1051–1056, 1969.
41. Davies RA et al.: Acquired hypertrichosis lanuginosa as a sign of internal malignant disease. Can Med Assoc J 118:1090–1096, 1978.
42. Jemec GBE: Hypertrichosis lanuginosa acquisita: Report of a case and review of the literature. Arch Dermatol 122:805–808, 1986.
43. Earhart RN, Ball J, Nuss DD, Aeling JL: Minoxidil-induced hypertrichosis: Treatment with calcium thioglycolate depilatory. South Med J 70(4):442–443, 1977.
44. Novak E, Franz TJ, Headington JT, Wester RC: Topically applied minoxidil in baldness. Int J Dermatol 24:83–87, 1985.
45. Dargie HJ, Dollery CT, Daniel J: Minoxidil in resistant hypertension. Lancet 2(1):515–518, 1977.
46. Headington JT, Novak E: Clinical and histological studies of male pattern baldness treated with topical minoxidil. Curr Ther Res Exp 36:1098–1106, 1984.
47. Uno H, Cappas A, Schlagel C: Cyclic dynamics of hair follicles and the effect of minoxidil on the bald scalp of stump tailed macaques. Am J Dermatopathol 7:283–297, 1985.
48. Wester RC, Maibach HI, Guy RH, Novak E: Minoxidil stimulates cutaneous blood flow in human balding scalps: Pharmacodynamics measured by laser Doppler velocimetry and photopulse plethysmography. J Invest Dermatol 82:505–517, 1984.
49. Buhl AE, Waldon DJ, Kawabe TT, Holland JM: Minoxidil stimulates mouse vibrissae follicles in organ culture. J Invest Dermatol 92(3):315–320, 1989.
50. Uno H, Cappas A, Brigham P: Increased DNA synthesis of the hair follicular and perifollicular cells by topical minoxidil in the macaque scalp (abstract). J Invest Dermatol 84:358, 1985.
51. Baden HP, Kubilus J: Effect of minoxidil on cultured keratinocytes. J Invest Dermatol 81:558–560, 1983.
52. Buhl AE: Minoxidil's action in hair follicles. J Invest Dermatol 96:73S–74S, 1991.
53. Burton JL, Schutt WH, Caldwell IW: Hypertrichosis due to diazoxide. Br J Dermatol 93:707–711, 1975.
54. Moore PF: The effects of diazoxide and benzothiadiazine diuretics upon phosphodiesterase. Ann NY Acad Sci 150:256–259, 1968.
55. Okun R, Russell RP, Wilson WR: Use of diazoxide with

trichlormethiazide for hypertension. Arch Intern Med 112:882–888, 1963.
56. Baker L, Kaye R, Root AW, Prasad ALN: Diazoxide treatment of idiopathic hypoglycemia of infancy. J Pediatr 71(4):494–505, 1967.
57. Menter MA (for Wells RS): Hypertrichosis lanuginosa and a lichenoid eruption due to diazoxide therapy. Proc R Soc Med 66:16–17, 1973.
58. Milner RDG, Chouksey SK: Effects of fetal exposure to diazoxide in man. Arch Dis Child 47:537–543, 1972.
59. Herberg K-P: Effects of diphenylhydantoin in 41 epileptics institutionalized since childhood. South Med J 70(1):19–24, 1977.
60. Livingston S, Pauli LL, Pruce I, Kramer II: Phenobarbital vs. phenytoin for grand mal epilepsy. Am Fam Physician 22(2):123–127, 1980.
61. Livingston S, Petersen D, Boks LL: Hypertrichosis occurring in association with dilantin therapy. J Pediatr 47:351–352, 1955.
62. Bartuska DG: Hypertrichosis in a brain damaged child. J Am Med Wom Assoc 18(9):711–713, 1963.
63. Benici PL et al.: Cutaneous lesions in 67 cyclosporine-treated renal transplant recipients. Dermatologica 172: 24–30, 1986.
64. European Multicentre Trial Group: Cyclosporin in cadaveric renal transplantation: One-year follow-up of a multicentre trial. Lancet 2(2):986–989, 1983.
65. Cohen DJ et al.: Cyclosporine: A new immunosuppressive agent for organ transplantation. Ann Intern Med 101:667–682, 1984.
66. Harper JI et al.: Dermatological aspects of the use of cyclosporin A for prophylaxis of graft-versus-host disease. Br J Dermatol 110:469–474, 1984.
67. Wysocki GP, Daley TD: Hypertrichosis in patients receiving cyclosporine therapy. Clin Exp Dermatol 12: 191–196, 1987.
68. Pendry A, Alexander P: Stimulation of hair growth on nude mice by cyclosporin A. In White DJG (ed): *Cyclosporin A.* New York, Elsevier Biomedical Press, 1982, pp 77–81.
69. Paus R, Stenn KS, Link RE: The induction of anagen hair growth in telogen mouse skin by cyclosporine A administration. Lab Invest 60(3):365–369, 1989.
70. Reznik VM, Jones KL, Durham BL, Mendoza SA: Changes in facial appearance during cyclosporin treatment. Lancet 1(2):1405–1407, 1987.
71. Elliott JA Jr: Clinical experiences with methoxsalen in the treatment of vitiligo. J Invest Dermatol 32:311–313, 1959.
72. Singh G, Lal S: Hypertrichosis and hyperpigmentation with systemic psoralen treatment (letter). Br J Dermatol 79:501–503, 1967.
73. Rampen FHJ: Hypertrichosis in PUVA-treated patients. Br J Dermatol 109:657–660, 1983.
74. Himathongkam T, Dasanabhairochana P, Pitchayayothin N, Sriphrapradang A: Florid Cushing's syndrome and hirsutism induced by desoximetasone. JAMA 239(5):430–431, 1978.
75. Fono R: Appearance of hypertrichosis during streptomycin treatment. Ann Paediatr 174:389–392, 1950.
76. Holzel A: Hypertrichosis in childhood. Acta Paediatrica 40:59–69, 1951.
77. Weiss IS: Hirsutism after chronic administration of acetazolamide. Am J Ophthalmol 78(2):327–328, 1974.
78. Bianchetti MG et al.: Comparative evaluation of the new vasodilator carprazidil and minoxidil in the treatment of moderate to severe hypertension. Eur J Clin Pharmacol 23:483–489, 1982.
79. Spätling L et al.: Verstärkter Haarwuchs unter Langzeittokolyse mit Fenoterol unter Berucksichtigung von Testosteron, Androstandiol, Cortisol und ACTH. Geburtshilfe Frauenheilkd 40:1022–1028, 1980.
80. Grossman ME et al.: Porphyria cutanea tarda: Clinical features and laboratory findings in 40 patients. Am J Med 67:277–285+, 1979.
81. Bleiberg J, Wallen M, Brodkin R, Applebaum IL: Industrially acquired prophyria. Arch Dermatol 89:793–797, 1964.
82. Cam C, Nigogosyan G: Acquired toxic porphyria cutanea tarda due to hexachlorobenzene. JAMA 183(2): 90–93, 1963.
83. Grossman ME, Bickers DR: Porphyria cutanea tarda: A rare cutaneous manifestation of hepatic tumors. Cutis 21:782–784, 1978.
84. Burry JN, Lawrence JR: Phototoxic blisters from high frusemide dosage. Br J Dermatol 94:495–499, 1976.
85. Birkett DA, Garretts M, Stevenson CJ: Phototoxic bullous eruptions due to nalidixic acid. Br J Dermatol 81:342–344, 1969.
86. Poh-Fitzpatrick MB, Masullo AS, Grossman ME: Porphyria cutanea tarda associated with chronic renal disease and hemodialysis. Arch Dermatol 116:191–195, 1980.
87. Epstein JH, Tuffanelli DL, Seibert JS, Epstein WL: Porphyria-like cutaneous changes induced by tetracycline hydrochloride photosensitization. Arch Dermatol 112:661–666, 1976.
88. Hanno R, Callen JP: Porphyria cutanea tarda as a cause of bullous dermatosis of hemodialysis. Cutis 28:261–263, 1981.
89. Corey TJ, DeLeo VA, Christianson H, Poh-Fitzpatrick MB: Variegate porphyria: Clinical and laboratory features. J Am Acad Dermatol 2:36–43, 1980.
90. Pathak MA, West JD: Porphyrias: Office procedures and laboratory tests for diagnosis of porphyrin abnormalities. Acta Dermatovener Suppl 100:91–105, 1982.
91. Magnus IA: The cutaneous porphyrias. Semin Hematol 5(4):380–408, 1968.
92. Nordmann Y, Deybach JC: Congenital erythropoietic porphyria. Semin Liver Dis 2(2):154–163, 1982.
93. Iwashita H et al.: Polyneuropathy, skin hyperpigmentation, edema, and hypertrichosis in localized osteosclerotic myeloma. Neurology 27:675–681, 1977.
94. Bosco J, Pathmanathan R: POEMS syndrome, osteosclerotic myeloma and Castleman's disease: A case report. Aust NZ J Med 21:454–456, 1991.
95. Feddersen RM et al.: Plasma cell dyscrasia: A case of POEMS syndrome with a unique dermatologic presentation. J Am Acad Dermatol 21:1061–1068, 1989.
96. Viard J-P et al.: POEMS syndrome presenting as systemic sclerosis. Am J Med 84:524–528, 1988.
97. Dix JH, Levy WJ, Fuenning C: Remission of acanthosis nigricans, hypertrichosis, and Hashimoto's thyroiditis with thyroxine replacement. Pediatr Dermatol 3(4): 323–326, 1986.
98. Stern SR, Kelnar CJH: Hypertrichosis due to primary hypothyroidism. Arch Dis Child 60:763–766, 1985.
99. Maekawa Y, Kito M, Hiramatsu R: Rolled hairs and hy-

pertrichosis: A manifestation of juvenile hypothyroidism. J Dermatol 10:157–160, 1983.
100. Harris HW, Miller OF: Midline cutaneous and spinal defects. Arch Dermatol 112:1724–1728, 1976.
101. Thursfield WRR, Ross AA: Faun tail (sacral hirsuties) and diastematomyelia. Br J Dermatol 73:328–336, 1961.
102. James CCM, Lassman LP: Spinal dysraphism: An orthopaedic syndrome in children accompanying occult forms. Arch Dis Child 35:315–327, 1960.
103. Lassman LP, James CCM: Meningocoele manqué. Child's Brain 3:1–11, 1977.
104. Perret G: Diagnosis and treatment of diastematomyelia. Surg Gynecol Obstet 105:69–83, 1957.
105. Andreev VC, Stransky L: Hairy elbows. Arch Dermatol 115:761, 1979.
106. Beighton P: Familial hypertrichosis cubiti: Hairy elbows syndrome. J Med Genet 7:158–160, 1970.
107. Rafaat M: Hypertrichosis pinnae in babies of diabetic mothers (letter). Pediatrics 65:745–746, 1981.
108. Singh M, Kumar A, Paul VK: Hairy pinna: A pathognomonic sign in infants of diabetic mothers. Indian Pediatr 24:87–89, 1987.
109. Woods DL, Malan AF, Coetzee EJ: Intra-uterine growth in infants of diabetic mothers. S Afr Med J 58:441–443, 1980.
110. Tosti A et al.: Acquired hairy pinnae in a patient infected with the human immunodeficiency virus. J Am Acad Dermatol 28(3):513, 1993.
111. Stern C, Centerwall WR, Sarkar SS: New data on the problem of Y-linkage of hairy pinnae. Am J Hum Genet 16(4):455–471, 1964.
112. Hamilton JB: A secondary sexual character that develops in men but not in women upon ageing of an organ present in both sexes. Anat Rec 94:466–467, 1946.
113. Slatis HM, Apelbaum A: Hairy pinna of the ear in Israeli populations. Am J Hum Genet 15:74–85, 1963.
114. Oliver GL, McFarlane DC: Congenital trichomegaly with associated pigmentary degeneration of the retina, dwarfism, and mental retardation. Arch Ophthalmol 74:169–174, 1965.
115. Glover MT, Malone M, Atherton DJ: Michelin-Tire baby syndrome resulting from diffuse smooth muscle hamartoma. Pediatr Dermatol 6(4):329–331, 1989.
116. Slifman NR, Harrist TJ, Rhodes AR: Congenital arrector pili hamartoma. Arch Dermatol 121:1034–1037, 1985.
117. Metzker A, Amir J, Rotem A, Merlob P: Congenital smooth muscle hamartoma of the skin. Pediatr Dermatol 2:45–48, 1094.
118. Cohen AH, Hollister DW, Reed WB: The skin in the Winchester syndrome. Arch Dermatol 111:230–236, 1975.
119. Jackson CE, Callies QC, Krull EA, Mehregan A: Hairy cutaneous malformations of palms and soles. Arch Dermatol 111:1146–1149, 1975.
120. Leung AKC, Kiefer GN: Localized acquired hypertrichosis associated with fracture and cast application. J Natl Med Assoc 81:65–67, 1989.
121. Becker SW: Concurrent melanosis and hypertrichosis in distribution of nevus unius lateris. Arch Dermatol Syphilol 60:155–160, 1949.
122. Bhawan J, Chang WH: Becker's melanosis: An ultrastructural study. Dermatologica 159:221–230, 1979.
123. Glinick SE, Alper JC, Bogaars H, Brown JA: Becker's melanosis: Associated abnormalities. J Am Acad Dermatol 9:509–514, 1983.
124. Haneke E: The dermal component in melanosis naeviformis Becker. J Cutan Pathol 6:53–58, 1979.
125. Poomeechaiwong S, Golitz LE: Hamartomas. Adv Dermatol 5:257–288, 1990.
126. Urbanek RD, Johnson WC: Smooth muscle hamartoma associated with Becker's nevus. Arch Dermatol 114:104–106, 1978.
127. Johnson MD, Jacobs AH: Congenital smooth muscle hamartoma. Arch Dermatol 125:820–822, 1989.
128. Person JR, Longcope C: Becker's nevus: An androgen-mediated hyperplasia with increased androgen receptors. J Am Acad Dermatol 10:235–238, 1984.
129. Szylit J-A et al.: Becker's nevus and an accessory scrotum. J Am Acad Dermatol 14:905–907, 1986.
130. Miyachi Y, Horio T, Yamada A, Ueo T: Linear melorheostotic scleroderma with hypertrichosis. Arch Dermatol 115:1233–1234, 1979.
131. Berglund EF, Burton GV, Mills GM, Nichols GM: Hypertrichosis of the eyelashes associated with interferon-α therapy for chronic granulocytic leukemia (letter). South Med J 83:363, 1990.
132. Foon KA: Increased growth of eyelashes in a patient given leukocyte A interferon. N Engl J Med 311(2):1259, 1984.
133. Weaver DT, Bartley GB: Cyclosporine-induced trichomegaly. Am J Ophthalmol 109(2):239, 1990.
134. Casanova JM, Puig T, Rubio M: Hypertrichosis of the eyelashes in acquired immunodeficiency syndrome (letter). Arch Dermatol 123:1599–1601, 1987.
135. Marks CG: Localized hirsuties following compression sclerotherapy with sodium tetradecyl sulphate. Br J Surg 61:127–128, 1974.
136. Trotter M: Hair growth and shaving. Anat Rec 37:373–379, 1928.
137. Richards RN, McKenzie MA, Meharg GE: Electroepilation (electrolysis) in hirsutism. J Am Acad Dermatol 15:693–697, 1986.
138. Feldmann EG (ed): *Handbook of Nonprescription Drugs,* 9th ed. Washington, DC, American Pharmaceutical Association, 1990.
139. Natow AJ: Chemical removal of hair. Cutis 38:91–92, 1986.
140. Barry RH: Depilatories. In Balsam MS, Sagarin E (eds): *Cosmetics: Science and Technology.* New York, Wiley-Interscience, 1957, pp 457–478.
141. Brauner GJ, Flandermeyer KL: Pseudofolliculitis barbae: Treatment. Int J Dermatol 16:520–525, 1977.
142. Holt MB: Hospital study of a depilatory cream for surgical patients. AORN J 2:66–71, 1964.
143. Seropian R, Reynolds BM: Wound infections after preoperative depilatory versus razor preparation. Am J Surg 121:251–254, 1971.
144. Prigot A, Garnes AL, Nwagbo U: Evaluation of a chemical depilatory for preoperative preparation of five hundred fifteen surgical patients. Am J Surg 104:900–906, 1962.
145. de La Guardia M: Facial depilatories on black skin. Cosmetics and Toiletries 91:37–38, 1976.
146. Wagner RF, Tomich JM, Grande DJ: Electrolysis and thermolysis for permanent hair removal. J Am Acad Dermatol 12:441–449, 1985.

147. Behrman HT: Diagnosis and management of hirsutism. JAMA 172(17):1924–1931, 1960.
148. Oliver RF: Whisker growth after removal of the dermal papilla and lengths of follicle in the hooded rat. J Embryol Exp Morphol 14(3):331–347, 1966.
149. Inaba M, Anthony J, Ezaki T, McKinstry C: Regeneration of axillary hair and related phenomena after removal of deep dermal and subcutaneous tissue by a special "shaving" technique. J Dermatol Surg Oncol 4:921–925, 1978.
150. Inaba M, Anthony J, McKinstry C: Histologic study of the regeneration of axillary hair after removal with subcutaneous tissue shaver. J Invest Dermatol 72:224–231, 1979.
151. McKinstry CT, Inaba M, Anthony JN: Epilation by electrocoagulation: Factors that result in regrowth of hair. J Dermatol Surg Oncol 5.407–411, 1979.
152. Montagna W, Parakkal PF: *The Structure and Function of the Skin,* 3d ed. New York, Academic Press, 1974, pp 182–185.
153. Cotsarelis G, Sun T, Lavker RM: Label-retaining cells reside in the bulge area of pilosebaceous unit: Implications for follicular stem cells, hair cycle, and skin carcinogenesis. Cell 61:1329–1337, 1990.
154. Byars LT, Sarnat BG: Congenital macrogingivae (fibromatosis gingivae) and hypertrichosis. Surgery 15:-964–970, 1944.
155. Nicholson DH, Goldberg MF: Ocular abnormalities in the de Lange syndrome. Arch Ophthalmol 76:214–220, 1966.
156. Jervis GA, Stimson CW: De Lange syndrome. J Pediatr 63:634–645, 1963.
157. Greaves MW, Inman PM: Cutaneous changes in the Morquio syndrome. Br J Dermatol 81:29–36, 1969.
158. Meinecke P, Engelbrecht R, Schaefer E: The Coffin Siris syndrome in a 5-year-old girl. Monatsschr Kinderheilkd 134:692–695, 1986.
159. Lucaya J, Garcia-Conesa JA, Bosch-Banyeras JM, Pons-Peradejordi G: The Coffin-Siris syndrome: A report of four cases and review of the literature. Pediatr Radiol 11:35–38, 1981.
160. Carey JC, Hall BD: The Coffin-Siris syndrome: Five new cases including two siblings. Am J Dis Child 132:667–671, 1978.
161. Haspelslagh M, Fryns JP, vanden Berghe H: The Coffin-Siris syndrome: Report of a family and further delineation. Clin Genet 26:374–378, 1984.
162. Gorlin RJ, Chaudhry AP, Moss ML: Craniofacial dysostosis, patent ductus arteriosus, hypertrichosis, hypoplasia of labia majora, dental and eye anomalies: A new syndrome? J Pediatr 56(6):778–785, 1960.
163. Freire-Maia N, Pinheiro M: *Ectodermal Dysplasias: A Clinical and Genetic Study.* New York, Alan R. Liss, 1984.
164. Rasmussen K, Storstein O: Hyperkinetic circulatory disorder after closure of persistent ductus arteriosus. Br Heart J 34:671–677, 1972.
165. Schinzel A, Giedion A: A syndrome of severe midface retraction, multiple skull anomalies, clubfeet, and cardiac and renal malformations in sibs. Am J Med Genet 1:361–375, 1978.
166. Donnai D, Harris R: A further case of a new syndrome including midface retraction, hypertrichosis, and skeletal anomalies. J Med Genet 16:483–486, 1979.
167. Janaki VR, Premalatha S, Rao NR, Thambiah AS: Lawrence-Seip syndrome. Br J Dermatol 103:693–696, 1980.
168. Reed WB, Dexter R, Corley C, Fish C: Congenital lipodystrophic diabetes with acanthosis nigricans. Arch Dermatol 91:326–334, 1965.
169. Cantu JM et al.: A distinct osteochondrodysplasia with hypertrichosis—Individualization of a probable autosomal recessive entity. Hum Genet 60:36–41, 1982.
170. Leung AKC: Hypertrichosis associated with topical hydrocortisone. Hong Kong J Paediatr 1:11–13, 1986.
171. Ressmann AC, Butterworth T: Localized acquired hypertrichosis. Arch Dermatol Syphilol 65:458–463, 1952.
172. Bergen D: Localized hirsutism following Colles' fracture. Can Med Assoc J 128:368, 1983.
173. Pillsbury DM, Shelley WB, Kligman AM: Hirsutism. In *Dermatology.* Philadelphia, W. B. Saunders, 1959, pp 1004–1005.
174. Tisocco LA, Del Campo DV, Bennin B, Barsky S: Acquired localized hypertrichosis (letter). Arch Dermatol 117:127–128, 1981.
175. Schraibman IG: Localized hirsuties. Postgrad Med J 43:545–547, 1967.
176. Allen EV, Barker NW, Hines EA Jr: Arteriovenous fistulas. In *Peripheral Vascular Diseases,* 2d ed. Philadelphia, W. B. Saunders, 1955, p 418.
177. Nielsen JS: Localized hirsutism following Colles' fracture (letter). Can Med Assoc J 129:229, 1983.
178. Kumar LR, Goyal BG: Pigmented hairy scar following smallpox vaccination. Indian J Pediatr 35:283–285, 1968.
179. Pembroke AC, Marten RH: Unusual cutaneous reactions following diphtheria and tetanus immunization. Clin Exp Dermatol 4:345–348, 1979.
180. Shafir R, Tsur H: Local hirsutism at the periphery of burned skin. Br J Plast Surg 32:93, 1979.

Chapter

14

HIRSUTISM

Claude L. Hughes, Jr.

INTRODUCTION

Hirsutism has been defined in various ways in the past. I wish to propose that as a biologic phenomenon, hirsutism is simply androgen-dependent differentiation and growth of hair in females. This biological sense is transformed into a clinical diagnosis when expert clinical judgment concurs that development and growth of hair in androgen-dependent areas are excessive. The clinical diagnosis of hirsutism implies underlying pathophysiology and necessitates a systematic evaluation. The assessment must be adequate to distinguish among causes that are (1) dangerous to life and health, (2) trivial for life and health, or (3) consequential for well-being over the short term and incur some significant health risks over the long term.

NORMAL AGE-RELATED ANDROGEN-MEDIATED HAIR GROWTH

As a biological process, hirsutism is simply androgen-dependent growth and development of hair in women. From this perspective, the conversion of follicles from vellus to terminal follows an expected, temporally defined sequence in "sexually dependent" body regions that manifests at puberty, is maintained during adult life, and commonly shows gradual diminution with reproductive senescence in both sexes.[1–3] As summarized in Table 14-1, general associations of androgen sources and levels can be made for each body location of terminal hair development. Simply put, low concentrations of androgens of primarily adrenal origin produce the adrenarchal development of axillary and pubic hair in both sexes, while higher concentrations of androgens of both adrenal and gonadal origin produce the characteristic male-pattern terminal hair growth of the beard, ears and nose, sternum, and upper pubic triangle. If male-pattern terminal hair growth occurs in a female, then the clinical symptom of hirsutism exists.

In the broadest sense, the age of onset of hirsutism serves as an important guide regarding the level of clinical concern and degree of required diagnostic testing. Hirsutism in a prepubertal child must be taken seriously and presumed to be the result of a hormone-secreting

Table 14-1
NORMAL ANDROGEN-DEPENDENT GROWTH AND DEVELOPMENT OF HAIR

	ANDROGENS ELICITING CONVERSION		
Body Regions	*Concentration*	*Source*	*Timing in Lifespan*
	Conversion of vellus to terminal hair		
Axilla	Low	Adrenal and gonads	Early puberty
Lower pubic triangle	Low	Adrenal and gonads	Puberty
Tanner stage			
2 (rare)	Low		11.7 years (9.3–14.1)
3 (sparse)	Low-moderate		12.4 years (10.2–14.6)
4 (moderate)	Moderate		13.0 years (10.8–15.1)
5 (adult)	Moderate		14.4 years (12.2–16.7)
Beard, ears and nose, sternum, upper pubic triangle	High	Testes	Late puberty and adulthood
	Conversion of terminal to vellus hair		
Temporal/frontal scalp	Low	Adrenal (male)	Puberty
	High	Testes	Adulthood
Axilla, pubic areas	Declining	Gonads	Reproductive senescence

Source: Adapted from Marshal and Tanner,[1] Root and Reiter,[2] and Grunfeld and Kase.[3]

tumor until sufficient evidence indicates an alternative explanation. In many instances, development of terminal hair in a prepubertal child will actually be the onset of adrenarche rather than hirsutism per se, whether appropriately timed (see Table 14-1) or precocious in onset. Perhaps as many as one in five girls will show growth of terminal pubertal and axillary hair prior to the other signs of puberty. These concerns regarding assessment of peripubertal events should generally be evaluated by pediatric endocrine specialists and, for practical purposes, are distinct from most of the issues surrounding hirsutism in adults.

Hirsutism in adults can be temporally divided into reproductive-age (premenopausal) and postmenopausal groups. The strategies for evaluation and management of hirsutism in these two groups generally follow the same logical course; however, some differences in emphasis are appropriate. Menopausal women who are not on hormonal replacement therapy with estrogen or estrogen plus progestin commonly show thinning of axillary and pubic hair but gradual development of hirsutism in other sites. This hirsutism seems to result from a functional change in the ratio of androgen to estrogen due to physiological ovarian failure. At menopause, the ovaries are depleted of follicles, which were the source of cyclic estradiol production during premenopausal adulthood. Thus, ovarian production of estradiol becomes essentially nil while ovarian androgen production continues unabated,[4] resulting in mild but often troubling hirsutism. In the postmenopausal group of patients, other functional diagnoses such as polycystic ovarian disease or late-onset congenital adrenal hyperplasia rarely manifest with a new onset of symptoms, so the possibility of an androgen-secreting tumor must be entertained for all patients exhibiting frank virilization or sudden-onset, rapidly progressive moderate to severe hirsutism.

Menopausal women with troublesome hirsutism unrelated to tumor sources do benefit from hormonal replacement therapy with estrogen plus or minus progestin. Conjugated equine estrogens (Premarin 0.625–1.25 mg per day), with or without medroxyprogesterone acetate (Provera), suppress testosterone levels by approximately 21 percent and androstenedione by 5 percent in menopausal women,[5] similar to oral contraceptive pill effects in younger women (see section titled "Ovarian Suppression"). However, the majority of patients who seek evaluation of hirsutism are of reproductive age and are the primary subjects for investigation and treatment.

ANDROGEN PRODUCTION, TRANSPORT, METABOLISM, AND CLEARANCE

There are three sources of androgens in women.[6] The ovaries and adrenal glands have steroidogenic enzymes that permit biosynthesis of androgens from cholesterol. The third important source of androgens is the "peripheral compartment," of which the skin is the major component. Although the peripheral compartment cannot synthesize androgens from cholesterol, the productive conversion of weak androgens to more potent androgens profoundly affects the serum level of androgenic bioactivity.[7]

Androgen Production

In quantitative terms, the rank order of plasma concentrations of androgens in women is dehydroepiandrosterone sulfate (DHEAS; 170,000 ng/dl), dehydroepiandrosterone (DHEA; 420 ng/dl), androstenedione (A; 176 ng/dl), androstenediol (75 ng/dl), testosterone (T; 39 ng/dl), and dihydrotestosterone (DHT; 19 ng/dl).[8] Figure 14-1 illustrates steroidogenesis in the ovaries and adrenal glands. The steroidogenic cascade is nearly identical in the adrenal and ovary, with the major differences in output resulting from prominence of aromatase (enzyme "F" in Fig. 14-1) activity in the ovary (but minimal activity in the adrenal) and prominence of 11β-hydroxylase (enzyme "H" in Fig. 14-1) activity in the adrenal (but minimal activity in the ovary). Although several tissues are capable of some aspects of androgen synthesis and metabolism, the full synthetic sequence of androgens from cholesterol can occur only where 3β-ol dehydrogenase (enzyme "C" in Fig. 14-1) is located; i.e., the ovaries and adrenals.

The rate-limiting step in steroidogenesis in both the adrenal gland and the ovary is the complex of enzymes known as the *side-chain cleavage enzymes.* This side-chain cleavage involves several chemical intermediates, but the net effect is conversion of the 27-carbon cholesterol to the 21-carbon pregnenolone by the enzymes at

Figure 14-1 Gonadal steroid and adrenal glucocorticoid biosynthesis. Enzymes in the sequence are (A) 20-hydroxylase; 20,22-desmolase; (B) 17α-hydroxylase; (C) 3β-ol dehydrogenase; (D) desmolase; (E) 17β-ol dehydrogenase; (F) aromatase (ovary only); (G) 21-hydroxylase; (H) 11β-hydroxylase (adrenal only). Note that arrow sizes do not imply quantitation.

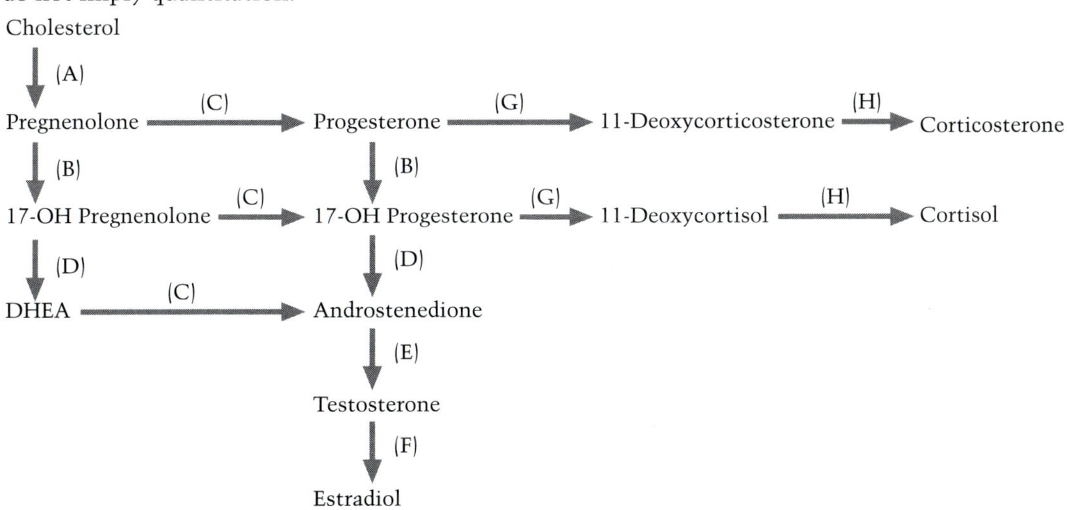

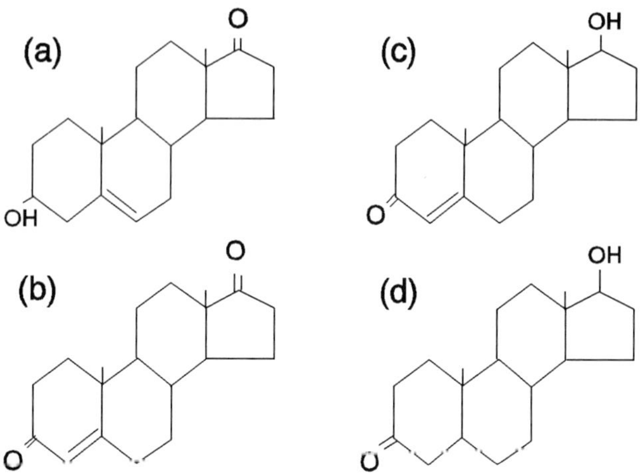

Figure 14-2 Structure of major androgens. Relative potencies based on receptor affinity, are (a) dehydroepiandrosterone (DHEA) < (b) androstenedione (A) < (c) testosterone (T) < (d) dihydrotestosterone (DHT).

the beginning of the pathway shown as (A) in Figure 14-1. This side-chain cleavage step is the most important site for regulation of the entire steroidogenic sequence. The principal regulators of steroidogenesis at the glandular level are the trophic pituitary hormones, adrenocorticotropic hormone (ACTH), and the gonadotropins [follicle-stimulating hormone (FSH) and especially luteinizing hormone (LH)]. ACTH in the adrenal and primarily LH in the ovary stimulate steroidogenesis at the rate-limiting side-chain cleavage step (*A* in Fig. 14-1).

In terms of target tissue action of androgens, the 19-carbon androgen structure requires a 17-OH group for binding to androgen receptors (Fig. 14-2). The enzyme 17β-ol dehydrogenase (enzyme "E" in Fig. 14-1) is present in many tissues and converts the 17-keto group (as in androstenedione) to a 17-OH group (as in testosterone). To convert T to DHT, a tissue must contain the enzyme 5α-reductase. Since DHT is the most potent endogenous androgen, those tissues such as skin, prostate, and liver that have 5α-reductase possess a local intracellular mechanism for amplification of androgen action (Fig. 14-3).[9,10] Although DHT is found in the circulation, presumably from hepatic production, the major impact of DHT has been presumed to be due to local synthesis and action. It is reasonable to speculate that local production of DHT and circulating DHT may both be important in androgenic bioactivity.

The hair follicle is a target tissue capable of responding in a dynamic way to any of several endogenous androgens. The requisite androgen receptors are present, but the local presence of enzymes permitting conversion of DHEA to A, then A to T and T to DHT means that several androgenic hormones from the circulation can elicit androgenic effects (Fig. 14-3). Diffusion of DHEA, A, or T into the follicle depends upon the amount of these androgens free in solution in the aqueous phase of the plasma and, in general, the compound's proximity to DHT in the metabolic sequence. Thus, the free-T level (that not bound by serum proteins) can serve as a usable marker for the amount of bioactive androgen delivered to the follicle.

Although the major metabolic role of the cortical portion of the adrenal gland is mediated by

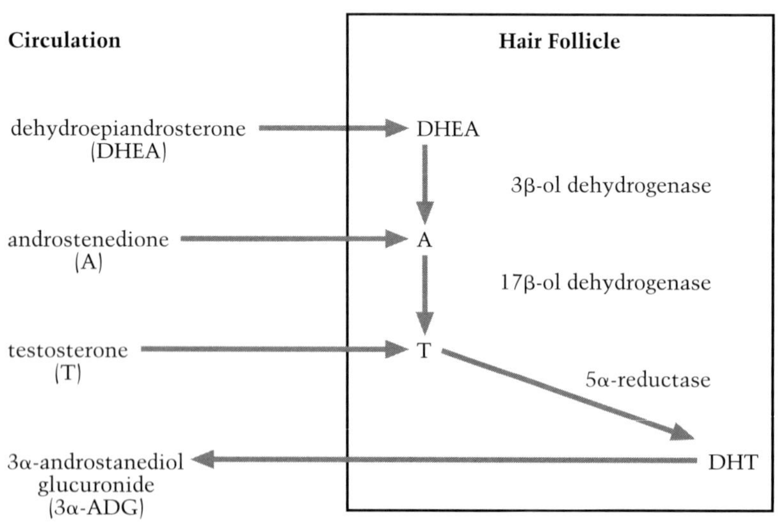

Figure 14-3 Intracellular production of dihydrotestosterone (DHT) within hair follicles from circulating androgenic precursors. DHT is the most potent intrafollicular androgen and is produced and acts locally by binding to androgen receptors.

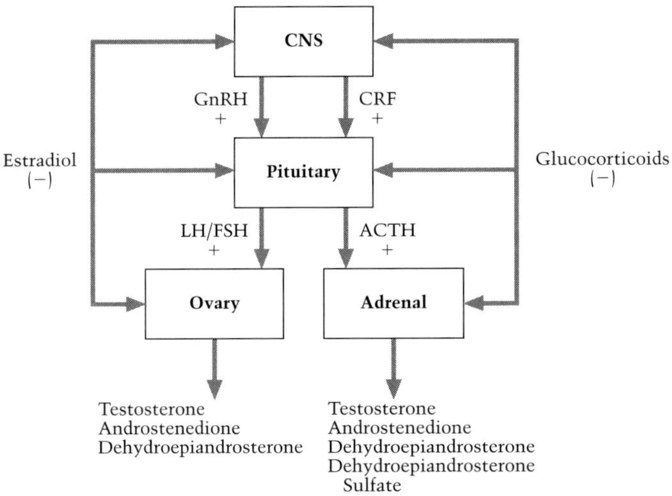

Figure 14-4 Basic inhibitory feedback by steroids on trophic hormone regulation of ovary and adrenal. Androgen production is stimulated by ACTH (adrenal) and LH (ovary), but circulating androgens are not important in the feedback inhibition of trophic hormone secretion in women. ACTH = adrenocorticotropic hormone; CNS = central nervous system; CRF = corticotropic-releasing factor; FSH = follicle-stimulating hormone; GnRH = gonadotropin-releasing hormone; LH = luteinizing hormone.

secretion of 21-carbon corticosteroid hormones, weak androgens are also produced in moderate amounts. As a result, the adrenal gland secretes approximately 90 percent of DHEAS and 90 percent of DHEA, with the remainder of each produced by the ovary. Regulation of adrenal androgen secretion is primarily influenced by ACTH,[11] but not all aspects of adrenal androgen secretion can be explained simply by that source of regulation.[12,13] Figure 14-4 illustrates the basic feedback relationships in the physiological control of the adrenal gland.

The central nervous system (CNS) control of pituitary output of ACTH depends upon hypophyseal-portal secretion of corticotropin-releasing factor (CRF). CRF stimulates ACTH synthesis and secretion, and ACTH from the pituitary stimulates adrenal steroidogenesis. It is important to note that the adrenal steroid products that provide both indirect inhibitory feedback control of CRF secretion from the CNS and direct inhibitory feedback control of ACTH secretion from the pituitary are the glucocorticoids rather than adrenal androgens. As a result, excess adrenal androgen production goes "unrecognized" by the central mechanisms that stimulate androgen output. In essence, feedback fails to constrain the disorder.

Central regulation of ovarian androgen secretion parallels that of the adrenal (Fig. 14-4). The CNS secretes gonadotropin-releasing hormone (GnRH) into the hypophyseal-portal system, and GnRH stimulates secretion of FSH and LH from the pituitary. Both FSH and LH stimulate ovarian function but in complementary ways. The phasic temporally complex patterns of gonadotropic hormones are necessary for normal ovulation and production of normal profiles of secretion of estradiol and progesterone (Fig. 14-5). In the simplest construct, FSH drives the follicular phase of growth of the follicle and concurrent estradiol secretion; the midcycle surge of LH causes ovulation and initiates progesterone production from the newly formed corpus luteum; and then in the luteal phase, LH maintains progesterone secretion from the corpus luteum either until conception occurs or until luteolysis occurs at the end of the cycle. Since estradiol is the major ovarian steroid product that provides both indirect inhibitory feedback control of GnRH secretion from the CNS and direct inhibitory feedback control of gonadotropins from the pituitary, ovarian androgens are nearly ineffectual in constraining central stimulation of ovarian steroidogenesis. Overall, the feedback of

Figure 14-5 Hormonal events in the normal menstrual cycle. E = estradiol; FSH = follicle-stimulating hormone; LH = luteinizing hormone; P = progesterone.

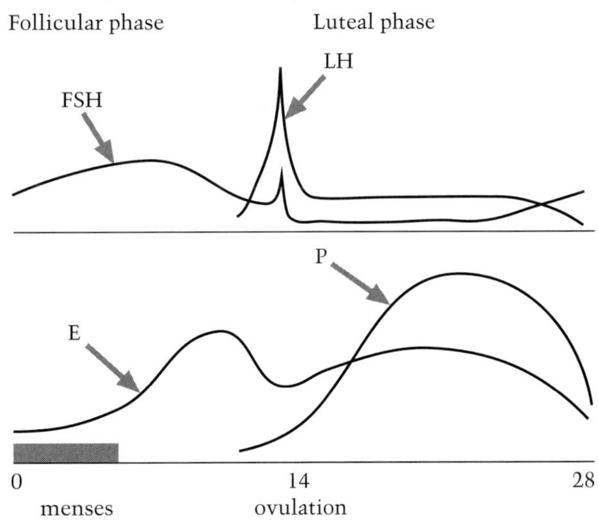

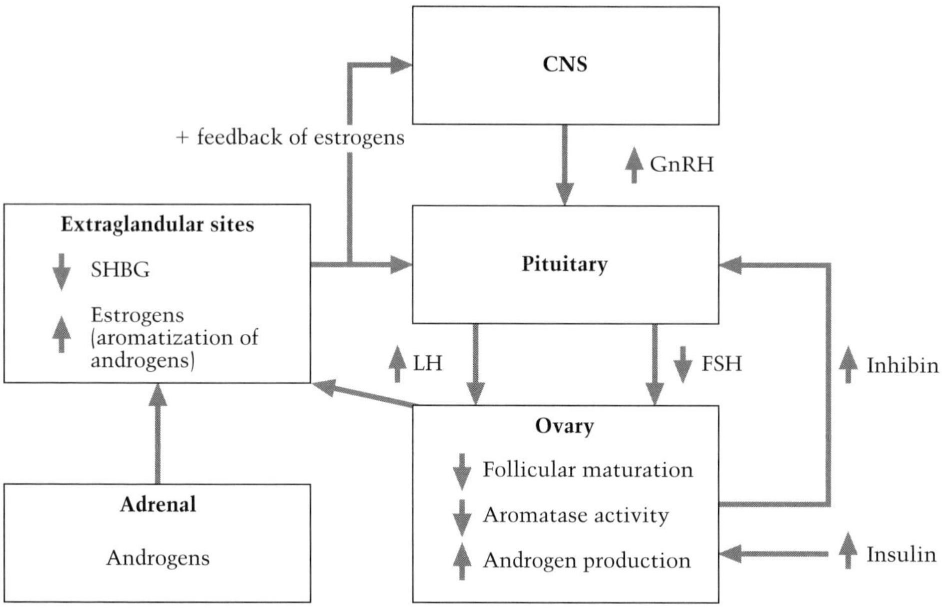

Figure 14-6 Disordered regulatory relationships in polycystic ovarian disease. Any one or several of the elements shown could be the initiating factor in some patients. Note that gonadotropin-releasing hormone (GnRH) is the signal from the CNS that causes pituitary secretion of FSH and LH. FSH primarily stimulates follicular growth in the 2 to 3 weeks prior to ovulation. LH as a midcycle surge causes rupture of the follicle with oocyte release and initiation of corpus luteum production of progesterone. During the 2 weeks after ovulation, several pulses of LH each day maintain progesterone output from the corpus luteum. The positive feedback effect of estradiol that normally elicits the midcycle surge appears to inappropriately enhance LH secretion in an untimely way in polycystic ovarian disease.

the ovary on the CNS and pituitary is quite complicated (Fig. 14-6), since other components of the system include positive feedback of estradiol to elicit the LH surge, progesterone augmentation of that positive feedback of estradiol, progesterone inhibition of LH secretion as the luteal phase progresses, and selective inhibition of FSH by the peptide hormone inhibin in the latter portions of the cycle.

Although of limited diagnostic value in the assessment of androgenic disorders, androstenedione (A) is quantitatively and functionally important in women.[7] A is approximately half ovarian and half adrenal in origin, and approximately half of the T in women is the product of peripheral conversion of A to T. Tissues capable of this conversion in women include liver, skin, fat, and muscle. Direct secretion of T into the circulation is approximately equally derived from ovary and adrenal, although during ovarian cycles, the relative contribution fluctuates with domination by the ovary of midcycle T and A secretion.

Circulatory Transport of Androgens

Androgens are hydrophobic compounds, and only a tiny fraction is in true aqueous solution in the plasma. Most androgens, like other classes of steroids, are predominantly protein-bound in the plasma.[14] Of the four plasma androgen–binding proteins, cortisol-binding globulin and acid α2-glycoprotein are of little importance, while sex hormone–binding globulin (SHBG) and albumin are critically important in androgen binding and transport. As an illustration, T in plasma is approximately 1 to 2 percent free, 20 percent bound to albumin, and 78 percent bound to SHBG.[8] In terms of bioavailability to tissues, the free T is the portion that is bioactive, while the albumin-bound T is loosely bound and can restore the free-T plasma pool as free T is sequestered, metabolized, and so forth, in target tissues. Since the SHBG-bound pool is large and the T-SHBG interaction is of high affinity, this pool of T serves as a more slowly available depot that may reduce the range of fluctuations in the other more dynamic pools of T. As a consequence, changes in SHBG concentration have a major influence on the free-T level and albumin-bound T pool.[15]

Regulation of hepatic synthesis of SHBG is, therefore, an important modulator of androgenicity. Since estrogens increase and androgens decrease SHBG synthesis, patients with a modest excess of androgen production experience disproportionate and accentuated effects of androgens in target tissues, because the decline in SHBG increases bioavailable free T.[15,16] SHBG is also reduced by obesity and hypothyroidism, so androgen activity tends to be increased in those conditions as well.

Peripheral Compartment Androgen Metabolism

Following diffusion of circulating T (also A and DHEA) into androgen-responsive target tissues, T is rapidly converted to DHT by 5α-reductase. DHT binds to the intracellular androgen receptor, and DNA binding of the receptor-steroid complex alters messenger RNA synthesis, thereby eliciting target tissue–specific changes that characterize androgen action.[10] At each step, this seemingly simple sequence of events within the target tissue is extremely complicated, and new data are being generated regarding the molecular details of steroidal regulation of gene expression.

Some aspects of the normal androgen-dependent development of hair (Table 14-1) can be explained by regional differences in androgen-metabolizing enzymes in skin. Basically, regions of skin that manifest androgen-dependent development of terminal hair have the local ability to produce DHT from T, A, and DHEA. During puberty, 5α-reductase activity increases in these androgen-responsive regions and is induced by T.[8] Thus, T increases the enzyme activity that, in turn, amplifies target tissue androgenicity by conversion of T to the more potent DHT.

Androgen Clearance

Ultimate disposition of androgens depends upon metabolic modifications that decrease potency and facilitate excretion. As is true for target tissue bioavailability for androgen action, the circulating androgen available for metabolic conversion, conjugation, and subsequent excretion is the free fraction. Thus, in general, metabolic clearance of androgens is increased if SHBG levels are reduced. The liver is the most important site of metabolic deactivation and conjugation of androgens.[17] Activity of the hepatic enzyme systems that produce this complicated series of steroidal conversions can be increased by oral intake of gonadal steroid analogues.[18] Hepatic metabolism of androgens produces several 17-ketosteroids; including androsterone, etiocholanolone, epiandrosterone, and epietiocholanolone. These 17-ketosteroids, plus others from earlier in the metabolic pathway, are conjugated in the liver to produce glucuronate and sulfate derivatives that are more water-soluble. These conjugated, and some unconjugated, androgen metabolites are then excreted in bile and urine.

PATHOLOGICAL CONDITIONS AND DIAGNOSTIC TESTING

Viewed as a clinical symptom, hirsutism is functionally an endogenous bioassay for androgen activity. This bioassay does not distinguish among exposure of the skin to modest amounts of excess potent androgen, exposure of the skin to large amounts of excess weak androgen, enhanced intrafollicular amplification of androgen effect by in situ production of more potent androgen (DHT), and intrinsically (i.e., genetically) more responsive follicular units. These alternative causes of hirsutism are distinguished by application of clinical judgment to information derived from the medical history, physical examination, and laboratory studies.[19] Critical to establishing the cause of hirsutism is assessment of the timing and severity of the condition and correlation with other signs or symptoms of androgen excess. Menstrual dysfunction is common in patients with even modest excess androgen production, while frank virilization with clitoromegaly, deepening of the voice, muscle enlargement, temporal balding, and breast atrophy virtually always implies significant excess androgen production. Various causes of androgenic syndromes are shown in Table 14-2.

The major division of diagnoses is between tumor and nontumor causes of androgenization.[20] The nontumor causes can be further subgrouped into functional androgen excess diagnoses or enhanced end-organ sensitivity (in the absence of

Table 14-2
CAUSES OF ANDROGENIC SYNDROMES

Androgen-secreting tumors
- Adrenal
  - Adenoma
  - Adenocarcinoma (rare)
  - Ectopic ACTH-secreting tumor (very rare; presents as adrenal androgen excess)
- Ovarian
  - Gonadal stromal tumor
  - Thecoma
  - Lipoid tumor

Functional androgen excess
- Adrenal enzyme deficiencies (congenital adrenal hyperplasia)
  - Early-onset 21-hydroxylase deficiency
  - Late-onset 21-hydroxylase deficiency
  - 11β-hydroxylase deficiency
  - 3β-ol dehydrogenase deficiency
- Cushing's syndrome
- Polycystic ovarian disease
  - With or without adrenal contribution
  - Hyperthecosis

"Idiopathic" hirsutism

Medication/drug use

Table 14-3
ASSESSMENT OF THE ANDROGENIZED PATIENT FOR ANDROGEN-SECRETING TUMOR

Initial suspicion derives from medical history and physical examination showing severe hirsutism, virilization, sudden onset and rapid progression of symptoms.

Primary tests are serum levels of total T and DHEAS. Marked elevations (twice normal or more) of either T or DHEAS make androgen-secreting tumor the likely diagnosis. In general, elevated T is associated with ovarian tumors and DHEAS is associated with adrenal tumors, but either or both hormones may be secreted by tumors of either ovary or adrenal origin.

Secondary tests that assess ovarian and adrenal anatomy include ultrasound and magnetic resonance imaging or computerized tomography. This level of investigation is usually adequate to confidently establish or exclude the diagnosis of androgen-secreting tumor. False-positive and false-negative diagnoses can occur, and the incidence of misdiagnosis is difficult to determine.

Tertiary tests can be considered in special circumstances and include selective catheterization of ovarian and adrenal veins, nuclear medicine imaging for focal uptake of radiolabeled cholesterol, or laparoscopy and/or exploratory laparotomy.

excess androgen production). Strategies for patient management hinge on distinguishing tumor from nontumor diagnoses. Typically, if hirsutism is accompanied by frank virilization and especially if the onset of symptoms is sudden or rapidly progressive, then circulating androgen levels will be markedly elevated and a tumor source (adrenal or ovary) is likely. The initial clinical suspicion of tumor is reinforced or diminished by the primary laboratory tests of elevated total serum T and DHEAS, with secondary tests directed toward confirming or excluding the existence and location of the tumor (Table 14-3).[19]

Functional disorders of adrenal and ovarian androgen excess are at once mechanistically fascinating and clinically frustrating. These entities include a fairly broad spectrum of presentations such that, at either extreme, the functional disorders (adrenal enzyme deficiencies and polycystic ovarian disease) must be distinguished from androgen-secreting tumors on one hand and from idiopathic (end-organ sensitivity) hirsutism (Table 14-4) on the other. The physiological features that underlie some of these diagnoses are well-established, as in the cases of classic early-onset (usually deficiency of 21-hydroxylase but rarely 3β-ol dehydrogenase or 11β-hydroxylase) and adult-onset (attenuated or partial deficiency of 21-hydroxylase) congenital adrenal hyperplasia.[21]

Adult-onset congenital adrenal hyperplasia usually results from partial deficiency of 21-hydroxylase. While elevated basal levels of 17-OH-progesterone (> 8 nmol/liter) strongly suggest partial 21-hydroxylase deficiency, ACTH-stimulation testing is usually considered definitive. Different protocols have been used, but a simple scheme is as follows: (1) perform the test between 8:00 A.M. and 1:00 P.M. when progesterone levels are < 8 nmol/liter; (2) draw a blood sample for serum 17-OH-progesterone and give 1 mg ACTH intravenously; (3) 30 minutes later draw a second blood sample for serum 17-OH-progesterone; (4) 21-hydroxylase deficiency is implied if the increase in 17-OH-progesterone is > 8 nmol/liter.[22] The vast majority of patients manifesting this spectrum of disease do not have demonstrable adrenal enzyme deficiency by such tests and are given the diagnostic label of polycystic ovarian disease.

Table 14-4
ASSESSMENT OF THE ANDROGENIZED PATIENT TO DISTINGUISH FUNCTIONAL ANDROGEN EXCESS FROM TUMOR AND IDIOPATHIC HIRSUTISM

Initial suspicion derives from medical history and physical examination showing mild to moderate hirsutism, little or no virilization, gradual onset, and slow progression of symptoms.
Primary tests of serum levels of total T and DHEAS show small to moderate elevations. Many patients with functional androgen excess will have normal serum levels of total T and DHEAS.
Secondary tests include serum levels of 17-hydroxyprogesterone, free T, 3α-ADG, androstenedione, LH, and FSH and an ACTH (Cortrosyn) stimulation test.

POLYCYSTIC OVARIAN DISEASE

Polycystic ovarian disease (PCOD) describes a disorder in reproductive-age women characterized most simply as estrogenic amenorrhea. That is, if a nonpregnant, premenopausal adult woman has amenorrhea or oligomenorrhea and responds to a 7- to 14-day course of exogenous progestins with menstrual-like uterine bleeding, then the presumptive diagnosis is PCOD. More rigorous criteria may be demanded by some clinicians or investigators and typically include amenorrhea or oligomenorrhea, physiological levels of estrogens, mild to moderate androgen excess, and a ratio of LH to FSH which is elevated to 2:1 or 3:1 or more. The ovaries are characterized by dysfunctional development of growing follicles while other cystic follicles are undergoing atresia. Proper selection of a dominant follicle from growing cohorts, timely occurrence of an LH surge, ovulatory release of an oocyte, and establishment of a normal luteal phase rarely occur in these patients. Decades of research by numerous investigators have failed to define cogently the cause of PCOD, although several disruptive interactions among sites in the CNS, pituitary, ovary, adrenal, and extraglandular tissues have been described (Fig. 14-6).[23] Whereas aberrations in any of the regulatory constituents can produce some or all of the features of PCOD, it may be necessary to consider the clinical diagnosis of PCOD to be an extant syndrome that encompasses an array of inadequately defined disorders that share similar clinical and laboratory characteristics but may result from different underlying causes. The alterations in physiological markers illustrated in Figure 14-6 have, in one way or another, each been proposed as causal for development and persistence of PCOD. There are data supporting each contending hypothesis, but no single explanation seems to account precisely for all of the changes observed in various patients. Although mechanistically noncommittal, it is probable that different initiating factors are causal in different subgroups of PCOD patients.

The *HAIR-AN syndrome* is perhaps the best-defined PCOD-type entity.[24] These patients manifest symptoms of hyperandrogenism (HA), insulin resistance (IR), and acanthosis nigricans (AN), and have PCOD-like ovarian dysfunction as described earlier. This syndrome results from hyperinsulinemia due to diminished number or activity of insulin receptors in target tissues.[25–27] Many of these patients eventually develop adult-onset diabetes mellitus. Beyond the profile of clinical features for identifying this syndrome, diagnostic confirmation requires a glucose tolerance test with insulin levels showing an accentuated rise even if glucose levels do not exceed the normal range.

Primary adrenal androgen excess, such as in patients with 21-hydroxylase deficiency, has been associated with PCOD-like ovarian dysfunction.[21] As expected, some patients normalize menstrual cyclicity and appear to have improved ovulatory function when excessive adrenal androgen is suppressed by exogenous glucocorticoids. However, the precise cause-and-effect relationships are not clear, since many properly diagnosed patients do not show clear-cut improvement in gonadal function once adrenal androgens are reduced. Since the phenomenon of suppression of adrenal androgen levels due to use of oral contraceptives has been observed, "cross talk" must occur between the adrenal axis and the ovarian axis. Conversely, effects of glucocorticoid treatment could be independent from adrenal androgen suppression per se. In spite of the complexity implied by the physiological interrelationship, an adrenal enzyme deficiency is a tangible, well-defined entity that is a credible cause of some cases of PCOD-like disorders.

Various ovarian causes of PCOD have been suggested, but it is very difficult to distinguish initiating causes from secondary epiphenomena. Certainly, excessive ovarian androgen production is a hallmark of many PCOD patients,[28] but excess androgen may be produced by stroma, theca, or both. It is not clear whether elevated intraovarian androgen is primarily a consequence of disordered follicular growth and atresia or if excess local synthesis of androgen interferes with normal folliculogenesis and causes anovulation and atresia of growing follicles. There appears to be subnormal aromatase activity in follicles in PCOD ovaries, but such changes in enzyme activity could reflect an intrinsic ovarian disorder or a secondary effect due to the influence of an abnormal pattern of gonadotropin secretion. Since the hyperinsulinemia in the HAIR-AN syndrome does seem to directly evoke excessive ovarian androgen synthesis, actions of other general metabolic hormones on the ovary are now under active investigation. Several reports suggest that growth hormone and insulinlike growth factor 1 (IGF-1) affect folliculogenesis in a positive way, so PCOD could result from subnormal levels of growth hormone or compromise of its intraovarian action.[29]

In human and in animal studies, patterns of gonadotropin secretion that modestly favor LH output with normal or diminished FSH output produce PCOD-like ovarian dysfunction.[30] These ovarian abnormalities include disordered folliculogenesis, premature luteinization of maturing follicles, inadequate or absent corpus luteum function, dysmature oocytes, decreased aromatase activity, and increased ovarian androgen secretion. In this construct, the ovary is the "victim" of inappropriate signaling from the pituitary, and most ovarian markers of PCOD can be explained on this basis. Since the pulsatile secretory pattern of gonadotropins is not due to an intrinsic pituitary pulse generator, disordered pituitary secretion of gonadotropins must be secondary to either altered feedback of circulating steroids or abnormal GnRH pulse frequency, amplitude, or pattern of secretion from the CNS. In either or both such instances, the pituitary could be considered a transducer but not a "cause" of PCOD in any satisfactory sense.

As implied previously, extraglandular sites of steroid metabolism could cause PCOD changes by enhanced conversion of weak androgens to estrogens with consequent positive feedback action on the pituitary tending to favor LH rather than FSH secretion.[30] Similarly, as SHBG levels decline, the bioavailable fraction of free gonadal steroids rises. Delivery of estradiol to pituitary tissue could thereby increase, pituitary sensitivity to GnRH would consequently increase, and LH secretion would be favored.

A sufficient explanation for PCOD in many cases may be changes in the CNS that result in increased GnRH pulse frequency and/or amplitude. Such alterations in GnRH secretion would increase LH secretion and diminish FSH secretion and produce most of the features of PCOD.[30] Studies in experimental animals show that normal androgenization of the male brain is due to estradiol via intraneuronal aromatization of testosterone and local estradiol action and that the fetal neonatal female brain can be similarly androgenized. Furthermore, since intrauterine or neonatal androgenization of the female brain causes early onset of acyclicity of a persistent estrus type (quite similar to PCOD in characteristics), early developmental events in the CNS might ultimately explain some subsets of PCOD in humans.[31] Since such CNS "androgenization" can be produced by exposure to naturally occurring dietary estrogens and xenobiotic environmental estrogens,[32] intrauterine, neonatal, or childhood exposures might ultimately explain a significant portion of PCOD cases.

THERAPY

After the possibility of an androgen-secreting tumor has been excluded, pharmaceutical treatment of hirsutism is directed toward lowering androgen bioactivity within the hair follicle. The logical strategies include diminution of exposure of the follicle to precursor androgens, reduction of intrafollicular synthesis of DHT, or blockade of follicular androgen receptors (Tables 14-5 and 14-6).

Ovarian Suppression

In reproductive-age patients, oral contraceptive pills (OCPs) are safe and effective treatment for symptomatic androgen excess.[6] OCPs have several effects that decrease delivery of androgens to the skin. The primary effect of OCPs is suppression of gonadotropins (LH and FSH) by action on the CNS (decreases GnRH pulses) and pituitary (decreases sensitivity to GnRH). The contraceptive efficacy of OCPs depends on the suppression of gonadotropins by which ovulation is blocked, and this same mechanism decreases the produc-

Table 14-5
TREATMENT OF HIRSUTISM: REDUCTION OF ANDROGEN BIOACTIVITY BY USE OF DRUGS WITH COMPLEMENTARY SITES OF ACTION

Site of Action	*Drug or Drug Class*	*Beneficial Effect*
Androgen receptors	Spironolactone, flutamide, and cyproterone acetate	Blocks androgen receptors
5α-Reductase	Finasteride	Inhibits DHT synthesis in follicles
SHBG	Oral contraceptives	Increased SHBG reduces free-T levels
Hepatic metabolism of androgens	Oral contraceptives	Induction of enzymes enhances androgen clearance
Ovarian androgens	Oral contraceptives or GnRH analogues	Suppression of LH/FSH reduces ovarian androgen production
Adrenal androgens	Glucocorticoids	Suppression of ACTH reduces adrenal androgen production
	Spironolactone	Mildly inhibits adrenal androgen synthesis
	Oral contraceptives	Lowers adrenal androgen levels by unknown mechanism

tion of all classes of gonadal steroids from the ovary. Since the OCPs provide de facto "replacement" levels of estrogen and progestin, the net consequence is diminished endogenous gonadal production of estrogen, progestin, and androgen in exchange for exogenous provision of only estrogen and progestin in approximately physiological doses. An important caveat is that some synthetic progestins are somewhat androgenic. Therefore, careful selection of certain formulations of OCPs with minimal androgenicity can improve the overall therapeutic response (see Table 14-6). Among these, the newest formulations include norgestimate, a nonandrogenic progestin. Expectations are that these formulations (Ortho-Cyclen and Ortho Tri-Cyclen) will supercede the older preparations in treatment of androgen-excess patients. In addition to this primary reduction in ovarian androgen secretion, OCPs mildly inhibit adrenal androgen secretion by unknown mechanisms.[6] Taken together, the suppressive action of OCPs on both androgen sources is a highly effective means of reducing overall endogenous androgen biosynthesis.

Two other actions of OCPs to diminish delivery of androgens to target tissues depend upon inductive effects on the liver. First, OCPs elicit increased hepatic production of SHBG.[6] Elevation of SHBG causes decreased free-T levels, and thus delivery of T to the skin is reduced. Second, since androgens are primarily cleared by biliary excretion after intrahepatic metabolism and conjugation, the inductive effect of oral steroids (OCPs) on hepatic enzyme activity can increase clearance of circulating androgens.[18] These secondary actions of OCPs are modest but contribute to the desirable end of diminished delivery of bioactive androgens to target tissues.

An additional benefit of OCP use in many pa-

Table 14-6
TREATMENT OF HIRSUTISM: A PHARMACEUTICAL SEQUENCE FOR REPRODUCTIVE-AGE WOMEN

1. Oral contraceptive pills (Ortho-Cyclen, Ortho Tri-Cyclen, Ovcon 50, Demulen 50, Demulen 1/35, Ovcon 35, or Brevicon/Modicon)
   If response is inadequate, add:
2. Spironolactone (50–100 mg b.i.d.)
   or
   Flutamide (125–250 mg b.i.d. or t.i.d.)
   If response is inadequate, consider adding:
3. Finasteride (5 mg/day)
   If response is inadequate and adrenal androgens are elevated, consider adding:
4. Dexamethasone (0.2–0.5 mg h.s.)
   or
   Prednisone (2.5–7.5 mg h.s.)

tients with functional disorders of androgen excess is regulation of endometrial growth.[23] Since many patients with PCOD-type disorders have normal or enhanced circulating levels of endogenous estrogens (estradiol and especially estrone) but inadequate or absent progesterone production, they are at significant risk of endometrial hyperplasia and thus increased risk of endometrial neoplasia. This risk can be reduced or negated by exogenous progestin administration in the form of cyclic or continuous medroxyprogesterone acetate (or another pharmaceutical progestin preparation) or via OCP use. Furthermore, since these patients are commonly infertile but not sterile, adequate contraception remains an important need. OCPs are obviously sufficient for that task. Finally, adequate contraception is a necessity in hirsute patients being treated with antiandrogens since there is the potential for fetal developmental abnormalities should exposure to these agents occur in early, middle, or even late gestation.

Several analogues of GnRH are available for clinical use and have found applications where suppression of gonadal hormone production is sought. These analogues mimic GnRH and bind to specific pituitary receptors with high affinity. The commonly used analogues are potent GnRH agonists, but prompt suppression of pituitary hormone secretion of gonadotropins results from down-regulation of GnRH receptors and consequent pituitary desensitization to further stimulation of gonadotropin output. While these agents are specific and highly effective pharmaceutical means to achieve a hypogonadal state, they are expensive and require injection [leuprolide (Lupron); 3.75 mg of the depot preparation intramuscularly once a month] or intranasal spray [nafarelin (Synarel); 200 μg twice a day intranasally] for administration. While it is clear that these agents are effective in selectively suppressing ovarian androgen production,[33] courses of therapy must be limited to only a few months secondary to the concomitant suppression of estrogen. Alternatively, hormonal replacement therapy with exogenous estrogen or estrogen plus progestin must be given concomitantly. Given that exogenous estrogen or estrogen plus progestin is highly efficacious therapy for androgen excess, the future role for GnRH analogues in patients with androgen excess is not clear.

Adrenal Suppression

Suppression of adrenal androgen production is another option for reducing circulating levels of androgens. Exogenous glucocorticoids (dexamethasone or prednisone) act upon the CNS and pituitary to suppress ACTH secretion and thereby decrease the major stimulus for adrenal steroid biosynthesis.[34] This adrenal suppression reduces endogenous glucocorticoid and adrenal androgen production, while the exogenous agent provides adequate basal glucocorticoid bioactivity. Commonly, a level of DHEA sulfate of > 5 μg/ml serum is sufficient to consider adrenal suppression with glucocorticoids.[21] Clearly, circulating androgen levels can be reduced by adrenal androgen suppression, but the symptomatic response to glucocorticoids alone does not generally match the response achieved by OCP use for three reasons. First, the efficacy of OCPs may be greater due to their multiple effects in reduction of androgen bioactivity. On the other hand, therapy with glucocorticoids may be less than optimal since the singular mechanism of action appears to be suppression of adrenal androgens. Second, the adrenal androgens are generally less potent than testosterone (predominantly from the ovary), so suppression of output of potent ovarian androgen should be more consequential than suppression of output of weak adrenal androgens. Third, due to the serious side effects of long-term supraphysiological glucocorticoid use, efforts must be made to keep the exogenous glucocorticoid dose as low as possible, and adrenal suppression may, as a result, be only modest or inadequate. These limitations in therapeutic management make adrenal suppression with glucocorticoids a secondary or tertiary treatment choice (see Table 14-6).

Antiandrogens

Blockade of androgen action within target tissues by androgen-receptor antagonists is a safe and effective strategy for treatment of hirsutism.[35] Several androgen-receptor antagonists exist, but spironolactone and flutamide are the most important agents available in the United States at present. These compounds are competitive inhibitors of androgen binding and have few side effects of significance. However, any androgen-dependent process, such as sebaceous secretion, libido, voice pitch, and hair growth, may be affected. The complementary action of these agents is particularly helpful in hirsute patients that have endogenous androgen production suppressed with OCPs and/or glucocorticoids. Such combined treatment (i.e., OCPs plus spironolactone) can be extremely effective in the management of hirsutism in many patients. This type of two-agent therapy is theoretically appealing because the points of intervention include suppression of ovarian (and adrenal) androgen synthesis, increased binding by SHBG, increased hepatic clearance of androgens, and androgen receptor blockade. In practice, this combination is well-tolerated by most patients, and compliance is high.

Androgen Receptor Antagonists

There is long-standing experience with treatment of androgen excess with spironolactone. The usual dose regimen is 50 to 100 mg orally b.i.d. with dosage selection based primarily on clinical assessment of patient size (higher doses for larger patients) and severity of symptoms (higher doses for more severe hirsutism). This is not highly quantitative, but the usual starting dose of 150 mg per day (100 mg in the morning and 50 mg at night) is appropriate for most hirsute women. Once the degree of response has been assessed after 6 to 12 months of therapy, doses can often be reduced to 75 to 100 mg per day but rarely lower. In general, doses greater than 100 mg b.i.d. (the usual maximum dose) do not seem to offer any improved response. In terms of side effects for hirsute patients, the diuretic effects of spironolactone (an aldosterone antagonist used for treating hypertension) is the most prominent and is generally well-tolerated. Effects on plasma electrolytes are typically inconsequential in the vast majority of patients, and any effect of elevating serum potassium would only be an issue in rare patients with hyperkalemia due to renal insufficiency. In premenopausal women who are not also on OCPs, approximately one in five will have increased menstrual frequency on spironolactone. This menstrual effect may be related to the weak progestational activity of spironolactone.

Flutamide is an antiandrogen approved for treatment of prostate cancer and there is only limited experience in the treatment of hirsutism in women. The initial suggestion is that at a dose of 250 mg twice a day, flutamide can markedly improve hirsutism in women[36] on OCPs and may work as a single agent as well.[36] Clinical experience and further studies will help clarify dose-response relationships in hirsute women and optimal regimens for use.

Cyproterone acetate is a potent persistent progestin which is also antiandrogenic and highly effective in the treatment of hirsutism. The contraceptive combination of 50 μg ethinyl estradiol (Dianette) with 2 mg cyproterone acetate is available in Europe. In Canada, cyproterone acetate is available (50 mg tablets) for treatment of prostate cancer and can be administered during the first 10 days of an OCP cycle as a reverse sequential scheme. Due to persistence and high progestin potency, such short intervals of administration of cyproterone acetate have been used in an effort to avoid disruption of menstrual pattern. In general, side effects of cyproterone acetate are those of progestational agents and include a modest incidence of symptoms such as disruption of menses, nausea, fluid retention, headache, and depressed mood.

5α-Reductase Inhibitors

The newest pharmaceutical tools for treating hirsutism, 5α-reductase inhibitors, are now becoming commercially available. Agents such as finasteride are potent inhibitors of 5α-reductase and diminish androgen action by drastically reducing the intrafollicular synthesis of DHT. Inhibition of local production of this most important effector androgen will certainly prove useful in the treatment of hirsutism. Finasteride is approved for use in men for the treatment of benign prostatic hypertrophy. At a dose of 5 mg per day in men, side effects are limited to a decrease in seminal volume, and < 4 percent incidence each of impotency, ejaculatory disorders, and decreased libido (Proscar product circular). With finasteride now available, markers of DHT production such as 3α-androstanediol glucuronide (3α-ADG) should gain substantial diagnostic value. Decisions to treat patients with the inhibitors will probably be predicated on levels of 3α-ADG as an indicator for potential efficacy of enzyme inhibition. The expectation is that follicular sensitivity will be reflected by the level of 3α-ADG and many cases of idiopathic hirsutism will become explicable. Reference values for 3α-ADG in serum as cited by the manufacturer of the assay kit (Diagnostic Systems Laboratories, Webster, TX) are as follows: premenopausal women, 2.47 ± 1.32 ng/ml; postmenopausal women, 1.51 ± 1.47 ng/ml; and hirsute women, 5.79 ± 1.98 ng/ml.

Comprehensive strategies for the medical treatment of hirsute patients will certainly evolve as experience with these new drugs accumulates, but the idea of complementary drug effects will remain a valuable guide as those new regimens are devised.

CONCLUDING REMARKS

The initial clinical challenge that a hirsute patient presents is the necessity to adequately assess her status so that the cause of this androgen excess symptom can be confidently classified. Once such a diagnostic impression has been developed, surgical management of tumor or medical management of nontumor patients can proceed. Currently available pharmaceuticals provide effective options for treatment of hirsutism, and the prospects are excellent for innovations in therapy with newer agents. Once the clinical response of hirsute patients is optimal and the process of conversion of vellus to terminal hairs is reduced or abrogated, then depilatory therapy such as electrolysis is quite rewarding. Combinations of systemic and local therapies can provide most of our patients with excellent control of the otherwise frustrating problem of hirsutism.

REFERENCES

1. Marshal WA, Tanner JM: Variations in pattern of pubertal changes in girls. Arch Dis Child 44:291–303, 1969.
2. Root AW, Reiter ED: Evaluation and management of the child with delayed pubertal development. Fertil Steril 27:745–755, 1976.
3. Grunfeld L, Kase NG: Hirsutism and virilization. In Kase NG, Weingold AB, Gershenson DM (eds): *Principles and Practice of Clinical Gynecology,* 2d ed. New York, Churchill Livingstone, 1990, pp 377–394.
4. Hughes CL, Wall LL, Creasman WT: Reproductive hormone levels in gynecologic oncology patients undergoing surgical castration after spontaneous menopause. Gynecol Oncol 40:42–45, 1991.
5. Judd HL, Lucas WE, Yen SSC: Effect of oophorectomy on circulating testosterone and androstenedione levels in patients with endometrial cancer. Am J Obstet Gynecol 118:793–798, 1974.
6. Lobo RA: Hirsutism. In Sciarra JJ (ed): *Gynecology and Obstetrics,* vol. 5, rev. ed. Philadelphia, J. B. Lippincott, 1992, chap. 28, pp 1–18.
7. Bardin CW, Lipsett MB: Testosterone and androstenedione blood production rates in normal women and women with idiopathic hirsutism or polycystic ovaries. J Clin Invest 46:891–902, 1967.
8. Givens JR: Hirsutism and hyperandrogenism. Adv Intern Med 21:221–247, 1976.
9. Mingriell J, Valladares L: Molecular aspects on the mechanism of action of testosterone in rat bone marrow cells. J Steroid Biochem 5:649–654, 1974.
10. Mainwaring WIP: *The Mechanism of Action of Androgens.* New York, Springer-Verlag, 1977.
11. Rosenfeld RS et al.: 24-Hour secretory pattern of dehydroisoandrosterone and dehydroisoandrosterone sulfate. J Clin Endocrinol Metab 40:850–855, 1975.
12. Parker LN, Lifrak ET, Odell WD: A 60,000 molecular weight human pituitary glycopeptide stimulates adrenal androgen secretion. Endocrinology 113:2092–2096, 1983.
13. Schiebinger RJ et al.: The effect of serum prolactin on plasma adrenal androgens and the production and metabolic clearance rate of dehydroepiandrosterone sulfate in normal and hyperprolactinemic subjects. J Clin Endocrinol Metab 62:202–209, 1986.
14. Vermeulen A: Plasma levels and origin of sexual hormones in postmenopausal women. In Martini L, Motta M (eds): *Androgens and Antiandrogens.* New York, Raven Press, 1977, pp 53–65.
15. Wyss HI, Huber PR: Transport and clearance of androgens in the woman. In Hammerstein J et al. (eds): *Androgenization in Women.* Amsterdam, Excerpta Medica, no. 493, 1980, pp 49–71.
16. Burke CW, Anderson DC: Sex-hormone-binding globulin is an oestrogen amplifier. Nature 240:38–40, 1972.
17. Vermeulen A: Androgen secretion by adrenals and gonads. In Mahesh VB, Greenblatt RB (eds): *Hirsutism and Virilism.* John Wright/PSG, Inc., Boston, 1983, pp 17–34.
18. Gordon GG et al.: Effect of medroxyprogesterone acetate (Provera) on the metabolism and biological activity of testosterone. J Clin Endocrinol Metab 30:449–456, 1970.
19. Faber K, Hughes CL: Laboratory evaluation of hyperandrogenic conditions. Infert Reprod Med Clin North Am 2:495–509, 1991.
20. Pittaway DE: Neoplastic causes of hyperandrogenism. Infert Reprod Med Clin North Am 2:531–545, 1991.
21. Scherzer WJ, Adashi EV: Adrenal hyperandrogenism. Infert Reprod Med Clin North Am 2:479–494, 1991.
22. Azziz R, Zacur HA: 21-Hydroxylase deficiency in female hyperandrogenism: Screening and diagnosis. J Clin Endocrinol Metab 69:577–584, 1989.
23. Kazer RR, Rebar RW: Polycystic ovary syndrome. In Sciarra JJ (ed): *Gynecology and Obstetrics,* rev. ed. Philadelphia, J. B. Lippincott, 1992, vol. 5, chap. 27, pp 1–10.
24. Schwartz LB, Diamond MP: The coexistence of hyperandrogenism and hyperinsulinemia. Infert Reprod Med Clin North Am 2:611–635, 1991.
25. Bar RS et al.: Characterization of insulin receptors in patients with the syndromes of insulin resistance and acanthosis nigricans. Diabetologia 18:209–216, 1980.

26. Kahn RC et al.: The syndromes of insulin resistance and acanthosis nigricans: Insulin receptor disorders in man. N Engl J Med 294:739–745, 1976.
27. Podskalny JM, Kahn CR: Cell culture studies on patients with extreme insulin resistance: Receptor defects on cultured fibroblasts. J Clin Endocrinol Metab 54:261–268, 1982.
28. Chang RJ et al.: Steroid secretion in polycystic ovarian disease after ovarian suppression by a long-acting gonadotropin-releasing agonist. J Clin Endocrinol Metab 56:897–903, 1983.
29. Kazer RR, Unterman TG, Glick RP: An abnormality of the growth hormone/insulin-like growth factor-I axis in women with polycystic ovary syndrome. J Clin Endocrinol Metab 71:958–962, 1990.
30. Insler V, Lunenfeld B: Pathophysiology of polycystic ovarian disease: New insights. Hum Reprod 6:1025–1029, 1991.
31. Finch CE et al.: Ovarian and steroidal influences on neuroendocrine aging processes in female rodents. Endocr Rev 5:467–497, 1984.
32. Faber KA, Hughes CL: The effect of neonatal exposure to diethylstilbestrol, genistein, and zearalenone on pituitary responsiveness and sexually dimorphic nucleus volume in the castrated adult rat. Biol Reprod 45:649–653, 1991.
33. Rittmaster RS, Thompson DL: Effect of leuprolide and dexamethasone on hair growth and hormone levels in hirsute women: The relative importance of the ovary and the adrenal in the pathogenesis of hirsutism. J Clin Endocrinol Metab 70:1096–1102, 1990.
34. Phipps WR, Tagatz GE: Physiology and tests of adrenal cortical function. In Sciarra JJ (ed): *Gynecology and Obstetrics,* rev. ed. Philadelphia, J. B. Lippincott, 1991, vol. 5, chap. 36, pp 1–16.
35. Rittmaster RS: Evaluation and treatment of hirsutism. Infert Reprod Med Clin North Am 2:511–530, 1991.
36. Cusan L et al.: Treatment of hirsutism with the pure antiandrogen flutamide. J Am Acad Dermatol 23:462–469, 1990.

Chapter

15

SURGICAL APPROACH TO HAIR LOSS

Walter P. Unger

INTRODUCTION

The surgical correction of alopecia may be conveniently divided into three general categories: hair transplantation, alopecia reduction, and flap surgery. Each of these has been modified to a major extent in the last decade, resulting in a marked improvement in results. Hair transplantation will be discussed under two major subheadings: (1) standard round grafting and (2) minigrafting. Alopecia reduction similarly will be subdivided into sections dealing with (1) standard alopecia reductions, (2) major alopecia reductions, and (3) alopecia reductions preceded by soft tissue expansion. Lastly, flap surgery will be subdivided into (1) standard "Juri" flaps and (2) other flaps.

HAIR TRANSPLANTATION

Standard Round Grafting

Standard round grafting consists of using a 4- to 5-mm trephine to remove round pieces of full-thickness skin grafts from a *donor area* in the temporal, parietal, or occipital scalp that is judged to be permanently hair-bearing. A round hole made with a slightly smaller trephine is then cut out of the area of alopecia or future alopecia (the *recipient site*), and an appropriately prepared graft is placed into it. Within 3 weeks, the hair in the graft is shed, and approximately 3 months later it begins to grow again. It will survive in its new site for as long as it would have in its original location.[1] Any area of total alopecia can be virtually solidly filled in three or four punch transplant sessions. In practice, only cosmetically strategic areas such as the hairline or the center of the whorl of the vertex are filled solidly, while others will be treated during one, two, or three sessions depending on the location and density required for that site.[2,3] Figure 15-1 illustrates common densities utilized.

For most practitioners, the "standard" round graft is one that is obtained with a 4-mm punch. In the first session, all grafts will be harvested with a 4-mm punch, but in subsequent sessions approximately 30 grafts will be taken using a 4.5-mm trephine. The purpose of the 30 larger grafts will be discussed later. Occasionally a 5-mm graft or a graft smaller than 4 mm is employed.

The basic pattern for the first session is a four- or five-row U-shaped recipient area (Fig. 15-2*A*).[3] Usually 80 to 110 grafts will be transplanted per session; however, this number can be increased to as many as 130 to 150 grafts by extending the U-shaped pattern posteriorly on one side to produce more of a J shape. The author prefers to avoid sessions of more than 110 grafts because of increased discomfort during surgery as well as postoperatively. Occasionally, if one is anticipating doing a U-shaped alopecia reduction later, an "island" of 15 to 25 grafts may also be inserted in the center of the peninsula between the arms of the "U."[3] An alopecia reduction is a surgical excision of part of the bald or balding area. (See later discussion.) Alternately, if the physician is planning a future elliptic or inverted Y-shaped alopecia reduction, a smaller-than-usual alopecia reduction or "minireduction" may be done concomitantly with the punch transplanting sessions.[5]

Figure 15-1 Any area of alopecia can be solidly filled in one of three different ways. The method shown in the superior part of this figure is the usual four-stage approach. Still-hair-bearing areas are treated as shown in the middle of the figure.[4] The approach shown at the bottom is the three-stage filling described by the Orentreichs.

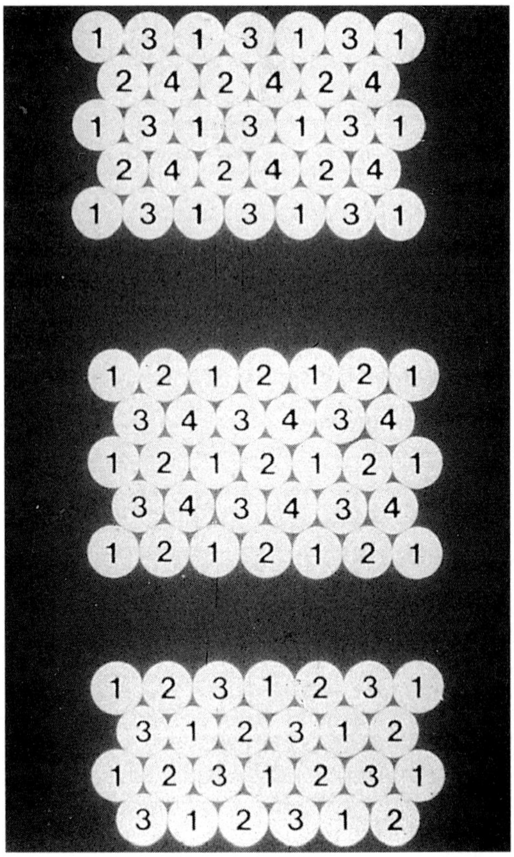

The same U-shaped pattern is repeated on the second session and, thereafter, is varied as will be described later. The second session is done 6 weeks after the first, while 3- to 4-month intervals are left between the second and third, and third and fourth sessions if dealing with the same area. These time intervals may be lengthened, but it is best not to shorten them as this may cause circulatory embarrassment to the grafts and a lesser yield of hair. One may, however, treat the anterior one-third to one-half of the scalp on one day and the posterior half of the scalp as soon as a day later because of the relative independence of the blood supply to both of those sites. This is generally done only if patients are traveling from great distances and prefer to minimize the number of times they must return for treatment.

Minigrafting

Minigrafting, a term that is used to describe the transplanting of grafts containing one to six hairs, has been increasingly incorporated into hair transplanting in the last 5 to 10 years. Minigrafting can be subclassified into three types of grafts:

MICROGRAFTING

In *micrografting,* round grafts or strips of donor hair are very carefully sliced into small pieces containing one to two hairs each and placed into holes made with a 16-gauge hypodermic nee-

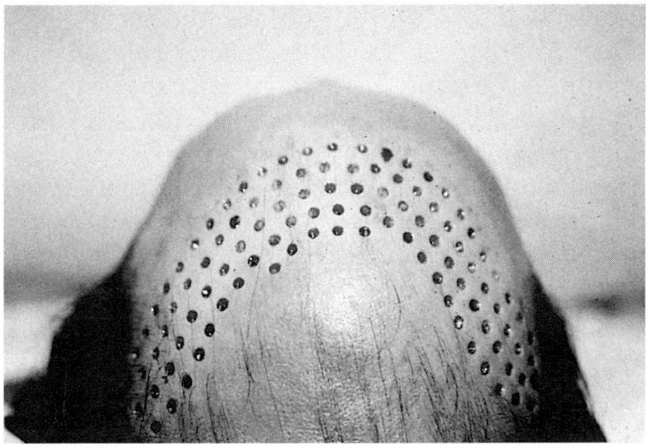

A

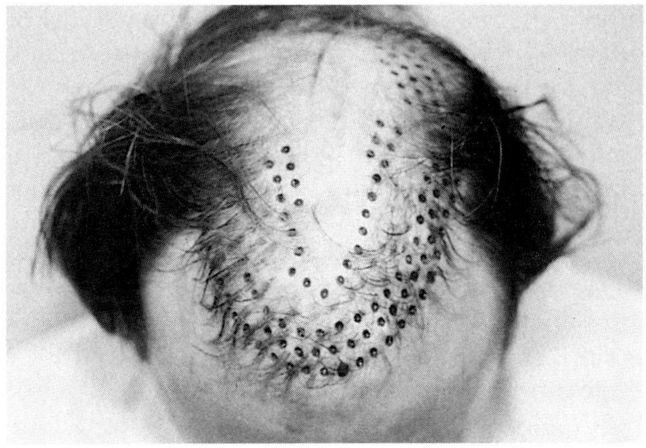

B

Figure 15-2 (*A*) The basic pattern for the first (and second) session is a four- or five-row U-shaped recipent area. (*B*) The distribution of grafts in the recipient area during the third session is somewhat different from the simple U-shape used on the first two. Three to four rows are punched out on the part side of the recipient site to just past the midline. On the nonpart side, only the anterior and most posterior rows are filled. The rest of the grafts that would have been used on the nonpart side are placed bilaterally more toward the midline.

dle.[6,7] They are placed anterior to the hairline in order to "soften" it, as well as to fill small hairless spaces between grafts and within an individual graft where hair has not grown evenly across its surface. The terms *unigrafts* and *mmunigrafts* have been used to describe single hair grafts obtained, inserted, and utilized in the same fashion.[8]

ROUND MINIGRAFTING

In *round minigrafting,* 1.5- to 2.5-mm grafts are obtained using very small trephines; alternately, strips of donor tissue or grafts of various sizes (usually 3.25 to 5 mm in diameter) are cut into sections containing approximately three or four, and five or six hairs, respectively. These are inserted into small, round holes prepared with a 1.0- to 2.5-mm-diameter trephine. They are used to fill small hairless spaces between or within previously transplanted grafts. In addition, however, they are employed extensively in females undergoing the procedure to replace the small hairless spaces that are interspersed within diffuse sparse hair growth that is characteristic in women with androgenetic alopecia.[9,10] They are also used exclusively by some operators to transplant entire areas in an effort to minimize the transitional "clumpiness" seen with punch grafting in sparse or bald areas.[11]

SLIT GRAFTING

In the procedure known as *slit grafting,* grafts similar to that described for round minigrafting are inserted into "slits" usually made by a no. 15 scalpel blade, rather than into round holes.[9,12,13] They are employed for the same purposes described for round minigrafts but, in the author's opinion, are more successful in minimizing transitional clumpiness. In addition, they are especially useful in thickening the areas of diffuse thinning in females as well as in males, in whom the objective is less dense filling (see later text). They are now used almost exclusively by the author for transplanting the vertex, and in combination with micrografts, for the anterior 2 to 3 cm of the hairline when some sparseness in this zone is acceptable or even preferred.[14] Because the incisions can be made between existing hairs, slit grafting has the advantage of minimizing or entirely eliminating the temporary thinning that was part of the "price" paid for using round grafts in patients with "early" androgenetic alopecia and females with diffuse thinning.

One can obtain three- to four-hair slit grafts by quartering or sometimes trisecting 4.0- to 5.0-mm round grafts. Similarly, bisecting a 3.5- to 4.0-mm round graft will most often result in five- to six-hair grafts that can be used for areas where greater density is preferred. More commonly they are produced by sectioning strips of donor hair (see section entitled "Donor Area"). The author prefers to utilize terms such as "small" (3–4 hair) and "large" (5–6 hair) "slit grafts" or "small" (3–4 hair) and "large" (5–6 hair) "round minigrafts" that tell the reader more precisely the number of hairs that are being transferred and into what type of recipient site than do terms such as *minigrafting, quarter grafts,* or *bisected grafts,* whose meaning is less precise and will vary from author to author.

Sessions of minigrafting or a combination of minigrafts and standard round grafts are done with the same time intervals described earlier for standard round grafting.

Planning

The anterior-superior-most points of what is judged to be the permanent temporal hair dictate the beginning and end of any hairline. Once an estimate is made of where these points will be, they are marked and a third point is chosen anteriorly in the midline, to which a line can be drawn, joining the two temporal points and producing a natural-looking ovoid or slightly bell-shaped hairline. The positioning of this midline point involves many factors including the length of the face, patient objectives, and the number of grafts available, but Stough has rightly pointed out that the hairline, when viewed laterally, should be more or less horizontal, or the effect will be aesthetically unsatisfactory.[15]

Whenever alopecia reductions are contemplated during the course of treatment, allowance must be made for how they will affect the chosen hairline and "part" line. In addition, grafts should not be put into areas that could be excised instead. Alopecia reductions not only decrease the size of the bald area, which thereby can be satisfactorily transplanted with fewer grafts, they also raise the superior border of the permanent fringe. Thus the future "part," which must nearly always go through the untransplanted permanent fringe, can be moved to a cosmetically more acceptable level.[2,16] Alopecia reductions are discussed in greater detail later in the text. Some idea of the number of grafts used to satisfactorily treat given areas can be gleaned from the clinical photos shown in this chapter and from previous publications.[3,17]

In general, the lighter the color and the finer the texture of hair, the better. White or salt-and-pepper hair is ideal, with blond the second-best color. The exception to the general rule on hair texture is a patient with very coarse or curly Negroid-type hair. These latter characteristics produce an appearance of greater than actual density, and one can adequately transplant any given recipient site with fewer grafts than would be required in a straight-haired Caucasian. In brief, three sessions instead of four are usually satisfactory for any given area, graft distribution is more symmetrical than in Caucasians since a curly hairstyle will be used (instead of the hair being parted from one side), and a U-shaped, "island" pattern (see earlier text) is nearly always used.[18]

Orientals tend to require significantly fewer grafts than the average Caucasian patient because the diameter of their hair shafts tends to be larger and therefore provides more coverage.[19]

Increasingly large numbers of individuals are being seen for surgery before they are totally bald. Such patients can and should be operated on as long as one is certain that the end result will be denser hair than they had at the onset of treatment. In the author's experience, "early" transplanting, that is, transplanting before the area is totally bald, does not accelerate the rate at which the patient is losing hair and in fact may retard it by lowering the overall tissue levels of dihydrotestosterone.[4] Starting "early" has the advantage of avoiding the embarrassment of total alopecia and of allowing the patient to camouflage the recipient area postoperatively much more easily and sometimes completely by the following day. It also enables the patient to proceed with transplanting at a more leisurely rate, simply keeping pace with the rate of hair loss.

Disadvantages of starting early include initial thinning of hair in the recipient area—if round grafts are being utilized. This is because the donor graft loses its hair for 3 months and is replacing an area that at least had some hair before it was excised to make room for the graft. When transplanting into areas of early male-pattern baldness, all sessions are usually spread 4 to 6 months or more apart, allowing each session to grow in and thicken the recipient sites before subsequent sessions are carried out.[4] "Slit" grafting in patients with early androgenetic alopecia, of course, avoids the problem of initial thinning but carries other disadvantages that will be described subsequently.

Another difficulty is accurately forecasting the eventual extent of the fully developed area of alopecia in order to avoid "chasing" an enlarging bald area and in order to make a valid assessment of how many grafts are actually available. A family history, careful examination, and experience go a long way toward minimizing this latter problem. It cannot be overemphasized that punch transplanting in patients who are not yet bald should be carried out only by physicians who have considerable experience.

As long as the patient's general health is satisfactory, age is not a contraindication to punch transplanting. The author has operated on a number of patients in their seventies, with results as good as or better than those seen in younger individuals. On the other hand, in general I avoid transplanting in those who are under 21 years of age because of the increased difficulty in estimating the eventual extent of alopecia and long-term patient motivation. Exceptions to this general rule are made to accommodate those who are seriously emotionally affected by their premature hair loss.

Patients who use hairpieces are advised that they should not be worn for a week after any transplant session and as little as possible for an additional week. The same applies for hats, though they can be worn for short intervals if they have holes allowing for the circulation of air. Hairpieces and hats produce warmth and moisture that are conducive to infection. Individuals who work in occupations or who have hobbies that expose them to dirt or debris are advised to avoid these circumstances for 1 week postoperatively.

Transplanting in Females

All of the earlier comments relating to early transplanting apply equally to operating on female patients with androgenetic alopecia. In addition, of course, one should be certain that such patients have good prospects for maintaining a relatively dense donor rim while thinning centrally. Some variations in approach are recommended in females. The most important are the treatment of only the left or right side of the recipient site at any given session, the use of smaller sessions, for example, 50 to 60 grafts per session (Fig. 15-3*A*), and spreading of sessions at least 6 months apart.[10,20] These differences allow for easier postsurgical camouflage, a lower dose of local anesthetic, and an accurate assessment of the results of each session; the latter aided by using the untreated side as a "control" (Fig. 15-3*B*).

Extensive use of "slit" grafts in areas of diffuse thinning and round minigrafts for small areas of total alopecia has become an integral part of transplanting in female patients.[9,10] Slit grafts will not remove any existing hairs (which may or may not be permanent), while the round minigrafts eliminate small totally alopecic areas and replace them with hair-bearing skin.

Preoperative Instructions and Anesthesia

Patients are started on prophylactic antibiotics—usually erythromycin 333 mg three times a day—beginning the night prior to, or 2 hours before, surgery. Antibiotics are discontinued 5 days postoperatively. Acetylsalicylic acid–containing drugs and vitamin E are avoided for 10 days and 3 weeks, respectively, prior to surgery in order to minimize surgical as well as postsurgical bleeding.[17] No alcohol should be consumed for 1 week preoperatively for the same reason.

A personal and family general medical history is taken to rule out any contraindication to surgery. Where indicated, further laboratory tests or consultations with other physicians are ordered. Unless the patient objects, we routinely notify the family physician and dentist and inquire about any factors they feel we should be aware of. All of our patients have a complete blood count, VDRL, routine urinalysis, and human immunodeficiency virus (HIV) and hepatitis B antigen testing performed prior to beginning treatment. These tests are repeated yearly should the course of treatment extend over more than a 12-month period. We also use gloves, masks, and protective glasses during surgery.

Diazepam 20 mg is administered orally 30 minutes prior to surgery, both for its sedative effects and for minimizing lidocaine neurotoxicity.[21] A solution composed of equal parts 1% lidocaine with 1/100,000 epinephrine and 0.5% bupivacaine (the latter to prolong the anesthetic effect) is used to produce a field block in the donor area, while 2% lidocaine with 1/100,000 epinephrine is usually used as a field block for the recipient site. The use of a 30-gauge needle as well as preoperative diazepam reduces the psychological and physical trauma of the anesthetic technique. A 1/200,000 solution of epinephrine is used superior to the field blocks to minimize

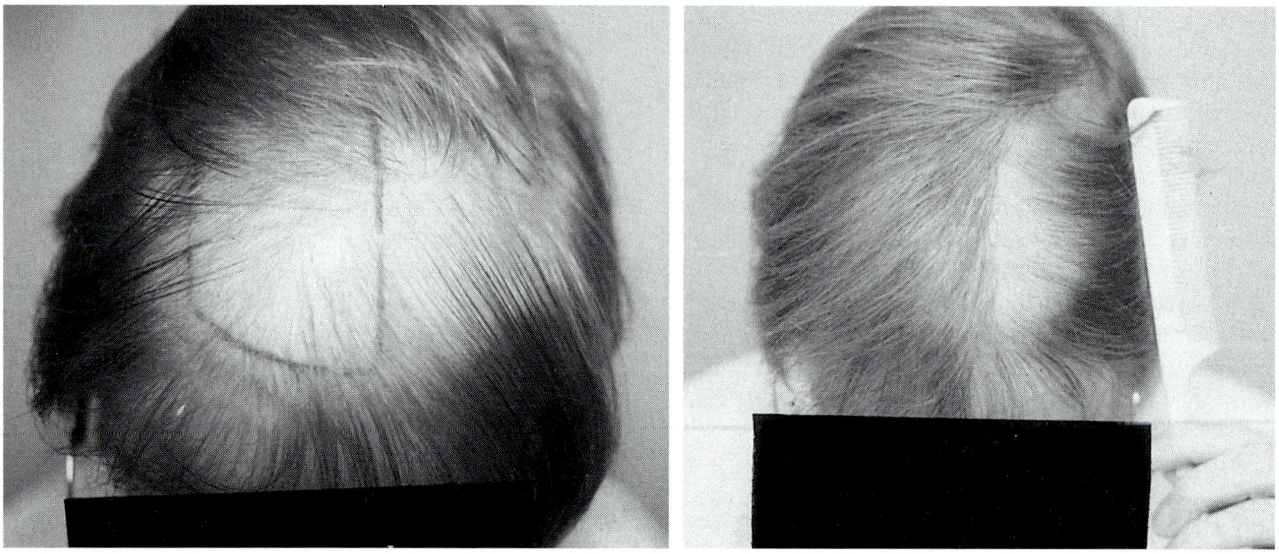

A B

Figure 15-3 (*A*) Before transplanting. This 42-year-old female had diffuse thinning of the anterior half of her scalp hair. The crayon mark denotes the limits of the area to be treated, which is primarily the right half of the affected zone but extends slightly over onto the medial aspect of the left half. A combination of slit grafts and round grafts 1 to 2 mm in diameter were obtained from sixty-five 4-mm round grafts and used in the area. (*B*) Six months after the first session. Notice the marked improvement when compared with the untreated left side of this site. Additional sessions to the treated area will be carried out in pace with further loss of original hair.

bleeding. Some operators employ nerve blocks in addition to the field blocks,[21] while others use a Dermajet instead of needles. The author has tried both of these variations and has not found either of them advantageous.

Occasionally patients require stronger solutions of anesthesia—for example, 3% or 4% lidocaine—in the recipient area. In the author's experience these individuals are often those with a Celtic background or with a past history of alcohol or drug abuse. Using sodium bicarbonate to buffer the pH of the lidocaine, as suggested by McKay et al.,[22] in order to minimize the pain of injections has been abandoned because of resultant increased bleeding.

Premixed 50% nitrous oxide with 50% oxygen (Entonox) is often used in our offices to alleviate the pain and anxiety associated with local anesthesia, sometimes converting this aspect of the procedure into a pleasant experience.

Complications of anesthesia can be minimized by preparing the donor site and recipient site in a step-by-step fashion rather than at the same time.[21] The management of complications that may occur secondary to local anesthesia has been described elsewhere.[23] Significant problems are very rare.

THE DONOR SITE

Donor grafts should be obtained from areas that are likely to maintain hair growth for the life of the patient. It is advisable to examine the scalp carefully with the hair wet in order to make as valid a delineation of the areas of thinning as is possible. In addition, a family history is also taken. If the patient is young, it is also wise to leave an extra 2.5 cm beyond any areas of forecasted hair loss as a margin of safety before the most superior line of donor grafts is harvested.

Patients are operated on in a prone position for the donor area. A "prone pillow" is especially useful when the occipital area is the donor site.[24] This pillow, with a central hole, allows the patient to breathe easily with his face directed straight into the operating table. Hand punches are usually used in the recipient area, but specially designed power punches (or parallel scalpel blades) are employed in the donor area. Hand punches are preferred to power punches in the recipient area because hand punches are less likely to entangle any existing hair present in the recipient area and because changing punch sizes is far faster if hand punches are being used instead of power punches.

Many types of donor harvesting have been described by various authors. The most commonly used options are paired rows of round grafts that are subsequently sutured closed[24] or strips of hair-bearing skin that are excised with the aid of parallel scalpel blades.[25] The latter technique is used whenever grafting is going to be confined to slit grafting and/or micrografting. A single fine scar is all that is left to mark the site of the harvest once healing has been completed. Theoretically, an "alopecia reduction in reverse" has been carried out when a strip of hair has been excised. Each excision results in a narrowing of the donor rim, the opposite of the goal of alopecia reduction. In practice, the author has not noticed this.

The donor area is prepared by first rubbing it with ethyl alcohol followed by the application of povidone iodine or chlorhexidene gluconate (Hibitane or Hibiclens) in order to provide continuing antibacterial activity.

The paired rows of round grafts are obtained after using curved scissors to clip the hair in the potential donor area to approximately a 2-mm length in 4- to 5-mm-wide lines separated by rows of uncut hair 2 to 3 mm wide. The clipped rows will provide the donor grafts, while those that are uncut are used to camouflage the donor site after the procedure. Anesthesia is then carried out as described previously. Grafts are cut, angling the punch in the same direction as the hair at that site. Two, or less commonly three, rows are harvested, and then a 14- to 15-mm-wide band of intact hair is skipped and another two rows are cut. The intact zone will be used for future donor rows. After the grafts are removed, the sites are closed with a running no. 2-0 Supramid suture (Fig. 15-4*A* and *B*). The loops should be kept quite superficial so as to minimize disruption of blood supply by deeper vessels. For the same reason, minimal tension should be present at the suture line. Where more brisk bleeding is present, the suture can be looped deeper and wider and tied tightly at that point. A new running suture is then started so as

Figure 15-4 (*A*) The donor site after removal of grafts. The superior "paired" rows have not yet been sutured, while the inferior "paired" rows have been closed with a running no. 2-0 Supramid suture. The intact hair between the paired rows will be used in the future to obtain additional grafts. (*B*) The donor area shown in (*A*) is now complete. Sixty-four grafts have been removed from this site, which can be easily camouflaged by surrounding hair. An additional 36 to 46 grafts can be obtained by extending the paired rows more anteriorly as well as by cutting one or two rows of grafts in the temporal area. The sutures are removed in 5 to 7 days.

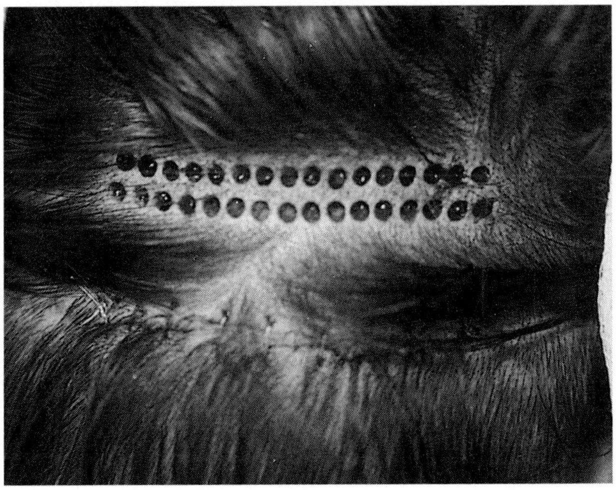

A

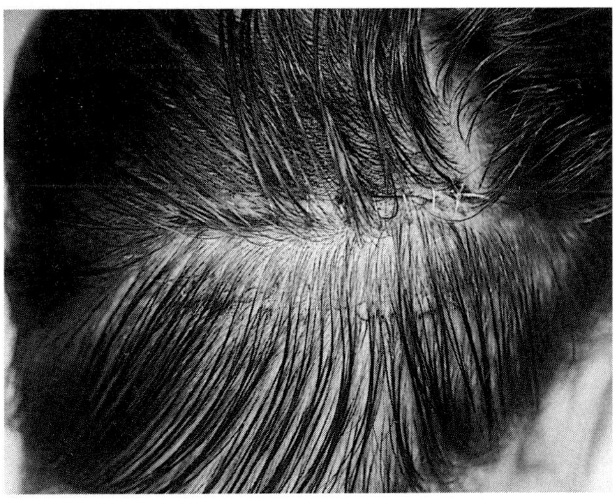

B

to avoid a tight closure along the entire incision line because of a single bleeding site. Sutures are removed 5 to 7 days postoperatively. A full description of this pattern and technique of donor site harvesting can be found in a previous publication.[14]

If the recipient area is the anterior scalp, an effort is made to take grafts containing fine-textured and low- to medium-dense hair that will be used in the anterior 2 to 2.5 cm. Such hair is most often obtained from temporal and inferior occipital areas. Coarser and denser hair can be harvested from more superior areas of the occiput and is used more posteriorly in the recipient area. Temporal grafts have an additional advantage in that they will gray as the patient ages at approximately the same time as this is occurring in the remaining temporal area, thus producing a natural and cosmetically consistent color change in the frontal recipient site in pace with adjacent temporal hair.

Punches are kept razor sharp at all times. In addition, the skin should ideally be kept taut with repeated injections of saline. This allows for more accurate angling of the punches as the tissue "gives" less when pressure is applied; consequently, there is less chance of inadvertently cutting off or fraying bent follicles at the periphery of the grafts. It is not unusual for many operators to use 30 to 100 ml of saline during the harvesting of donor grafts. Most 4-mm grafts will yield between 8 and 20 intact hair follicles, though some may contain as many as 30.

When "strip harvesting" is used, once again saline is injected to produce tissue turgor, and the blades are angled so as to conform to hair direction at the donor site (Fig. 15-5). After the strip is totally excised, bleeders are treated with electrocautery, the superior edge is undermined, and the wound is closed with a single-layer running no. 2-0 Supramid suture.[25]

Of all the advantages claimed by those who prefer scalpel-excised rows, two are certainly true: harvesting and preparation time for slit grafts will usually be significantly reduced and grafts prepared this way fit better into incisional slits.

THE RECIPIENT SITE

Patients are operated on in a supine position with the head of the bed raised to a 45° angle for the recipient area unless the vertex is the recipient site, in which case the patient is usually placed in a sitting position. A majority of patients today are treated with a combination of various graft types. Micrografts containing one to two hairs are used anterior to the proposed hairline, and then a zone of slit grafts, which is usually 2 to 3 cm wide, is used posterior to these before standard round grafts are employed posterior to the slit grafts (Fig. 15-6*A* through *C*). The anterior slit grafts will contain three to four hairs, while the posterior slit grafts will contain five to six hairs each. It is worth repeating that the donor areas used for the micrografts as well as slit grafts are those with finer-textured hair. The zone of micrografts and slit grafts may be widened if the patient is particularly concerned about postoperative camouflage, rapid healing and hair growth, and the absence of transitional tuftiness.

Patients with very large present or future areas of alopecia and correspondingly narrow donor rims, or those who have lower hair density objectives, may prefer transplanting a larger proportion of the area less densely by employing slit grafts for most of the entire area (Fig. 15-7*A*). Individuals who have or will have relatively sparse temporal hair should also be strongly advised to do all or most of their transplanting with slit grafts, as the dense filling that would be required to eliminate the transitional tuftiness produced

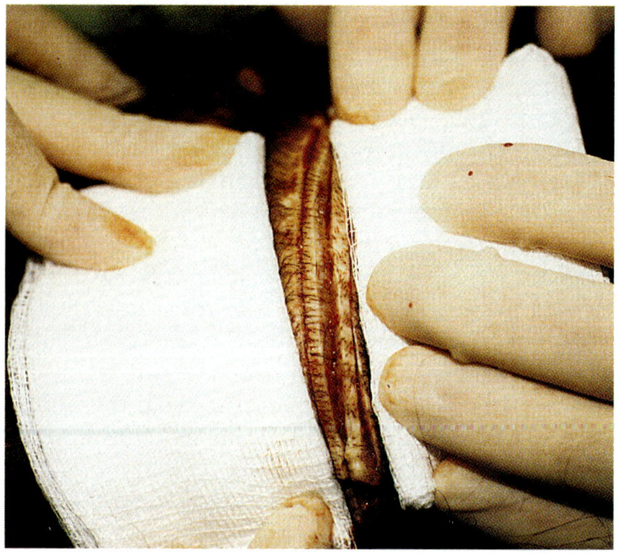

Figure 15-5 "Strip harvesting" is accomplished by utilizing special double- or triple-bladed instruments.

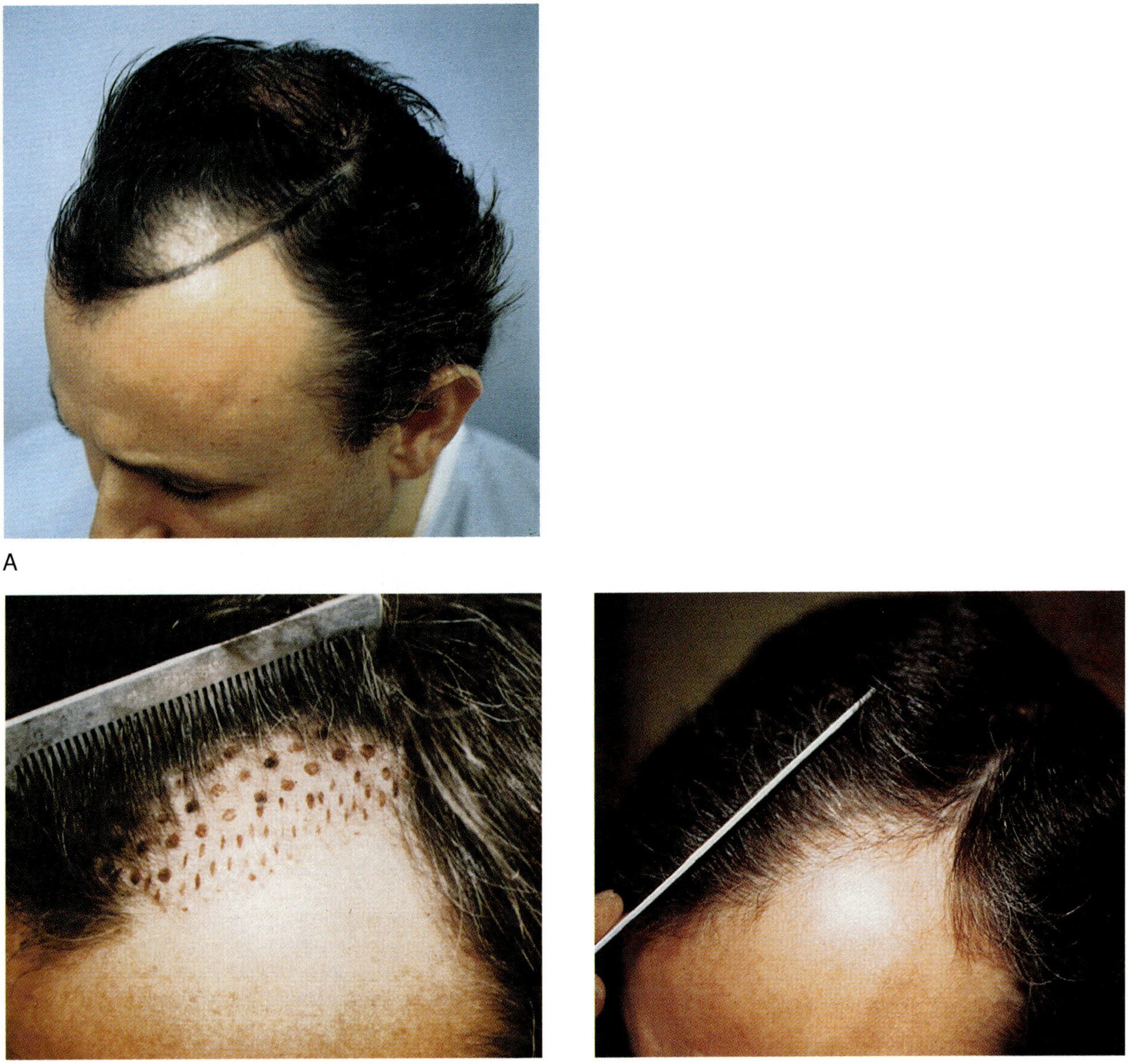

A B C

Figure 15-6 (*A*) Before transplanting. Black crayon mark is proposed new hairline. (*B*) One week after the first hair transplant. Micrografts containing one to two hairs each have been inserted into holes made with a 16-gauge needle anteriorly. "Slit" grafts containing three to four hairs each have been placed into slits just posterior to the micrografts, while those grafts containing five to six hairs each have been planted in the most posterior rows of slits, producing a gradually increasing density of hair in the hairline zone. Standard-sized round grafts have been used posterior to the slit grafts, not only because they will produce denser hair growth but also because the transitional "clumpiness" that will result from their use will be more easily camouflaged at this level. (*C*) Six months after the second transplant, with the hair combed back for critical evaluation. The smaller grafts used for micrografting and slit grafting were taken from donor sites where the hair was quite fine. Thus, not only was a natural-looking, gradually increasing density produced, but also the texture of the hair changed from fine to coarser as one moved posteriorly just as occurs in the natural hairline.

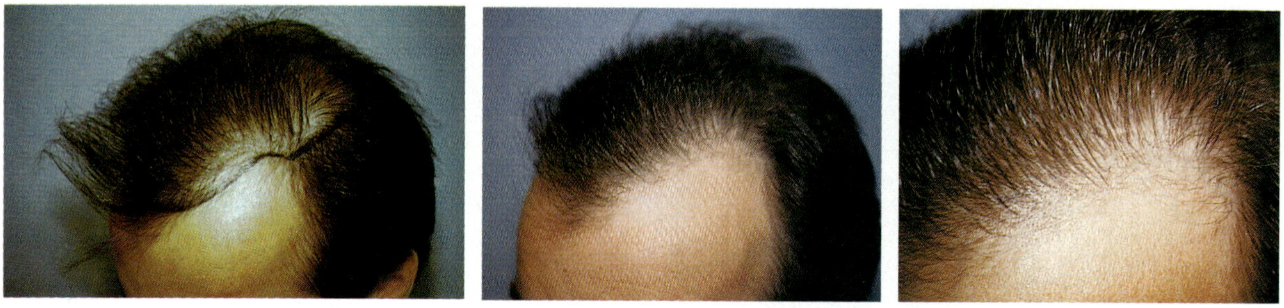

A B C

Figure 15-7 (*A*) Before first transplant. Patient had moderately advanced baldness. His goal was hair no more than twice as thick as current density. (*B*) Six months after a single session of 200 "slit" grafts. No temporary thinning occurred immediately after the first operation as happens when round grafts are used. There was none of the usual tendency to a clumpy appearance normally seen with only one session of round grafts. (*C*) Close-up of photo shown in (*B*). One or two additional sessions will be required to maintain this hair density when the patient loses more of his original hair.

with round grafts results in hair growth that is usually denser than in their temporal areas and consequently is less cosmetically satisfactory (Fig. 15-7*B*).

The presence of a reasonable amount of fine-textured hair is in fact almost a qualifying characteristic if one is to attempt transplanting an entire frontal zone with slit grafting. If the hair is coarse, and especially if it is dark and/or dense, even slit grafting will produce a tufted appearance unless only two- to four-hair grafts are utilized. The most important advantage of slit grafting would thereby be eliminated—a more natural look with fewer grafts consumed (Fig. 15-7*C*). More will be said about this subsequently.

Where a combination of graft types is being used, twenty 4.5-mm grafts with relatively fine hair and 12 to 20 hairs per graft can be divided to produce three- to four-hair grafts. An additional twenty 3.75-mm grafts containing 10 to 12 hairs can be taken from similar areas and usually bisected to produce five- to six-hair grafts. The size of the original round graft, of course, can be varied so that bisecting, trisecting, or quartering them will produce slit grafts with the desired numbers of hairs. Alternately, and preferably, a strip of donor tissue is sectioned to produce an equal number and type of slit grafts. Approximately 50 to 70 round grafts in two to three rows will most often be used in conjunction with the slit grafts and micrografts. If the hair is particularly coarse, dark, and/or dense, or if the objective is relatively dense hair, it is usually preferable to transplant micrografts followed by round grafts immediately posterior to them, eliminating the zone of slit grafting (Fig. 15-8).

Figure 15-8 The hairline shown here was constructed with four sessions of round grafts and a single session of micrografts. Note how natural the hairline appears even though only one set of micrografts and no slit grafts were used. This patient was operated on nearly 10 years ago, when we were just starting to do micrografts. He demonstrates that good results can be obtained in individuals with darker, coarser hair without the use of slit grafts if one intentionally uses sparser, finer-haired grafts for the anterior two to three rows of grafts combined with even one session of micrografts. Today micrografts would be done as part of every session, producing even better results.

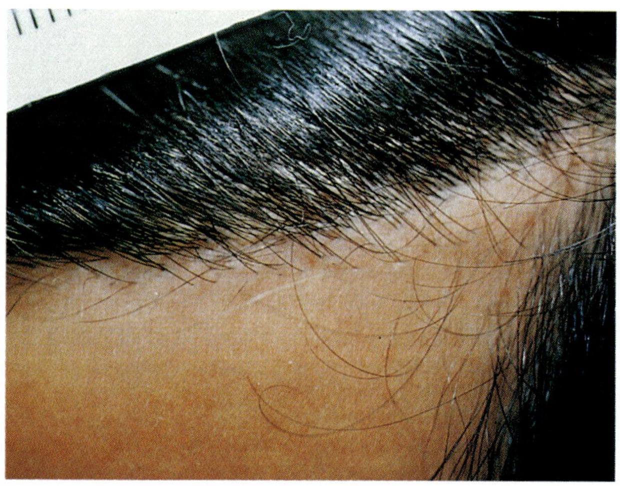

Recipient sites for grafts obtained with a 4-mm trephine will generally be made with a 3.25-mm trephine, while those obtained with a 4.5-mm trephine will generally be prepared with a 3.5-mm one. The size of the recipient-area punch can be increased or decreased in order to achieve complete filling of the recipient hole without bulging of the graft above the surrounding skin.[17] One should try to angle hair in the recipient areas as closely as possible to the original hair direction at that site.

As noted earlier, a U-shaped pattern that is four to five rows deep is generally used for the first and second session. An interval of 6 weeks will be left between the first two sessions, while 4 months or longer will be left between all further treatments. The exception to this general rule is when there is a significant amount of hair left in the recipient area. In such cases, intervals of 4 to 6 months are left between all sessions.[4]

The distribution of grafts in the recipient area during the third session is somewhat different from the simple U used on the first two. In addition to more micrografts, three to four rows are punched out on the part side of the recipient site to just past the midline. On the nonpart side, only the anterior and most posterior rows are filled. The rest of the grafts that would have been used on the nonpart side are placed bilaterally more toward the midline (Fig. 15-2*B*). The exception to this general distribution pattern is when the hairstyle envisioned for the individual is going to be a nonparted one, such as a short curly or more Negroid style.[18] In such cases, grafts are distributed in an even and bilateral fashion, often with grafts put into rows 1, 3, 7, and 9 (with row 5 being skipped).

On the fourth session, the distribution of grafts is primarily on the part side in rows 2, 4, and 6, and then wherever needed aesthetically. Very few grafts are placed into the nonpart side during this session, the majority of them being used more medially in the area started on the third session as well as occasionally in new areas toward the vertex. Once again, if a short, curly hairstyle is planned, the grafts are distributed symmetrically and only in those few areas where increased hair density is necessary. Micrografts, round minigrafts, and slit grafts will be used during this last session to fill any small hairless spaces between or within previously transplanted grafts. All of the preceding, of course, refers to when the entire recipient area is being treated in the first three sessions only with standard-sized round grafts and micrografts. If a combination of graft types is employed, although the emphasis of graft placement mimics that described earlier, approximately the first three rows of round grafts are treated instead with slit grafts.

As was pointed out previously, whenever grafts are placed toward the midline, room is always left for alopecia reductions if it is anticipated that they will be used in that individual. Alopecia reductions will usually be carried out between the second and third and the third and fourth transplant sessions, preferably with a 3-week or longer interval between transplant sessions and alopecia reductions.[16] Occasionally, if a patient is coming from a distant location, an alopecia reduction can be done the day before the transplant session in order to minimize the number of trips. This individual will have tighter sutures in the donor area and therefore more discomfort, as well as a somewhat increased chance of getting slightly wider donor site scars. In addition, grafts cannot be used on alopecia reduction scars until the scars are at least 3 weeks old. Occasionally, one or two alopecia reductions will be done before any transplanting is carried out. This is discussed more fully under the section of this chapter dealing with alopecia reductions.

For several years now, we have been transplanting most vertex areas exclusively with three- to four-hair and five- to six-hair slit grafts, that is, *not* in combination with regular size grafts (Fig. 15-9*A* through *C*). Alternately, slit grafts may be used only for the part side of the vertex area to produce a subtle gradual blending of sparser hair into denser hair as one moves away from the "part." One of the drawbacks in transplanting the vertex with standard grafts has always been that the part side of the crown is in essence the "hairline" of the crown that must be transplanted almost solidly if a clumpy appearance is to be avoided. Solid transplanting, however, produces a relatively dense growth of hair, which is usually substantially thicker than the hair on the adjacent superior temporoparietal area. The result has been a sudden artificial change from relatively sparse superior temporoparietal hair to relatively dense transplanted vertex hair. The use of three- to four-hair and five- to six-hair slit grafts in this area, either on the part side alone or throughout the whole site, has essentially solved this problem. If the

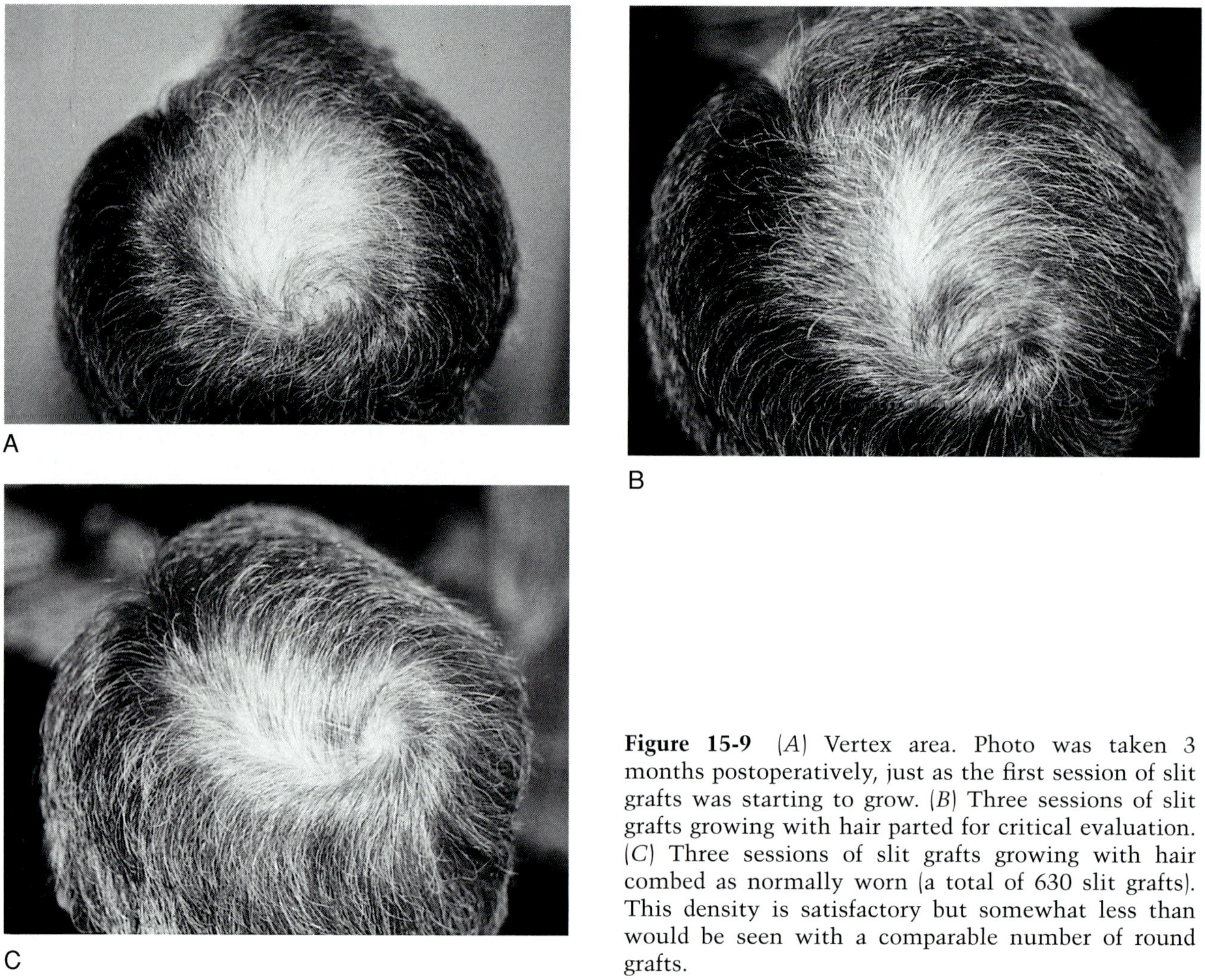

Figure 15-9 (*A*) Vertex area. Photo was taken 3 months postoperatively, just as the first session of slit grafts was starting to grow. (*B*) Three sessions of slit grafts growing with hair parted for critical evaluation. (*C*) Three sessions of slit grafts growing with hair combed as normally worn (a total of 630 slit grafts). This density is satisfactory but somewhat less than would be seen with a comparable number of round grafts.

hair is particularly dense, coarse, or dark, three- to four-hair slit grafts are used throughout the vertex.

Because of the advantages noted previously, there has been a recent tendency by hair transplant surgeons to utilize more and more slit grafts. This has reached the point where some operators have actually begun to feel that round grafts are going to become obsolete. It therefore seems worthwhile at this point to summarize clearly the advantages as well as the disadvantages of slit grafts.

ADVANTAGES OF SLIT GRAFTS

1. Slit grafts minimize the transitional "clumpiness" seen with round grafts.
2. Slit grafts can produce less-dense coverage that looks more natural than when a similar amount of donor tissue is used for round grafts.
3. Slit grafts therefore have more potential for reducing the depletion of the donor area (number of grafts and sessions required in the recipient area), as well as the cost, *in properly selected patients.*
4. Slit grafts produce minimal injury to existing hair in the recipient area and therefore are particularly useful for transplanting in men with "early" androgenetic alopecia and in females with androgenetic alopecia.
5. Postoperative crusting is shed faster than when round grafts are utilized.
6. Hair regrowth occurs in approximately 2 months, and temporary hair loss is more

likely to be minimized or aborted with the use of 2% minoxidil postoperatively.

7. Slit grafts produce minimal scarring and hypopigmentation.

DISADVANTAGES OF SLIT GRAFTS

1. The same amount of transplanted tissue in slit graphs can never produce the same density as when round grafts are used, as no bald or potentially bald skin is removed. *This should always be pointed out to patients with early male-pattern baldness who choose slit grafting over round grafting.*
2. Individuals with dark and/or coarse and/or dense hair may actually require *more* sessions and grafts to produce natural-looking results than if standard round grafting had been done. This is especially true if there is a marked difference between hair and skin color. The hair in three- to four-hair or five- to six-hair slit grafts becomes "compressed" into a slit, producing rather dense lines of coarse, dark hair in such individuals. The coarser, denser, and darker the hair, the more one should utilize two- to four-hair slit grafts vs. five- to six-hair slit grafts, and the more care one should take in locating donor areas with less dense and finer hair for sectioning for the anterior hairline and part side of the vertex. If a sufficient supply of such donor hair is not available, slit grafting should probably not even be utilized. The removal of the epidermis of the grafts may also help minimize compression by allowing a more linear orientation of hair. *The problem of "compression" will be less noticeable in patients with coarse and/or dense and/or dark hair who still have some of their original hair in the recipient area. Such individuals will have a "time bomb" ticking away that will explode slowly as they lose the rest of this hair.*
3. Ingrown hairs occur more frequently with slit grafts than with standard round grafts. This is usually a temporary problem.
4. In some individuals, slit grafts become depressed below the level of adjacent skin. This is sometimes marked enough that adjacent epidermis grows over the grafts, resulting in persistent ingrown hairs and associated problems. This can be corrected by punching out the troublesome areas.
5. Preparing grafts for slits is a time-consuming process, though it can be greatly facilitated by using strips of donor hair that are sectioned rather than round grafts (see section entitled "Donor Area").

From the preceding, it should now be obvious that the best candidates for slit grafting and round minigrafting have the same characteristics as the best candidates for standard round grafting; that is, they have hair with a fine texture, light color, and moderate to good density, and they have minimal contrast between the color of their hair and skin. If the patient has good hair characteristics, why use slit grafting instead of standard round grafting? The reasons are to minimize transitional clumpiness and to accomplish a less dense but still natural-looking result because: (1) this is what the patient wants, (2) a more gradual transition from hairless forehead to dense frontal hair is the objective, (3) there is a poor ratio of donor to recipient area, (4) the vertex is the recipient site, and (5) the patient has or will have relatively sparse temporal hair.

In this latter case, the dense transplanting required to overcome the transitional plugginess of round grafting would result in the hair in the transplanted area being substantially denser than the hair in the adjacent temporal areas—an unnatural-looking state of affairs.

CLEANING AND INSERTION OF GRAFTS

Once the grafts have been removed from the donor area, they are placed in a dish containing a 4 × 4 mm gauze and normal saline. It is imperative that they not be permitted to dry out at any time. Excess amounts of subcutaneous tissue as well as any spicules of hair or hair follicles without matrices are removed carefully, using small sharp scissors and fine jeweler's forceps. The grafts are then lined up in rows in a second similar dish, segregating the most ideal grafts for various purposes. When strip grafts are harvested with, for example, parallel scalpel blades 3 mm apart, the same blades may be used to divide the strips into 3-mm-wide sections. The 3 × 3 mm square grafts can then be further divided into halves or quarters or trisected to yield sections with the desired number of hairs.

Grafts should be handled as little as possible

during cleaning as well as during their insertion into recipient sites. One should be careful that no adjacent hair has been accidentally trapped beneath the graft and its recipient hole or slit, and that the graft has been placed in such a way that the angle of hair is directed properly. In our office, a standard turbanlike bandage is applied overnight.[26] The bandage is used more to keep the grafts oriented properly and to absorb any small amount of bleeding that might occur postoperatively than to actually stop bleeding with pressure. A somewhat modified bandage that does not cover the ears can also be employed and is more comfortable for this reason.[26] The only problem with the latter is that it is more prone to become dislodged or to slip upward.

The bandage is removed the morning after surgery and the areas cleansed with hydrogen peroxide. The hair is then carefully shampooed and blown dry to produce the most optimal camouflage of the surgery as is possible. Patients begin washing their hair on their own 2 to 3 days postoperatively. They are asked not to do any heavy exercise or anything that would cause sweating, and to avoid exposure to air that might contain dirt or debris for 1 week.

The use of alkyl-2 cyanoacrylate to "glue" the grafts in place has been advocated as a way to avoid overnight bandaging.[27] Unfortunately, the glue also tends to mat surrounding hair and fixes the crust in place, significantly delaying its shedding. Orentreich and Orentreich have described suturing grafts in place in order to avoid bandaging.[28] This is useful if relatively small numbers of grafts are being transplanted but even then results in a foreign body (the sutures) being left in the nonsterile recipient site, thus increasing the possibility of infection at that site.

Pouteaux has for many years used no alkyl-2 cyanoacrylate, sutures, or overnight bandage.[29] He asks patients to stay in his office for the full working day. Gauze soaked lightly with saline is applied to the recipient and donor areas, and a tensorlike bandage is used to apply pressure and keep the gauze in place. The dressing is changed periodically and at the end of the day is removed entirely before the patient is sent home. Pouteaux states that he has never had a graft fall out or been called for bleeding overnight, as any potential problems make themselves known during the day and have been attended to before the patient leaves the office. We occasionally use the same procedure to avoid overnight bandaging in individuals who are prepared to stay in the office for 3 hours, without the patients experiencing any postoperative difficulties.

For the past 9 years, we have been applying a solution of 2% minoxidil in an alcohol base just after the recipient area has been cleansed. In addition, patients continue twice-daily applications of the solution for a period of 5 weeks. Most patients, though not all, note a later effluvium of hair from the transplanted grafts and a more rapid regrowth of hair than occurred before minoxidil was used.[30] Intramuscular betamethasone sodium phosphate and betamethasone acetate (Celestone Soluspan) 12 mg and/or a 1-week course of prednisone are offered to patients after the first session, as well as to those who are anxious about postoperative edema because of previous problems with it.[31] The usual contraindications to corticosteroids are respected.

A single intramuscular injection of ketorolac tromethamine (Toradol) 30 to 60 mg at the conclusion of surgery has dramatically decreased the need for postoperative oral analgesics in our patients. It is, however, not offered to patients who prefer prednisone, who are bleeding more than the average patient during surgery, or who have a history of asthma. When required, acetaminophen with 30 mg codeine (Tylenol No. 3), oxycodone hydrochloride (Percocet), oral ketorolac tromethamine, or meperidine (Demerol) may also be used.[32]

POSTOPERATIVE COMPLICATIONS

This subject has been covered in detail in previous publications[31–33] and includes the following: (1) mild pruritus, which may be treated with a combination corticosteroid-antibiotic, e.g., Valisone G cream (betamethasone valerate–gentamicin sulfate), applied one to three times per day; (2) edema, which occurs in most though not all patients beginning usually between 1 and 3 days after surgery and lasting for 7 to 10 days; (3) discoloration of grafts that are either mildly erythematous to violaceous for a period of several weeks to several months, after which the discoloration resolves spontaneously; (4) graft elevation, which can be corrected by simple hyfercation; (5) hypoesthesia, which results from the severing of nerves in the donor and/or recipient areas and which normally is temporary; (6)

hematoma, which has been reported but has never occurred in over 20,000 operative sessions in my experience; (7) hypertrophic scarring, which may occur in predisposed individuals; and (8) arteriovenous fistulae, which may develop in some individuals either in the donor area or more rarely in the recipient area and which will resolve spontaneously over a period of several months.

More serious complications include (1) keloidal healing in predisposed individuals; (2) infection, which occurs in the donor area in approximately 0.1 percent of patients and which responds quickly to appropriate antibiotic therapy such as erythromycin 250 mg q.i.d. or cloxacillin 250 mg q.i.d.; (3) osteomyelitis, one case of which has been reported in the medical literature;[34] and (4) postoperative bleeding (virtually zero incidence in the recipient area, < 0.3 percent incidence in the donor area). Usually all that is required to control the bleeding is an additional suture at the site of origin.

To put matters into perspective, all of these complications are rare and mild when the procedure is carried out with skill and care.

ALOPECIA REDUCTION

Standard Alopecia Reduction

Alopecia reduction or scalp reduction can be defined as the excision of an area of alopecia or prospective alopecia. The size of the area that can be excised is dependent on two factors: (1) the degree of natural scalp laxity and (2) the extent of surgical undermining. The larger the area that can be removed, the smaller the remaining area of alopecia will be, with the result that fewer grafts will be required to adequately transplant hair into it. In general, the author recommends that alopecia reductions be employed any time the objective of the patient is complete coverage of frontal and vertex alopecia. The more alopecia reductions that are done, the more likely it becomes that one will not run out of available donor tissue before the entire area of alopecia is treated.

In some individuals, a second very important function of alopecia reductions is the raising of the superior border of the hair-bearing temporoparietal area that accompanies each alopecia reduction procedure. If the patient intends to use a "part," for aesthetic reasons it should begin at a line drawn vertically from the lateral canthus of the eye or at some point medial to this.[2] If the anterior-superior-most point of permanent temporal hair is inferior to where the part line should aesthetically begin, the part will therefore pass through transplanted areas.

Unfortunately, in most individuals one cannot part through a transplanted zone without it being obvious that transplanting has been carried out, as the hair is not perfectly evenly distributed. Ideally, therefore, one would want to somehow move the superior border of the temporoparietal hair (and the anterior-superior-most point of the temporal hair) more superiorly so that if a part is made, it will pass through intact original temporoparietal hair. In individuals with relatively narrow persistent rims of hair, alopecia reductions therefore become almost a necessity rather than an option if an optimal cosmetic result is being sought.

There has been much debate in the medical community as to whether a good portion of the gain obtained with an alopecia reduction is subsequently lost as the scalp laxity returns postoperatively. This is frequently referred to as "stretch-back" and has led many practitioners to all but abandon alopecia reductions. In a study reported on by M. Unger, such stretch-back resulted in an average loss of less than 10 percent in the 60 patients he followed.[35] Nordstrom has reported stretch-back loss of approximately 34 percent (at the widest point of the alopecia reduction) in the 13 patients he studied, but this difference is probably because of differing surgical techniques and still leaves one with a substantial gain.[36,37] This author cannot state strongly enough that although some stretch-back is a component of every alopecia reduction, the ultimate benefits obtained will almost always far outweigh the stretch-back that may occur postoperatively *if the alopecia reduction has been carried out properly* (Fig. 15-10*A* and *B*).

A variety of alopecia reduction patterns have been described,[16] but the most common patterns employed are the ellipse, inverted Y and, more recently, flattened "S" shape. The "inverted Y" pattern should be used if one anticipates insufficient donor tissue to transplant the entire bald area even after alopecia reductions. This design prevents the production of scar in areas that cannot later be covered with transplanted hair. As previously stated, usually the alopecia reduc-

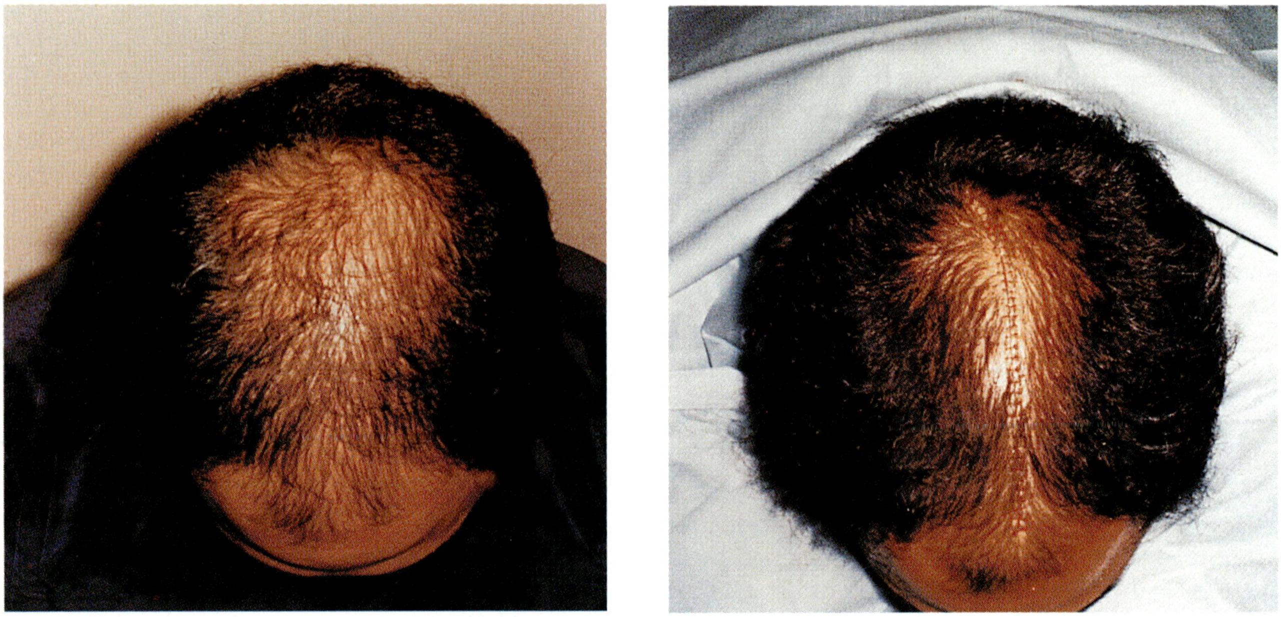

A B

Figure 15-10 (*A*) Before an alopecia reduction. (*B*) Immediately after an elliptic alopecia reduction. Virtually all of the thinning area has been removed with a single alopecia reduction because this patient had an unusually lax scalp. Most patients would require two or three alopecia reductions to obtain the same results. (*Courtesy of Dr. Martin Unger.*)

tions are carried out after the first two transplants have been completed. Additional reductions may be done every 2 to 3 months. Occasionally an alopecia reduction will be done before any transplanting is started. This will occur most often in the following situations: (1) there is a great deal of scalp laxity, making it likely that the shape of the hairline will be significantly altered by the alopecia reductions, (2) the area of alopecia is particularly large and therefore requires several alopecia reductions to raise the superior border of the temporoparietal hair to an appropriate level; the shape of the hairline would be significantly changed in such a patient if the transplanting had begun prior to the first alopecia reduction, (3) the crown is the recipient area and the patient is relatively young and might need the grafts saved by the alopecia reduction for other areas of future alopecia, or (4) one is correcting poorly planned transplanting in which new areas of alopecia have developed without sufficient donor grafts having been left to treat them, and (5) one is treating large areas of cicatricial alopecia.[17,38]

TECHNIQUE

Alopecia reduction is usually carried out on an outpatient basis under sterile conditions. The patient is given 15 to 20 mg of oral Valium 30 minutes before surgery with or without meperidine 50 mg intramuscularly at the same time. The procedure begins with drawing in the described pattern using a marker such as a Micropoint Super Marker (Micropoint Inc., Sunnyvale, CA).

Two percent lidocaine with 1/100,000 epinephrine is utilized to produce a circle of anesthesia around the circumference of the head inferior to the expected extent of undermining. In addition, it is injected along the proposed lines of incision to minimize bleeding.

If the pattern is an ellipse or a variant of an ellipse, an incision is made down to and through the galea along one side of its entire length, usually in a staged fashion, stopping to control bleeding with cautery where required. Care is taken to angle the blade so as not to injure any adjacent follicles, and if previously transplanted grafts are nearby, a 2-mm margin of safety is observed.

Mayo scissors are used to begin the undermining between the periosteum and galea aponeurotica, which is then completed to at least 10 cm or more on either side by blunt finger dissection. There is usually little bleeding encountered during this stage of the surgery except in the vertex area, where two or more perforators are frequently transected and must be cauterized or ligated.

The amount of redundant scalp tissue is estimated by overlapping the tissues, followed by perpendicular incisions made through the top flap, stopping at the points where the flaps meet. The perpendicular cuts are then joined and the excess tissue is thereby removed. If the alopecia reduction is done in the shape of an inverted Y—a far more commonly utilized pattern than the ellipse—each "arm" of the Y is treated as a separate ellipse.[16]

Alopecia reductions are closed in two layers, using interrupted no. 2-0 Dexon or Vicryl sutures for the galea and running 4-0 chromic catgut sutures for the skin. The postoperative dressing consists of three or four layers of gauze covered by a 6-inch stockinette shaped into a cap to hold the gauze in place. The patient removes this himself the following day. Postoperative and preoperative instructions and medications are essentially the same as described for punch transplanting.

Major Reductions

"Major" reductions have been described by Marzola, Bradshaw, and Brandy.[40,41] Many names have been used for these reductions, including *bilateral occipital parietal flaps* and *bilateral temporal flaps*. Major reductions are distinguished from standard alopecia reductions by more extensive undermining involving the severing of temporal, postauricular, and occipital arteries bilaterally as part of the undermining process. Although the efficacy of these procedures in excising substantial areas of alopecia is beyond question, the relative safety of carrying them out has caused a great deal of discussion among physicians.[16] It is the author's view that potential complications including wound dehiscense, permanent hair loss in the occipital and temporoparietal area, and necrosis of large areas of scalp tissue, although infrequent, are significant enough that this type of reduction is not recommended. Vertical scars in the temporal area and raising of the inferior border of supra-auricular and nape hair which always accompanies major alopecia reductions can also lead to cosmetic difficulties. Marzola and Bradshaw, who were the first physicians to employ major reductions, have discontinued their use as well.[42] Recently Brandy has been employing ligation of occipital arteries weeks before his procedure to increase collateral circulation and minimize complications. This is a logical innovation that will likely make the procedure more acceptable to more physicians.

Alopecia Reduction Preceded by Soft Tissue Expansion

Radovan first described the use of tissue expansion prior to excision of tissue. This has been applied to alopecia reductions in some individuals for at least the last decade.[39,43–45] In brief, specially designed balloonlike tissue expanders are inserted as a separate procedure, usually approximately $1^1/_2$ to 3 months prior to a planned alopecia reduction. They are then gradually inflated with injections of saline every 1 or 2 weeks. At the end of approximately $1^1/_2$ to 3 months, the expanders are removed and an alopecia reduction is carried out at the same time. The use of such expanders has enabled physicians to excise as much as 10 to 12 cm of alopecia in one alopecia reduction. The cosmetic disability caused by the gradually inflated expanders, which results in a hydrocephalic-like appearance toward the end of the inflation, has almost completely limited tissue expansion prior to alopecia reduction to individuals with cicatricial alopecia. Very few patients with male-pattern baldness will tolerate the cosmetic disability which is a component of tissue expansion.

COMPLICATIONS

Complications of alopecia reductions include postoperative bleeding, hypotension, infection, nerve damage, persistent hair loss in the fringe areas, and poor scars.[46] All of these occur infrequently or not at all if the procedure is carried out properly.

FLAP SURGERY

At least four different types of flaps have been extensively used for the correction of alopecia:

temporoparieto-occipital flaps, lateral scalp flaps, long and short temporal vertical flaps, and microsurgical free scalp flaps.[47] Our discussion will deal primarily with what is by far the most common type of flap employed—the temporoparieto-occipital flap—frequently referred to as the *Juri flap* because of its originator, Dr. Jose Juri.

The Juri Flap

A flap is designed starting in the temporal area running through the parietal zone and descending into the occipital area without crossing the midline. The design is intended to have the terminal parietal branch of the superficial temporal artery running down its midline (a Doppler flowmeter is often used to facilitate this); to be approximately 4 cm wide; to stay within permanent hair-bearing areas and inferior enough to the superior border of the fringe hair to camouflage any scars; and to be long enough—by employing a greater or lesser curvature of the flap—to reach the fringe hair on the opposite side of the scalp[48] (Fig. 15-11). Two "delays" are employed:

The first operation is often carried out under local anesthesia in a properly equipped office. During this procedure, the hair is clipped short along the proposed incision lines but left its original length within the body of the proposed flap—the longer hair can be braided and taped out of the way. The clipped lines are then anesthetized with 1% lidocaine with 1/100,000 epinephrine to minimize bleeding as well as to provide anesthesia. The inferior and superior borders of the flap are incised, taking care to angle the blade in the direction of hair growth, down and through the galea aponeurotica. After appropriate hemostasis is obtained with cautery, the incision lines are sutured with running Prolene, for example, and a 24-hour dressing is applied. The posterior 6 cm of the flap is incised *and raised* 1 week later. Once again, the incision lines are sutured after any bleeders are cauterized or ligated.

A week later, under general anesthesia and in a fully equipped operatory, but again using local anesthesia along the incision lines to minimize bleeding, the entire flap is raised and transposed to the preselected new anterior hairline. An incision is made along this line and is angled anteriorly while cutting toward the galea to produce a better "fit" for the flap. This results in hair growing through the scar at the anterior edge of the flap.[48]

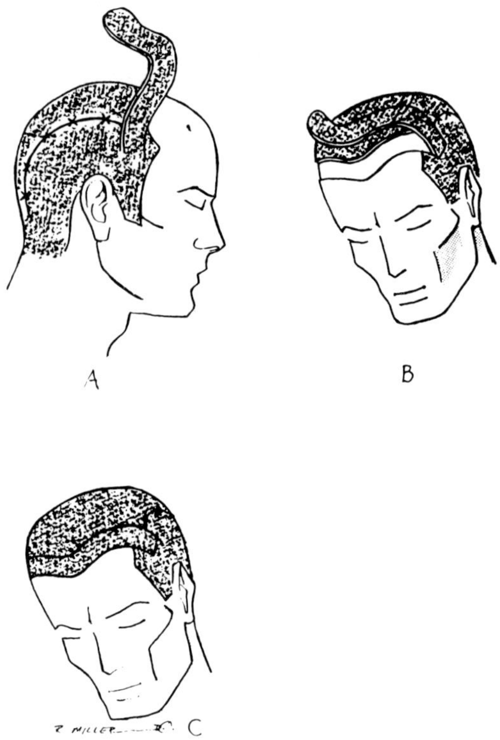

Figure 15-11 The Juri flap. (*A*) Closure of the donor wound following undermining. (*B*) Resecting of the glabrous frontal zone. (*C*) Placing and suturing of the flap.

Extensive undermining of the anterior scalp and the retroauricular area as low as the nape of the neck is followed by suturing of the donor site on two levels: galea and skin. Usually no. 3-0 interrupted Dexon sutures are employed for the galea and no. 5-0 interrupted nylon for the skin, with suturing beginning at the proximal end of the donor bed. Closing the donor site first minimizes the amount of skin that must be removed at the recipient site to accommodate the flap. Any fibrotic material on the undersurface of the distal end of the flap is removed; after bleeding has been controlled, it is then transposed and sutured into place with no. 5-0 nylon. A second similar flap from the other side of the scalp may be transposed 1 month later if the area of alopecia requires this. A 2-cm-wide gap of intact skin should be left between the flaps and can be excised 2 months or more later. Still larger areas of alopecia can be treated with a third flap employing a retroauricular or occipital pedicle (Fig. 15-12).

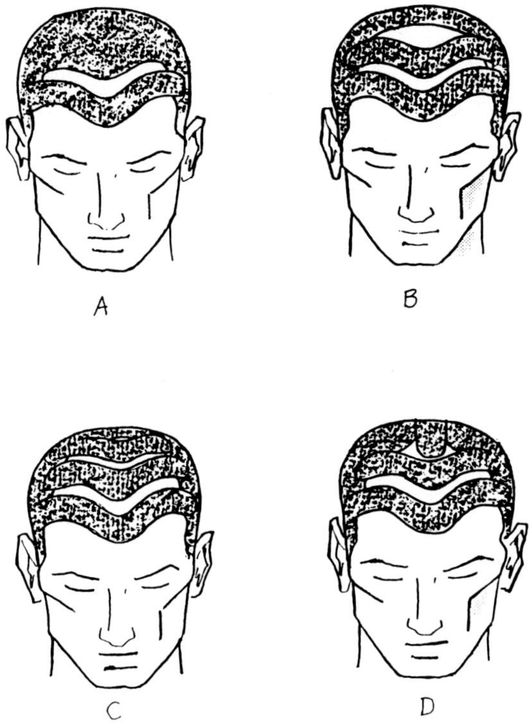

Figure 15-12 The Juri flap. (*A*) One flap with temporoparieto-occipital pedicle. (*B*) Two flaps with temporoparieto-occipital pedicles (one from each side of the head). (*C*) Three flaps, two with temporoparieto-occipital pedicles and one with retroauricular pedicle. (*D*) Three flaps, two with temporoparieto-occipital pedicles and one with occipital pedicle.

ADVANTAGES

The most important advantage of transplanting flaps is the absence of significant postoperative telogen effluvium. The hair in the flaps continues to grow immediately after surgery. This produces immediate results that contrast very favorably with punch transplanting, which often requires 6 to 12 months to produce good cosmetic results.

The second most important advantage of flaps as opposed to punch grafts is the achievement of a perfectly diffuse pattern of hair growth without first traversing a stage in which the patient's scalp looks like that of a "Barbie-doll." Slit grafting and micrografting have, to a large degree, eliminated these advantages of flaps over smaller grafts.

A third advantage of flaps is the production of very dense hair in the recipient site. This advantage is a "double-edged sword," however, because in patients who have or will have large areas of alopecia, it represents an uneconomic use of a limited supply of donor tissue. This will be elaborated on subsequently.

Finally, because skin in the recipient area is excised, flaps have the potential advantage of removing large areas of scar or diseased tissue in the recipient area as part of its replacement with hair-bearing tissue.

DISADVANTAGES

The most important disadvantage of the Juri flap is its uneconomic use of a limited supply of donor tissue. The price of using so much donor material in the transposed flap is a significant depletion of donor tissue. The chance of using up all the potential donor material before completely treating the entire area of alopecia is thereby substantially increased. Smaller grafts allow for treating cosmetically important areas densely and less important areas less densely, thereby increasing the likelihood of being able to treat the whole bald area. In addition, as has been described previously, small grafts taken from donor areas optimal for the purpose allow for the creation of transplanted hairlines in which the hair changes gradually from sparse and fine to dense and coarse as one moves posteriorly—as in a natural hairline. Flap surgery does not allow for this elegant transitional zone, not only with regard to density but also with regard to texture.

The second important disadvantage of Juri flaps is that the hair within them is always directed posteriorly. This not only is contrary to the normal hair direction seen in 99 percent of patients, it also results in complete exposure of any anterior line scar and the hairline. As noted previously, this is nearly always too dense and coarse to look natural. The unnaturalness may not be as obvious in a young man whose permanent rim is still dense and relatively coarse, but it will gradually become more unnatural-looking as the patient ages and the hair in the temporal area becomes finer and sparser.

Potential complications sometimes include very wide donor site scars and partial or complete necrosis of a portion of the flap, resulting not only in a significant cosmetic problem but, in the case of the latter, a sizable loss of limited donor tissue.[46] The more experience the operator has, the smaller the risk, but such risks do not exist with punch grafting. The gain-to-potential-loss ratio is therefore better with punch grafting.

Transposition flaps always result in "dog-ears" at the base of the flap that not uncommonly must be excised as a separate procedure. The gaps of intact skin between two or more flaps must be excised as separate surgeries if complete coverage is to be accomplished. Again, additional procedures are required. When these are added to the surgery to correct dog-ears, the difference between the number of operations required to treat an area of alopecia with small grafts vs. flaps is narrowed considerably. More importantly, the hairless gaps frequently cannot be entirely excised because there is far less scalp laxity and mobility anteroposteriorly than from left to right. The result is alternating bands of dense hair and total alopecia.

Because of the above disadvantages, the author does not recommend flap surgery except in patients who have and will have relatively small bald areas and who have naturally curly hair or who are prepared to "perm" their hair indefinitely. The exception to these guidelines is an individual who has extensive scarring or diseased scalp tissue that should be replaced in its entirety and cannot be treated with alopecia reduction with or without soft tissue expansion.

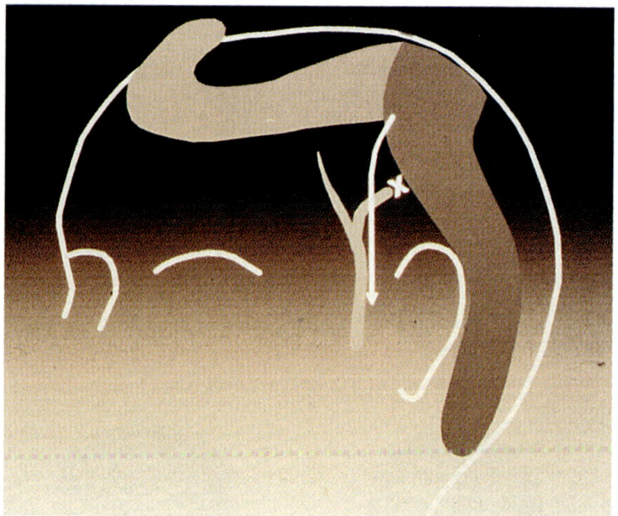

Figure 15-13 The retroauricular version of the temporovertical flap is preferred over Elliott-type flaps for three reasons. Firstly, its greater length, secondly, the fine quality of the retroauricular hair, and lastly, complete sparing of the temporal hairy zone, which is more visible, and which can hide a possible alopecic junction of the edges after closure of the donor zone.

Other Flaps

In addition to the Juri flap described earlier, a variety of shorter and narrower types of flaps have been described by others, and include the following:

The Elliot-type *lateral scalp flap* has a temporal base similar to the Juri flap.[49] Because it is shorter and narrower than the Juri flap, it is less difficult to execute and has a lower morbidity, but at least two such flaps (from contralateral sides) are necessary to bridge completely an average-sized area of alopecia. It is, however, a single-step operation without delays.

The *Long Temporal Vertical Flap* described by Nataf[50] has approximately the same width as an Elliot-type flap but has three advantages over it because of its clever design: (1) It can be as long as 25 cm, which allows it to bridge a major part (but not all) of most average-sized bald areas; (2) the quality of the retroauricular hair it contains is excellent for most hairlines; and (3) the direction of hair in the flap closely mimics that of most normal hairlines. It also leaves the temporal area intact, as the base of the flap is superior and posterior to the temple (Fig. 15-13). It is carried out in three stages.

The *Short Temporal Vertical Flap* described by Nataf as well as Marzola[51] (*preauricular flap*) is a shorter and narrower flap than the long temporal vertical flap discussed earlier; it uses the temporal area for donor tissue but is otherwise quite similar to its larger "brother." It is used primarily for correcting frontotemporal thinning in females and producing small frontal areas of hair (Marzola) after alopecia reductions have removed the rest of a previously alopecic area.

A microsurgical free scalp flap has been described by Ohmori and others in which 4-cm-wide flaps as much as 24 cm long are totally excised from various donor areas and placed into properly prepared recipient beds.[52] Using specialized microsurgical instruments and microscopes developed for replantation of amputated fingers and transplanting of free tissues and organs with a vascular pedicle, blood vessels present in the flap are anastomosed to those adjacent to their new site, e.g., branches of the superficial temporal artery. This technique allows for a single-step procedure that produces natural hair direction and dense growth. On the other hand, it has some of the disadvantages associated with Juri flaps, including dense hair where this is not desirable, and is technically extremely demanding.

CICATRICIAL ALOPECIA

Patients with cicatricial alopecia may be treated with flap surgery or alopecia reduction with or without preceding soft tissue expansion. In addition, punch grafting and minigrafting can be successfully utilized in such individuals.[53,54] Because the blood supply within the scar is not as good as in normal skin we will often: (1) try to excise as much of the scar as possible prior to utilizing grafting; (2) first transplant the periphery of the scar, which is closest to the normal blood supply; (3) do fewer grafts per session and spread them farther apart than usual; and (4) spread sessions farther apart, for example every 3 to 6 months.

The author has found it useful to reach into each recipient hole and make an extra cut into the galea aponeurotica before attempting to put a graft into it. Grafts tend to sit more flush to the surface and more snugly when this is done. Roenigk also advises a more careful trimming of fat on the grafts to minimize graft elevation and the elimination of a vasoconstrictor from the local anesthesia used in the local site (H. Roenigk, personal communication).

CONCLUDING REMARKS

Among the more important advances in hair transplant surgery over the last decade has been the increasing use of strip harvesting for the donor area and the development and perfection of the use of smaller grafts. Strip harvesting results in finer and fewer scars in the donor area and, therefore, allows for a significant increase in the amount of usable donor tissue. Smaller grafts of various sizes enable patients to gradually grow more hair without going through the unsightly interim "pluggy look" that is seen with larger grafts. In addition, in patients who begin hair transplantation before they are bald, essentially no temporary hair loss is experienced postoperatively. It is now possible to produce very natural looking hair of medium to low density and hairlines that are virtually indistinguishable from natural ones.

A promising new development is the use of lasers for preparing recipient sites for smaller grafts. This technique is currently being investigated by an international group of cosmetic laser surgeons, and the author expects that lasers, such as the Ultrapulse CO_2, will eventually play a more important role in hair transplanting.

Improvements in alopecia reduction have likewise broadened the spectrum of patients who are acceptable for the procedure and increased the number of individuals who can expect total or near total treatment of the area affected by male pattern baldness.

REFERENCES

1. Orentreich N: Autografts in alopecias and other selected dermatological conditions. Ann NY Acad Sci 83:462, 1959.
2. Unger WP, Marritt M: General principles of recipient site organization and planning. In Unger W, Nordstrom R (eds): *Hair Transplantation,* 2d ed. New York/Basel, Marcel Dekker, 1988, pp 105–128.
3. Unger WP: The recipient area. In Unger W, Nordstrom R (eds): *Hair Transplantation,* 2d ed. New York/Basel, Marcel Dekker, 1988, pp 211–285.
4. Unger WP: Hair transplantation in "early" androgenetic alopecia. In Unger W, Nordstrom R (eds): *Hair Transplantation,* 2d ed. New York/Basel, Marcel Dekker, 1988, pp 285–294.
5. Unger WP: Concomitant minireductions and punch hair transplanting. J Dermatol Surg Oncol 9(5):388–392, 1983.
6. Fujita K: Hair transplantation in Japan. In Kobori T, Montagna W (eds): *Biology and Disease of the Hair.* Baltimore, University Park Press, 1976, pp 519–527.
7. Marritt E: Single hair transplantation for hairline refinement: A practical solution. J Dermatol Surg Oncol 10:962–965, 1984.
8. Unger WP: Hair transplantation: "Mmunigrafts." In Robins P (ed): *Surgical Gems in Dermatology,* vol. 2. New York/Tokyo, Igaku-Shoin, 1991, pp 68–69.
9. Stough B, Stough D: Incisional (slit) grafting. J Dermatol Surg Oncol 17:53–60, 1991.
10. Cotterill P, Unger W: Hair transplantation in females. J Dermatol Surg Oncol 18:477–481, 1992.
11. Lucas M: German surgeon favours small grafts, holes. Hair Transplant Forum 2(1):1–3, 1991.
12. Bradshaw W: Quarter grafts: A technique for minigrafts. In Unger W, Nordstrom R (eds): *Hair Transplantation,* 2d ed. New York/Basel, Marcel Dekker, 1988, pp 333–351.
13. Bradshaw W: Slit grafts. Hair Transplant Forum 2:7, 1991.
14. Unger WP: Hair transplantation. In Moy R, Lask G (eds): *The Principles and Techniques of Dermatologic Surgery.* New York, McGraw-Hill, in press.
15. Stough DB IV: Hair transplantation by the feathering zone technique: New tools for the nineties. Am J Cosm Surg 9(3):243–248, 1992.
16. Unger MG: Scalp reduction. In Unger W, Nordstrom R (eds): *Hair Transplantation,* 2d ed. New York/Basel, Marcel Dekker, 1988, pp 435–497.
17. Unger WP: Hair: Surgical aspects. In Parrish LE, Lask GP

(eds): *Aesthetic Dermatology*. New York, McGraw-Hill, 1991, pp 210–227.
18. Unger WP: Hair replacement surgery in the black male and female. In Pierce HE (ed): *Plastic Surgery in Non-white Patients*. New York, Grune and Stratton, 1982, pp 51–69.
19. Unger WP: Hair transplantation in Orientals. In Unger W, Nordstrom R (eds): *Hair Transplantation*, 2d ed. New York/Basel, Marcel Dekker, 1988, pp 306–307.
20. Unger WP: Hair transplantation in females. In Unger W, Nordstrom R (eds): *Hair Transplantation*, 2d ed. New York/Basel, Marcel Dekker, 1988, pp 295–300.
21. Monheit G: Anesthesia. In Unger W, Nordstrom R (eds): *Hair Transplantation*, 2d ed. New York/Basel, Marcel Dekker, 1988, pp 133–143.
22. McKay W et al: Sodium bicarbonate attenuates pain on skin infiltration with lidocaine, with or without epinephrine. Anesth Analg 66:572–574, 1987.
23. Abadir AR: Use of local anesthetics in dermatology. J Dermatol Surg Oncol 1:65–70, 1975.
24. Alt T: The donor site. In Unger W, Nordstrom R (eds): *Hair Transplantation*, 2d ed. New York/Basel, Marcel Dekker, 1988, pp 145–209.
25. Bissacia E, Scarborough D: A technique for square plug hair transplantation. Am J Cosm Surg 7(4):219–222, 1990.
26. Unger WP, Nordstrom R: Bandaging. In Unger W, Nordstrom R (eds): *Hair Transplantation*, 2d ed. New York/Basel, Marcel Dekker, 1988, pp 375–380.
27. Morrison I: Tissue adhesive in hair transplant surgery. Plast Reconstr Surg 68(4):491–497, 1981.
28. Orentreich N, Orentreich D: "Cross-stitch" suture technique for hair transplantation. J Dermatol Surg Oncol 10(12):970–971, 1984.
29. Pouteaux P: Other alternatives. In Unger W, Nordstrom R (eds): *Hair Transplantation*, 2d ed. New York/Basel, Marcel Dekker, 1988, pp 581–589.
30. Unger WP: Punch hair transplantation. Dermatol Clin 2(2):303–317, 1984.
31. Tromovitch TA, Stegman SJ, Glogau RG: Sequelae and complications of hair transplantation. In Unger W, Nordstrom R (eds): *Hair Transplantation*, 2d ed. New York/Basel, Marcel Dekker, 1988, pp 399–408.
32. Stegman SJ, Tromovitch TA: Punch grafts for alopecia. In *Cosmetic Dermatologic Surgery*. Chicago/London, Year Book Medical Publishers, 1984, pp 77–100.
33. Unger WP: Complications in hair transplantation. In Harahap M, Gebhardt V (eds): *Complications of Dermatologic Surgery*. New York/Berlin, Springer-Verlag, in press.
34. Jones J et al.: Osteomyolitis of the skull following scalp reduction and hair plug transplantation. Ann Plast Surg 5:480–482, 1980.
35. Unger MG: Scalp reduction. In Epstein E (ed): *Recent Advances in Skin Surgery. Clinics in Dermatology*, New York, Elsevier, in press.
36. Nordstrom R: Post A.R. relaxation of gain. In Unger W, Nordstrom R (eds): *Hair Transplantation*, 2d ed. New York/Basel, Marcel Dekker, 1988, pp 504–510.
37. Nordstrom RE: Stretchback in scalp reductions for male pattern baldness. Plast Reconstr Surg 73:422, 1984.
38. Unger WP, Unger MG: Alopecia reduction. In Epstein E (ed): *Skin Surgery*, 5th ed. Springfield, IL, Charles C Thomas, 1982, pp 530–545.
39. Maders EK, Graham WP III: Alopecia reduction by scalp reduction. J Dermatol Surg Oncol 10(12):967–969, 1984.
40. Brandy DA: The Brandy bitemporal flap. Cosmet Surg 3:11–15, 1986.
41. Brandy DA: The bilateral occipito-parietal flap. J Dermatol Surg Oncol 12:1062–1066, 1986.
42. Norwood O'T: Treatment of extensive baldness. J Dermatol Surg Oncol 13(5):465–466, 1987.
43. Argenta LC, Watanabe MJ, Grabb WC: The use of tissue expansion in head and neck reconstruction. Ann Plast Surg 11:31, 1983.
44. Nordstrom RE, Devine JW: Scalp stretching with a tissue expander for closure of scalp defects. Plast Reconstr Surg 75:578, 1985.
45. Manders EK, Graham WP, Shenden MJ, Davis TS: Skin expansion to eliminate large scalp defects. Ann Plast Surg 12:305, 1984.
46. Bell M: Complications of alopecia reduction and their management. In Unger W, Nordstrom R (eds): *Hair Transplantation*, 2d ed. New York/Basel, Marcel Dekker, 1988, pp 497–504.
47. Kabaker S et al.: Various scalp flaps. In Unger W, Nordstrom R (eds): *Hair Transplantation*, 2d ed. New York/Basel, Marcel Dekker, 1988, pp 621–722.
48. Juri J, Juri C: Use of pedicle flaps in surgical treatment of alopecia. In Unger W, Nordstrom R (eds): *Hair Transplantation*, 2d ed. New York/Basel, Marcel Dekker, 1988, pp 635–645.
49. Elliot RA: Lateral scalp flaps for instant results in male pattern baldness. Plast Reconstr Surg 60:699, 1977.
50. Nataf J: The long temporal vertical flap and various other scalp flaps. In Unger W, Nordstrom R (eds): *Hair Transplantation*, 2d ed. New York/Basel, Marcel Dekker, 1988, pp 675–690.
51. Marzola M: Combination of lateral scalp reductions and preauricular flaps: Hair replacement without punch grafts. In Unger W, Nordstrom R (eds): *Hair Transplantation*, 2d ed. New York/Basel, Marcel Dekker, 1988, pp 691–705.
52. Ohmori K: Microsurgical free scalp flap and androgenetic alopecia. In Unger W, Nordstrom R (eds): *Hair Transplantation*, 2d ed. New York/Basel, Marcel Dekker, 1988, pp 661–674.
53. Burke JW et al: Surgical treatment of cicatricial baldness. South Med J 59:662, 1966.
54. Stough DB, Berger RA, Orentreich N: Surgical improvement of cicatricial alopecia of diverse etiology. Arch Dermatol 97:331, 1968.

Chapter

16

HAIR CARE PRODUCTS

Marianne Nelson O'Donoghue

HAIR ANATOMY

Hair is a cylinder of impacted keratinized cells. The detailed embryology and anatomy of hair are discussed elsewhere. When hair care products are discussed, a simple model of a hair shaft is appropriate (Fig. 16-1).

A cross section of the hair shaft reveals the three major structures of a fully mature and keratinized hair. The outside layer is called the *cuticle.* The next layer is the *cortex,* and the centralmost layer is the *medulla.*

Medulla

This section of the hair contains melanin granules and is present only in thick terminal hair. It is the least important part of the hair as pertains to hair care products. Ultrastructurally, the loosely aggregated cells of the hair medulla contain melanosomes, empty vacuoles, citrulline-red granules, and immature filaments embedded in an electron-dense material.[1]

Cortex

Most of the changes that occur in the hair shaft occur in the cortex, the thickened part of the hair shaft. The cortex consists of elongated cells containing tonofilaments and interfilamentous matrix materials which are rich in cystine. The keratin in the cortex is different from that in epidermal keratinocytes, primarily in the increased numbers of disulfide bonds in hair. This composition gives hair its great tensile strength.[2]

Cuticle

The integrity of the hair shaft is maintained by the cuticle. The cuticle consists of flattened cells along the hair shaft arranged like shingles on a roof. The overlapping is extremely tight, preventing damage to the underlying cortex. The scale-

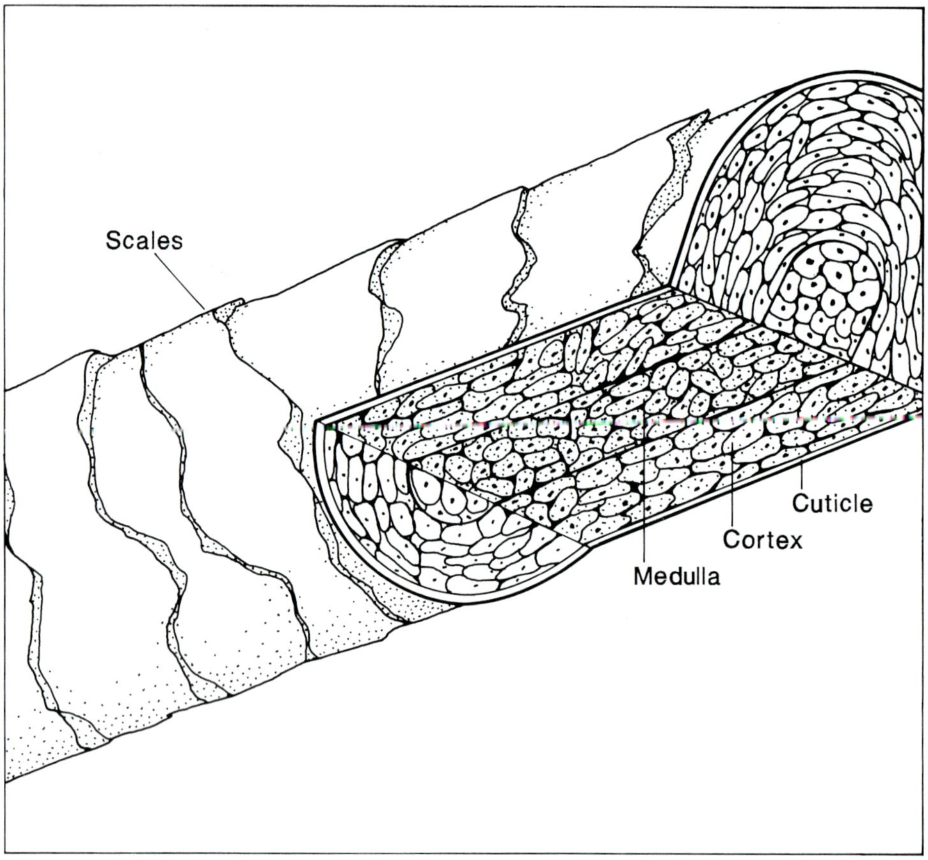

Figure 16-1 The hair shaft.

like cells overlap in a proximal-to-distal direction along the hair shaft. When the cuticle is intact, the scales are smooth, reflect light, and provide a shiny, healthy look to the hair.

HAIR PHYSIOLOGY

Having briefly described the anatomy of the hair shaft, let us proceed to its physiology. The three major characteristics of the hair shaft that affect its function and appearance are porosity, elasticity, and texture.

Porosity

The porosity of the hair is its ability to absorb moisture. In a normal hair shaft with no cuticular damage, only a minimal amount of water or other substances can penetrate through the cuticle into the cortex. When permanent wave or color reactions take place in the cortex, they do so because the cuticle has been rendered vulnerable or open. By increasing the temperature or by changing the pH of the environment around the shaft, the scales of the cuticle are separated and chemicals are allowed inside the cortex. When the processing of hair is finished, these cuticular scales gradually close again. If the hair is processed too many times, the cuticle never quite returns to its original tightness and the barrier becomes imperfect. Figure 16-2 is a diagrammatic representation of the porosity of the hair shaft.

Hair that is overporous is dry, contains split ends, fractures easily, and feels gummy or spongy when wet. Besides chemical processing, other methods that damage the cuticle, such as blow-drying, wind, sun, and curling irons, can also become factors in the porosity of hair. If the cuticle becomes damaged, the shaft swells with water whenever the hair is washed. Repeated expansion and contraction of the hair shaft gradually weakens it.

Some hair is resistant to the chemicals needed to open and close the cuticular cells. This resistance is usually genetic. In these cases, stronger chemicals are often needed to effect cosmetic

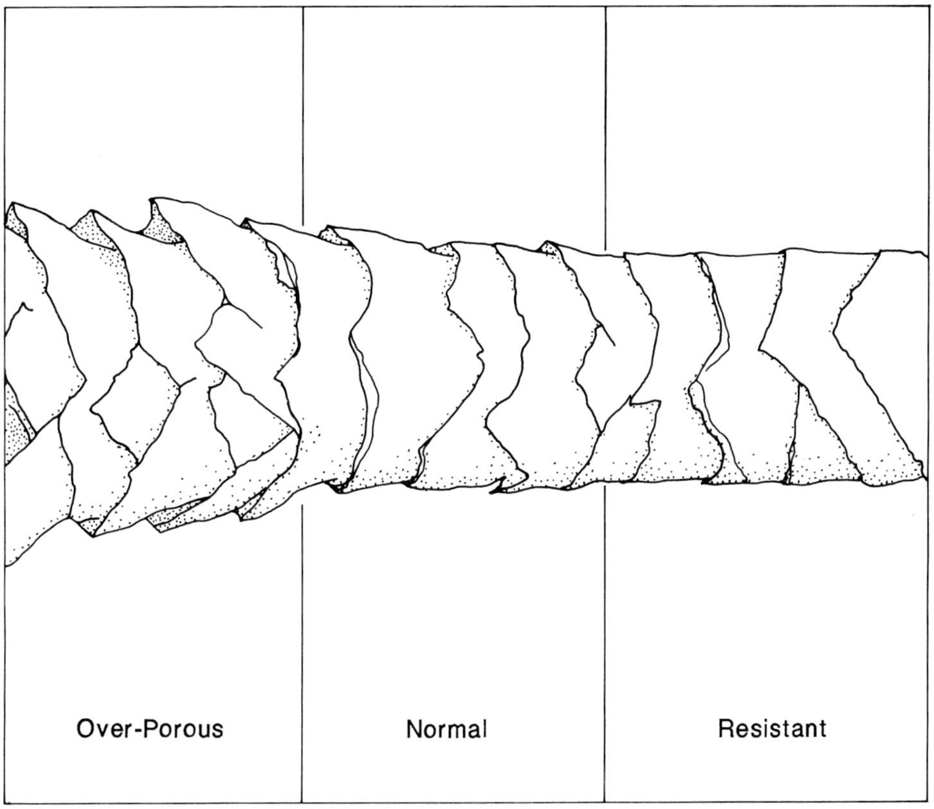

Figure 16-2 Porosity of the hair shaft.

changes, but these may lead to breakage of the hair shaft.

Elasticity

The second major characteristic of the hair shaft is its elasticity. Elasticity, or the measure of the tensile strength of the hair, can be quantitated by either stretching or assessing the weight it can support. Healthy hair can stretch to $1^1/_3$ times its original length when wet and return to its original length when dry.[3] Dry hair can usually support a 100-g weight without breaking.

Hair passes through three phases while being extended under increasing force (Fig. 16-3). The first phase,[2] the *elastic region,* is characterized by reversible extension. The second phase is characterized by a partially reversible transformation; this phase is known as the *yield region.* The third phase is the *postyield region* or *breaking point.* Manufacturers of hair cosmetics and sunscreens use these qualities of the hair shaft to evaluate their products.

Hair with poor elasticity will have no curl, will break easily when groomed, and will be unable to withstand the routine permanent wave solutions. The tensile strength is dependent upon a healthy cortex which, in turn, is dependent upon protection by a healthy cuticle.

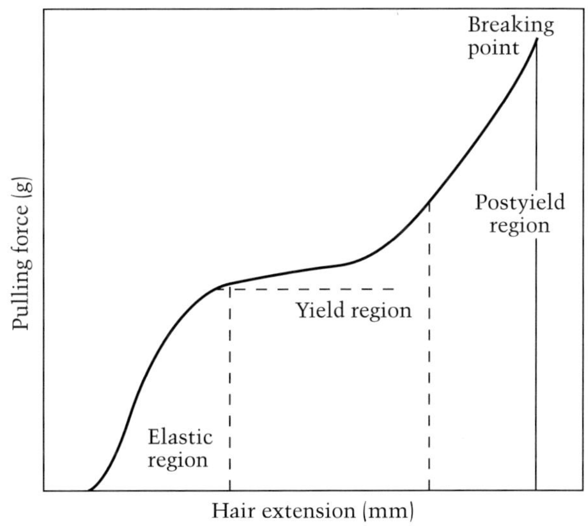

Figure 16-3 Typical stress-strain curve of single hair fiber as obtained with an Instrom tensile strength tester.

Texture

The third major characteristic of hair is its texture. Texture is dependent on two factors: (1) the diameter of the individual hair fiber, which affects its degree of coarseness or fineness, and (2) the feel of the hair, whether harsh, soft, or wiry. If hair is fine, it may process quickly or break off, simply because the chemicals are too strong for it. If hair is wiry, the cuticular scales lie flat and firm next to the cortex and may be resistant to chemical changes. Texture is a major factor in the wooly hair syndrome, spun-glass syndrome, and many of the aminoaciduria syndromes.

Permeability

These three major characteristics of the hair shaft—porosity, elasticity, and texture—will affect the overall permeability of hair to chemicals. Texture and porosity are judged together in determining the processing time. Although porosity is more significant, texture is also important. Fine hair, having a small diameter, will become saturated with waving lotion more quickly than hair with a large diameter if both are equally porous. Coarse hair that is very porous, however, will process faster than fine hair that is not porous. The hair texture will also contribute to its elasticity. The stronger the hair shaft, the greater its elasticity.

As physicians, we may be asked to advise patients on the possibility of processing their hair. My usual advice is to have the patient locate a cosmetician who is capable of working with people with unusual or difficult-to-manage hair. This may be someone in one of the major cosmetic companies in New York, or it may be a technician near the patient's home. He or she should first apply a test dose of color or permanent solution to the hair at the base of the occiput. This area is selected because if an adverse reaction occurs, it can be concealed. If the test hairs are processed without complications, then the technician can proceed to treat the entire scalp a week or so later.

SHAMPOO

The major hair care product used by patients is shampoo. Shampoos have undergone a metamorphosis from agents which were simply products to remove sebum, perspiration, environmental dirt, and desquamated stratum corneum to agents which cleanse, beautify, and thicken hair. There are many types of shampoos; their characteristics are outlined below.

Soap Shampoo

Soap shampoo is the original hair cleanser. It consists of an alkali such as sodium hydroxide or an alkanolamine, plus oil, plus the salts of fatty acids. The type of oil used to compound a shampoo may be vegetable, almond, peanut, coconut, olive, castor, or palm nut. Fats that may be used are animal fats, lanolin, tallow, or synthetic fats. The advantages of a soap shampoo are that it cleans the hair and is very inexpensive. The major disadvantage of soap shampoo is that it forms a scum precipitate on the hair shaft in hard water because of the calcium, magnesium, and iron salts in the water. Since hard water is universal, soap shampoos are used infrequently today.

Detergent Shampoo

Since many people live in areas with hard water, new formulations of shampoo using sulfonated oil started to become popular in the 1950s. These shampoos consist of three major components: (1) principal surfactants for detergency and foaming power, (2) secondary surfactants to improve and condition the hair, and (3) additives which complete the formulation and add special effects. The surfactants or detergents act by removing the dirt from the hair with a lipophilic component and transferring it to the rinse water with a hydrophilic component. The three types of surfactants or detergents found in shampoos are anionic, nonionic, and amphoteric.

ANIONIC SURFACTANTS

The principal surfactants in detergent shampoos are the anionic substances. These are named for their negatively charged hydrophilic components and are made from alcohol obtained from the fatty acid of coconut and palm leaves. Sodium lauryl sulfate and ammonium lauryl sulfate have the strongest cleaning and lathering qualities. These occasionally can be too strong and irritating. This could be because of the pH, or because there is too much detergent action on the hair, which causes too much sebum to be removed.

Triethanolamine (TEA) salts of alkyl sulfates

are more easily tolerated and are usually mixed with the stronger surfactants. Two other anionic detergents are sarcosines and sulfosuccinates. The sarcosines clean poorly but leave the hair in good condition. The sulfosuccinates are strong degreasers but leave the hair in poor condition.[4] The laureth sulfates are less irritating than the lauryl sulfates and contribute more to the shine of the hair. In order for an ingredient to leave the hair shinier, it must leave more sebum on the hair shaft.

NONIONIC SURFACTANTS

Some of the nonionic surfactants are ethoxylated fatty alcohols, ethoxylated alkyl phenols, ethoxylated fatty amines, and ethoxylated fatty amides. These compounds condition the hair and perform gentle cleansing. These substances can increase the quality of lather in a shampoo, as well as its viscosity and solubility. Sorbitol esters (known as Tweens) are very good emulsifiers and solubilizers. These are mild compounds and do not irritate or sting.[5] Other nonionic surfactants are polyglyceryl ether and amine oxide. All of these surfactants can be added to attenuate the harshness or improve the antistatic qualities of a shampoo.

AMPHOTERIC SURFACTANTS

Amphoteric surfactants contain a balance of positive and negative charges. They are very gentle cleansers and the major components of baby shampoos. They condition the hair but do not overly clean it. They are also nonirritating to the eyes. Examples of these surfactants are N-alkylamino acids, betaines, and alkyl imidazoline compounds.

OTHER ADDITIVES

As noted earlier, the first two components of a detergent shampoo—primary and secondary surfactants—are made up of the strong anionic surfactants tempered by some of the milder anionic surfactants, the nonionic surfactants, and the amphoteric surfactants. The third component of the detergent shampoos consists of other additives. These additives serve to beautify and thicken the hair; sequester heavy metals; keep the shampoo free of bacteria; give aesthetic qualities; and treat seborrheic dermatitis, psoriasis, and eczema.

BEAUTIFIERS

Hydrolyzed animal proteins are used in shampoo to repair split ends or damage to the cuticle. These proteins are attached to the damaged hair by electric charges. These will be discussed later when conditioners are addressed.

THICKENERS

Sodium chloride is probably the most common thickener used to give shampoo products more viscosity. Other thickeners are natural gum (karaya, tragacanth), alginates, cellulose derivatives, and carboxyvinyl polymers.

SEQUESTERING AGENTS

Polyphosphates and ethylenediaminetetra acetic acid keep calcium, iron, and magnesium salts from precipitating on the hair shaft.

PRESERVATIVES

Because of the water content in shampoos, preservatives are absolutely necessary to prevent infection, especially around the eyes and ears. Formaldehyde, formaldehyde donors (e.g., Dowicil 200), parabens, Bronidox, and methyl chloroisothiazolinones (Kathon CG) are common preservatives in shampoos. Contact dermatitis is caused less frequently by formaldehyde in shampoos than by that in other cosmetics because the shampoo is rinsed off quickly. If a patient is exquisitely sensitive to formaldehyde, however, shampoos must be selected carefully.

In beauty salons, shampoos are usually purchased in a concentrated form, and water (without antibacterial agents) is added at the salon. Fainstein et al.[6] reported the induction of *Pseudomonas* infections in two leukemic patients who went to the same salon within one week. Physicians should advise patients who are neutropenic to bring their own bottled shampoo with them if they go to a salon for procedures. The preservatives in individually purchased bottles of shampoo are usually sufficient to protect the patient from infection.

When advising beauty salons on how to prevent such infections, there are four recommendations: (1) All solutions should be mixed fresh each day, with unused solutions discarded at the end of the day; (2) containers for diluted products should be widemouthed and easy to clean; (3) the containers should be washed, rinsed, and dried at least once during the day; (4) the containers should be rinsed with 70% alcohol and allowed to dry at the end of each day.

AESTHETIC ADDITIVES

Color and fragrance are two aesthetic additives which can cause an allergic reaction. Fragrance of any kind and preservatives head the list of ingredients from the North American Contact Dermatitis Society that can cause allergic reactions to cosmetics.[7]

ANTISEBORRHEIC, ANTIPSORIATIC, AND OTHER THERAPEUTIC ADDITIVES

The major therapeutic compounds added to detergent shampoos are tar, selenium disulfide, zinc pyrithione, salicylic acid, sulfur, and ketoconazole. The first five additives act by decreasing mitoses[8] and, thus, corneocyte count. A group from the University of Pennsylvania has demonstrated quite adequately that there is increased epidermal cell turnover in seborrheic dermatitis.[9] They liken seborrheic dermatitis to a forme fruste of psoriasis. When an antiseborrheic shampoo is used at least every 4 days, the corneocyte count (which is elevated in seborrheic dermatitis) is kept at a normal range. Because all of the ingredients (e.g., zinc pyrithione, tar, salicylic acid) can be added to any basic shampoo formulation, there is no need to think that a dandruff shampoo by definition needs to be harsh on the hair. Of all the antiseborrheic ingredients, zinc pyrithione seems to be the least damaging to the hair shaft. Selenium sulfide is probably the most effective ingredient, however.[9] There are many excellent formulations which can control seborrheic dermatitis and psoriasis and beautify the hair at the same time.

For the school of dermatologists who believe *Pityrosporon ovale* plays a part in seborrhea, ketoconazole (Nizoral) shampoo is a good alternative.

Shampoos for Different Hair Types

A shampoo formulated for oily hair generally consists of a greater fraction of a strong anionic detergent and a lesser fraction of conditioning properties. A shampoo for dry hair usually has some of the weaker anionic surfactants, which are less effective cleansers. Shampoos for limp or fine hair contain fewer conditioners because they will inhibit curling or fluffing. These latter shampoos contain, instead, more protein additives to give the hair extra body. Permed or damaged hair needs amphoteric surfactants or nonionic surfactants to preserve the cuticle because damaged hair has little nicks in the cuticle; anionic surfactants may enlarge those nicks or breaks in the continuity of the cuticle, thus causing the hair shaft to break or split.

In the formulations of all these shampoos, there needs to be a balance between strong cleansing and more electrical charge, and less cleansing but more manageable hair.

CONDITIONERS

Conditioners, or substances which increase the manageability and shine of the hair, can be divided into four major categories: rinses, cationic detergent conditioners, film-forming conditioners, and protein-based conditioners.

Rinses

The earliest substances used to promote the manageability and shine of hair needed to combat the soap film left on the hair after shampooing. The chief substances used were vinegar and lemon. These had a low pH which balanced the high pH of soap and soap shampoos. Usually $^1/_4$ cup of vinegar to $^3/_4$ cup of water was adequate to neutralize the soap film.

The next available types of rinses were those containing wax and paraffin. These substances coated the cuticle and allowed each strand of hair to lie next to the other without static cling. Balsam, an exudate from birch trees, was the best ingredient in this category.

Cationic Detergent Conditioners

Quaternary ammonium compounds, specifically stearalkonium ammonium chloride, have been used since the 1950s to improve the manageability and shine of the hair. This substance is "highly substantive to keratin fibers, normally positively charged because of the negative charge of the fatty portion of its molecule. When acidic cationic solutions are passed through the hair, a fatty shiny layer of such materials is deposited, and many hair problems are promptly solved."[10] These products are needed by people who process their hair with color or permanent waves. Cationic detergents can be damaging to the eye, so an appropriate concentration must be used, and careful application of such products on children's hair is important.

Film-Forming Conditioners

Some of the polymers, such as polyvinylpyrrolidone (PVP), Polymer J.R. (Union Carbide), and others, can be attached to the quaternary ammonium compounds. These conditioners add body, or viscosity, and shine to the hair and also prevent tangling. They attach to the hair shaft where the cuticle is damaged, because of the negative charge on the shaft where the cuticle is broken. Occasionally, if these conditioners are used for too long a period, a buildup of protein can occur on the hair shaft. The hair can be "stripped" of this buildup with a good anionic detergent shampoo.

Protein-Based Conditioners

Protein-based conditioners are the most popular type of conditioner because of their ability to penetrate the hair shaft. When hair has just been processed—with color, permanent wave solution, or heat—the cuticular cells are still slightly separated. Amino acids and small polypeptide fragments of hydrolyzed protein become linked within the keratin of damaged hair shafts and can mend cuticular breaks and split ends. Some of the sources for these proteins are animal proteins, eggs, placenta, collagen, and keratin.

All of these conditioners can be applied after the shampoo as a quick rinse or under a heated plastic cap for 20 minutes. The heat allows the cuticular scales to open, thereby allowing the protein to enter the cortex. The heat can be supplied by a hair dryer, or it may be solely from the person's own body heat, which increases locally while under the plastic cap. Adding the heat to a conditioner does enhance its efficacy and does not harm the hair. In the experience of most cosmetic chemists, two steps—shampoo plus conditioner—are usually superior to the single step of using a product containing both conditioner and shampoo. Because the ingredients may cancel each other out, the combination product neither cleans nor conditions the hair well enough.

STYLING AIDS

Styling aids are products which serve to keep the hair in place, allow for unusual hairstyles, and waterproof the hair.

Styling Lotions and Gels

Styling lotions are applied to towel-dried or dry hair prior to the use of a blow dryer, curlers, or hairpins. These substances usually contain water, copolymers, PVP, some quaternium salts, and fragrance. These products have a thin consistency but may add body to the hair.

Styling gels are usually thicker and contain more polymers and hydrolyzed animal protein. The gels are used for stiffer hair arrangements such as making the hair stand up straight on the head, defying the laws of gravity. Because these are so substantive to the hair, users generally shampoo their hair daily to avoid unattractive buildup.

Mousses

Mousses are foaming hairstyling aids. They, too, contain copolymers to style the hair but are not as heavy as gels. Often they are used to supply a "wet" look to the hair.

Mousses, if allowed to cake around the hairline, may contribute to a type of pomade acne. If the ingredients are confined to humectants such as propylene glycol, panthenol, and glycerin, acneiform eruptions can be prevented.

Hair Spray

The old formulas for hair spray contained shellac, synthetic resins, parabens, karaya gum, lanolin, gum acacia, and gum tragacanth. These substances were very hard to remove from the hair and have been replaced with modern formulations. These new formulations contain "plasticizers, humectants, solvents, conditioners, and fragrance. The copolymer concentration in the spray determines the amount of hold, and styling fixes and spritzes generally have a stronger hold than do hair sprays."[4] There is a certain amount of alcohol in all the formulations of hair spray, and this may dry out the cuticle. Most sprays are now formulated with an air-pump dispenser rather than an aerosol spray; these eliminate the fluorocarbons, which can damage the earth's ozone layer.

Finally, vinyl acetate can be added to waterproof the hair. This eliminates the sagging and drooping of a hairstyle if the person is perspiring or is caught in a minor rain shower. Vinyl acetate decreases the hygroscopic nature of PVP but makes the product more difficult to shampoo off of the hair.

PERMANENT WAVES AND RELAXERS

There are three types of naturally occurring wave patterns to hair—straight, wavy, and kinky (Fig. 16-4). These patterns are genetically inherited and can be changed by breaking the disulfide bonds. Straight hair, which is almost perfectly round in cross section, is the prototype of Oriental hair. Wavy hair, with its mild tendency to curl, is oval in cross section and is most typical of Caucasian hair. Kinky hair, with its tendency to break easily and curl tightly, is the prototype of Negroid hair.

Disulfide bonds can be broken and reshaped with heat and chemicals. The first permanent wave machine was invented by Charles Nessler in 1905.[5] This procedure reshaped the hair with very high heat, but the hair was often broken in the process.

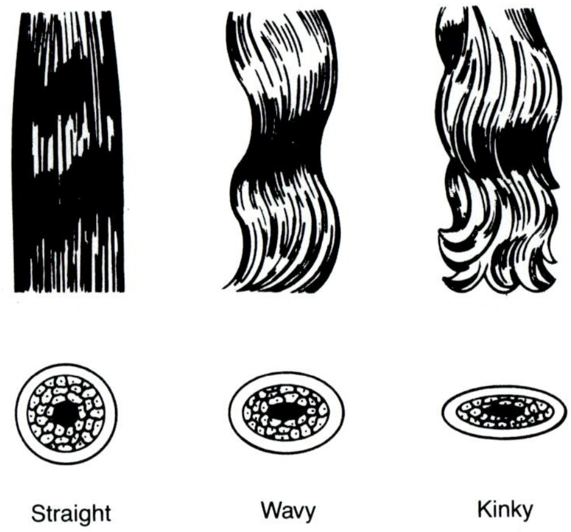

Figure 16-4 Wave patterns in hair. *(Reprinted with permission from O'Donoghue MN: Hair Cosmetics. Dermatol Clin 5 (3): 619–626,1987.)*

Mercaptan Permanent Waves

The next two types of permanent waves, the base and acid perms, are the most popular types used today.[11] Thiol compounds are used in either a base pH or an acid pH to change the shape of the hair. The prototype chemical reaction is as shown in Figure 16-5.

BASE PERMANENTS

In the 1930s, a cold wave process was invented. A solution of ammonium thioglycolate was applied to the hair, the disulfide bonds were broken, and the substance was neutralized with hydrogen peroxide, sodium perborate, or sodium or potassium bromate. The mechanics of a permanent wave are these: (1) The hair is shampooed to permit water to enter the hydrogen bonds within the hair shaft to allow flexibility; (2) the hair is then wrapped over rods or curlers; (3) the hair is saturated with ammonium thioglycolate; (4) after 5 to 20 minutes, the hair becomes limp, is neutralized, and hardens into the new shape around the rollers. Every time a permanent wave is performed, some of the disulfide bonds do not

K-S-S-K	+	2 R-SH	⟶	2K-SH	+	R-S-S-R
Keratin		Thiol compound (mercaptan)		Reduced keratin		Disulfide of thiol compound
2 K-SH	+	Oxidizing agent	⟶	K-S-S-K	+	H_20
				Reconstituted keratin		

Figure 16-5 Prototypical chemical reaction of thiol compounds in permanent waves. (Adapted from Zviak C: *Permanent waving and hair straightening. In Zviak C (ed):* The Science of Hair Care. *New York, Marcel Dekker,* 1986, p. 189.)

reform. For this reason, hair that has had a permanent wave applied or has been processed might not be as strong, resilient, or elastic as untreated hair. The cuticular scales do not always go back tightly in place, thus leaving the hair a little more porous with each procedure.

The ammonium thioglycolate permanent is highly successful. It has the following advantages: (1) it curls the hair very tightly, (2) it produces a curl that lasts at least 3 to 5 months, and (3) it can be used safely at home.

ACID PERMANENTS

Because men and women color, blow-dry, and frequently shampoo their hair, a more gentle permanent wave product was needed. In 1970, an acid-based glycerol monothioglycolate (GMTG) permanent wave was invented. Glycerol monothioglycolate, because of its lower pH, is less harmful to the cuticle than ammonium thioglycolate: the cuticular scales are separated to a lesser degree with a lower pH and are more likely to return to the original state after treatment. People who used to have frizzy hair after a permanent wave can now have hair that is more natural-looking. The acid-based permanent is particularly advantageous to individuals who have color-processed hair.

The acid-based permanent requires heat to activate it. This can be accomplished with a hair dryer or a plastic bag placed over the curlers. The mechanics of this permanent wave are the same as for the base perm except for a few cautions. The acid waving solution can be thioglycolic acid buffered with ammonium bicarbonate or the more common GMTG. The pH of these permanents is 7 to 8.5. These substances can cause a severe contact dermatitis if not applied carefully. The hairdresser must wear gloves, and he or she must place cotton around the edges of the rods or curlers. This cotton should be changed at least once to prevent dripping of the solution down the neck of the client.

A study was performed to evaluate the persistence of allergic contact dermatitis 3 months after a patient had received a GMTG permanent.[12] Patch testing was done with samples of the patient's treated hair. Positive reactions were seen to treated hair particles for up to 3 months after the permanent, thus explaining the persistent dermatitis. It is wise for patients with prior adverse reactions to permanent wave solutions to have a small patch test performed with treated hair 1 week before the entire head is permed, in order to detect an allergic reaction. A 1% ammonium thioglycolate or GMTG solution in petrolatum can be used in a patch test to document an allergy to the base or acid perm, respectively. These may be obtained from Omni Derm (8400 Darnley Rd. Montreal, Quebec, Canada H4T1M4) or from the manufacturers of the permanent wave solutions themselves.

The disadvantages of the acid perm, besides the incidence (approximately 20 percent) of contact dermatitis,[7] are that the wave is not strong enough to affect resistant hair such as Negroid hair, the curl is not as tight, and it does not last as long. An acid perm may last 2 to 3 months, whereas a base perm may last 3 to 5 months.

Relaxers

There will be an extensive discussion of these in Chapter 17, but a brief discussion of relaxers is appropriate here.

HOT COMB

The most common type of relaxation procedure involves applying an oil to the hair shaft, combing the hair shaft straight with a hot comb (300–500°F) until there is no more curl, and then optionally reshaping that hair shaft over large rollers. This procedure may be done every 2 weeks and will last until the hair is shampooed. The major disadvantage of this procedure, besides its short-lived effect, is the triggering of hot-comb alopecia. The hair can break off, and there can be true destruction of the hair follicle by the hot oil going down the shaft, especially on the top of the head.

PERMANENT WAVE RELAXERS

The two major types of relaxers are the sodium hydroxide type and the guanidine hydroxide type. The pH of the sodium hydroxide or lye type of straighteners can vary between 13 and 14. These relaxers contain up to 3% sodium hydroxide and must be applied very carefully. If the cream gets on the face or ears, severe burning occurs and the reaction must be neutralized with vinegar immediately. If the chemical is left on the hair too long, the hair shaft can break. The reason this strong solution is needed is that Negroid hair can be quite resistant to chemicals. This is a genetic trait.

Newer lye-free straightening products contain guanidine hydroxide and lithium hydroxide. These can still burn the scalp, eyes, and ears, however, and must be applied with care.

Most of the hair care products for Negroid hair combine a shampoo and a conditioner with each permanent wave. This will be further discussed in Chapter 17.

COLORING AGENTS

There are five major types of coloring agents which can be used to modify or change hair color. These include temporary color, metallic dyes, natural coloring, semipermanent dyes, and permanent dyes.

Temporary Hair Color

The easiest approach for a patient who desires either to color gray hair or to change his or her image is to use a temporary dye. These dyes became available for human use after extensive use in the textile industry. They are high-molecular-weight acidic textile dyes that are deposited on the outside of the cuticle without penetrating the hair shaft.

These products are available as rinses, gels, mousses, and sprays, and can allow for a fun or party look for people with gray or blond hair; they would probably not make a significant change in brown or red hair. These products have a low risk of irritant or allergic contact dermatitis. The major disadvantage to temporary hair color is the fact that it lasts only until the next shampoo. The dye can also get on a person's clothing when it rains and can temporarily stain the cover on a pillow.

Metallic Dyes

For a gradual color change from gray to brown or black, metallic salts can be applied to the hair. These are most commonly lead acetate and silver nitrate. The most common formula is an aqueous solution of lead acetate and glycerin with a small quantity of suspended sulfur. This mixture is applied to the hair daily and shades of brown or black gradually appear. The colorless lead salt converts to brownish oxides and sulfides. Silver dyes have a greenish cast, which may tone down brassy hair, and those containing copper dyes turn red. This change takes about 2 months and appears from a distance to look natural.

There are several disadvantages to these preparations. The metallic dyes precipitate on the outside of the cuticle, making the hair appear dull and lifeless. The smell of the sulfides on the hair can be most unpleasant. Finally, because the metals are deposited on the cuticle, the use of permanent waves or permanent color is precluded.

Natural Coloring

In the days of Cleopatra, henna from the plant *Lawsonia inermis* was used to impart red highlights to brown hair. This is the only all-natural hair coloring agent and therefore is guaranteed to be noncarcinogenic. Because of the pulmonary problems, namely asthma, and allergies related to this substance, it is rarely, if ever, used today. The *Journal of Occupational Medicine*[13] contains an excellent discussion of occupational asthma in a beautician from the use of persulfate salts and henna. This substance also turns gray hair an unsightly shade of orange. It does not, however, preclude permanent waving.

Semipermanent Dyes

To color gray hair or add highlights, low-molecular-weight dyes were specifically synthesized for hair coloring. These dyes are able to penetrate the cuticle and go into the cortex of the hair fiber because of their small size. Semipermanent dyes are available in lotions or foam and are a mixture of red, yellow, blue, and orange. Because they contain no hydrogen peroxide, they cannot lighten hair. They can give a rich, dark color to hair, however. The dyes are N-substituted nitrophenylene dimers and aminoanthraquinones.

The semipermanent dyes can last for almost six shampoos. However, just as the dye molecules are able to enter into the hair shaft, they can also diffuse out. The red molecules seem to slip out most easily, so that by the sixth shampoo the hair can be drab-looking. These dyes are quite safe and can be easily applied at home. Certainly, they are an excellent first step for a person contemplating a change of hair color.

Cellophanes are blends of primary colors with an acidic pH. These are elegant semipermanent dyes. They are elegant because of their unusual packaging in a cellophane sleeve, and they can be temporary or semipermanent depending upon how long they are left on the hair during processing. The usual function of these products is to highlight hair rather than to change the basic color.

Highlighting hair involves processing only a portion of the strands of hair. This is performed by either pulling the hair through a crocheted cap placed on the head or wrapping sections of the hair in foil. This causes a more natural appearance, since monochromatic hair can look artificial.

Permanent Color

The most common type of color used throughout the world is permanent hair color. In permanent or oxidative hair coloring, the formation of colorless molecules from their precursors occurs inside the cortex as a result of oxidation by hydrogen peroxide.

Bleaching occurs when 30 or 40 volume percent hydrogen peroxide is applied to strip the hair of all its color. This can be boosted by the addition of ammonium persulfate or potassium persulfate. Eumelanin pigments are more easily removed from the cortex than are pheomelanin pigments, which means it is harder to lighten reddish hair. Taking out all the color is the harshest of all the procedures on the hair because the bleaching process destroys more of the keratin proteins than the process of darkening the hair. Also, the hair color is lifeless after the bleaching procedure so that another chemical reaction with a new color is necessary: this is therefore referred to as a two-step process. Allergic contact dermatitis and asthmatic bronchitis have been reported following exposure to ammonium persulfate.[14]

The more typical coloring of hair is the use of 20 volume percent hydrogen peroxide with a dye precursor in an alkaline soap or synthetic surfactant solution. "Three classes of chemical reaction are required: the primary intermediates, the couplers, and the oxidant. The primary intermediates are the so-called para dyes, particularly p-phenylenediamine, p-toluenediamine, and p-aminophenol. These materials are capable of undergoing oxidation by the oxidant, normally hydrogen peroxide, to give reactive imines. The imines react rapidly with the couplers to produce indo dyes. The most frequently used couplers are *m*-phenylenediamine, 2,4-diaminophenoxyethanol, and a 1-naphthol; resorcinols; *m*-aminophenol; 1,5-dihydroxynaphthalene; and 2-hydroxy-4-aminotoluene."[15]

$$\text{p-phenylenediamine} + H_2O_2 \rightarrow \text{amines}$$
$$\text{amines} + \text{couplers} \rightarrow \text{indo dyes}$$

After the reaction, the molecules are too large to slip out through the cuticle again, so the change is permanent. This color usually does not fade unless the person has badly damaged hair, allowing molecules to escape through the broken cuticle. To keep the new color presentable, the person must color the outgrowth of hair from the scalp. This is usually necessary about every 5 or 6 weeks.

Paraphenylenediamine binds to keratin and, hence, reactions with the skin are possible. However, few reactions are seen because paraphenylenediamine has a greater affinity for the keratin in the hair fiber than in the epidermis and because there is more keratin in the hair shaft than in the epidermis. Usually the chemical reaction lasts only about 20 minutes, so unless the chemicals get on the neck or the ears, there are few problems. If there is any question, a patient should have a small area of hair tested at the base of the occiput 1 week before an all-over color is attempted.

Highlighting or coloring part of the hair can be done for people who are allergic to hair dye. The dermatologist can work with a competent cosmetician to help patients who have difficulty.

After any processing of hair—coloring or waving—a milder shampoo with an acidic pH should be used to assist the cuticle in closing. These shampoos are usually labeled as "low pH" or mild. The hairdresser should be able to recommend a specific shampoo.

Finally, the screening patch-test series for hairdressers outlined by Fisher and Adams includes all the chemicals that the dermatologist needs to evaluate a potential allergic reaction[16] (Table 16-1).

No cosmetic or cosmetic procedure should be used in or on dermatitic skin. Patients should avoid applying hair color or having a permanent wave at the time they have severe seborrheic dermatitis or scalp trauma from extensive brush-

Table 16-1
A "SCREENING" PATCH-TEST SERIES FOR HAIRDRESSERS

Bleaches	
	Ammonium persulfate 2.0% (Caution: may cause syncope)
Fragrance†	
	Fragrance mix No. 3 (standard tray)
Hair dyes*	
	O-nitro-p-phenylenediamine 1%
	P-aminophenol 1%
	P-phenylenediamine 1%
	P-toluylenediamine 1%
	Pyrogallol 1%
	Resorcinol
Metals†	
	Nickel 5% (standard tray)
Perfumes	
	Balsam of Peru 25%
Permanent waving	
	Ammonium thioglycolate 2.5%
	Glyceryl monothioglycolate 2.5%
Preservatives	
	Formaldehyde 1% aqueous
	Proteins
	Quaternium 15 (Dowicil 200)
Rubber chemicals	
	Carbamate mix
	Mercaptobenzothiazole 2%
	Thiram mix

†Standard tray.
*All these may cross-react with paraphenylenediamine except resorcinol and pyrogallol.
Note: All are tested with petrolatum except formaldehyde (1% aqueous).
Source: From Fisher and Adams.[16]

ing of the hair. They should also avoid two chemical procedures within the same week, such as coloring the hair and permanent waves; this could lead to hair breakage.

SUN, SUNSCREENS, AND HAIR

Sunlight can produce many undesirable changes in the hair shaft. These consist of dryness, reduced strength, rough surface texture, loss of color and luster, stiffness, and brittleness. Hair that has lost its luster does not reflect light. Damage to the cuticle starts the parade of problems, and damage to the cortex finishes it.

The changes that occur to brown hair color from the sun are a result of the photooxidative bleaching of the eumelanin hair pigment. The changes in blond hair are a result of photodegradation of cystine, tyrosine, and tryptophan residues, producing yellow and brown reaction products. Other amino acids broken down in blond hair are histidine, lysine, and proline. Superoxides are formed when pheomelanin is degraded by irradiation with long-wavelength ultraviolet and visible light. This sensitivity of pheomelanin explains why more color changes are noticed in blond and red hair. This often causes a brassy look in blonds.

The other mechanism of hair damage is the formation of free radicals when ultraviolet radiation is absorbed by cystine, tyrosine, phenylalanine, and tryptophan. The absorption produces free radicals and then homolytic scission of disulfide bonds, as occurs in permanent waving, resulting in damaged keratin. The tensile strength and the quality of the hair diminish after ultraviolet exposure.

The ideal sunscreen for hair must be substantive to the hair cuticle without causing loss of sheen or adding a sticky or gummy feel to the hair. This substance must be able to withstand the action of surfactants in shampoos and conditioners. Octyl-dimethyl para-aminobenzoic acid (PABA) has been found to be a good sunscreen, and it has at least some substantivity to hair.

Sergio Nacht, in his evaluation of hair sunscreens, suggests a scale termed *hair protective factor* (HPF): "A practical HPF can be determined by measuring ultraviolet damage to hair as detected by yield slope analyses of tensile strength assessments."[2] There is a fairly good correlation with loss of tensile strength and ultraviolet radiation. Nacht has chosen to arbitrarily number the products 2 through 15, with the higher number representing no damage at all to the hair tensile strength. Several strengths of a shampoo containing octyl-dimethyl PABA were tested, and the conclusions were that 0.5% to 1.0% is an appropriate concentration of octyl-dimethyl PABA for an HPF of 9.8 to 12.0. The effectiveness of these shampoos as sunscreens can be enhanced by conditioners. The conditioners can disperse the sunscreen more evenly on the shaft, and they can also have sunscreen incorporated in them. Hair that is badly damaged, however, needs the protection of a stronger sunscreen. Many shampoos and conditioners today list the sunscreen on their labels. Chemically treated hair should certainly be protected.

CONCLUDING REMARKS

As physicians we should be able to assist our patients in preserving a good self-image. With the understanding of these hair care products and the knowledge of skilled cosmeticians in our area of practice, this goal can be accomplished.

REFERENCES

1. Moschella SL, Hurley HJ: *Dermatology,* 2d ed. Philadelphia, W. B. Saunders, 1985, p 49.
2. Nacht S: Sunscreen and hair. In Lowe NJ (ed): *Physician's Guide to Sunscreens.* New York, Marcel Dekker, 1991, pp 123–136.
3. Corbett J: Coloring and bleaching. Paper presented at the International Conference on Skin Therapy and Cosmetics, Cannes, France, 1985.
4. Draelos ZK: Hair cosmetics. In O'Donoghue MN (ed): *Cosmetics and Cosmetic Surgery in Dermatology.* Dermatol Clin 9(1):19–27, 1991.
5. Predeteanu C: *The ABC's of Cosmetics.* Bloomfield Hills, MI, Institute Predete Publishing Company, 1987, p 224.
6. Fainstein V, Andres N, Umphrey J, Hopfer **R**: Hair clipping: Another hazard for granulocytopenic patients? J Infect Dis 158(3):655–656, 1988.
7. Adams RM, Maibach HI: A five-year study of cosmetic reactions. J Am Acad Dermatol 13:1062–1069, 1985.
8. Leyden JJ: Presentation to the FDA Miscellaneous Panel OTC, 1984.
9. Leyden JJ, McGinley KJ, Kligman AM: Dandruff: Pathogenesis and treatment. In Frost P, Horowitz S (eds): *Principles of Cosmetics for the Dermatologist.* St. Louis, C. V. Mosby, 1982, pp 167–172.
10. Goldemberg RL: Hair conditioners: The rationale for modern formulations. In Frost P, Horowitz S (eds): *Principles of Cosmetics for the Dermatologist.* St. Louis, C. V. Mosby, 1982, p 157.
11. Cannell DW: Permanent waving and hair straightening. Clin Dermatol 6:71, 1988.
12. Morrison LH, Storrs FJ: Persistence of an allergen in hair after glyceryl monothioglycolate-containing permanent wave solution. J Am Acad Dermatol 20(4):688–690, 1989.
13. Schwartz HJ: Effect of chronic chromolyn sodium therapy in a beautician with occupational asthma. J Occup Med 31(2):112–114, 1989.
14. Fisher AA, Dooms-Goossens A: Persulfate hair bleach reactions. Arch Dermatol 112:1407, 1976.
15. Corbett JF: Changing the color of hair. In Frost P, Horowitz S (eds): *Principles of Cosmetics for the Dermatologist.* St. Louis, C. V. Mosby, 1982, p 162.
16. Fisher AA, Adams RM: Occupational dermatitis. In Fisher AA (ed): *Contact Dermatitis,* 3d ed. Philadelphia, Lea & Febiger, 1986, p 511.

Chapter

17

DISORDERS OF HAIR GROWTH IN AFRICAN AMERICANS

Wesley S. Wilborn

INTRODUCTION

When referring to individuals as African American, one must realize that he or she is referring to a very heterogeneous group of individuals. During the author's lifetime, he has seen this designation change from colored, to Negro, to black, and in 1992, to African American. African Americans may be uniracial, biracial, or multiracial. Very few are of pure African Negroid descent, but rather are mostly of African European ancestry. For the purposes of this writing, hair in African Americans will be defined as cranial and facial hair that has more African Negroid than Caucasoid or Mongoloid characteristics.

RACIAL VARIATIONS IN HAIR

Morphologically, hair is classified along racial lines, although phenotypic variation may occur within groups. Mongoloid or Oriental hair is straight, round in cross section, and greater in diameter than the hair of other population groups. Caucasoid hair is usually straight, wavy, or helical, and round to oval in cross section. Negroid hair is tightly coiled, helical, or spiraled, and elliptic or flattened in cross section[1,2] (Fig. 17-1). Hair in African Americans may exhibit characteristics of all three population groups.

Despite the obvious differences in phenotype, there are few biochemical differences found to date that explain the differences between the hair of different racial groups in general. There have been no significant differences in the amino acid composition of hair in the Caucasoid, Negroid, and Mongoloid races,[3,4] but this does not imply amino acid homology. The most commonly used method for keratin fiber analysis uses hydrochloric acid; this method degrades tryptophan and partially decomposes cystine, threonine, tyrosine, phenylalanine, and arginine during the process.[5,6] There are no significant differences between groups in low-sulfur protein

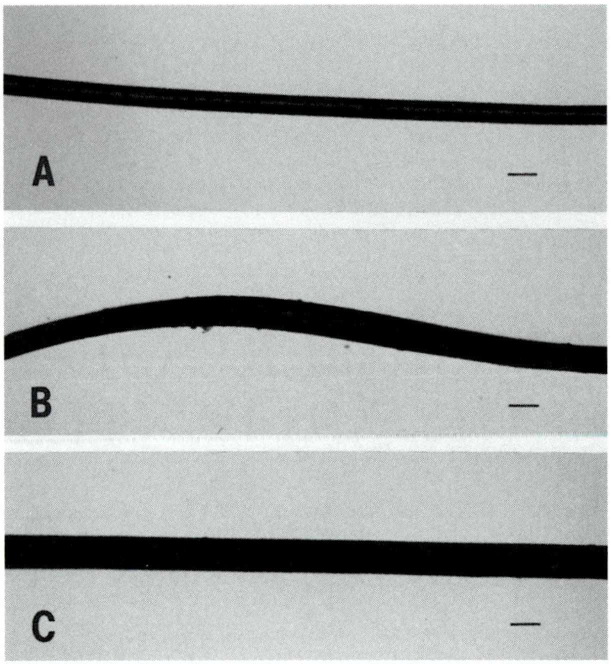

Figure 17-1 Racial variations in hair (light micrographs). (*A*) White male: slightly curved, medium-thickness hair shaft. (*B*) Black male: ribbonlike, slightly flattened, medium-thickness hair shaft. (*C*) Asiatic male: straight, thick hair shaft. (Scale bars = 100 μm) (Courtesy of Dr. A. P. Bertolino).

composition by two-dimensional electrophoresis,[7] acrylamide gel electrophoresis, stress-strain, or x-ray diffraction analysis.[3] Deiko and Jidoi, however, looked at the differential centrifugation of S-carboxymethylated (SCM) fibrous protein derivatives vs. SCM matrix protein derivatives.[6] Solubilization by S-carboxymethylation breaks disulfide bonds by reduction into low-sulfur and high-sulfur groups with the high-sulfur proteins predominantly in the matrix and low-sulfur proteins in filamentous proteins.[6] Negroid hair has a lower ratio of SCM fibrous protein to SCM matrix protein (0.18 ± 0.02) than Mongoloid hair (0.45 ± 0.03) or Caucasoid hair (0.29 ± 0.02).[8] Thus, the differential expression of low-sulfur protein to high-sulfur protein may be involved in phenotypic racial variations.

The excessive curliness or crimping of Negroid hair is somewhat analogous to wool. The crimping of wool fibers has been related to the physical arrangement of ortho- and paracortical cells in the hair cortex, but this has not been substantiated in human hair.[9]

A better understanding of the Negroid hair follicle has been gained through the work of Lindelof, Forslind, Hedblad, and Kareus,[10] who have shown that the piliary canal in African Americans is actually spiraled in shape. Utilizing a computer to obtain a three-dimensional reconstruction of hair follicle morphology, they showed that the shape of the hair conformed to the shape of the follicle in all three major racial hair types. The physical characteristics of shape and degree of kink and curl, then, are probably reflections of cross-links in the cortex that develop during the molding of the hair shaft.

Negroid hair is typically very dry, and the cuticle weathers more readily than that of other racial hair phenotypes.[11] Most published data suggest that Negroids produce more sebum than Caucasians, and that most of the hair lipids are derived from the scalp lipids.[7,12] However, because of the extreme curliness of Negroid hair, the natural oils may not be distributed along the shaft. Negroid hair responds differently than Caucasian hair to certain oils such as lecithin, soybean oil, wheat germ oil, peanut oil, linolenic acid, phospholipid complexes, and several other plant oils (W. Wilborn, unpublished data). Negroid hair tends to become even curlier and drier when these agents are applied.

HAIR GROOMING IN AFRICAN AMERICANS

Hairstyles

If one has ever tried to comb tightly coiled Negroid hair, then one can certainly understand why most African Americans use some type of product or appliance to assist in grooming their hair. The choice of product depends on the desired hairstyle, which often is dictated by current trends. Currently, chemical restructuring agents are predominantly used by African American women and not by African American men or preadolescent children. African American men usually keep their hair trimmed to a particular length: currently, the close-cut sides with the back cut progressively shorter from top to bottom (commonly referred to as a "fade"; Fig. 17-2), and very short sides with a high, square-top "box" are most popular. Many men prefer to keep all of the cranial hair closely cut. In females and children, chemically unaltered hair is usually styled in one of the following ways: a nat-

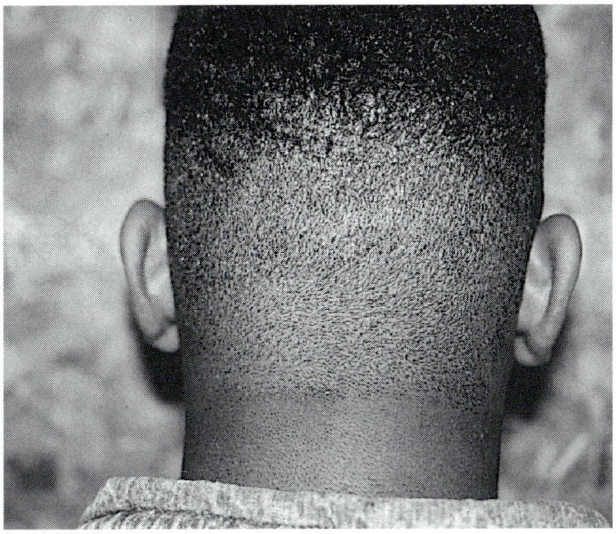

Figure 17-2 The "fade." Popular hairstyle among young African American males. Note progressively shorter cut from vertex to nape of neck.

ural, or "fro," ponytail and/or braids, or cornrow braids.

Very few African American females wear a natural, or fro, style at present. With this style, the hair must be kept less than 4 to 5 inches in length to allow for ease of grooming. Moisturizers are generally used, and, depending on the phenotype of the hair, activators or pomades may also be used to aid in combing and conditioning.

With ponytails or braids, the hair is pulled back tightly into one mass and either braided or held together by rubber bands or elastic band ornaments, or it is parted into two or more sections and usually braided on the ends. The braided ends may also be reinforced by rubber bands or elastic band ornaments. The hair is usually most taut at the temples. The frontal area is often styled in bangs: this hair is sometimes "hot-pressed," or chemically relaxed (straightened). This style is currently used most often by young African American females.

Figure 17-3 Cornrow braids. The hair is braided in rows very close to each other with considerable tension on the roots. Note decorative ornaments.

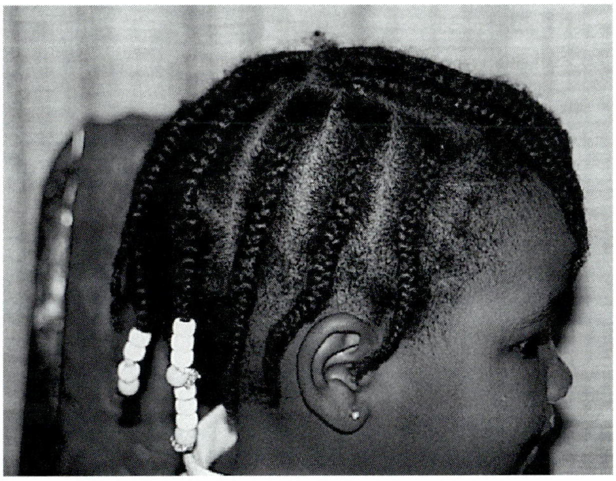

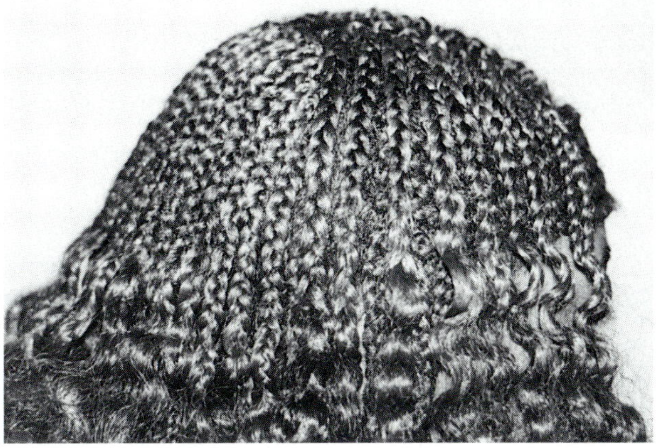

Figure 17-4 Cornrow braiding with synthetic extensions. This style is frequently used to give hair a respite from hair restructuring agents.

Cornrows begin the hair braiding as close to the scalp as possible. Barrettes and small comb ornaments are often attached to the hair (Fig. 17-3). This style requires less upkeep and can be left in place for 1 or more weeks. Synthetic extensions to add length are braided onto the natural hair at times (Fig. 17-4).

HAIR GROOMING PRODUCTS

Shampoos

Too-frequent shampooing of Negroid hair will result in excessive dryness and brittleness unless the hair is adequately remoisturized after each shampoo. Shampoos that contain anoinic agents are particularly drying to the hair: an example is sodium lauryl sulfate.[13] The sodium laureth sulfate–containing shampoos are not as harsh, but Negroid hair needs shampoos that contain humectants and milder cleansing agents, such as amphoteric and nonionic blends (Table 17-1). Antidandruff and antiseborrheic shampoos are

Table 17-1
HAIR GROOMING PRODUCTS FOR AFRICAN-AMERICAN HAIR

Uses of Product	*Brand Name*	*Manufacturer*
Dry brittle hair, natural or curly perm, hot-pressed or chemically relaxed hair	Back Alive Moisturizing Shampoo	Essence of Quality, Atlanta, GA
	Back Alive Curl Shampoo	Essence of Quality, Atlanta, GA
	Optimum Care Moisture Shampoo	Soft Sheen Products, Chicago, IL
Hard-to-comb hair, any style	Creme of Nature Shampoo	Roux Laboratories, Jacksonville, FL
	Back Alive Curl Shampoo	Essence of Quality, Atlanta, GA
Chemically relaxed hair	Optimum Care	Soft Sheen Products, Chicago, IL
	Mizani	Soft Sheen Products, Chicago, IL
	Nexus	Nexus Products, Santa Barbara, CA
Split ends; hair chemically damaged from relaxers	Nexus	Nexus Products, Santa Barbara, CA
	Optimum Care	Soft Sheen Products, Chicago, IL
	Mizani	Soft Sheen Products, Chicago, IL
Unusually dry hair with breakage from chemicals and dyes	Back Alive Curl Revitalizer	Essence of Quality, Atlanta, GA
	Moisture Max	Lustrasilk, Minneapolis, MN
	Luster's Pink Lotion	Luster Products, Chicago, IL
	Nexus Humectress	Nexus Products, Santa Barbara, CA
	Optimum Care	Soft Sheen Products, Chicago, IL
	Mizani	Soft Sheen Products, Chicago, IL
	Carefree Gold	Soft Sheen Products, Chicago, IL
	Cholesterol	Any brand
	Preset (Rodding Cream)	Essence of Quality, Atlanta, GA
For those with seborrheic dermatitis; free of lanolin and other contributing agents	Murray's Superior Hair Dressing	Murray's Superior Hair Products, Detroit, MI
	White petrolatum	Multiple Manufacturers
	Back Alive Line	Essence of Quality, Atlanta, GA
	Curl Revitalizer	
	Instant Moisturizer	
	Gel Curl Activator	
	Jojoba oil	Any brand
	Mineral oil	Any brand

especially harsh on Negroid hair: selenium sulfide shampoos, in particular, make the hair very dry and brittle. If there are no alternatives to using these medicated shampoos, then it is best to at least limit their use to the scalp and to shampoo the hair with a milder agent followed by an effective moisturizer.

Oils and Pomades

African Americans often employ some type of heavy emollient or oil to assist in grooming their hair or to treat a dry, scaly scalp. Castor oil, wheat germ oil, olive oil, and mineral oil are some of the most popular oils used (Table 17-2). Of this group, only mineral oil will not aggravate an underlying seborrheic dermatitis. Jojoba oil and its synthetic counterpart, oleyl erucate, do not appear to aggravate dandruff or seborrheic dermatitis and, in fact, may actually help to alleviate them (W. Wilborn, unpublished data).

A *pomade* was originally defined as the residual fatty material from the enfleurage process of extracting floral odors.[13] Pomades sold today consist primarily of petrolatum, lanolin, mineral oil, olive oil, and perfume, whereas solid *brilliantines* are vegetable or mineral oils stiffened with waxes.[13] Various combinations of these ingredients can be found in commercial products, along with vitamins, aloe vera, isopropyl myristate, ethoxylated glycols, and other plant oils. Both of these agents coat the hair, thereby reducing the static electric charges between the hairs and allowing for ease of combing and styling.

Table 17-2
OILS AND POMADES

Ingredients	*Products Containing*	*Manufacturer*
Petrolatum, mineral oil, fragrance	Murray's Superior Hair Dressing Pomade	Murray's Superior Hair Products, Detroit, MI
Petrolatum, olive oil, fragrance	Royal Crown Hair Dress	J. Strickland Co., Memphis, TN
Petrolatum, mineral oil, lanolin, fragrance	Dax—Wave and Groom Hair Dress	Imperial Dax Co., Fairfield, NJ
Petrolatum, lanolin, lecithin, mineral oil, fragrances, D&C green No. 6, D&C violet No. 2	Blue Magic Conditioner Hair Dress	J. Strickland Co., Memphis, TN
Petrolatum, coconut oil, castor oil, mineral oil, fragrance	Dax—Short and Neat	Imperial Dax Co., Fairfield, NJ
Petrolatum, lanolin, mineral oil, fragrance, D&C green No. 6, D&C violet No. 2	Blue Magic Pressing Oil	J. Strickland Co., Memphis, TN
Petrolatum, lanolin, olive oil, lecithin, fragrances, isopropyl myristate, D&C yellow No. 11, D&C green No. 6	Blue Magic Bergamot Hair and Scalp Conditioner Queen Bergamot Hair and Scalp Conditioner	J. Strickland Co., Memphis, Tn Beauty Creations, Memphis, TN
Petrolatum, mineral oil, lanolin, aluminum stearate, microcrystalline wax, fragrance, lauric acid, propylparaben, D&C green No. 6	Ultra Sheen Conditioner and Hair Dress	Johnson Products Co., Chicago, IL
Petrolatum, water, glycerin, ceteth-20, propylene glycol, polysorbate-60, mineral oil, oleth-5, paraffin, hydroxylated lanolin, oleth-10, fragrance, methylparaben, propylparaben	Sporting Waves Gel Pomade with Navistrol III	Soft Sheen Products, Chicago, IL
Water, mineral oil, lanolin derivatives, beeswax, petrolatum, borax, pathenol, sorbitan monoleate, octyl dimethyl PABA, preservatives, fragrance, FD&C red No. 31	Luster's Pink Oil Moisturizer Hair Lotion Plus Vitamins and Sunscreen	Luster Products, Chicago, IL
Petrolatum, mineral oil, lanolin, paraffin, Peg-8 dilaurate, isopropyl myristate, wheat germ oil, dicetylydimonium chloride, fragrance, quarternium-33, ethyl hexenediol, tocopherol, isostearyl hydrolyzed animal protein, microcrystalline wax, ergocalciferol, corn oil, BHA, butyl paraben	TCB Hair Food Daily Intensive Hair Lubricant	Alberto Culver, USA, Melrose Park, IL

They also are used to keep the hair in place by plastering it down.

Some pomades or brilliantines contain ingredients that may induce acne or folliculitis or aggravate seborrheic dermatitis.[14] Lanolin, castor oil, wheat germ oil, and soybean oil are the main culprits. Contrary to other published reports, unadulterated petrolatum and mineral oil do not appear to cause these problems, and glycerin, propylene glycol, jojoba oil, or oleyl erucate are also safe alternatives (W. Wilborn, unpublished data; Table 17-1). Avoidance of causative agents is the best method of controlling these problems.

Moisturizers

Moisturizers contain humectants that attract and hold water in the keratin fibers. Unaltered Negroid hair that is kept adequately moisturized will comb more easily and not break from the combing, hence allowing a longer length of hair to develop. Hair that has been chemically curled or waved will require more moisturizing than non–chemically treated hair. Most of the popular moisturizers on the market today contain lanolin or one or more of its derivatives (Table 17-1). Glycerin in concentrations of 20 to 50% in water and propylene glycol are good moisturizers with few or no side effects. However, they cannot be left on hair that has been straightened with chemical relaxers or a hot comb, because the relaxed hair will go limp and the hot-pressed hair will revert to its preprocessed state. However, glycerin-based products may be used as a preshampoo moisturizer and/or conditioner for relaxed hair if they are washed out.

Activators

Activators are products specifically designed for curls. They contain surface active agents such as proteins, cationic agents, and/or plant oils (soybean, wheat germ oil). These surface active agents will cause tightening of the curl pattern. Originally, curls required the use of both a moisturizer and an activator because humectants alone tended to loosen the curl pattern. Today, many commercial products contain both humectants and surface active agents, thus eliminating the need for separate products (Table 17-1).

Conditioners

Hair conditioners here are defined as any products that enhance the appearance, manageability, and growth of the hair. A conditioner may be simply an emollient or a very complex mixture of proteins, quaternary ammonium compounds, oils, gums, and humectants (Table 17-1). The type of conditioning agent needed will depend on the hair phenotype and the type of chemicals or other styling aids used. Non–chemically treated hair may be conditioned simply by using a good moisturizer. Hot-pressed hair may require an agent that contains proteins and quaternary ammonium compounds, such as stearyl benzyl dimethyl ammonium chloride (stearalkonium chloride), the quaternized cellulose polymers (e.g., Polymer JR), and the copolymers of dimethyl diallyl ammonium chloride plus acrylamide (e.g., polyquaternium 6 + 7).[12] These agents aid in preventing breakage by adding a protective coating to the hair as well by creating ionic attractions to the negatively charged fibers. Chemically relaxed hair would benefit from the same type of conditioner or one that is relatively rich in protein. Curled or waved hair is kept conditioned by moisturizers and activators, or by combination products.

Styling Gels and Spritzes

Styling gels and spritzes are becoming increasingly popular among African Americans. The gels contain carbomer 940 (2% or more) and hydrolyzed animal protein (5% or more): this combination forms a thick, tacky gel that dries on the hair, leaving it very stiff and fixed in the style sculptured into the hair. The spritzes usually contain a copolymer of polyvinyl-pyrrolidone and vinyl acetate (PVP-VA). Some of the styling gels also contain this copolymer. Once on the, hair, these products dry rapidly, and fixation may be enhanced with heat from a hair dryer.

HAIR RESTRUCTURING AGENTS

Hot-Combing

Hair-pressing, as it is called, was invented by Mme. C. J. Walker, who was awarded a patent for the hot (pressing) comb. This method employs the use of an emollient followed by the combing of the hair with a hot metal comb heated in a small kiln, over a hot flame, or electrically. The temperature may at times exceed 400°F. Petrolatum, or an oil that tends to emit little smoke when heated, is used most commonly. The treated hair subsequently remains straight until moisture causes reversion. Pomades are applied as needed to help prevent this reversion and to add sheen to the hair. The hair may later be set either on rollers or with a hot curling iron.

This process can be damaging to both the hair and the scalp. Scalp burns are frequent, and burns on the face and other areas are sometimes seen if the iron is accidentally dropped. Another sequela of this process is hot-comb alopecia.

Relaxers (Chemical Straighteners)

Presently the most popular method of hair straightening among African Americans is the chemical relaxer. Two types of relaxers currently dominate the market: sodium hydroxide (*lye*) relaxers and the guanidine hydroxide (*no-lye*) relaxers. There are also potassium and lithium hydroxide relaxers, the latter promoted as "no-lye," "no-mix" relaxers to compete with the guanidine hydroxide relaxers. Because guanidine hydroxide is highly unstable, it has to be formed in vitro at the time of use by mixing a calcium hydroxide base with a guanidine carbonate solution. The latter is referred to as the activator and should not be confused with "activators" used on "curls" as previously described. Guanidine hydroxide relaxers are sometimes referred to as calcium relaxers by many professionals, but one must not be misled by this, because calcium hydroxide alone is not used in relaxer products. Technically, any product not made with sodium hydroxide may be called a no-lye relaxer, but potassium and lithium hydroxide products have the same caustic effects as those based on sodium hydroxide. Guanidine hydroxide, however, is an organic base and is less caustic than the other relaxers. Because of their mildness, the guanidine hydroxide relaxers have become increasingly popular among professional hairstylists and currently dominate retail sales. Table 17-3 lists the most popular brands of relaxers and their principal active ingredients.

Ammonium bisulfite has also been used in commercial relaxers but is relatively ineffective as a straightening agent. Hair that is more Caucasoid than Negroid in texture responds best to these agents. The bisulfites work best at a pH near 7 and have a similar, yet less harsh, effect on hair as the thioglycolates (Fig. 17-5). Ammonium bisulfite relaxers usually require heat to accelerate the relaxing process, an alkali to decompose the formed thiosulfates, or "Bunte salts," and a neutralization step.[15] One major advantage of the bisulfite relaxers is that one potentially could perform a curl over bisulfite-treated hair: this cannot be done with the caustic alkali relaxers.

Relaxers may be further classified as *base* or

Table 17-3
RELAXERS (CHEMICAL STRAIGHTENING AGENTS)

Active Ingredients	*pH*	*Brand Name*	*Manufacturer*
Sodium hydroxide	13–14	Affirm	Avlon Industries
		Bantu	Johnson Products
		Revlon's Realistic	Revlon
		Designer's Touch	Luster Products
		Precise	Johnson Products
		Optimum	Soft Sheen Products
		Cream of Nature	Revlon
Potassium and sodium hydroxide	13–14	Gentille	Kelley Chemicals
Lithium hydroxide	13–14	TCB No-Lye Conditioning Relaxer	Alberto Culver, USA
Guanidine hydroxide (no lye); formed by mixing calcium hydroxide and guanidine carbonate at time of use	12–13	Dark and Lovely	Carson Products
		Fabulaxer	Revlon
		Soft 'N' Beautiful	Proline
		Soft 'N' Free	Johnson Products
		Optimum	Soft Sheen Products
		Gentle Treatment	Johnson Products
Ammonium bisulfite	7	New Era Gel Perm.	Scientific Research Products

$$\underset{\text{cystine residues}}{R-CH_2S-SCH_2-R} + \underset{\substack{\text{bisulfite}\\ \text{relaxer}}}{X_2SO_3} <=====> \underset{\text{mercaptan}}{R-CH_2-SX} + \underset{\text{Bunte salt}}{R-CH_2-S-SO_3X}$$

Figure 17-5 The reaction of the bisulfite ion with the formation of a "Bunte salt." This reaction is reversed by air oxidation and is enhanced in an alkaline medium. (*Adapted from* Robins[12])

no base. With a base relaxer, an emollient such as petrolatum is applied to the skin along the scalp hair margins prior to application of the relaxer to protect the skin from anticipated chemical burns. A no-base relaxer supposedly contains ingredients that negate the need for the added protection of a base. Although the no-base formulations may cause less burning than the base preparations, they are not as effective in straightening the hair. Table 17-4 lists the components of a typical relaxer system and their functions.

Mild caustic burns of the scalp and neck secondary to relaxers are relatively common, especially with the alkali relaxers, but are usually not severe enough to require medical attention. More severe burns may result in blistering, but scarring rarely occurs and palliative treatment is usually all that is required. Permanent hair loss is highly unlikely with hair restructuring chemicals because the burns are generally only superficial and do not destroy the follicular unit. Residual postinflammatory hyperpigmentation is the only prolonged sequela the author has ever seen from even the most severe burns. A bland emollient and/or a topical corticosteroid may be used in an attempt to reduce the postinflammatory hyperpigmentation.

Hair breakage is the most common side effect from chemical relaxers. Factors that influence the degree of breakage include the strength of the relaxer, the speed of application, the effectiveness of its removal, and the phenotype of the hair. Hair breakage is most common in the nape area (Fig. 17-6), with the anterior scalp margin being next in frequency of involvement (Fig. 17-7). The prime location of damage is related to where the hairstylist first applies the relaxer and,

Table 17-4
COMPONENTS OF A RELAXER SYSTEM AND THEIR FUNCTION

Product	*Ingredients*	*Function*
Base	Petrolatum or other emollient	Protects skin from caustic effects of chemicals; applied to scalp and skin along hairline
Relaxer	Sodium, potassium, or lithium hydroxide in an emollient base	Permanently straightens hair by destroying disulfide bonds; applied only to previously untreated hair
No-lye relaxer	Guanidine hydroxide formed in situ by the reaction of calcium hydroxide with guanidine carbonate in a cream base	Same as sodium hydroxide relaxer but less structural damage to hair
Neutralizing shampoo	Ammonium lauryl sulfate or nonionic amphoteric blend, acidified with citric or hydrochloric acids	Stops action of chemical and removes excess chemical from hair and scalp
Conditioner	Quaternary ammonium compounds, proteins, emollients, oils, and humectants	Softens and detangles hair; also mends split ends and seals breaks in cuticle
Setting lotion	Quaternary ammonium compounds, proteins, gums, water, and fixatives	Seals cuticle and promotes set retention
Oil sheen	Mineral oil, natural and synthetic oils, and silicones	Adds sheen to hair

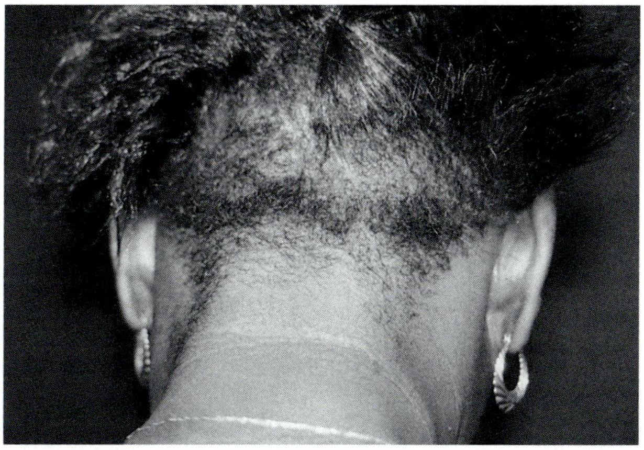

Figure 17-6 Hair breakage from chemical relaxer in suboccipital and nape area. This area is where the relaxer is usually applied first.

hence, to the duration of exposure to the relaxer. Usually, the nape area is treated first and then the front, but often the more obvious new growth in the frontal and temporal margins is treated or "touched up next." A "touch-up" is the application of the relaxer to the new hair growth that has developed since the last treatment. Some women get a touch-up every 3 to 4 weeks. This is too frequent since with only a small amount of new growth, the relaxer invariably will overlap onto previously treated hair, causing resultant irreparable damage to the hair shaft and subsequent breakage.

Figure 17-7 Hair breakage along frontal hairline from relaxer being left on too long in this area.

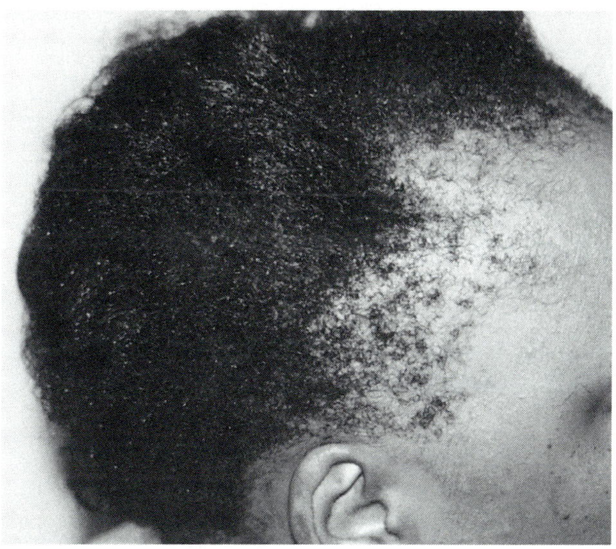

Unfortunately, most hairstylists fail to choose the correct relaxer based on the hair phenotype or condition, and/or fail to properly monitor the process. A depilatory effect may occur from improper use of a chemical relaxer. Since there are no stringent standards for these hair restructuring agents, lack of quality control is also a significant problem and may contribute to hair damage.

Prevention is obviously the best treatment for hair breakage caused by chemicals. Products that work rapidly should be used only by the most highly skilled hairstylists. In recent years, more professional hairstylists have begun using the guanidine hydroxide relaxers (no-lye), which have a greater margin of safety. However, the no-lye products leave the hair much drier than the lye relaxers, and hair so treated will need moisturizing treatments on a regular basis.

Chemically relaxed hair should be handled very gently when wet because it is more susceptible to breakage when wet than when dry. Combing, brushing, rolling, and hot-curling should be kept to a minimum. In general, hair that has been damaged by relaxers will benefit from a protein, gum, or cationic gum conditioner. If the damage is more distally localized, simply cutting off the damaged portion of the hair is an excellent remedy. Many African American women, however, never achieve any significant length of their hair until they use a chemical restructuring agent, and they may be very reluctant to cut their hair for fear that it will not grow back again. In such cases, the hair can be pulled back into a ponytail or gently braided to minimize further trauma. For patchy hair breakage, a hair weave can be used to fill in the gaps. This is expensive, however, and it would be much more economical to use a properly fitted wig. Women who have enough self-esteem to wear their hair short will usually accept the suggestion to cut the hair down to the new growth and allow it to grow out again.

CURLS AND WAVES (THIOGLYCOLATE PERMS)

Chemical curls were popular among African American women in the 1970s and 1980s. Initially referred to as the *Jheri curl* after Jheri Redding, the inventor of the process, the chemical curl is simply a modification of the Caucasian

$$\underset{\text{cystine residues}}{R - CH_2S - SCH_2 - R} + \underset{\text{thioglycolic acid}}{2HS - CH_2 - COOH} \Longleftrightarrow \underset{\text{cysteine residues}}{2RCH_2 - SH} + \underset{\text{dithioglycolic acid}}{HOOC - CH_2S - S - CH_2 - COOH}$$

Figure 17-8 The reaction of thioglycolates with the disulfide bonds of cystine in the hair. This process is reversible through oxidation with hydrogen peroxide or sodium bromate or more slowly by air. The by-product dithioglycolic acid would presumably continue to reduce the keratin protein if not removed during rinsing or shampooing. (*Adapted from* Cosmetics: Science and Technology, *2nd. ed., vol. 2, 1979, p. 189.*)

perm. The primary difference is that the tightly coiled Negroid hair first has to be chemically straightened before it can be rolled and reshaped. Although the curling process initially is more time-consuming than chemical relaxing, curls do not require a skilled professional for maintenance. They usually last 2 to 3 months and, when properly executed, hair breakage can be avoided.

The wave, which is a modification of the curl process, was popular in the mid-1980s because it promoted a looser curl, achieved by setting the hair on a larger roller similar to the type used for setting relaxed hair. However, the formulations used were too strong and the hair was kept too dry for this type of chemical processing. It became apparent within a few years that this process was very damaging to the hair, and its popularity waned.

The curl or wave process is a two-step procedure requiring that the chemically unaltered new growth be straightened first with a rearranger, straightener, or presoftening gel and then set on rollers with a booster. Both the rearranger and booster steps are based on thioglycolates, the latter of a lesser concentration than the former (Fig. 17-8). After rinsing, the hair is saturated with an oxidizing agent (neutralizer), usually sodium bromate. This process is repeated every 2 to 3 months and is very harsh on the hair. The second and third steps of this process are essentially identical to the Caucasian perm. Structural bonds are impaired, and the hair loses much of its water-retaining capacity. Damage can result from either the reduction step (rearranger and booster) or the oxidation step (neutralizer). Table 17-5 lists the principal ingredients of a curl or wave system and some of the more popular brands. Table 17-6 lists the functions of the components of a curl or wave system.

Curls and waves, like relaxers, can cause severe hair breakage, but the breakage will usually be more widespread and limited to the distal ends of the hair shafts. With curls and waves, the entire hair shaft is treated with the booster each time the hair is redone, which can lead to severe hair shaft damage. Managing hair breakage from curls or waves is the same as that for chemical relaxers, with one notable exception. The hair must be kept hydrated because curled or waved hair is stronger when wet, as opposed to chemically relaxed hair, which is stronger when dry.

Table 17-5
CURLS AND WAVES

Active Ingredients	*pH*	*Brand Name*	*Manufacturer*
Ammonium thioglycolate	9.2–9.6	Carefree Curl	Soft Sheen Products
		Worlds of Curls	Worlds of Curls
		BB Cosmopolitan Curl	Bronner Bros
		Donnies	American Beauty
		Leisure Curl	D'Orum Products
		Wave Nouveau	Soft Sheen Products
		Lustrasilk	Lustrasilk Products
		Soft and Free	Johnson Products
		Elasta	Elasta Products
Monoethanolamine thioglycolate and diisopropanolamine	9.3–9.4	The X-ceptional Back Alive Curl	Essence of Quality

Table 17-6
THE COMPONENTS OF A CURL OR WAVE SYSTEM

Product	*Ingredients*	*Function*
Rearranger	Ammonium thioglycolate and ammonium hydroxide in a gel or cream base. Monoethanolamine and diethanolamine or diisopropanolamine.	Straightens virgin Negroid hair. Applied to portion of hair not previously treated. Rinsed out after desired straightening has been achieved.
Booster	Same as above but with about one-half to two-thirds of the active ingredients. May be in a lotion or liquid base.	Softens hair by cleaving disulfide bonds. Applied to entire hair shaft. Hair is then rodded in this. After desired softening, hair is rinsed thoroughly while still on rods.
Neutralizer	Sodium bromate or hydrogen peroxide in a liquid or lotion base. May contain urea, humectants, proteins, and other biofunctional agents.	Oxidizes sulfhydryl groups of cysteine to reform cystine. Applied to hair on rods and allowed to remain long enough to reset hair in new configuration. Hair is then rinsed and rods removed.
Shampoo	Anionic, nonionic, and amphoteric surfactants, quaternary ammonium compounds, oils, gums, humectants, and silicones.	Removes residual chemical but less drying than relaxer-type shampoos. Many hairstylists omit this step.
Moisturizer	Glycerin, propylene glycol, oils, lanolin and its derivatives, wheat germ oil, castor oil, corn oil, soybean oil, mineral oil, silicones, jojoba oil, and synthetic humectants.	Restores moisture and helps restore curl or wave pattern.
Activator	Glycerin and other humectants.	Restores and tightens curl or wave pattern.

With curled hair, products with high concentrations of protein should be avoided because they prevent absorption of moisture by the hair.

Alternative Techniques

Alternative hair grooming techniques have been designed to lengthen the effect of hot-combing alone while minimizing the use of chemical restructuring agents. Some alternative techniques rely on the use of quaternary ammonium agents, but others contain a mild thioglycolate that produces a permanent straightening effect when used with the hot comb. With the latter, the hair will usually become very dry and require additional moisturizing. As one might surmise, severe breakage can result from these combination techniques: heat and thioglycolates are a very destructive combination if improperly used. Treatment is the same as for hair breakage caused by other thioglycolate products.

DISORDERS OF THE SCALP

Some scalp disorders in African Americans are related specifically to the phenotype of their hair and the grooming techniques and aids they employ. Some scalp disorders in African Americans require a different approach to management, as presented here and in Table 17-7.

Traction Folliculitis and Traction Alopecia

Traction folliculitis occurs primarily in children (Fig. 17-9). Clinically, one may see erythema and scaling, papules, or pustules. Cultures of the pustules consistently have yielded no growth or normal bacterial flora.[16] The hair dressing used or other factors may play a role in the development of folliculitis.[14]

In traction alopecia related to braids or ponytails, hair loss usually occurs in the temporal

Table 17-7
MANAGEMENT OF HAIR AND SCALP DISORDERS IN AFRICAN AMERICANS

Condition or Disease Entity	*Causative Agent(s) or Factors*	*Therapy and Management*
Traction alopecia	Tight ponytails and braids Sponge or other tight rollers	Avoid tension on hair. Topical monixidil in severe cases.
Hair breakage in nape and suboccipital regions, generally from relaxers; breakage in crown area usually associated with scratching	Hydroxide relaxers Scratching	Protein and cationic conditioners, leave-in conditioners or emollients. Use milder relaxer. Treat cause of itching.
Hair shaft very weak distally and crumbles with minimal trauma; severe breakage in parietal area	Thioglycolates	Lipid moisturizers. Avoid protein conditioners. Use milder formulation or booster alone to curl or wave hair.
Severe breakage that cannot be masked by own hair	All causes	Hair weave or wig
Seborrheic dermatitis	Lanolin, squalene, wheat germ oil, castor oil, stress	Topical corticosteroids with a) propylene glycol or ointment base for curls, waves and natural hairstyles, b) an ointment base for hot-pressed hair, and c) any vehicle for chemically relaxed hair.
Hot-comb alopecia (follicular degeneration syndrome)	Use of hot combs, curling irons, and hood dryers	Avoid heat where possible. Use spacer between hot comb and hot curling iron. Decrease time spent under hood dryers.
Pseudofolliculitis barbae	Close shaving or plucking in males; plucking or electrolysis in females	Avoid shaving if possible or shave in direction of hair growth. Use clipper with 3(0) blade or depilatory if tolerated. Topical retinoic acid and corticosteroid.
Folliculitis keloidalis	Genetic predisposition; shaving or close-cutting of hair in nape and posterior scalp	Avoid close-cutting of hair in affected areas. Topical or systemic antibiotics. Liquid nitrogen cryotherapy, intralesional corticosteroids. Surgical or CO_2 laser excision.
Dissecting cellulitis	Genetic predisposition; part of follicular occlusion triad	Systemic antibiotics. Systemic corticosteroids. Surgical drainage. Isotretinoin, Dapsone, zinc, and x-ray epilation in recalcitrant cases.

areas, anterior and superior to the ears, but the frontal and occipital areas are occasionally affected (Fig. 17-10). If the traction is continued long-term, a permanent scarring alopecia may develop: this appears to require 3 to 5 years to develop and is usually evident by early adolescence in children so affected. Frontal and temporal alopecia is most commonly seen in adulthood and occurs almost exclusively from hair rollers (Fig. 17-11). One will usually see a rather dense growth of intermediate hairs at the periphery and sparse vellus hairs in the center of the affected areas.[17] Sponge rollers are the worse offenders because once wound, they do not "give." Biopsy of areas of traction alopecia in the early stages generally reveals a subacute perifollicular inflammation with occasional overlying parakeratosis. Long-standing cases show a normal overlying epidermis but absent or very sparse small follicles.[18]

Traction alopecia can be prevented. All health care professionals and cosmeticians need to be

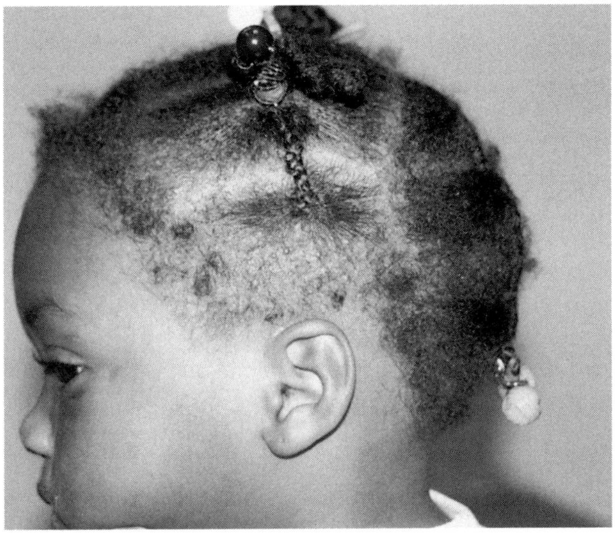

Figure 17-9 Young African American female with braids secured with rubber band ornaments. Note follicular pustules in supraauricular area (traction folliculitis).

aware of this condition and must educate the parent or individuals grooming the affected person's hair not to pull it so tight. Even if traction alopecia is obvious, however, topical minoxidil in a 1 to 2% concentration has led to dramatic improvement in a few patients (W. Wilborn, unpublished data), with new vellus growth appearing as early as 3 months after use. Earles has used hair transplants and rotation flaps to surgically correct traction alopecia, but the scarring associated with these procedures may be unacceptable.[17] If superinfection is suspected, as evidenced by widespread crusting and inflammation, a 10-day course of systemic antibiotics directed at pathogenic staphylococci is recommended.

Figure 17-10 Traction alopecia. Marked hair loss in frontal and temporal regions. Note persistence of short hair along anterior margins.

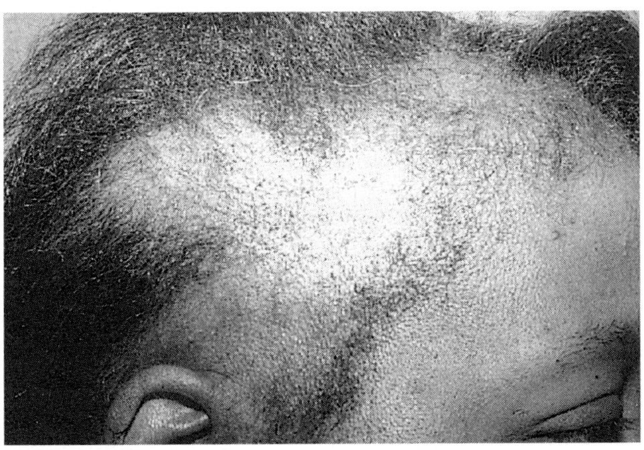

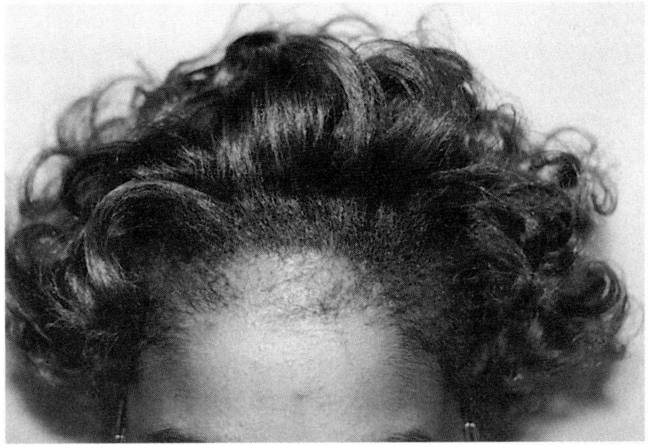

Figure 17-11 Traction alopecia from sponge hair rollers. The frontal location is typical in adults.

Seborrheic Dermatitis

Seborrheic dermatitis may be aggravated by some of the ingredients in hair products that are commonly used by African Americans. Lanolin is, by far, the one ingredient most likely to aggravate the condition, but soybean oil, wheat germ oil, lecithin, castor oil, and squalene may also cause problems. In many cases, simply avoiding products with these ingredients will alleviate the problem. Moisturizers that generally can be used without problems in patients with seborrheic dermatitis include glycerine and propylene glycol for natural styles or curls, and white petrolatum, jojoba oil, or some of the simpler pomade formulations for hot-pressed or chemically relaxed hair.

Because daily shampooing is too drying for Negroid hair or too impractical for most African American females with hot-pressed hair, African Americans with seborrheic dermatitis can reasonably only be asked to shampoo once a week. The shampoo should be applied to the scalp for 20 to 30 minutes, followed by a nonmedicated shampoo for the hair and the patient's usual moisturizers or conditioners. In essence, the shampoo is used as a scalp treatment only and not as a cleanser for the hair. If there is considerable inflammation and/or lack of response to the shampoo, a low- to mid-potency topical corticosteroid is prescribed. The choice of steroid vehicle will depend on the hairstyle and type of chemical processing used on the hair. Natural or thioglycolate-treated hair (curls and waves) dry very easily and, thus, alcoholic vehicles should be avoided: a propylene glycol or ointment vehicle may be prescribed instead. Women with hot-pressed hair need an ointment vehicle. Women with chemically relaxed hair tolerate alcoholic solutions very well and thus may safely use any vehicle.

Hot-Comb Alopecia

Clinically, *hot-comb alopecia* is characterized by a well-defined area of partial hair loss over the top of the head (Fig. 17-12). There is obvious loss of follicular orifices on clinical inspection of involved areas, and clusters of hair are scattered in the area of scarring alopecia.[18] Polytrichia is mentioned as a feature of this condition, but this finding may be a more common natural occurrence in African Americans than is generally recognized. The predilection for the top of the head in hot-comb alopecia is presumably secondary to the hot petrolatum running down the hair shaft and onto the scalp. On the sides and back of the head, the petrolatum would tend to run down toward the scalp margins when the hair shafts are extended horizontally away from the scalp.[18]

Recently, the direct causal relationship of this clinical condition and hot combs has been questioned. Sperling and Sau described a similar clinical scarring alopecia in African American women who had not used, or infrequently used, hot combs and thus have proposed the term *follicular degeneration syndrome* to replace the term hot-comb alopecia.[19] In their study, they noted that the earliest observable histological abnormality present in all patients was the premature degeneration of the inner root sheath of certain follicles scattered amid histologically normal hairs.

The author has observed that one common denominator in women with the clinical appearance of this follicular degeneration syndrome is the excessive use of heat in affected areas, whether from a hot comb, curling iron, or hooded hair dryer. The excessive use of heat can and should be avoided. Use of a comb as a spacer to prevent the hot comb and curling iron from getting too close to the scalp is advised. Also, if the hair is dried under a hair dryer, the length of time spent under the dryer needs to be markedly reduced. The temperature at the apex of the dryer has been measured at above 200°F: shielding of the top of the head with a folded towel after the first 20 to 25 minutes under the dryer may potentially help to prevent or at least diminish the intensity of this problem.

Figure 17-12 Advanced stage of follicular degeneration syndrome (hot-comb alopecia). Only sparse hairs remain.

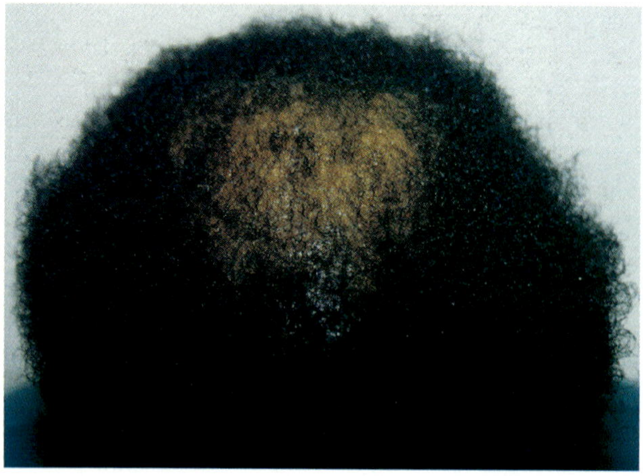

Pseudofolliculitis Barbae and Folliculitis Barbae

Pseudofolliculitis barbae consists of perifollicular and follicular papules and papulopustules in shaved areas of those people with inherently kinky or curly hair (Fig. 17-13). The culprit is the curved follicle and consequently the curved hair shaft which grows back into the skin surface or pierces the follicular wall when the hair is cut very short. Severe scarring may result (Fig. 17-14). Shaving is the usual precipitating stimulus of the condition, and pseudofolliculitis barbae has been noted in 45 to 83 percent of black men secondary to societal standards for a clean-shaven face.[20,21] In a recent product brochure by a manufacturer of depilatories (Carson Products, Savannah, GA), however, the incidence was estimated at 25 percent.

Extrafollicular penetration occurs when the hair shaft completes an arc with the sharp-pointed cut hair tip invaginating the epidermis 1 to 2 mm from the follicular opening as it grows back toward the skin. Transfollicular penetration

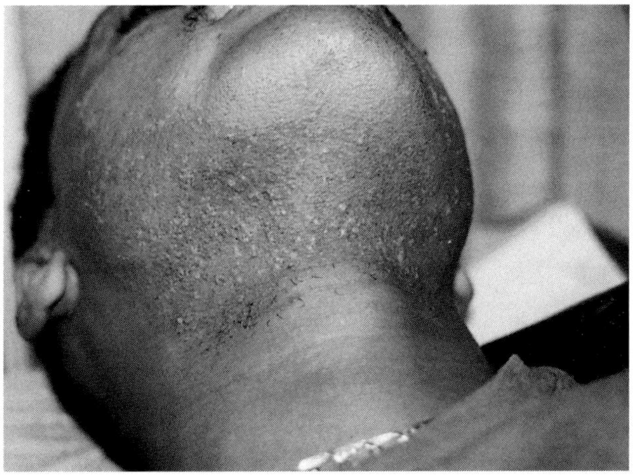

Figure 17-13 Pseudofolliculitis barbae from use of a close-cutting clipper.

occurs when the skin is pulled taut prior to shaving, causing the pointed tip to retract under the skin as tension is released. This can also occur with electrolysis or when hairs are plucked with tweezers and break off short within the follicle.[20,22] This may create a marked inflammatory response and a foreign body–type reaction.[22,23]

The extrafollicular form of pseudofolliculitis barbae is the more difficult of the two to manage. Growing a beard is the only certain cure, but many men with this condition feel that they must conform to the practice of being clean-shaven, especially in certain professions. Members of the military services,[21,24,25] public safety personnel (policemen and firemen), airline employees, and bankers have stringent dress codes, official or not. Physician notes stating the medical need to grow a beard may not be accepted by employers. Thus, physicians must work both to change these rigid standards for those affected with pseudofolliculitis barbae and to use existing measures to lessen the problem.

Figure 17-14 Scarring from pseudofolliculitis barbae.

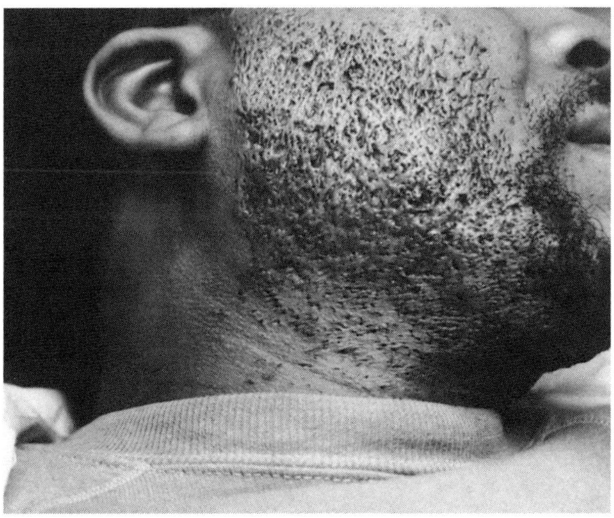

For those individuals who can tolerate them, depilatories are very effective in controlling pseudofolliculitis barbae. A barium sulfide (Magic Shave, Royal Crown Shave Powder) vs. calcium thioglycolate (Magic Shave Gold Powder, Surgex cream) depilatory is usually more effective in dissolving beard hair, but the latter emits a foul odor and has the potential for irritation if used too frequently.[20] In general, depilatory lotions act more slowly than pastes and creams but are less irritating and can be used more often.[20]

If the individual prefers to shave, the key to successful treatment is to allow the hair to grow long enough to prevent reentry into the skin. Krause and Kligman suggest that an initial 30-day respite from shaving is necessary before attempting to shave the hair again.[22] New hair should then not be cut shorter than 0.5 to 1 mm and should be shaved in the direction of hair growth. Cutting the beard with a clipper that has a triple zero (000) blade is very effective.[25] Use of the more close-cutting liners, however, can be as bad as using a sharp razor. The old adjustable razor, properly set to leave a short stubble, was also very effective but has since become outdated. Alexander evaluated the use of a foil-guarded razor, later marketed as the "PFB" razor, and showed that the majority of respondents rated it superior to other methods.[26] However, these special shavers and razors for pseudofolliculitis barbae have not proved in practice to be as effective as claimed (W. Wilborn, unpublished data). Some nonprescription items with resorcinol, salicylic acid, and other mild keratolytics, or a brisk rub with a coarse washcloth or sponge prior to shaving may elevate and soften hair.

Kligman and Mills studied the effects of a 0.05% topical retinoic acid solution and found that, in early cases of pseudofolliculitis barbae, there was some improvement after 3 to 4 weeks of treatment and good to excellent results after 8 weeks of treatment.[27] Long-standing and severe cases did not improve. Brown has reported limited success with this therapy but found that a mild corticosteroid had to be used to counter the irritation.[23]

Plucking is a very prominent contributory cause of pseudofolliculitis barbae: many men who have ingrown hairs not only free them but pluck them as well, and almost all women with this problem pluck hairs instead of shaving. Plucking must be absolutely forbidden, and where a beard is permissible and desired, it should be encouraged. Shaving waivers should be given to those individuals whose employers are not so stringent about shaving and, in some instances, a change in occupation may be necessary.

Postinflammatory hyperpigmentation from this condition is often the presenting complaint. Brauner and Flandermeyer reported good results in treating the pigmentation with the alternate use of topical retinoic acid, 5% hydroquinone, and a topical fluorinated steroid.[24] The retinoic acid is applied at night, the hydroquinone twice a day, and the corticosteroid in the morning. The retinoic acid and hydroquinone can be discontinued temporarily if excessive irritation develops. The author prefers a compounded mixture of 0.1% retinoic acid, 0.1% triamcinolone, and 5% hydroquinone in unibase with ascorbic acid as an antioxidant: this formulation may be used once or twice a day and alternated with 1% hydrocortisone if excessive irritation develops. The use of a potent topical steroid on the face must be limited to days, not weeks.

Some men who shave get a true folliculitis, especially when a dull razor is used. Many patients experience a true folliculitis after having their nape area trimmed very close or shaved (lined) by a barber. A few women are also being seen with the same condition because of the shorter hairstyles. Avoiding contaminated equipment, changing the razor blades more often, and wearing the hair longer can all help to alleviate the problem in most patients. Topical and/or systemic antibiotics where appropriate will control this folliculitis. For chronic cases, daily use of topical erythromycin, clindamycin, or benzoyl peroxide can prevent recurrences.

Folliculitis Keloidalis

Also termed *acne keloidalis* or *dermatitis papularis capillitii, folliculitis keloidalis* is a chronic inflammatory and potentially scarring process that occurs primarily over the posterior neck and scalp, mainly in African American men.[28] The lesions are usually distributed in areas where a razor or "liner" is used to shape the hairline, thus causing folliculitis and pseudofolliculitis in susceptible individuals. The early soft papules become more firm with time, and susceptible individuals can form keloidal papules and plaques (Figs. 17-15 and 17-16). With the close-cut hairstyles currently preferred by young African American men, there has been an increase in the incidence of these problems.

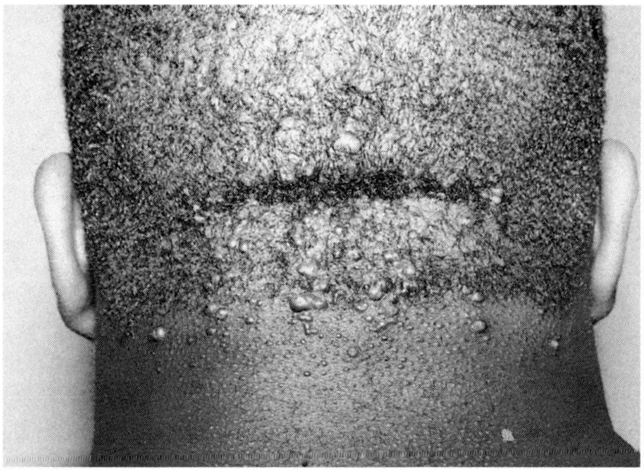

Figure 17-15 Folliculitis keloidalis in an early nonscarring stage, with soft papules and a single hair in the center of a lesion.

Figure 17-16 Folliculitis keloidalis. Large keloidal mass at base of occiput, a typical location for these lesions.

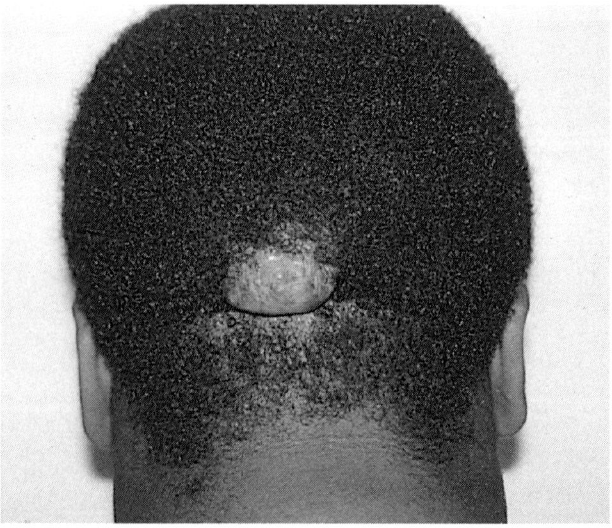

Histologically, early papules represent terminal hairs engulfed in a mixed inflammatory infiltrate at the infundibulum and midisthmus levels, which later develops into a chronic granulomatous infiltrate in the lower follicle. Sebaceous gland atrophy is present, as well as a mixed plasma cell–lymphocytic perivascular infiltrate. With time, the smoldering granulomatous inflammation leads to scar formation.[29]

In order for any treatment of folliculitis keloidalis to be effective, one must avoid all of the predisposing factors that can lead to follicular damage. Patients should be advised not to allow their necks to be lined with either a razor or a liner: the hair should be left at least 2 to 3 mm above the surface. If patients are wearing a natural style, they should not comb the hair without the aid of a moisturizer or lubricant. Where an active folliculitis exists, a topical or systemic antibiotic is required. Tetracycline 0.5 to 1 g, doxycycline 100 to 200 mg, minocycline 100 mg, and erythromycin 0.5 to 1 g per day have all been effective. Topical erythromycin, clindamycin, mupirocin, and chloramphenicol have also proved to be effective in milder cases. These should be continued as long as the problem persists.

In the soft papular stages of this condition, the application of liquid nitrogen with a cotton-tip applicator is preferred to use of a spray. This will usually abort the early lesions, but one must be careful not to overfreeze or permanent depigmentation will result. Curettage of small lesions followed by intralesional corticosteroids has also been quite effective. Intralesional corticosteroids can shrink even the most stubborn lesions. However, this requires time and patience, and patients must be continually encouraged to comply with the treatment regimen. The author has found triamcinolone hexacetonide (Aristospan) 5 mg/ml to be quite effective; it is easy to administer with a 1-ml insulin syringe. Triamcinolone acetonide 10 mg/ml is also commonly used. Very thick lesions may be presoftened by injecting xylocaine before the steroid. When the lesion begins to soften, resolution may be enhanced by using a concentration of ~20 mg/ml triamcinolone. Once the lesion is soft enough to receive triamcinolone acetonide 40 mg/ml undiluted, this will further enhance resolution. These injections are performed at biweekly to monthly intervals. Although atrophy and depigmentation may initially result, the color will eventually be restored once the treatment is completed. Patients should be forewarned of this but made to understand that strong measures are necessary to flatten the papules and keloidal tissue and to maintain the desired effect. Excision vs. vaporization with the carbon dioxide laser has been shown by Kantor, Ratz, and Wheeland to produce good results:[30] two of their patients developed hypertrophic scarring that was controlled with triamcinolone acetonide 20 to 40 mg/ml intralesionally.

Dissecting Cellulitis (Perifolliculitis Capitis Abscedens et Suffodiens)

It is difficult to effectively manage patients with dissecting cellulitis. No clear etiology has been delineated, but the condition is considered to be a part of the follicular occlusion triad that also includes acne conglobata and hidradenitis suppurativa. All three of these conditions may exist at the same time in susceptible individuals and are more common in African American males. Dissecting cellulitis is characterized by multiple large abscesses, chronic draining sinuses, follicular occlusion, and scarring alopecia (Fig. 17-17). Hypertrophic scars and, at times, keloids may develop. Lesions often coalesce to form massive carbuncles. Cultures are usually negative or grow out normal bacterial flora or *Staphylococcus aureus*. In recent years, most of the cul-

Figure 17-17 Dissecting cellulitis. Patient has multiple small pustules and many large connecting abscesses.

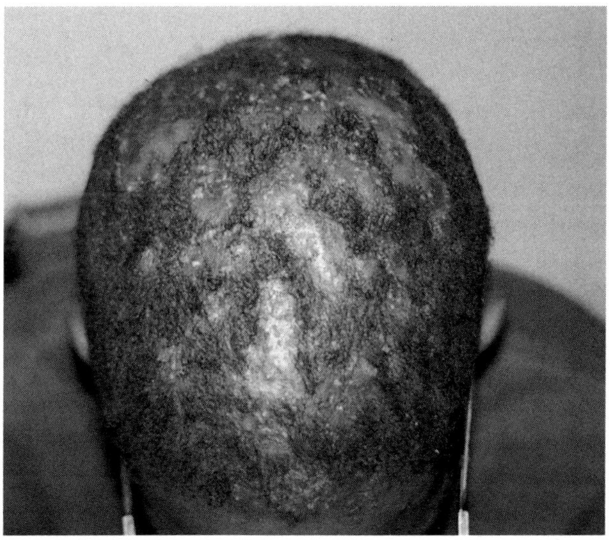

tures performed by the author have grown out a coagulase-negative staphylococcus.

Systemic antibiotics, systemic corticosteroids, and extensive surgical removal have all been used in the past with varying degrees of success.[31–33] Isotretinoin has been reported to be effective,[34] and the author has seen dramatic resolution with isotretinoin in at least three cases. Berne, Venge, and Ohman reported a case of dissecting cellulitis that cleared dramatically on oral zinc sulfate 400 mg t.i.d., corresponding to 90 mg elemental zinc.[35] Dapsone in doses of 100 mg two to three times per day has also been beneficial in some cases.[36] More recently, the author has found that a combination of ciprofloxacin or cephalexin 500 mg b.i.d. with rifampin 600 mg q.d. may be very beneficial. Initially, a 2-week course is prescribed, followed by successive 2-week courses if necessary. Persistent cases are then treated with isotretinoin 40 mg per day for 4 to 5 months. Incision and drainage of fluctuant abscesses with insertion of a drain may also help to speed resolution. Excellent results have been reported with x-ray epilation, and, when all else fails, this certainly must be entertained.[32,33] It is obvious that clinicians treating this condition must have a good deal of patience and must provide encouragement to their patients.

CONCLUDING REMARKS

Although the morphological differences of the hair of the three major races are well-defined, definitive data on the chemical differences are still lacking. Some hair and scalp disorders are unique to African Americans because of genetic differences, while others are related more to cultural differences in hair grooming and styling. The type of hair cosmetics needed and used on Negroid hair differs greatly from that of other racial groups: use of these cosmetics can induce or aggravate preexisting conditions. African Americans are particularly prone to pseudofolliculitis barbae, acne keloidalis, and dissecting cellulitis. These conditions are very difficult to manage and at times require multiple therapeutic approaches. It is hoped that future research will provide insight not only into the chemical and structural variations in human hair but also into clinical problems, such as the follicular degeneration syndrome.

REFERENCES

1. Steggerda M, Seiber HC: Size and shape of head hairs from six racial groups. J Hered 32:315–318, 1942.
2. Hrdy D: Quantitative hair form variation in several populations. Am J Phys Anthropol 39:7–18, 1973.
3. Hrdy D, Baden HP: Biochemical variation of hair keratins in man and non-human primates. Am J Phys Anthropol 39:19–24, 1973.
4. Gold RJM, Schriver CR: The amino acid composition of hair from different racial origins. Clin Chim Acta 33:465–466, 1971.
5. Baum JD, Hughes EA, Harris DA: Neonatal hair as a record of intra-uterine nutrition. Biol Neonate 25:208–218, 1974.
6. Dawber RPR. Hair follicle structure, keratinization and the physical properties of hair. In Rook A, Dawber RPR (eds): *Diseases of the Hair and Scalp.* Oxford, Blackwell Scientific Publications, 1982, pp 18–40.
7. Deiko S, Jidio J: Hair low-sulfur protein composition does not differ electrophoretically among races. J Dermatol 15:393–396, 1988.
8. Deiko S, Jidio J: Amounts of fibrous proteins and matrix substances in hairs of different races. J Dermatol 17:62–64, 1990.
9. Orwin DFG: Variations in wool follicle morphology. In Rogers GE, Reis PJ, Ward KA, Marshall RC (eds): *The Biology of Wool and Hair.* New York, Chapman and Hall, 1989, pp 227–241.
10. Lindelof B, Forslind B, Hedblad M, Kaveus U: Human hair form: Morphology revealed by light and scanning electron microscopy and computer aided three-dimensional reconstruction. Arch Dermatol 124:1359–1363, 1988.
11. Bradfield RB, Montagna W: Scanning electron microscopy in assessment of protein calorie malnutrition. Lancet 2:1026, 1974.
12. Robins CR: *Chemical and Physical Behavior of Human Hair,* 2d ed. New York, Springer-Verlag, 1988, pp 58–60.
13. Lehne RK: Hair grooming preparations. In Sagarin E, Goulden HD, Klarmann EG, Powers DH (eds): *Cosmetics: Science and Technology.* New York, Interscience Publishers, 1957, pp 550–582.
14. Plewig G, Fulton JE, Kligman AM: Pomade acne. Arch Dermatol 101:580–584, 1970.
15. Cannell DW: Permanent waving and hair straightening. Clin Dermatol 6(3):71–82, 1988.
16. Slepyan AH: Traction alopecia. Arch Dermatol 78:395–398, 1958.
17. Earles RM: Surgical correction of traumatic alopecia marginalis or traction alopecia in black women. J Dermatol Surg Oncol 12(1):78–81, 1986.
18. LoPresti P, Papa CM, Kligman AM: Hot comb alopecia. Arch Dermatol 98:234, 1968.
19. Sperling LC, Sau P: The follicular degeneration syndrome in black patients: "Hot comb alopecia" revisited and revised. Arch Dermatol 128:68–74, 1992.
20. Halder RM: Pseudofolliculitis barbae and related disorders. Dermatol Clin 6:407–412, 1988.
21. Alexander AM: Pseudofolliculitis barbae in the military: A medical administrative and social problem. J Natl Med Assoc 66:459–479, 1974.

22. Strauss JS, Kligman AM: Pseudofolliculitis of the beard. Arch Dermatol 74:533–542, 1956.
23. Brown LA: Pathogenesis and treatment of pseudofolliculitis barbae. Cutis 32:373–375, 1983.
24. Brauner CJ, Flandermeyer KL: Pseudofolliculitis barbae: II. Treatment. Int J Dermatol 16:520–525, 1977.
25. Conte MS, Lawrence JE: Pseudofolliculitis barbae no "pseudoproblem." JAMA 241(1):53–54, 1979.
26. Alexander AM: Evaluation of the foil-guarded shaver in the management of pseudofolliculitis barbae. Cutis 27:534–542, 1981.
27. Kligman AM, Mills OH: Pseudofolliculitis of the beard and topically applied tretinoin. Arch Dermatol 107:551–552, 1973.
28. Dinehart SM, Herzberg AJ, Kerns BJ, Pollack SV: Acne keloidalis: A review. J Dermatol Surg Oncol 15:642–647, 1989.
29. Herzberg AJ, Dinehart SM, Kerns BY, Pollack SV: Acne keloidalis: Transverse microscopy, immunohistochemistry, and electron microscopy. Am J Dermatopathol 12(2):109–121, 1990.
30. Kantor GR, Ratz JL, Wheeland RG: Treatment of acne keloidalis nuchae with carbon dioxide laser. J Am Acad Dermatol 14:263–267, 1986.
31. Scott DA: Disorders of the hair and scalp in blacks. Dermatol Clin 6(3):387–395, 1988.
32. Moyer DG, Williams RM: Perifolliculitis capitis abscedens et suffodiens. Arch Dermatol 85:118–124, 1962.
33. McMullen FH, Zeligman I: Perifolliculitis capitis abscedens et suffodiens. Arch Dermatol Syphilol 73:256–263, 1956.
34. Schewach-Millet M, Fiv R, Shapira D: Perifolliculitis capitis abscedens et suffodiens treated with isotretinoin (13 cis-retinoic acid). J Am Acad Dermatol 15:1291–1292, 1986.
35. Berne B, Venge P, Ohman S: Perifolliculitis capitis abscedens et suffodiens (Hoffman): Complete healing associated with oral zinc therapy. Arch Dermatol 121:1028–1030, 1985.
36. Halder RM: Hair and scalp disorders in blacks. Cutis 32:378–380, 1983.

INDEX

Numbers followed by the letter f refer to illustrations; numbers followed by the letter t refer to tables.

A

B

C

D

E

I

J

K

P